COMPUTED TOMOGRAPHY

OF THE BODY

With Magnetic Resonance Imaging

COMPUTED TOMOGRAPHY OF THE BODY

With Magnetic Resonance Imaging

Second Edition

Albert A. Moss, M.D.
Professor and Chairman, Department of Radiology
University of Washington School of Medicine
Seattle, Washington

Gordon Gamsu, M.D.
Professor of Radiology and Medicine
University of California, San Francisco, School of Medicine
San Francisco, California

Harry K. Genant, M.D.
Professor of Radiology, Medicine, and Orthopaedic Surgery; Chief of the
Musculoskeletal Section; Director of the Osteoporosis Research Group
University of California, San Francisco, School of Medicine
San Francisco, California

Volume One
Thorax and Neck

W.B. SAUNDERS COMPANY
A Division of Harcourt Brace & Company
Philadelphia   London   Toronto   Montreal   Sydney   Tokyo

W.B. SAUNDERS COMPANY
A Division of
Harcourt Brace & Company

The Curtis Center
Independence Square West
Philadelphia, Pennsylvania 19106

Library of Congress Cataloging-in-Publication Data

Moss, Albert A.
Computed tomography of the body with magnetic resonance
imaging / Albert A. Moss, Gordon Gamsu, Harry K. Genant.
— 2nd ed.

 p. cm.

Rev. ed. of: Computed tomography of the body / Albert A.
Moss, Gordon Gamsu, Harry K. Genant.

Includes bibliographical references and index.

ISBN 0–7216–2415–4 (set)

1. Tomography. 2. Magnetic resonance imaging.
I. Gamsu, Gordon. II. Genant, Harry K.
III. Moss, Albert A. Computed tomography of the body.
IV. Title.

[DNLM: 1. Anatomy, Regional. 2. Magnetic
Resonance Imaging. 3. Tomography, X-Ray Computed.
WN 160 M913c]

RC78.7.T6M68 1992

DNLM/DLC 91–32837

Editor: Lisette Bralow
Designer: W.B. Saunders Staff
Production Manager: Peter Faber
Manuscript Editors: Lorraine Zawodny and Kendall Sterling
Illustration Coordinator: Walter Verbitski
Indexer: Nancy Newman
Cover Designer: Michelle Maloney

Computed Tomography of the Body With
Magnetic Resonance Imaging, 2/e.

ISBN Volume I 0–7216–4358–2
Volume II 0–7216–4359–0
Volume III 0–7216–4503–8
Three Volume Set 0–7216–2415–4

Last digit is the print number: 9 8 7 6 5

DEDICATION FOR VOLUME ONE

This volume is dedicated to Gay, Jessica,
colleagues at the University of California, San Francisco,
and the numerous investigators whose efforts
have shaped our knowledge of thoracic imaging and disease.

GORDON GAMSU

CONTRIBUTORS FOR VOLUME ONE

WILLIAM P. DILLON, M.D.
Associate Professor of Radiology and Neurology, University of California,
San Francisco, School of Medicine; Attending Neuroradiologist, The Medical
Center at the University of California, San Francisco; San Francisco, CA
  THE NECK

BERTRAND DUVOISIN, M.D.
Médecin-Adjoint, University Hospital, Lausanne, Switzerland
  TRAUMA

AXEL ESSINGER, M.D.
Associate Professor of Radiology, Department of Diagnostic Radiology,
University Hospital, Lausanne, Switzerland
  TRAUMA

GORDON GAMSU, M.D.
Professor of Radiology and Medicine, University of California, San Francisco,
School of Medicine, San Francisco, CA
    THE TRACHEA AND CENTRAL BRONCHI
    THE MEDIASTINUM
    THE PULMONARY HILA
    THE LUNGS
    THE CHEST WALL, AXILLARY SPACE, PLEURAE, AND DIAPHRAGM
    TRAUMA
    THE LARYNX AND PIRIFORM SINUSES

CHARLES B. HIGGINS, M.D.
Professor of Radiology, University of California, San Francisco, School of
Medicine; Chief, Magnetic Resonance Imaging, Medical Center at the
University of California, San Francisco; San Francisco, CA
  HEART AND PERICARDIUM

JEFFREY S. KLEIN, M.D.
Assistant Professor of Radiology in Residence, Medical Center at the
University of California, San Francisco; Staff Radiologist, San Francisco
General Hospital; San Francisco, CA
  INTERVENTIONAL TECHNIQUES

ANTHONY A. MANCUSO, M.D.
Associate Professor of Radiology, University of Utah School of Medicine, Salt Lake City, UT
THE NECK

PIERRE SCHNYDER, M.D.
Chairman and Professor of Radiology, University Hospital, Lausanne, Switzerland
TRAUMA

W. RICHARD WEBB, M.D.
Professor of Radiology, University of California, San Francisco, School of Medicine, San Francisco, CA
THE CHEST WALL, AXILLARY SPACE, PLEURAE, AND DIAPHRAGM

PREFACE

The second edition of *Computed Tomography of the Body* has been extensively updated and is presented as a comprehensive, state-of-the-art text on computed tomography (CT) of the body that now includes an integration of magnetic resonance (MR) imaging in all sections of the book. Since the first edition, there have been great advances in CT and its application to patient care. Although the impact of CT has been enormous, magnetic resonance imaging is undergoing explosive growth and is having an ever-increasing impact on body imaging.

As in the first edition, this text is organized so that basic anatomy and CT and MR techniques are discussed for each region of the body. The features of disease entities in these two imaging modalities are described and illustrated, and the relationship of CT to MR and other imaging techniques is discussed in depth. Recommendations are offered as to the role of each modality in specific clinical situations. The book presents an integrated approach, reflecting our current standard of practice. Knowledge of CT and MR imaging will continue to expand, and recommendations, techniques, and patterns of use will undoubtedly change in the future.

In writing this book, now expanded to three volumes, there have been many people without whose support, guidance, insight, and help this work could not have been completed. We thank our colleagues who contributed their time and case material, and we acknowledge the illustration departments at the University of California, San Francisco, and the University of Washington, as well as the secretarial and editorial support of Jan Taylor, Isabel Rosenthal, and Denice Nakano.

ALBERT A. MOSS, M.D.
GORDON GAMSU, M.D.
HARRY K. GENANT, M.D.

INTRODUCTION TO VOLUME ONE

Computed tomography (CT) was developed for brain imaging in the late 1960s. Technical improvements rapidly allowed its application to the entire body. CT is now universally applied for imaging most thoracic pathologies and has all but replaced such procedures as conventional tomography and bronchography. Although advances in CT have tended to stabilize over the past several years, investigation of its uses and efficacy continues. The impact of CT on thoracic radiology and medicine has been enormous, and it is difficult to conceive of the practicing of these specialties without daily use of CT.

Magnetic resonance (MR) was introduced for human imaging in the mid-1970s. It has gained widespread acceptance for imaging the brain, spinal column, and musculoskeletal system. Within the thorax, however, its role has been less easily established. Cardiac, vascular, and neck imaging with MR are widely seen. In most other areas, such as the mediastinum, CT can provide comparable or more precise information. Thoracic MR with the imaging techniques currently available is limited by the physicomagnetic properties of lung tissue. The conceptual and technical developments required for successful pulmonary imaging with MR are several years away.

This volume is a comprehensive and practical update and expansion of the thorax and neck sections of the previous edition of this text. Since the publication of the first edition in 1983, thoracic CT and MR imaging have been greatly expanded and refined. For instance, recent studies on the staging of lung cancer have provided new information about the imaging of the most common fatal malignancy. High-resolution CT has been a significant advance for imaging parenchymal lung disease, and we have an important section on recent developments in this area. New chapters on interventional thoracic techniques and trauma are presented. Chapters on the physics of CT and MR imaging are included in Volume III.

The insight and guidance of many have shaped this text. We thank our co-authors and colleagues who have contributed time and effort. We also thank Isabel Rosenthal and Barbara Fougier for their editorial and secretarial support. Finally, we offer thanks to those mentors who taught us respect for patients, medicine, and scientific integrity: Doctors David Gamsu, George Simon, Leo Rigler, Ben Felson, Robert Fraser, Richard Greenspan, and Alexander Margulis.

GORDON GAMSU, M.D.

CONTENTS

TRACHEA AND CENTRAL BRONCHI

GORDON GAMSU

Computed tomography (CT) is an excellent method for visualizing mediastinal and hilar structures, including the central airways. The normal CT anatomy of the trachea and bronchi has been described.[1-4] CT scanning of abnormalities of the trachea and bronchi has also been reported in several articles. The trachea and major bronchi generally lie in a plane perpendicular to the CT image, and their lumina are well displayed in cross-sectional images. The tracheobronchial tree is visible in continuity on CT as far peripherally as segmental and subsegmental bronchi.[5-7] This chapter deals with these airways and almost exclusively with CT scanning. The present temporal and spatial resolution of magnetic resonance (MR) imaging precludes its clinical use for imaging of the trachea and central bronchi. Those circumstances in which mediastinal and hilar masses encroach on the trachea and bronchi are discussed in Chapters 2 and 3.

Anatomy

Trachea

The trachea is a fibromuscular and cartilaginous tube 10 to 12 cm long (Fig. 1–1).[8] It extends from the lower border of the cricoid cartilage in the neck to its bifurcation at the tracheal carina in the mediastinum. The trachea is a midline structure except for its few inferior centimeters, which incline slightly to the right. Its walls are parallel except for two minor indentations. The impression of the aortic arch on the left anterolateral wall of the trachea can be seen on CT scans in many normal individuals. An indentation on the right from the arch of the azygos vein is seen less frequently.

The tracheal wall comprises 20 to 22 horseshoe-shaped cartilages connected posteriorly by a thick fibromuscular membrane. The diameter of the trachea is normally 10 to 27 mm in adults (mean: 19.5 mm in males; 17.5 mm in females).[9, 10] Griscom[11] and Effmann and colleagues[12] have studied the CT dimensions of the trachea in infants and children. They found that the tracheal cross-sectional area correlated most closely with body height. Effmann and colleagues[12] found about 20 per cent variation in tracheal dimensions at different levels of the intrathoracic trachea in children. The diameter of the trachea increased with age up to 16 or 18 years.

Six to 9 cm after entering the thorax, the trachea divides into the two main bronchi.[2] The shorter right main bronchus is about 2.2 cm long, whereas the left is about 5 cm in length.[13] The diameter of the right main bronchus averages 15.3 mm, and that of the left 13 mm when measured on chest radiographs at full inspiration.[14] The trachea can change its dimensions and shape with various respiratory maneuvers.

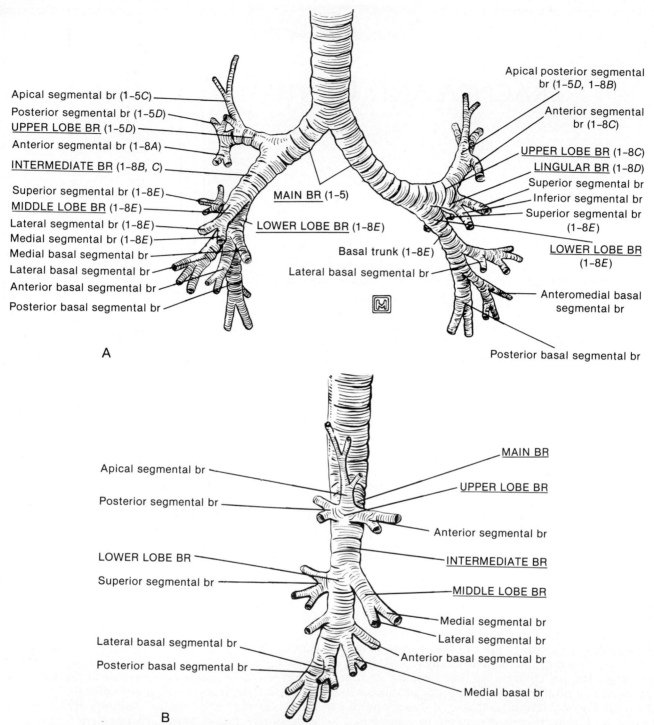

Apical segmental br (1–5C)
Posterior segmental br (1–5D)
UPPER LOBE BR (1–5D)
Anterior segmental br (1–8A)
INTERMEDIATE BR (1–8B, C)
Superior segmental br (1–8E)
MIDDLE LOBE BR (1–8E)
Lateral segmental br (1–8E)
Medial segmental br (1–8E)
Medial basal segmental br
Lateral basal segmental br
Anterior basal segmental br
Posterior basal segmental br

MAIN BR (1–5)
LOWER LOBE BR (1–8E)
Basal trunk (1–8E)
Lateral basal segmental br

Apical posterior segmental br (1–5D, 1–8B)
Anterior segmental br (1–8C)
UPPER LOBE BR (1–8C)
LINGULAR BR (1–8D)
Superior segmental br
Inferior segmental br
Superior segmental br (1–8E)
LOWER LOBE BR (1–8E)
Anteromedial basal segmental br
Posterior basal segmental br

A

Apical segmental br
Posterior segmental br
LOWER LOBE BR
Superior segmental br
Lateral basal segmental br
Posterior basal segmental br

MAIN BR
UPPER LOBE BR
Anterior segmental br
INTERMEDIATE BR
MIDDLE LOBE BR
Medial segmental br
Lateral segmental br
Anterior basal segmental br
Medial basal br

B

FIGURE 1–1 ■ Schema of lower trachea and central bronchi. The bronchial tree is shown in frontal projection *(A)*, right lateral projection *(B)*, and left lateral projection *(C)*. In *A*, numbers in parentheses refer to figures showing the relevant anatomic features. (See also Chapter 3, Figs. 3–1 through 3–9).

At end-expiration the trachea narrows slightly. During a Valsalva maneuver, the extrathoracic trachea increases its diameter 2 to 4 mm while the intrathoracic trachea remains unchanged in size. During a forced expiratory maneuver or coughing, the posterior tracheal membrane invaginates to greatly reduce the cross-sectional area of the trachea, whereas the lateral and anterior walls are minimally altered.

Right Lung Bronchi

On the right, the short main bronchus divides into an upper lobe bronchus and an intermediate bronchus (Fig. 1–1). The right upper lobe bronchus courses laterally for 1 to 2 cm before dividing into its three segmental bronchi.[3, 4] The branching pattern is moderately variable, but on CT scans, all three seg-

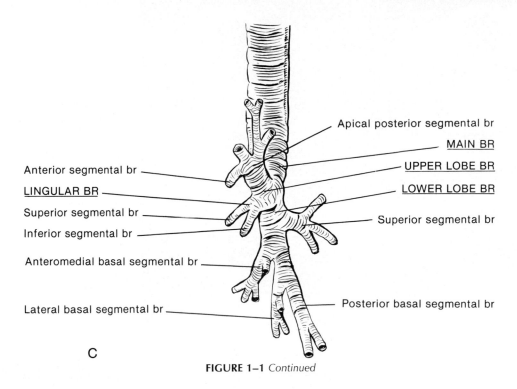

Apical posterior segmental br

MAIN BR

UPPER LOBE BR

LOWER LOBE BR

Superior segmental br

Posterior basal segmental br

Anterior segmental br

LINGULAR BR

Superior segmental br

Inferior segmental br

Anteromedial basal segmental br

Lateral basal segmental br

C

FIGURE 1–1 *Continued*

mental bronchi are usually visible. The intermediate bronchus is 3 to 4 cm long and courses slightly laterally in a superior-inferior direction. The posterior wall of the intermediate bronchus can be seen on CT scans outlined by the right lower lobe from its origin to its bifurcation in virtually all normal subjects.[15] It is a uniformly thin line measuring 0.5 to 2 mm in thickness. Rarely, an anomalous pulmonary vein courses posteriorly behind the intermediate bronchus and should not be mistaken for an abnormal mass. The middle lobe bronchus arises from the right anterolateral wall of the intermediate bronchus and passes inferiorly, laterally, and anteriorly at about a 45° obliquity for 1 to 2 cm before dividing into its medial and lateral segmental bronchi. After giving rise to the middle lobe bronchus, the intermediate bronchus continues as the right lower lobe bronchus. A distinct spur at the junction of the middle and lower lobe bronchi frequently is visible. The first segmental branch of the right lower lobe is the superior segmental bronchus, which arises from the posterior wall of the lower lobe bronchus. Beyond the origin of the superior segmental bronchus, the right basal trunk continues for 1 to 2 cm before dividing into medial, anterior, lateral, and posterior basal segments.

Left Lung Bronchi

The branching pattern of the left bronchial tree is different from that of the right (see Fig. 1–1). The long left main bronchus divides directly into upper and lower lobe bronchi. The upper lobe bronchus gives off a lingular branch from its anteroinferior surface and usually continues as a short common trunk before dividing into anterior and apical-posterior branches.[16] Less commonly, the left upper lobe bronchus trifurcates into anterior, lingular, and apical-posterior bronchi. The lingular bronchus, which is the least frequently visualized major airway on CT, is directed anteroinferiorly for 2 to 3 cm and then bifurcates into superior and inferior segmental bronchi. The absence of an intermediate bronchus on the left results in the left lower lobe bronchus arising at a level 1 to 2 cm cephalad to the right lower lobe bronchus. As on the right, the first branch of the lower lobe is the superior segmental bronchus directed posteriorly. The anteromedial, lateral, and posterior basal segments arise 1 to 2 cm distal to the origin of the superior segmental bronchus.

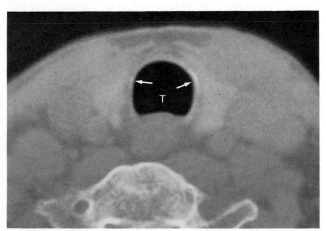

FIGURE 1–2 ■ Normal extrathoracic trachea. CT shows a normal horseshoe-shaped trachea (T). The posterior tracheal membrane bulges slightly into the tracheal air column. Anteriorly, a calcified tracheal cartilage is visible *(arrows)*.

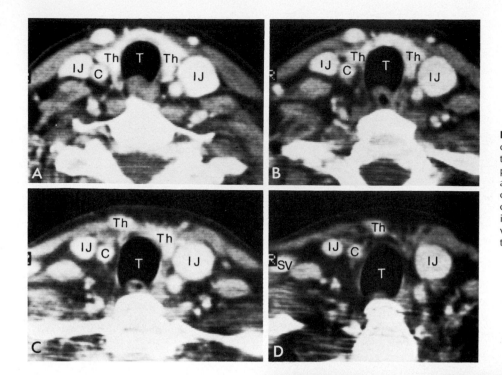

FIGURE 1–3 ■ Normal extrathoracic trachea. *A* to *D*, Sequential scans through the lower neck. The middle and lower poles of the thyroid gland (Th) are anterior and lateral to the horseshoe-shaped trachea (T). The right carotid artery (C) courses from anterior to posterior. The internal jugular veins (IJ) and right subclavian vein (SV) are anterolateral to the trachea.

FIGURE 1–4 ■ Normal thoracic inlet. *A* to *D*, Sequential CT scans 5 mm thick through the thoracic inlet from above downward. The trachea (T) is midline, and the esophagus (E) is to the left. On the right side, the subclavian artery (SA) is behind the anterior scalene muscle (SM) in *A*, and is behind the right subclavian vein (SV) and internal jugular vein (IJ) in *B* through *D*. The right common carotid artery (CA) stays close to the trachea. In *A* to *D*, the right highest intercostal vein (HIV) is behind the subclavian artery. On the left, the common carotid artery (CA) is lateral to the esophagus. The left subclavian artery courses from posterior to anterior. The internal jugular vein (IJV) and subclavian vein join anteriorly and laterally to the common carotid artery. In *A* to *C*, the left vertebral artery (VA) is posterior and lateral to the common carotid artery.

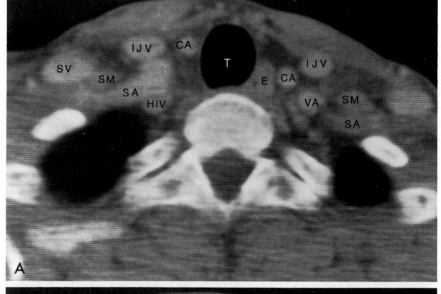

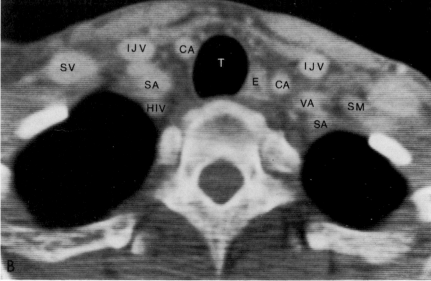

CT Appearances

TRACHEA

The extrathoracic trachea begins at the lower border of the cricoid cartilage and ends at the thoracic inlet, a distance of 2 to 4 cm.[2] The subglottic larynx, within the cricoid cartilage, is always circular on CT scans, and the airway is in close proximity to the underlying perichondrium. Immediately below the cricoid cartilage, the extrathoracic trachea assumes a horseshoe, elliptical, or circular configuration (Fig. 1–2). In about 50 per cent of normal people, the posterior tracheal membrane protrudes slightly into the tracheal air column.

The thyroid gland encases the anterior and lateral walls of the extrathoracic trachea (Fig. 1–3). It is always visible on CT scans and extends vertically for 2 to 4 cm. The thyroid gland is usually denser than the surrounding soft tissues because of its iodine content. The sternohyoid and sternothyroid muscles, together with a variable quantity of fat, also border the anterior wall of the extrathoracic trachea.

The common carotid arteries and jugular veins are usually lateral to the extrathoracic trachea (Fig. 1–3) but are occasionally slightly behind a coronal plane through the trachea. The right common carotid artery is usually more anterior than the left. The right internal jugular vein lies lateral to the right common carotid artery and is usually larger than the left internal jugular vein, which is anterolateral to the left common carotid artery.

The thoracic inlet is a sloping plane at the junction of the thorax and neck. It extends from the suprasternal (jugular) notch anteriorly, to the first thoracic vertebral body posteriorly. Below this level, the trachea is intrathoracic and makes its first contact with the right lung 1 to 3 cm above the suprasternal notch. The relationship of the great arteries and veins to the trachea changes rapidly at the thoracic inlet (Fig. 1–4). The innominate artery is visible on CT scans on the right, next to the anterior third of the trachea, where it divides to form the right subclavian and common carotid arteries. The right internal jugular

FIGURE 1–4 Continued

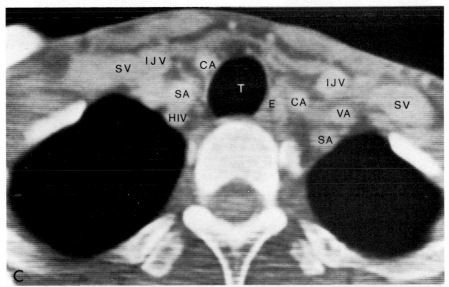

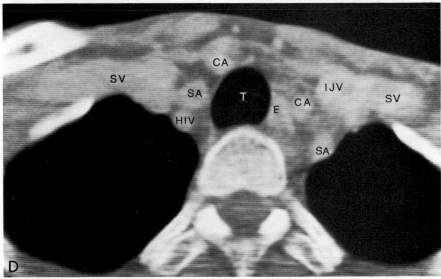

and subclavian veins join to form the right brachio-cephalic vein lateral to the innominate artery. The left common carotid artery is next to the middle or posterior third of the tracheal wall on the left. The left subclavian artery is initially posterior to the trachea and then courses anterolaterally toward the left first rib. The esophagus at the level of the thoracic inlet is always directly behind the trachea at or slightly to the left of the midline. The inferior extensions of the strap muscles are directly anterior to the trachea.

The apices of the lungs are seen on CT on the level at which the trachea becomes intrathoracic. The in-trathoracic trachea is 6 to 9 cm long (mean: 7.5 ± 0.8 cm).[2] The shape of the normal intrathoracic trachea on CT scans varies from person to person and at different levels in the same person. The usual shape is circular or slightly oval (Fig. 1–5A–D). It may be horseshoe-shaped with a flat posterior wall. Less commonly, it has the shape of an inverted pear or can be almost square. In children the trachea is almost always circular or nearly circular.[17] Mild variations in shape occur at different levels, but the posterior indentation produced by the tracheal membrane is not found in children. The child's trachea is remarkably uniform over its length.

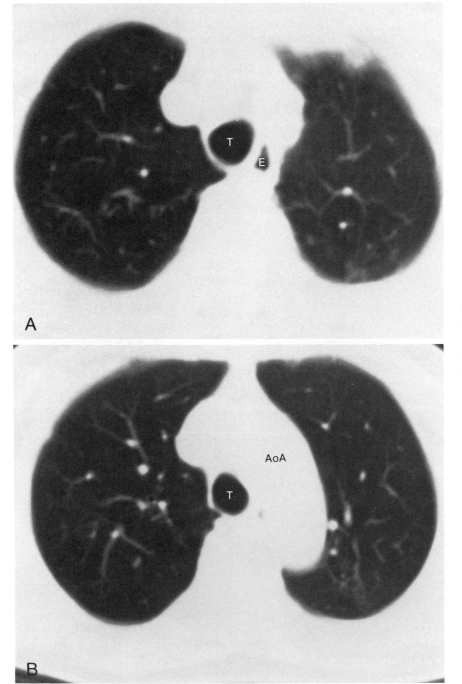

FIGURE 1–5 ■ Normal intrathoracic trachea in a young adult male. CT at 2-cm intervals demonstrate changes in the trachea (T) at various levels. *A*, The right lung contacts the right lateral wall of the trachea. The esophagus (E) is to the left. *B*, At the level of the aortic arch (AoA), the left anterior wall of the trachea is slightly flat.

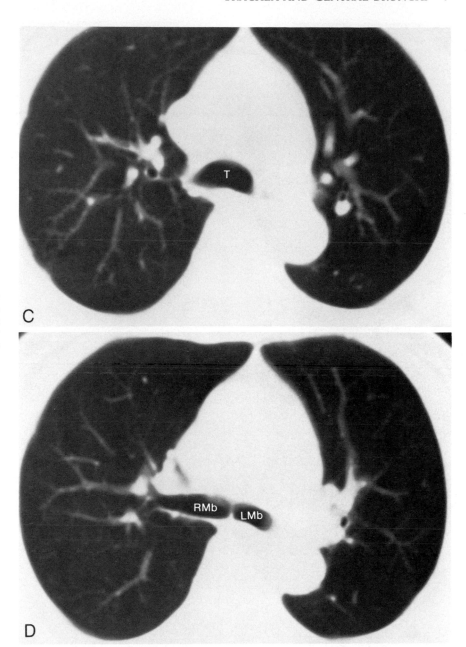

FIGURE 1–5 *Continued* ■ *C,* Immediately above the tracheal carina, the trachea assumes a horizontal oval shape. *D,* At the level of the tracheal carina, the right main bronchus (RMb) and left main bronchus (LMb) are demonstrated.

The tracheal wall is usually visible on CT scans as a distinct thin line against a background of low-density mediastinal fat, except where lung parenchyma or vessels contact its wall. Calcification of the tracheal cartilages is usually seen only in people over the age of 40 (see Fig. 1–2). It is visible as small, discontinuous foci of high density within the tracheal wall. Soft tissue is not normally present within the outline of the tracheal wall. In about 2 per cent of patients, a glob of mucus can be seen in the trachea or major bronchi and should not be mistaken for a mass (Fig. 1–6).[18]

The relationship of the intrathoracic trachea to the vessels around it and to the esophagus depends on the level of the scan. The great vessels are in front and to the left of the upper 2 to 4 cm of the intrathoracic trachea. The innominate artery is directly anterior to the trachea in about 40 per cent of normal people. In the remainder, it is either slightly to the left or the right of the midline (Fig. 1–7). The left common carotid artery is seen to the left of and anterior to the trachea in its lower portion and to the left of and lateral to the trachea in its upper portion. The left subclavian artery has a variable anteroposterior relationship to the upper intrathoracic trachea. In about half of normal people, it is directly lateral to the middle third of the trachea. In most of the remainder, it is lateral to the anterior third, whereas in a small minority, it is lateral to the posterior third. Mediastinal fat usually separates the upper trachea from the left lung and surrounds the left subclavian artery to a variable degree.

On the right side of the upper mediastinum, the right lung first contacts the posterolateral surface of

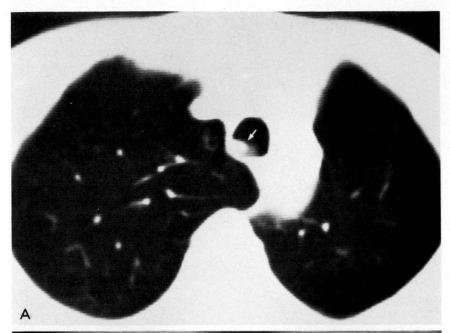

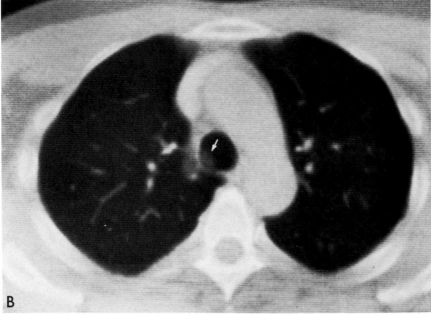

FIGURE 1–6 ■ Mucus in the tracheal lumen. A, CT shows a glob of mucus in the trachea (arrow). B, In a second patient, CT at extended window settings shows the relationship of a glob of mucus (arrow) to the tracheal wall.

the trachea. For the next 1 to 2 cm, contact is with the posterior one half to two thirds of the right tracheal wall (see Fig. 1–5A). The superior vena cava is always anterior to and to the right of the trachea; only near the thoracic inlet does the right brachiocephalic vein assume a position lateral to the trachea. In the supine position, CT shows one third to two thirds of the posterior wall of the trachea is in contact with the right lung (see Fig. 1–7).[19–21] In most subjects, the rest of the posterior wall of the trachea is bordered by the esophagus or mediastinal fat. In about 15 per cent of subjects, the retrotracheal space is small, and the trachea is in direct contact with the spine. Under these conditions, the esophagus is entirely to the left of the trachea.

Below the level of the great vessels, the aortic arch is visible over a vertical distance of 1 to 2 cm, anterior and to the left of the trachea. On CT scans, the aortic arch frequently produces a slight flattening of the left anterolateral wall of the trachea but does not otherwise distort the normal trachea (see Fig. 1–5B). Inferior to the thoracic inlet, the only vascular structure bordering the right tracheal wall is the azygos arch, which is visible on CT scans at a level between 1 and 3 cm above the tracheal carina and may produce a slight indentation on the right tracheal wall.[22]

The trachea assumes a horizontal oval shape in its most inferior 1 to 2 cm (see Fig. 1–5C). The fat-containing pretracheal space separates the lower trachea from the ascending aorta.[23] The left side of the lower trachea forms the medial boundary of the aortic-pulmonic window. However, on CT scans obtained with the scanner gantry in the vertical position and using 10 mm collimation, a distinctive aortic-pulmonic window is seen in only about a third of subjects. In the remainder, the inferior surface of the aortic arch or the superior surface of the left pulmonary artery obscures this window.

A tracheal bronchus is an uncommon anomaly consisting of an ectopic bronchus arising from the right lower trachea. It may predispose to infection in the supplied segment of the right lung. A tracheal bronchus appears on CT as a tubular, air-containing structure arising from the trachea above the level of the carina.[24, 25]

CENTRAL BRONCHI

The frequency with which a central bronchus is seen on CT scans depends on the size of the bronchus, its orientation relative to the plane of the scan, and the scan thickness.[3, 5, 7] Normally, the main bronchi, intermediate bronchus, and lobar bronchi are visible. Segmental bronchi that are in cross-section or imaged along their major axes are also usually demonstrated. The middle lobe and the lingular and basal bronchi course obliquely to the CT plane and are well seen on scans 1 cm thick about 80 per cent of the time. On thinner sections, these bronchi are seen more frequently. Bronchi beyond segmental branches are not routinely seen with CT. (The relationships of the bronchi to the pulmonary arteries and veins are discussed in Chapter 3.)

The short right main bronchus can be seen coursing inferiorly and laterally on one or two adjacent scans (Fig. 1–8A). It then divides into a right upper lobe bronchus and an intermediate bronchus. The upper lobe bronchus normally courses laterally for 1 to 2 cm and can be seen on one or two contiguous scans (Fig. 1–8A). The anterior and posterior segmental bronchi are often demonstrated on the same scan as the lobar bronchus. They are oriented in a near-horizontal plane and pass anterolaterally and posterolaterally, respectively. On 10-mm sections, the right upper lobe bronchus may be imaged in slight obliquity and may appear to taper laterally (Fig. 1–8B). The anterior segmental bronchus is more horizontal than the posterior segmental bronchus and is visible over a greater length. The apical bronchus is almost always seen in cross section, at levels 1 to 2 cm cephalad to the lobar bronchus.

The intermediate bronchus is visible in almost perfect cross section as it courses almost vertically from the origin of the right upper lobe bronchus to the origin of the middle lobe bronchus. On three to four contiguous images, it appears as a ring bordered by lung posteriorly and the interlobar branch of the right pulmonary artery anterolaterally (Figs. 1–8C, D).

The origin and length of the middle lobe bronchus are seen on one to two contiguous scans, arising from the anterolateral surface of the intermediate bronchus (Fig. 1–8E). It courses anteriorly, laterally, and inferiorly for 1 to 3 cm before dividing into its medial and lateral segmental bronchi. In about 60 per cent of normal subjects, the segmental bronchi are of equal size. In the remainder, the medial segmental bronchus predominates and can be recognized on CT scans as the larger of the two.[3] The lateral segmental bronchus is in a more horizontal plane and is frequently demonstrated over a greater length than the medial segmental bronchus. The segmental bronchi of the middle lobe are those most often poorly demonstrated on 1-cm CT slices.[5]

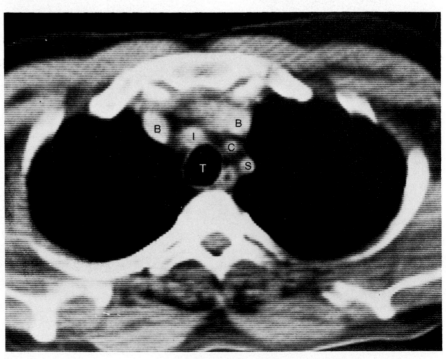

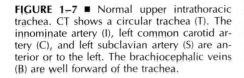

FIGURE 1–7 ■ Normal upper intrathoracic trachea. CT shows a circular trachea (T). The innominate artery (I), left common carotid artery (C), and left subclavian artery (S) are anterior or to the left. The brachiocephalic veins (B) are well forward of the trachea.

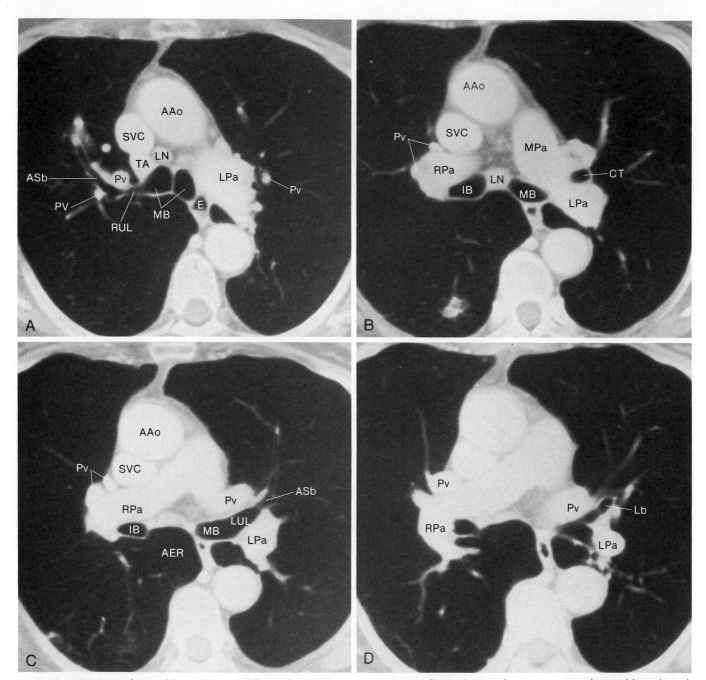

FIGURE 1–8 ■ Normal central bronchi in a mildly emphysematous man. Five-mm collimated scans demonstrate normal central bronchi and their vascular relationship. AAo = ascending aorta; LPa = left pulmonary artery; SVC = superior vena cava; Pv = pulmonary vein; MB = main bronchus; RUL = right upper lobe bronchus; ASb = anterior segmental bronchus; E = esophagus; TA = anterior trunk; MPa = main pulmonary artery; LN = lymph node; RPa = right pulmonary artery; LT = left upper lobe common trunk; IB = intermediate bronchus; AER = azygoesophageal recess; Lb = lingula bronchus; LA = left atrium; MLb = middle lobe bronchus; SSb = superior segmental bronchus; BT = basal trunk; BSb = basal segmental bronchi; LAa = left atrial appendage; LUL = left upper lobe bronchus.

The bronchus to the superior segment of the right lower lobe is directed posteriorly and slightly laterally (Fig. 1–8E). Its proximal 1 to 3 cm is usually seen, frequently accompanied by a branch of the pulmonary artery on its lateral side. The superior segmental bronchus originates at the level of the right middle lobe bronchus; 1 cm caudad to it; or because of the orientation of the lung in the chest, it can even appear 1 cm cephalad. Lung borders the posterior

hilum at this level and is in contact with the posterior and, often, the medial walls of the intermediate bronchus, as well as the medial wall of the superior segmental bronchus.

The short right lower lobe basal trunk distal to the superior segmental bronchus courses in a vertical plane and is usually visible on only one CT scan (Fig. 1–8F). The right pulmonary artery is lateral to the basal trunk, and the right inferior pulmonary vein is

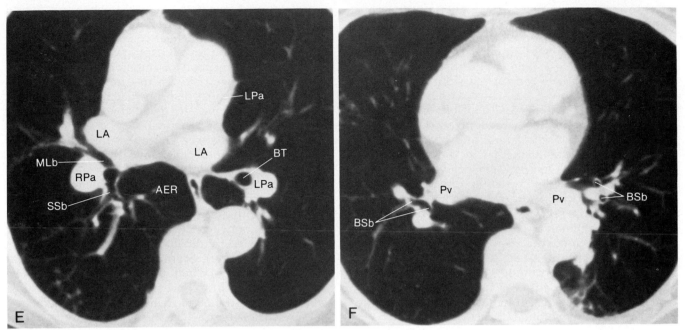

FIGURE 1–8 *Continued*

posterior. The lung parenchyma of the right lower lobe lies anterior to the basal trunk. The basal segmental bronchi originate approximately 1 cm distal to the right middle lobe bronchus and course in oblique directions. Frequently, only two to three of the basal bronchi are demonstrated on 1 cm–collimated CT. The inferior pulmonary vein courses from lateral to medial, behind the dividing basal segmental bronchi, and is always visible on CT. In many subjects the segmental pulmonary arteries accompanying the bronchi are variable and may be duplicated or even triplicated. The pulmonary arteries are situated toward the periphery of the lung in their relationship to the bronchi. In about 20 per cent of individuals, the usual lower lobe branching pattern is not found, owing to anatomic variation.[6] Naidich and colleagues[7] used thin-section (1.5 or 5 mm) collimation to image the basal bronchi. All basal segmental bronchi were demonstrated and showed six patterns of variation in division in the right lower lobe. Absence of one or more basal bronchi was also encountered. Using thin sections, subsegmental bronchi were also identified in 56 per cent of individuals.

The left main bronchus is considerably longer than the right main bronchus and is visible on three to four contiguous 1 cm thick CT scans (Fig. 1–8A–C). Its orifice and proximal segment, immediately distal to the tracheal carina, are directly medial to the left pulmonary artery, anterior to the descending aorta, and posterior to the left superior pulmonary vein (Fig. 1–8C). The distal left main bronchus and the left upper lobe bronchus are visible at two contiguous levels 2 to 4 cm below the tracheal carina. On the more cephalad of these two scans, the posterior wall of the left upper lobe bronchus may appear slightly concave where it is in contact with the descending

left pulmonary artery (Fig. 1–8C). In almost 90 per cent of individuals, the left lung extends medial to the descending left pulmonary artery and anterior and lateral to the descending aorta.[26] This tongue of lung contacts the posterior wall of the distal left main bronchus and proximal left upper lobe bronchus, forming the left "retrobronchial stripe," visible on one to three successive CT scans. In the remaining patients, lung is precluded from this retrobronchial recess by a tortuous aorta or the narrow anteroposterior diameter of the chest.

The left upper lobe bronchus terminates in one of two branching patterns. In 75 per cent of subjects, a single airway is visible distal to the origin of the lingular bronchus, coursing in a cephalad direction. This is the common trunk for the anterior and apical-posterior segmental bronchi. In the remaining 25 per cent, the left upper lobe bronchus trifurcates into anterior, apical-posterior, and lingular bronchi. The anterior segmental bronchus of the left upper lobe courses in an anterior and slightly lateral direction. In most people, the course is horizontal and is visible for 1 to 3 cm (Fig. 1–8C). The apical-posterior segmental bronchus is seen 1 to 2 cm above the left upper lobe bronchus, at the level of the proximal left main bronchus (Fig. 1–8B). The lingular bronchus is demonstrated with 10-mm slices in about 80 per cent of people, whereas its two segmental bronchi can be seen in only about 40 per cent of individuals. It is immediately caudad to the anterior segmental bronchus and courses in an anterior, lateral, and inferior direction, oblique to the plane of the CT scan (Fig. 1–8D).

The origin of the left lower lobe bronchus is demonstrated on the lower of the two scans through the distal left main bronchus and proximal left upper lobe bronchus (Fig. 1–8D). Frequently, a spur delineates the orifices of the left lower and left upper lobe bronchi. The left lower lobe bronchus is usually demonstrated on the same scan as the lingular bronchus. Its orifice is anteromedial to the descending left pulmonary artery. The superior segmental bronchus of the left lower lobe arises from the posterior wall of the left lower bronchus within 1 cm of its origin (Fig. 1–8D). It is usually visible on CT and its posterior direction is easily recognized. The descending pulmonary artery is lateral and a portion of the left lower lobe usually medial to the superior segmental bronchus. One to 2 cm below the origin of the superior segmental bronchus, one to three of the three basal bronchi to the left lower lobe are demonstrated in cross section (Fig. 1–8F). As on the right, tributaries of the inferior pulmonary vein courses from lateral to medial across the back of the hilum at this level. With high resolution (HR) CT, all basal segmental bronchi on the left are demonstrated and show five separate patterns of division.[7] In 35 per cent of instances subsegmental bronchi can be detected with thinly collimated sections.

Techniques of Examination

Computed tomography of the trachea and bronchi is generally performed in a manner similar to that of the rest of the thorax (see also Chapters 2 through 4). When it is known that the patient is being studied for a tracheal or central bronchial abnormality, 3- or 5-mm collimation through the site of the lesion can give better spatial resolution, and endotracheal or endobronchial masses can be more easily appreciated. The patient is usually in the supine position. When the region of primary concern is the extrathoracic trachea, the patient's arms are positioned at the side, with the shoulders pulled down as far as possible. If the intrathoracic, mediastinal portion of the trachea or the central bronchi are the regions of interest, the patient's arms are usually positioned above the head to eliminate streak artifacts from the shoulder girdle and arms. A computed projection radiograph (scout view, projection view) can be obtained at the beginning of the examination to localize the area that will be scanned.

In most circumstances, CT scans of the trachea and bronchi are performed while the patient suspends respiration at full inspiration. A few deep breaths before scanning can aid the patient in suspending respiration for the required time. In older patients who are unable to hold their breath, scanning can be undertaken during quiet mouth breathing. Occasionally, scans during a specific respiratory maneuver can assist in the diagnosis of tracheal abnormality. For example, a Valsalva maneuver will increase intratracheal pressure and distend the extrathoracic trachea, allowing segments of abnormal tracheal compliance to be demonstrated. Forced expiratory maneuvers cause a marked reduction in the cross-sectional area of the normal trachea and central bronchi. When ultrafast scanners are available, segments of abnormal tracheal collapse can sometimes be detected during forced expiration.

Intravenous injection or infusion of contrast medium has not been shown to directly assist in the diagnosis of tracheal or bronchial masses. Contrast medium does, however, detail the mediastinal and cervical vessels and demonstrate the relationship of a mass to these vessels. During scanning, 125 to 150 ml of 60 or 76 per cent contrast material can be administered by slow infusion or by a series of bolus injections. A mass impinging on the trachea or a bronchus can be a large vessel or soft tissue tumor. CT scans with intravascular contrast material will differentiate between the two. High levels of contrast can be achieved by obtaining rapid sequential scans (dynamic scanning). Scanning can be carried out at a single level or, when the scanner table can be incremented with a short interscan delay, multiple levels through the abnormality can be scanned.

CT scans of the trachea and bronchi are viewed at several window levels and widths. Narrowing of the trachea and bronchi is best detected at a window level of -250 to -500 Hounsfield units (H) and a window width of 500 to 1000 H. At these settings, normal and abnormal airways have a smaller caliber than at soft tissue window settings. The most precise setting for measurement of airway size depends on the tissue around the airway.[27] For an airway surrounded by soft tissue, it is a window level of about -150 H. For an airway surrounded by lung, it is a window level midway between the density of air in the lung and the soft tissue of the airway wall, or approximately -450 H. A narrow window width should be used. The hilar contours are viewed at window settings usually used for the lungs (level -500 to -700 H, width 1000 to 1500 H). Masses within the trachea or invading the tracheal wall are viewed at soft tissue window settings normally used for the mediastinum (level 40 to 60 H, width 150 to 300 H).

Pathology

Generalized Tracheal Abnormalities

INCREASED TRACHEAL CALIBER

Tracheobronchomegaly (Trachiectasis, Mounier-Kuhn Syndrome) ■ This is a distinctive condition consisting of marked dilation of the trachea and central bronchi, in association with chronic respiratory tract infections.[28, 29] The clinical features are ineffective chronic cough and recurrent bronchitis or pneumonia. Tracheobronchomegaly probably results from a congenital defect of the elastic and muscle fibers within the tracheal and bronchial walls. Typically, the trachea and central bronchi are involved, but occasionally bronchial involvement alone is found. Studies of pedigrees suggest a genetic disease, and an association with the Ehlers-Danlos syndrome has been described.[30]

Radiographically, the condition is characterized by a greatly increased tracheal caliber, measuring 35 to 50 mm or more in diameter.[29] The tracheal air column has an irregular, corrugated appearance caused by the protrusion of redundant mucosa between the cartilaginous rings. CT scans can show the enlarged trachea and central bronchi as well as the saccular outpouchings between the bronchial cartilages.[31] Detection of concomitant lung disease is possible. Bronchiectasis, bronchiolectasis, bullous emphysema, diffuse emphysema, chronic bronchitis, and pulmonary fibrosis can all be present and can be demonstrated with CT.

Tracheobronchomalacia ■ Described by Williams and Campbell,[32] this condition is characterized by a deficiency of cartilage in the tracheobronchial tree. It is a developmental defect and can be associated with other congenital anomalies such as cleft palate and laryngomalacia. As with tracheobronchomegaly, there is excessive flaccidity of the tracheal wall and recurrent pneumonia and bronchiectasis. The trachea and central bronchi are dilated on radiographs during inspiration and collapse with expiration. The CT findings should be similar to those of tracheobronchomegaly, although tracheobronchomalacia is a more severe condition and most patients die from respiratory failure in childhood.

DECREASED TRACHEAL CALIBER

Diffuse narrowing of the trachea is uncommon and is usually due to a specific cause. Symptoms are often nonspecific, consisting of dyspnea, cough, wheezing, and sometimes hoarseness, or stridor. Five entities should be considered when dealing with diffuse tracheal narrowing: saber-sheath trachea, amyloidosis, relapsing polychondritis, tracheobronchopathia osteochondroplastica, and scleroma.

Saber-Sheath Trachea ■ In some patients with chronic obstructive pulmonary disease, the intrathoracic trachea has a saber-sheath configuration.[33, 34] The coronal dimension is narrow and is less than two thirds of the sagittal diameter at the same level (Fig. 1–9). In one study, 95 per cent of patients with a saber-sheath trachea had clinical evidence of chronic obstructive lung disease, 100 per cent had a history of smoking, and 80 per cent had symptoms of chronic bronchitis.[33]

Chest radiographs show the abnormal configuration of the trachea, and the tracheal wall may appear thickened. CT scans do not demonstrate abnormal soft tissue within the tracheal lumen and do not confirm thickening of the tracheal wall.[2] On CT the tracheal cartilages are usually densely calcified, and the coronal narrowing of the intrathoracic trachea is due to an abnormal shape of the tracheal cartilages, which have a narrow anterior arch. CT scans during forced expiration have shown that the intrathoracic trachea narrows abnormally.[2] Instead of the posterior tracheal membrane invaginating to reduce the lumen

of the trachea, as in normal subjects, the lateral walls of the trachea collapse inward (Fig. 1–9B).

Amyloidosis ■ Deposition of the protein-polysaccharide complex known as amyloid within the respiratory system can occur in both the primary and secondary forms of the disease.[35, 36] Deposition can involve the lungs, resulting in pulmonary nodules, or can be limited to the trachea and bronchi. In the latter form, amyloid is in the submucosal and muscular layers of the airway wall. Irregular, lard-like masses encroach on the lumen of the trachea and central bronchi, and produce focal or diffuse narrowing of the airway. Mediastinal and hilar lymphadenopathy can be present. The airway narrowing can be seen on conventional chest radiographs or CT. CT will also show thickening of the tracheal wall, sometimes with foci of calcium within the amyloid deposits (Fig. 1–10). Diagnosis is usually made by bronchoscopy and biopsy of the tracheal or central bronchial masses.

Relapsing Polychondritis ■ Relapsing polychondritis is an unusual systemic disease that affects cartilage at many sites throughout the body, including the ears, nose, joints, and tracheobronchial tree.[37, 38] Cartilage is destroyed and replaced by fibrous tissue. Respiratory distress is common and death from respiratory failure can occur. The cause of relapsing polychondritis is unknown. The cartilage destruction appears to be mediated by lysosomal enzymes that destroy connective tissue and release chondroitin sulfate from the cartilage matrix.[39] Anticartilage antibodies have been found in some patients.[38, 39]

The diagnosis can be suspected from recurrent episodes of inflammation of cartilage, most commonly of the nose and ear. Deafness and arthritis are frequently present. When the airways are involved, radiographs and CT can show generalized or focal, fixed narrowing of the trachea and bronchi (Fig. 1–11A, B).[40] Flaccidity of the airway has been described in one case.[41]

Tracheobronchopathia Osteochondroplastica ■ Occurring almost exclusively in older men, tracheobronchopathia osteochondroplastica is a degenerative disease characterized by the formation of nodules of bone and cartilage within the submucosa of the trachea and bronchi.[42–44] These nodules produce sessile and polypoid masses that irregularly narrow the lumen of the trachea and central bronchi. The airways appear beaded on conventional tomograms and positive-contrast studies. On CT, plaques and calcifications are seen in the anterior and lateral walls of the trachea (Fig. 1–12). The lesions are confined to parts of the trachea and bronchi that normally contain cartilage, and thus the posterior tracheal membrane is spared. Peripheral bronchial lesions can cause obstruction of segmental and lobar bronchi, giving rise to atelectasis and obstructive pneumonitis. The condition may not be suspected during life, and the diagnosis may be made only at necropsy.[45] The beaded appearance seen at bronchoscopy is typical, and the diagnosis is readily confirmed.[44]

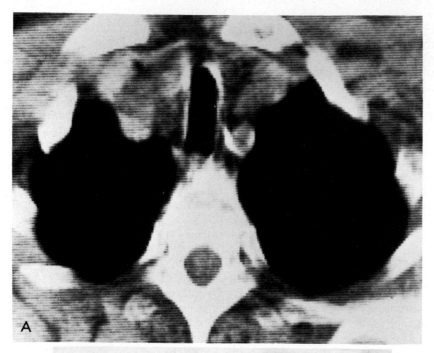

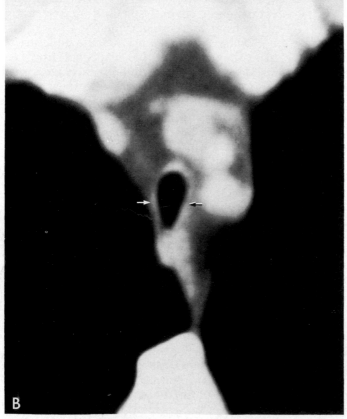

FIGURE 1–9 ■ Saber-sheath trachea. *A,* CT shows the typical configuration of a saber-sheath trachea. The anteroposterior dimension is increased, and the lateral dimension is decreased. The anterior arch is narrow. *B,* During forced expiration, a saber-sheath trachea shows abnormal inward collapse of its lateral walls *(arrows).*

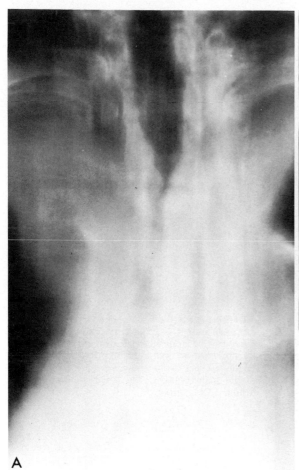

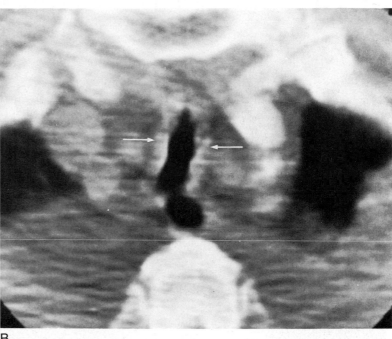

FIGURE 1–10 ■ Amyloid of the trachea. *A,* Conventional tomogram demonstrates diffuse, irregular narrowing of the tracheal air column. *B,* CT through the upper intrathoracic trachea shows irregular thickening of the tracheal wall *(arrows).*

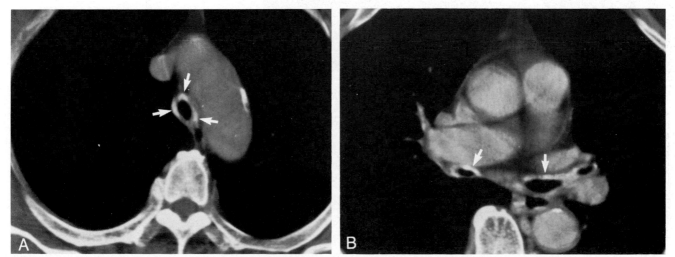

FIGURE 1–11 ■ A 54-year-old male with relapsing polychondritis. *A,* CT through the mid-trachea and *B,* proximal bronchi demonstrate diffuse narrowing of the airways with thickening and calcification of the bronchial and tracheal walls *(arrows).*

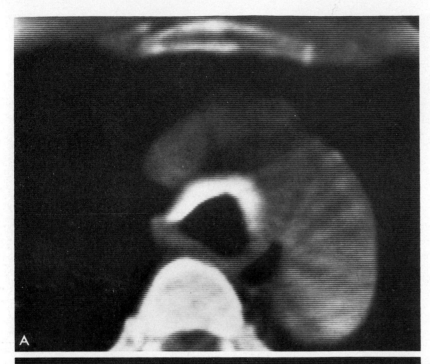

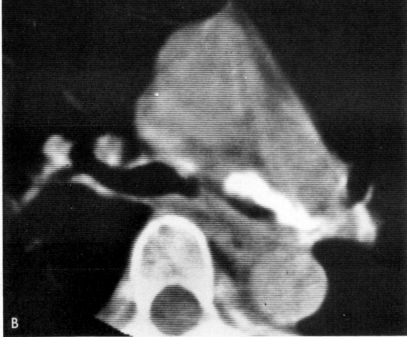

FIGURE 1–12 ■ Tracheobronchopathia osteochondroplastica. *A,* CT through the midtrachea shows dense calcification of tracheal cartilage. The tracheal lumen is near normal in caliber. *B,* CT at the level of the tracheal carina shows irregular calcification of the main bronchi. The left main bronchus is distorted and narrowed.

Scleroma ■ Scleroma is a specific chronic granulomatous condition caused by a strain of *Klebsiella pneumoniae (Klebsiella rhinoscleromatis).*[46] It is endemic in parts of Eastern Europe, Russia, South America, and Asia and is being seen with increasing frequency in North America. The nose is the main site of infection, but the larynx, trachea, and bronchi can be involved. Continuity between the nasal granulomas and the lower airway may or may not be present. The age distribution ranges from childhood to old age. Symptoms include nasal obstruction, hoarseness, dyspnea, and cough. The trachea is not involved unless lar-

yngoscleroma is present. Subglottic stenosis is the most common tracheal abnormality. Diffuse, uniform tracheal narrowing from mucosal thickening or multiple masses may be seen with CT.

Localized Tracheal Abnormalities

NEOPLASMS

Localized lesions of the trachea can be primary benign or malignant neoplasms, inflammatory masses, pseudotumors caused by a variety of conditions, secondary invasion from malignant neoplasms arising in adjacent organs, or metastases (Table 1–1) (Fig. 1–13A–C). Extrinsic compression of the trachea can manifest clinically and radiographically as a tracheal mass. Tracheal stenosis and granulomas after intubation, tracheotomy, or tracheal injury can also appear as masslike lesions of the trachea.

The symptoms of focal tracheal lesions are frequently nonspecific and mimic various pulmonary diseases, such as asthma. Most symptoms are related to airway obstruction. Many patients are treated for asthma or chronic bronchitis before the focal tracheal lesion is suspected.

Benign Neoplasms ■ Benign neoplasms are a minority of benign tracheal masses. Inflammatory, posttraumatic, and infiltrative lesions are all more common. Most benign tracheal neoplasms are found in the pediatric age group: squamous cell papilloma, fibroma, and hemangioma are the most common.[47, 48] In adults, the most common benign tumors are chondroma, papilloma, fibroma, hemangioma, and granular cell myoblastoma.[48]

Chondromas of the trachea, however, are rare neoplasms.[49–51] In one report, three chondromas were

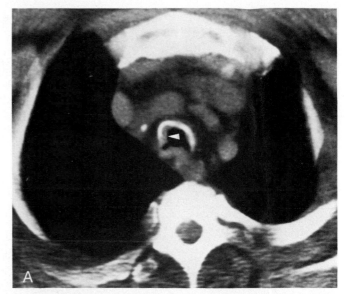

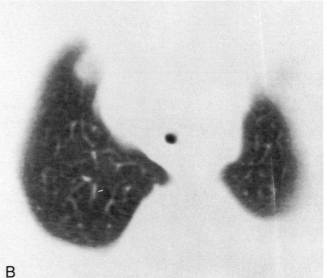

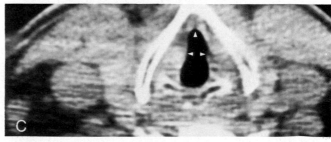

FIGURE 1–13 ■ A 36-year-old man with Wegener's granulomatosis involving the larynx and trachea. A and B, CT of the trachea demonstrates dense tracheal cartilages, soft tissue within the trachea (arrowhead), and marked reduction in the tracheal lumen. C, CT through the larynx demonstrates swelling of both vocal cords and of the anterior commissure (arrowheads).

TABLE 1–1 ■ **Causes of a Tracheal Mass**

Inflammatory granuloma	Posttraumatic
	Tuberculosis
	Fungus
	Wegener's granulomatosis
	Scleroma
	Laryngeal papillomatosis
Benign neoplasms	Chondroma, hamartoma
	Squamous cell papilloma
	Fibroma
	Hemangioma
	Granular cell myoblastoma
	Leiomyoma
	Others (neurilemoma, lipoma, fibrous histiocytoma, benign mixed tumors)
Malignant neoplasms	Squamous cell carcinoma
	Adenoid cystic carcinoma (cylindroma)
	Adenocarcinoma
	Sarcoma
	Carcinoid
	Other (pseudosarcoma, oat cell carcinoma, lymphoma, plasmacytoma, melanoma, hemangioendothelioma)
Invasion from adjacent neoplasm	Thyroid
	Lung
	Esophagus
Metastasis from distant site	Breast
	Colon
	Genitourinary
	Melanoma
Extrinsic compression	Neoplasm
	Aneurysm
	Vascular ring
Idiopathic	Goiter
	Amyloid
	Tracheopathia osteochondroplastica

found among 84 primary and secondary neoplasms of the trachea.[52] The tumor appears at bronchoscopy as a smooth, well-circumscribed, hard mass covered by normal epithelium. Chondromas tend to recur if inadequately excised.

Squamous cell papillomas are sessile or papillary nodular masses limited to the tracheal mucosa. They

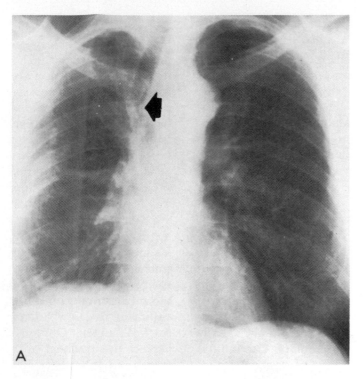

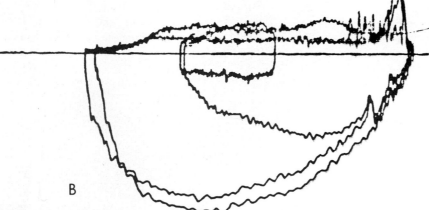

FIGURE 1–14 ■ Primary adenocarcinoma of the trachea. *A*, Frontal chest radiograph shows a mass projection into the intrathoracic tracheal air column *(arrow)*. *B*, Flow:volume loop, with flow on the vertical axis and volume on the horizontal axis, demonstrates marked limitation of expiratory flow with a plateau on the expiratory curve.

can be single or multiple. Multiple papillomas of the trachea can occur from the spread of laryngeal papillomatosis. Recurrence is frequent, and repeated surgical excisions may be necessary.

Fibromas of the trachea occur as a mixture of fibrous tissue with other tissue elements to produce fibroadenomas, neurofibromas, myxofibromas, and chondrofibromas. None of these shows specific characteristics on imaging studies.

Other benign neoplasms and non-neoplastic masses occur in the trachea (see Table 1–1). They are usually well defined and sessile or pedunculated. They do not invade deeply into the tracheal wall. Their diagnosis is based on histologic characteristics from biopsy specimens or from the excised tumor.

Most benign neoplasms can be demonstrated with well-penetrated chest radiographs if they are suspected clinically. Benign lesions are usually less than 2 cm in size and are well circumscribed.[52] They invariably project into the lumen of the trachea. Malignant tracheal neoplasms can have similar radio-

graphic features and can be indistinguishable from benign tumors. Calcification is frequently visible in cartilaginous tumors such as chondroma and hamartoma. CT scans should be obtained in patients with suspected tracheal neoplasms to detect invasion of the tumor through the tracheal wall and the craniocaudad extent of the tumor.[2] CT will demonstrate the intratracheal component of a benign tracheal neoplasm and can accurately localize the position and extent of the lesion. The tracheal wall is visible on collimated CT scans, and benign tumors should be clearly confined to the tracheal wall. CT scans are more sensitive than conventional radiographs in detecting calcification within lung and mediastinal masses. Calcification within benign tracheal tumors such as chondromas is readily visible on CT. CT scans can also assess the severity of airway narrowing by a mass, and the cross-sectional area of the airway can be measured.

Primary Malignant Neoplasms ■ These are uncommon, accounting for less than 0.1 per cent of malignancies.[53, 54] Malignant tumors of laryngeal and bronchial origin are, respectively, at least 75 and 180 times more common than those arising in the trachea.[52] In adults, primary malignant tumors of the trachea are slightly more common than benign tumors, and carcinomas account for 80 to 90 per cent of these malignancies.[48, 53] Squamous cell carcinoma derived from tracheal epithelium is the most frequent, and adenoid cystic carcinoma (cylindroma) arising from mucous glands in the tracheal wall is next in frequency. In a study by Houston and colleagues,[53] 51 per cent of malignant tracheal neoplasms were squamous cell carcinoma, and 40 per cent adenoid cystic carcinoma. Sarcoma, lymphoma, plasmacytoma, adenocarcinoma, chondrosarcoma, malignant carcinoid, and oat cell carcinoma have been reported but are rare tumors.

The most common location for tracheal neoplasms is the lower third of the trachea, with 35 to 44 per cent arising in this location.[48, 53, 55, 56] Squamous cell carcinoma is particularly common in the distal trachea, and over half arise within 3 to 4 cm of the tracheal carina. The extrathoracic, proximal trachea is the next most frequent site for squamous cell carcinoma and the most common site for other malignant tumors.

The symptoms of tracheal malignancies are frequently nonspecific, leading to a delay in diagnosis that averages 10 months.[56] About 50 per cent of the diameter of the trachea must be occluded before symptoms of obstruction occur. Cough is present in 33 to 85 per cent of patients, hemoptysis in 27 to 66 per cent, and dyspnea in 20 to 75 per cent.[53, 55, 56] Weight loss and dysphagia are late symptoms. Proximal tracheal tumors can interfere with vocal cord function or cause recurrent laryngeal nerve paralysis, both resulting in hoarseness. Distal tracheal tumors can prolapse into a main bronchus and produce symptoms of bronchial obstruction.[48] Both squamous cell carcinoma and adenoid cystic carcinoma of the trachea may metastasize widely to the lungs, liver, bone, and lymph nodes. Pulmonary function studies are useful in localizing airway obstruction above the tracheal carina.[57] In particular, the shape of the flow-volume loop can show the presence of tracheal stenosis when the airway is reduced to less than about 8 mm in diameter.

Chest radiographs are limited in detecting tracheal tumors.[56, 58, 59] Karlan and colleagues[56] found that in only 4 of 11 patients with tracheal tumors was the chest radiograph prospectively interpreted as abnormal. Penetration of the mediastinum on most chest radiographs is insufficient to allow adequate visualization of the tracheal lumen. Oblique views of the chest project the tracheal air column away from the spine and are often helpful in visualizing suspected endotracheal masses. Coned-down radiographs of the thoracic inlet and of the soft tissues of the neck can also assist in demonstrating a tracheal tumor. Conventional tomograms formerly were the standard radiographic technique for localizing tracheal masses (Fig. 1–14A–D).[56, 59, 60] Contrast tracheograms can

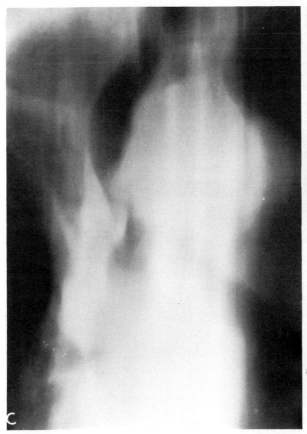

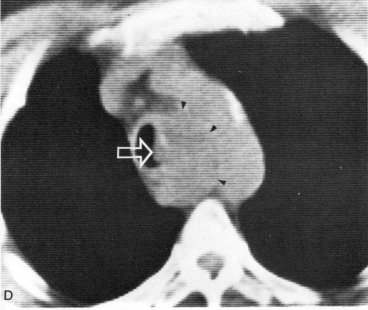

FIGURE 1–14 *Continued C,* Conventional tomogram demonstrates the intratracheal tumor. The widened mediastinal contour suggests a component extratracheal to the mass. *D,* CT demonstrates the mass (open arrow) within a tracheal cartilage and the mediastinal extension (arrowheads) of the carcinoma.

demonstrate an endotracheal mass and its site of origin.[61, 62] The contour of the area of narrowing usually differentiated neoplasms from benign structures. Tracheograms, however, cannot define extratracheal extension of a tumor and the technique has largely been replaced by high resolution (HR) CT for imaging suspected tracheal neoplasms.[2] Tracheography is also potentially hazardous and deaths have been reported from the procedure.[59]

Malignant tracheal tumor appears on CT scan as a mass of soft-tissue density arising from the tracheal wall. The posterior and lateral walls of the trachea are the most frequent sites of origin for tracheal tumors. Tumors are most often sessile and eccentric, producing an asymmetric narrowing of the tracheal lumen (Fig. 1–15). They can, however, be polypoid and entirely intraluminal.[53, 59] Approximately 10 per cent of malignant tracheal neoplasms are circumfer-

ential, a finding that is not seen with benign tumors. Malignant tracheal tumors extend directly into the mediastinum in 30 to 40 per cent of patients.[55, 56] In some patients, a mediastinal mass can be seen on chest radiographs or conventional tomograms. CT however is more accurate than other imaging modalities in demonstrating the extent of mediastinal invasion of tracheal neoplasms.[2, 63, 64] CT can show extension through the tracheal wall as well as encasement of mediastinal structures. Benign tumors rarely show extension through the tracheal wall into the mediastinum. The two morphologic factors that will determine surgical resectability of a tracheal malignancy are the length of tracheal wall that will require resection and the extent of extratracheal invasion. Spizarny and colleagues[64] showed that CT underestimates the longitudinal extension of the tumor when submucosal extension is present and also

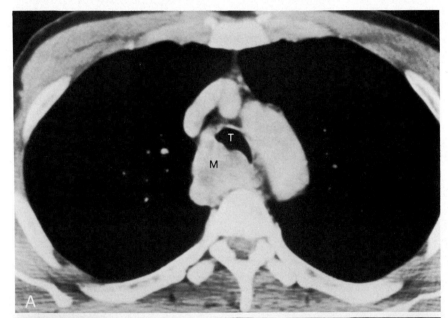

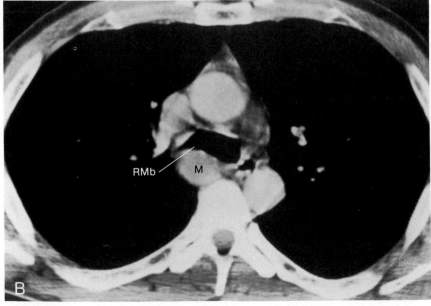

FIGURE 1–15 ■ Adenoid cystic carcinoma of the trachea in a middle-aged man with wheezing and hemoptysis. *A,* CT at the level of the aortic arch shows an inhomogeneous mass (M), causing asymmetric narrowing of the tracheal lumen (T). A large extratracheal component is present. *B,* Four cm inferiorly, at the level of the tracheal carina, the mass (M) involves the right main bronchus (RMb). The carcinoma is nonresectable because of the large extratracheal component, the length of tracheal involvement, and the involvement of the right main bronchus.

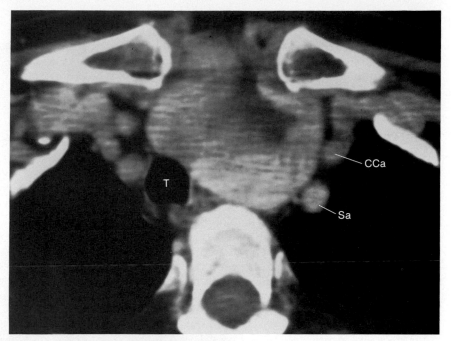

FIGURE 1–16 ■ Tracheal displacement by a goiter. CT scan through the upper mediastinum demonstrates a large, inhomogeneous goiter involving the left lobe of the thyroid, displacing the trachea (T) to the right and the left subclavian (Sa) and common carotid (CCa) arteries to the left. The mass shows enhancement with intravascular contrast material.

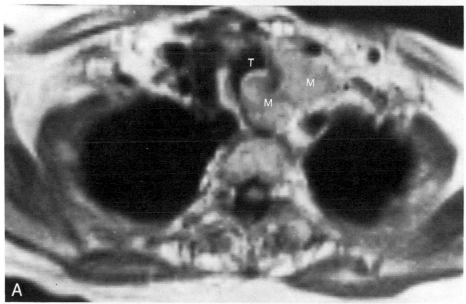

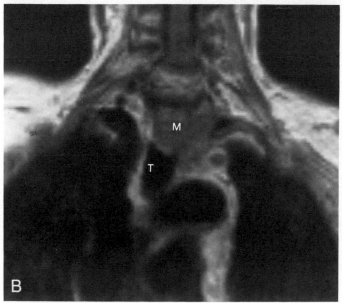

FIGURE 1–17 ■ Thyroid carcinoma invading the trachea. *A,* Axial and *B,* Coronal T1-weighted spin-echo MR images demonstrate an intermediate signal intensity mass (M) invading the trachea (T). The MR findings could equally well be from a primary tumor of the trachea.

may not detect mediastinal organ invasion. MR should thus be considered for additional imaging of these patients.

Secondary Malignant Neoplasms ■ Mediastinal masses, anomalous vessels, or aneurysms commonly compress the trachea without invading the tracheal wall. These produce a smooth, concentric impression on the tracheal lumen and frequently displace the trachea toward the contralateral side. CT scans can usually demonstrate the cause of tracheal compression. The most common cause in adults is a dilated innominate artery or aortic arch. A goiter in the neck or superior mediastinum is also a frequent cause (Fig. 1–16). CT scans after infusion of contrast material show enhancement of a dilated vessel. Most goiters demonstrate marked and prolonged enhancement after infusion of contrast material.[65] In children, masses causing extrinsic tracheal compression are lymphoma, neurofibroma, metastasis, benign lymph node hyperplasia, and vascular anomalies.[66, 67] Vascular rings are readily identified on CT or MR.[68]

Malignant neoplasms can either directly invade the trachea or, less commonly, metastasize to the tracheal mucosa. Carcinoma arising in the thyroid gland, esophagus, larynx, and lung is responsible for most cases of invasion of the trachea (Fig. 1–17A, B).[2, 52, 69, 70] CT scans show asymmetric tracheal narrowing and a soft-tissue mass directly extending to within the tracheal cartilages. When a dominant extrinsic mass is not apparent, a secondary tumor of the trachea can mimic a primary tracheal tumor. In most circumstances, endoscopy with biopsy is required for diagnosis.

Subglottic extension of laryngeal carcinoma to the proximal trachea is most accurately demonstrated on CT.[71] The true vocal cords are readily identified, and a mass involving the airway wall below the inferior margin of the cricoid cartilage indicates proximal tracheal extension of the neoplasm. Carcinoma of the larynx not infrequently recurs at the tracheal stoma and adjacent tracheal wall in patients who have had a laryngectomy.[72] In stoma recurrence of a laryngeal carcinoma, CT can assist by demonstrating the extent of the tumor involvement of the tracheal wall and the size of the mass around the trachea. The severity of tracheal narrowing can also be assessed from CT scans.

Esophageal neoplasms that arise in the upper third of the esophagus can encase and invade the trachea. CT scans can show tumor around the trachea and direct extension through the tracheal wall (Fig. 1–18).[70, 73] Esophageal carcinoma can, however, invaginate the unsupported posterior tracheal membrane without extending through the tracheal wall (Fig. 1–19). Blurring of the boundary between the esophagus and trachea has been described as a sensitive CT finding, indicating tracheal invasion by esophageal carcinoma.[70, 73] A plane of separation between the esophagus and trachea however is not always visible on CT scans, and invasion of tumor into the outer

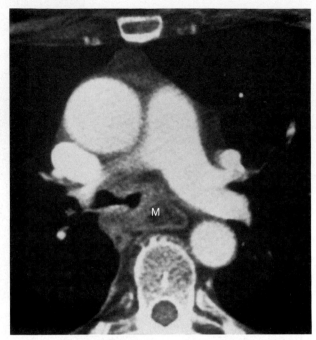

FIGURE 1–18 ■ Esophageal carcinoma invading the lower trachea and left main bronchus. CT scan at the level of the left pulmonary artery demonstrates a posterior mediastinal mass (M) thickening the tracheal carina and narrowing the left main bronchus.

layers of the tracheal wall cannot be determined accurately with CT.

Hematogenous metastases to the tracheal mucosa are rare. They are most commonly from breast carcinoma, melanoma, and genitourinary tract malignancies. CT scans show a polypoid mass within the tracheal wall that can simulate a primary tracheal tumor (Fig. 1–20) or irregular thickening of the tracheal wall (Fig. 1–21).

STRICTURES

Intubation or tracheostomy for assisted ventilation is used with increasing frequency but can damage the tracheal wall, leading to stenosis.[74–76] Neck trauma is the second commonest cause of tracheal injury. The trachea can become scarred, resulting in a segment of fixed stenosis. Alternatively, trauma can result in a tracheal segment becoming flaccid (tracheomalacia) and functionally stenotic. Advances in tracheal surgery have made resection of long tracheal segments possible.[77, 78] Imaging studies of the injured trachea must not only detect the site of abnormality, but must also precisely determine the severity and length of the stenosis and the compliance of the airway. CT scans can demonstrate the site of narrowing in most patients with fixed tracheal stenosis.[2] It can also differentiate heaped up granulation and scar tissue within the tracheal cartilages that may be amenable to laser resection (Fig. 1–22), from collapse of the tracheal cartilages (Fig. 1–23).[79]

In patients with a tracheal web or a short stenotic

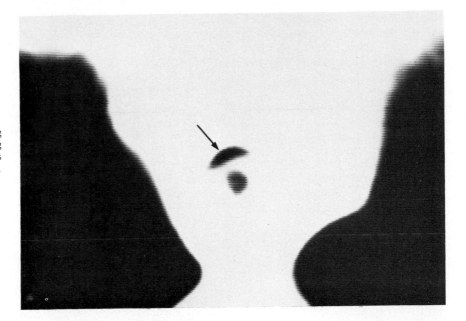

FIGURE 1–19 ■ Esophageal cancer mimicking tracheal stenosis. CT shows marked narrowing of the trachea *(arrow)*. The esophageal cancer is invaginating the posterior tracheal membrane. Bronchoscopy showed no tumor in the trachea.

segment, CT scans using 1-cm collimation may not show the airway narrowing, because the stenosis is obscured by volume averaging with air in the tracheal lumen. For this reason, 1.5- or 3-mm collimation is required through sites of suspected stenosis. CT obtained in the recumbent patient tends to overestimate the severity of stenosis when compared with tracheograms. When evaluating the trachea for resection of a stenosis, the narrowed segment and any adjacent abnormal mucosa must be removed. CT scans cannot evaluate the tracheal mucosa, and the length of abnormal trachea is usually longer than the wall abnormality detected on CT. CT scans normally obtained during suspended respiration cannot demonstrate flaccid segments of tracheomalacia. At present, tracheograms are often required in addition to CT for definitive evaluation of non-neoplastic tracheal stenosis, prior to surgery.

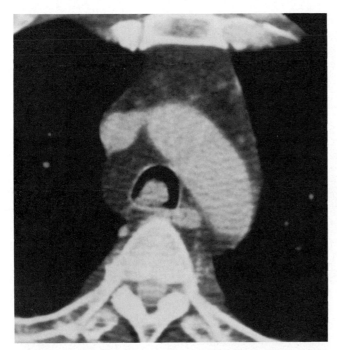

FIGURE 1–20 ■ Melanoma metastasis to the trachea. CT scan at the level of the aortic arch demonstrates a polypoid mass within the trachea arising from the posterior tracheal membrane. Biopsy of the lesion showed a melanoma. (Courtesy of Colleen Bergen, MD, Palo Alto, CA.)

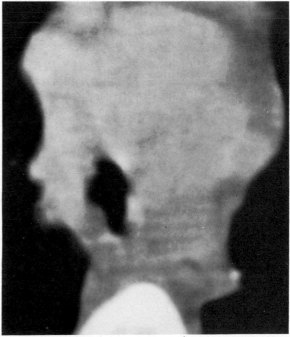

FIGURE 1–21 ■ Metastasis to the trachea from breast carcinoma. CT demonstrates irregular circumferential narrowing of the trachea by tumor. The right wall of the trachea is thickened. Tumor confirmed by bronchoscopy and biopsy.

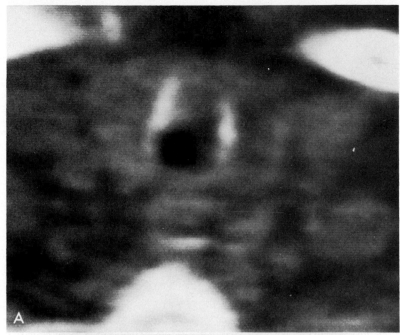

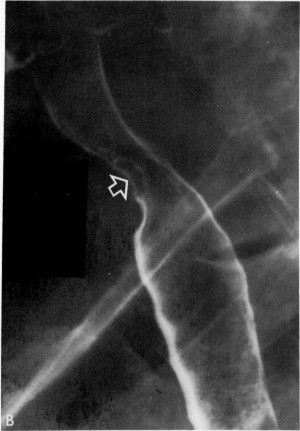

FIGURE 1–22 ■ Tracheal stenosis from previous tracheotomy. *A*, CT through the stenotic segment shows soft tissue anteriorly within the tracheal cartilage. The tracheal lumen is 4.9 × 6.0 mm in diameter. The length of stenosis as determined from sequential scans was 2 cm. *B*, Oblique view from tracheogram shows tracheal stenosis with heaped-up granulation tissue anteriorly *(arrow)*. The minimum diameter of the stenosis is 4.5 × 5.5 mm. The abnormal segment is 3.5 to 4.0 cm long. At surgery, 4 cm of trachea was resected. (From Gamsu G, Webb WR: Computed tomography of the trachea: normal and abnormal. AJR 139:321, © 1982, American Roentgen Ray Society. Used with permission.)

Bronchial Abnormalities

Lesions of the central bronchi (tracheal carina to segmental bronchi) encompass a variety of diseases. Tumors are by far the most common masses and occur much more frequently in the central bronchi than in the trachea. Bronchogenic carcinoma ac-counts for more than 90 per cent of central bronchial neoplasms, whereas benign tumors are uncommon.[80] In one series covering a 10-year period, 11,626 bronchoscopies discovered 2000 bronchogenic carcinomas and only 11 benign neoplasms.[81] Non-neoplastic benign masses do occur in the central bronchi but are uncommon.

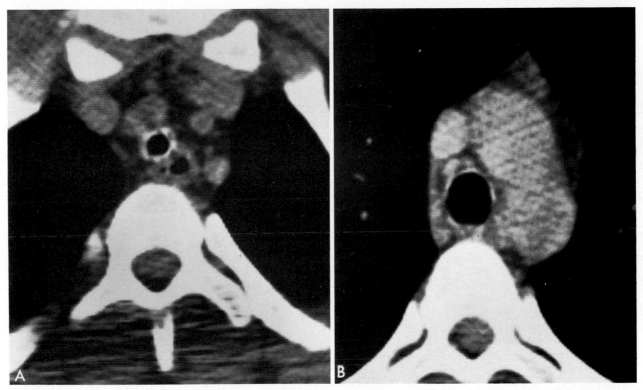

FIGURE 1–23 ■ Tracheal stenosis following prolonged intubation. *A,* CT shows collapse of a tracheal cartilage around the stenosed trachea. (Significance of tracheal cartilage extending circumferentially is unknown.) *B,* CT 4 cm caudad shows the normal tracheal size for comparison.

INFLAMMATORY STRICTURES AND GRANULOMAS

Bronchial disease is common in both primary and reinfection tuberculosis. In primary tuberculosis, bronchial narrowing is usually the result of compression of bronchi by enlarged lymph nodes.[82] Tuberculosis granulation tissue of the bronchial mucosa is uncommon in primary tuberculosis.

Occasionally, infection in a lymph node will erode the bronchial wall, causing stenosis or occlusion of the bronchus.[82, 83] The bronchi of the anterior segment of an upper lobe or the medial segment of the middle lobe are most commonly involved. In reinfection tuberculosis, endobronchial involvement results in mucosal ulcerations, scarring, and bronchostenosis. Bronchial disease is usually within the bronchi, subtending a tuberculous cavity or focal area of caseation. The diagnosis of endobronchial tuberculosis is usually made by bronchoscopy and biopsy of the abnormal mucosa. CT scans can localize areas of bronchial wall thickening and stenosis prior to bronchoscopy.[83a] The CT findings are often of concentric narrowing and frequently mimic those of bronchogenic carcinoma.

Bronchostenosis is rare in most mycotic granulomatous diseases such as histoplasmosis, coccidioidomycosis, or blastomycosis. Central bronchial obstruction occurs uncommonly in cryptococcosis. When present, the radiographic appearances are also frequently mistaken for bronchogenic carcinoma.[84] The CT findings have not been described but presumably also mimic those of a lung carcinoma. Sarcoidosis can cause bronchostenosis in the advanced stages of

the disease.[85–87] One or more segmental or lobar bronchi are involved. CT can be used in these circumstances to localize areas of narrowing before bronchoscopy and biopsy.

The CT findings of inflammatory strictures of the bronchi have had limited description. In our experience, sites of airway narrowing as far distally as the segmental bronchi can readily be detected with CT. Bronchial wall thickening, mediastinal and hilar adenopathy, and unsuspected parenchymal disease that are not apparent from radiographs may be discovered with CT. In instances in which a mass surrounds and narrows a bronchus, CT cannot predict mucosal involvement. It can, however, localize sites for transbronchial biopsy.[88, 89]

BRONCHIECTASIS

Bronchiectasis is a permanent abnormal dilatation of bronchi resulting from destruction of the elastic and muscular components of the bronchial wall. The most common form of bronchiectasis results from necrotizing bacterial infections in childhood.[90] Antibiotics and vaccines have markedly decreased the incidence of bronchiectasis in the developed countries. The condition does however remain a major problem in medically less developed regions of the world. Congenital forms of bronchiectasis exist, although they are uncommon.[91]

Congenital anomalies of the bronchi such as bronchomalacia are frequently associated with bronchiectasis. About 20 per cent of patients with dextrocardia

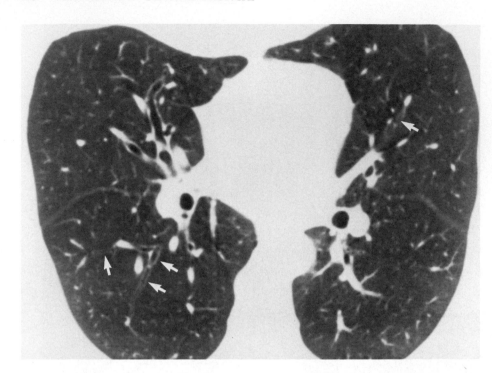

FIGURE 1–24 ■ Focal cylindric bronchiectasis in a 26-year-old woman with cough and recurrent fever. Chest radiograph was normal. HRCT demonstrates cylindric dilatation and thickening of the bronchi in the middle lobe. Mild bronchial wall thickening in the right lower lobe and left upper lobe *(arrows)* should not be mistaken for bronchiectasis.

have associated bronchiectasis (Kartagener's syndrome). This syndrome is one variety of a genetically determined group of disorders known as the immotile cilia syndrome.[92] Other hereditary or familial conditions such as cystic fibrosis have a breakdown in local defense mechanisms of the lung.[93] Deficiency in systemic defense mechanisms such as immunodeficiency states and allergic conditions such as bronchopulmonary aspergillosis can also be complicated by bronchiectasis.[93a]

Patients with bronchiectasis may have an abnormal chest radiograph, reflecting the pathologic changes.[94] Bronchi are increased in size, and their walls more prominent than normal. The vessels in the involved areas of the lung appear ill-defined and are crowded together, reflecting volume loss of the affected lung segments. Cystic spaces, sometimes containing fluid levels, are indicative of advanced disease. Our recent experience with CT and HRCT has shown that focal but symptomatic bronchiectasis is probably more common than previously thought and frequently does not show abnormalities on conventional radiographs. Bronchography, previously the method for establishing the diagnosis and determining the extent of bronchiectasis, has been replaced by HRCT.

Naidich and colleagues[95] described the CT findings in six cases of bronchiectasis. In all patients, CT scans revealed abnormalities indicative of the disease. In patients with cylindrical or varicose bronchiectasis, the normally invisible intraparenchymal bronchi are thick-walled and dilated (Fig. 1–24). In patients with cystic bronchiectasis, the characteristic CT findings are thick-walled cystic spaces that are either grouped together in a cluster or strung together in a linear fashion (Fig. 1–25). Fluid levels within the cysts are readily demonstrated on CT scans. When segmental

or lobar collapse accompanies bronchiectasis, the crowded dilated bronchi are seen against a background of increased CT density. Motion artifacts superficially may simulate mild bronchiectasis, but should be easily differentiated.[96] The dilated bronchi of bronchiectasis are easily differentiated from bullae and blebs. Bullae and blebs are thin-walled and peripheral and are not accompanied by branches of the pulmonary artery. Several articles have confirmed the diagnostic accuracy of CT in detecting and demonstrating the extent of bronchiectasis.[97–100] Although medium collimation (4 mm) has been suggested for assessment of bronchiectasis,[99] we advocate the technique described by Grenier and colleagues.[97] Thin (1.5 mm) sections are obtained with 8- to 10-mm intersection spacing from the lung apices to the bases. Intravascular contrast material is not required. As long as the study is technically satisfactory, the information is equal to or better than that from bronchograms in most instances.

On HRCT, mild bronchial dilatation and wall thickening can be seen diffusely through the lungs (Fig. 1–26) in patients with the clinical symptoms of chronic bronchitis. These findings probably are those of chronic bronchitis and should not be mistaken for bronchiectasis.

The bronchi within regions of marked lung fibrosis are characteristically dilated and appear bronchiectatic. This form of cicatricial bronchiectasis is distinctive and is limited to the sites of fibrosis. It should not be mistaken for the commoner infectious bronchiectasis and is probably due to the increased retractile focus of the fibrotic lung acting on the bronchi. Cicatricial bronchiectasis is also a prominent feature of chronic radiation damage to the lung (see Chapter 4).[101]

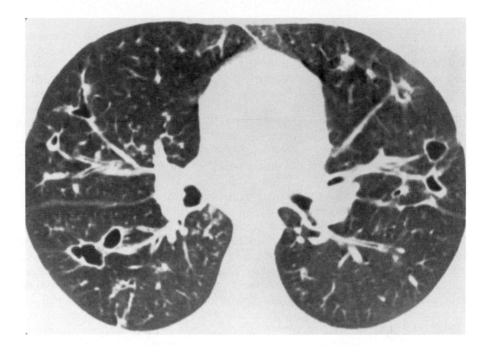

FIGURE 1–25 ■ Cystic bronchiectasis in a patient with recurrent fever. HRCT demonstrates multiple bilateral sites of thick-walled cystic bronchiectasis. Serial scans demonstrated continuity of all of these cystic spaces with the airways.

ATELECTASIS AND BRONCHIAL OBSTRUCTION

Atelectasis, or collapse of lung, denotes an abnormal loss in volume of that portion of lung relative to the other lobes or segments. Atelectasis is necessarily associated with diminished air within the affected lung and impaired function in the form of decreased gas exchange. Ventilation is diminished, whereas perfusion may or may not be maintained. The factors maintaining normal expansion of the lung are a finely tuned balance of mechanical and surface forces. The chest wall, physicomechanically coupled by surface forces through the pleurae, is essential for normal lung expansion. The normal retractile properties of the lungs will cause them to collapse if dissociated from the chest wall. The elastic properties of the lung are distributed throughout the lungs by interdepend-

ence of the elastic properties of bronchi, lung parenchyma, and pleura.[102, 103] These interconnections tend to stabilize the lung and prevent collapse. Surfactant lining the alveoli of the lung parenchyma forms a third important mechanism by which the lung resists collapse. Ventilation, via both the normal pathways and those allowing collateral ventilation, is also essential for maintaining lung inflation.

Disruption of these properties can lead to lung instability and collapse. The mechanisms of lung collapse can thus be described in terms of interference with the stabilizing mechanism. Resorption of the gas distal to an airway obstruction is the most common cause of atelectasis and an important clinical problem. Relaxation atelectasis results from uncoupling of the lung and chest wall by fluid or gas in

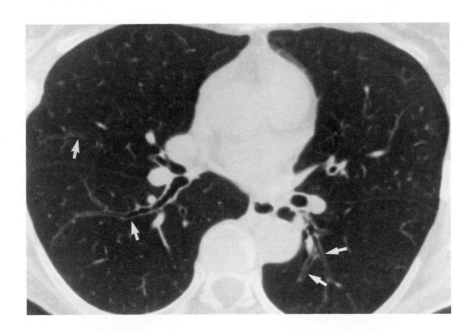

FIGURE 1–26 ■ Chronic bronchitis. HRCT demonstrates diffuse mild bronchial dilatation and bronchial wall thickening *(arrows)*. The patient is a middle-aged smoker with chronic cough and sputum production. These findings probably represent chronic bronchitis.

the pleural space. Scarring of the lung interferes with several stabilizing mechanisms and produces cicatricial atelectasis. The fourth form of atelectasis occurs when the surfactant system is disrupted by such causes as radiation or in respiratory distress syndrome, causing adhesive atelectasis.

For descriptive purposes, we will deal with obstructive and nonobstructive atelectasis. Although this division works well for descriptive CT purposes, in both circumstances, several mechanisms are operational in destabilizing the lung and causing it to reduce its volume.

Obstructive Atelectasis ■ Obstruction of a bronchus promotes atelectasis or collapse of the subtended lung, owing to resorption of air distal to the obstruction. This is not, however, an inevitable occurrence. The lung distal to the site of obstruction may experience several responses. If the other stabilizing mechanisms are still operational and collateral ventilation can occur, the obstructed lobe or segments can maintain normal volume. Alternatively, the distal lung parenchyma and airways may become filled with fluid and secretions and may become densely consolidated, but lose little or no volume (the "drowned lung"). Occasionally, the obstructed lung will become overdistended with air, producing an appearance of hyperinflation. The causes of bronchial obstruction are varied and can be from intrinsic bronchial disease or extrinsic compression (Table 1–2). The resultant CT appearance will vary with the site of obstruction, the rapidity of the collapse, and the cause of obstruction. The most common circumstance under which lung collapse occurs in the postoperative period is when mucus collects in the fourth

TABLE 1–2 ■ Causes of Bronchial Compression

Inflammatory lymphadenopathy
   Tuberculosis
   Histoplasmosis
   Sarcoidosis
   Nonspecific
Neoplastic lesions
   Benign
      Bronchogenic cyst
      Gastroenterogenous cyst
      Neurogenic tumors
   Malignant
      Metastatic lymphadenopathy
      Primary malignancy
         Carcinoma of the lung
         Lymphomas
Sclerosing mediastinitis
Enlarged vessels in normal position
   Enlarged left atrium
   Pulmonary valve atresia—large pulmonary artery
   Pulmonary artery aneurysm
Abnormally positioned vessels
   Aberrant left pulmonary artery—pulmonary sling
   Pulmonary agenesis—abnormal position of aorta
   Patent ductus with pulmonary atresia
   Transposition of the great vessels—postoperative
      pulmonary artery dilatation
Acquired aortic disease
   Traumatic false aneurysm of the descending arch

or fifth generation and more distal bronchi.[104] The more central airways then remain air-filled.

The radiographic appearances of lobar and segmental collapse are well described.[105–108] Several authors have described the CT appearances in detail and CT has a major role in evaluation of the patient with suspected lobar or segmental atelectasis.[109–112] Woodring[113] and Mayr and colleagues[114] have shown that CT is highly sensitive in detecting the site of obstruction and whether a neoplasm is responsible for the obstruction.

Naidich and co-workers[109] were the first to describe the CT features of obstructive lobar atelectasis. The CT findings are similar to those for chest radiographs, the differences being in the transaxial display of CT. In general, the obstructed and variably collapsed lobe demonstrates increased density that will obliterate the normal vessels. Most frequently, the bronchi fill with material that is indistinguishable in density from the material filling the lung. After the intravascular injection of contrast material, the inspissated mucus often present in the dilated bronchi behind the site of obstruction will be lower in density than the surrounding enhanced lung parenchyma (Fig. 1–27).[115] On CT, following injection of contrast material, a nonenhancing central mass causing the obstruction can sometimes be distinguished from the enhancing distal lung. When the obstructed bronchus is surrounded by a mass on CT, the cause of the obstruction is invariably a malignant tumor.

Upper Lobe Collapse ■ The upper lobes collapse upward, medially and anteriorly. On the right side, the collapsed lobe shifts to a position against the upper anterior mediastinum. When airless and small, it may resemble a paramediastinal mass.[110] It also usually maintains some contact with the right anterior chest wall. The distinctive smooth contours of the fissures delineate the interphase between the collapsed lobe and the expanded normal lobes (Fig. 1–28). The middle lobe extends upward and fills the space lateral to the collapsed right upper lobe. The lower lobe expands upward and posteriorly, often extending to the apex of the thorax. Occasionally, the upper lobe is separated from the posterior mediastinum by a portion of the lower lobe that insinuates itself between the collapsed lobe and the mediastinum. A fan-shaped medial portion of the collapsed lobe connecting it to the hilum persists and is evident on CT.

Left upper lobe collapse is similar to that on the right, with the differences produced by the lingula at lower levels (Fig. 1–29). The apicoposterior and anterior segments collapse medially and anteriorly, frequently vacating the lung apex. The lingula tends to maintain its contact with the pericardium, producing a wedge-shaped density, adjacent to the heart. As on the right, CT and often MR can demonstrate central masses and the site of obstruction (Fig. 1–29).

Middle Lobe Collapse ■ The middle lobe collapses as a wedge of density that may be visible over only

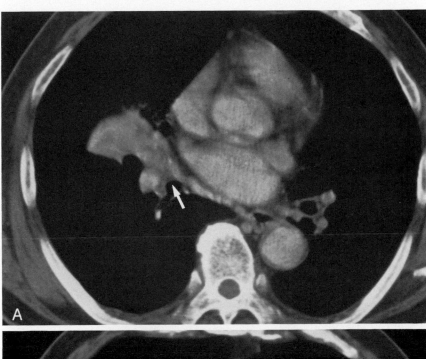

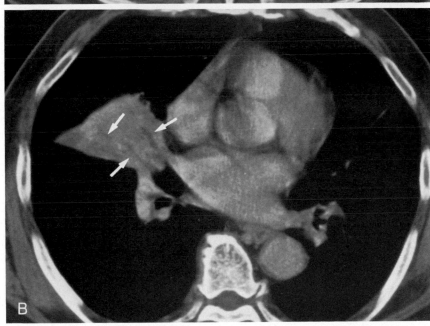

FIGURE 1–27 ■ Middle lobe bronchial obstruction with mucous bronchograms. *A*, CT demonstrates obstruction of the orifice of the middle lobe bronchus *(arrow)*. No central mass is identified. The middle lobe is partially collapsed. *B*, One cm caudad, distinct mucous bronchograms *(arrows)* are seen within the middle lobe, which has been enhanced with intravascular contrast material.

2 or 3 cm. As with the upper lobes, the middle lobe tends to maintain its connection to the mediastinum but most frequently moves away from the anterolateral chest walls. Since it is the smallest lobe, the middle lobe is the most mobile, and as it collapses, its position varies in relationship to its normal site. With collapse, one of the two bordering fissures tends to be more displaced than the other, producing either a vertically or horizontally collapsed configuration. On CT the collapsed middle lobe usually has a triangular wedge-shaped appearance.

Lower Lobe Collapse ■ Both lower lobes tend to collapse in a similar fashion, producing similar CT appearances. Both collapse medially and inferiorly, maintaining contact with the posterior mediastinum

and adjacent hemidiaphragm. With marked reduction in volume, the lower lobe appears to lose its contact with the diaphragm. The major fissure is displaced posteriorly and rotates to assume a more anteroposterior orientation.

Secondary findings of lobar atelectasis may not be as readily appreciated on CT as chest radiographs. The hilar structures, especially the bronchi, are displaced in the direction of the collapsed lobe and are elevated or depressed. The vessels in the unaffected lobe(s) on the side of the collapse become spread out compared with the normal side. The density of the hyperinflated lobe is decreased, a finding that is often striking on CT. Mediastinal displacement to the side of collapse may be apparent. With left lower

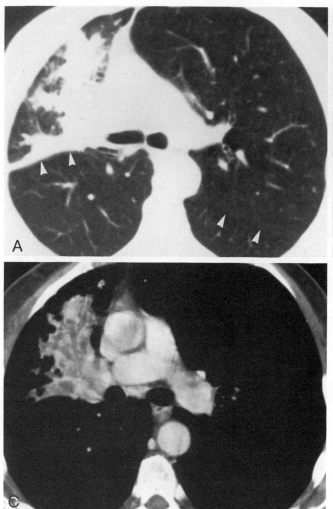

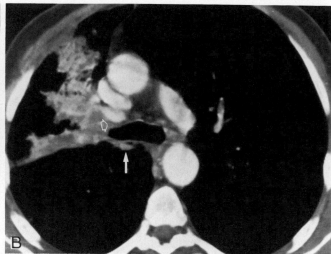

FIGURE 1–28 ■ Squamous cell carcinoma, right upper lobe. CT at the level of the tracheal carina, using lung window settings *(A)* and soft tissue window settings *(B)* demonstrate occlusion of the right upper lobe bronchus with partial atelectasis of the right upper lobe. The right major fissure *(arrowheads)* is displaced anteriorly compared with the left major fissure *(arrowheads)*. The mediastinum and anterior junction line are displaced to the right. Partial ventilation of the right upper lobe is by collateral ventilation. Tumor causing thickening of the posterior wall of the right main bronchus *(arrow)* is shown. Tumor also extends between the right upper lobe pulmonary artery and the right main bronchus (open arrow). *C*, CT 2 cm caudad demonstrates extensive mucous bronchograms within the partially collapsed right upper lobe.

lobe collapse, the heart may rotate as it displaces towards the left.

MR has been described in two situations involving bronchial obstruction. Mayr and colleagues[116] compared the ability of CT and MR to demonstrate endobronchial masses in 29 patients. In this study, using a 0.35 T MR imager and spin-echo images, CT proved superior to MR in defining both normal and abnormal bronchi. Tobler and co-workers[117] studied the ability of MR and CT to distinguish between a central tumor mass and subtended collapsed lung. Images with T2-weighting were the best MR technique. However, CT after contrast material injection was superior to MR for this purpose, confirming the findings of Naidich and colleagues.[111]

Herold and colleagues studied 43 patients with atelectasis using MR.[117a] They found a distinct difference between obstructive and nonobstructive atelectasis on T2-weighted images. Obstructive atelectasis was hyperintense on T2-weighted sequences, whereas 22 of 25 cases of nonobstructive atelectasis showed low signal intensity. This observation needs further investigation.

Nonobstructive Atelectasis ■ Nonobstructive atelectasis is encountered in many situations such as pneumothorax. In most of these circumstances CT and MR are not indicated. However, they may be obtained for nonobstructive lung collapse, in conjunction with a large pleural effusion. In this instance, the collapsed lobe assumes a different configuration from that found with obstructive atelectasis.[118] The CT features of a large pleural effusion are typical. In the supine position, free pleural fluid collects posteriorly, laterally, and medially. The lobes collapse anteriorly and toward the hilum. Larger quantities of freely flowing pleural fluid surround the lobes, including their medial surfaces, and are visible within the fissures (Fig. 1–30). The CT density of the pleural fluid is distinctly different from that of the collapsed lung. In most instances, the parenchyma of the lung is of greater density than the fluid, especially after infusion of intravascular contrast material. The lung parenchyma in the atelectatic segments or lobes is invariably airless with large effusions. Air, however, is evident within the central bronchi, extending into the lung for several generations. On CT scans, unlike chest radiographs, air-bronchograms may be visible to within several centimeters of the pleural surfaces.

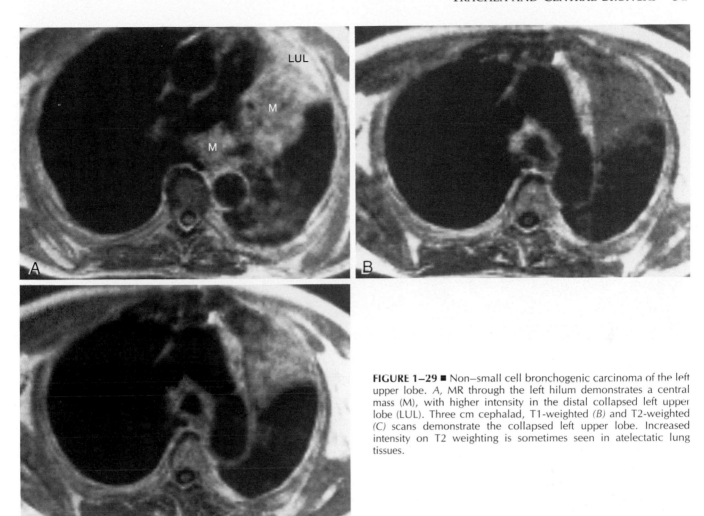

FIGURE 1–29 ■ Non–small cell bronchogenic carcinoma of the left upper lobe. *A,* MR through the left hilum demonstrates a central mass (M), with higher intensity in the distal collapsed left upper lobe (LUL). Three cm cephalad, T1-weighted *(B)* and T2-weighted *(C)* scans demonstrate the collapsed left upper lobe. Increased intensity on T2 weighting is sometimes seen in atelectatic lung tissues.

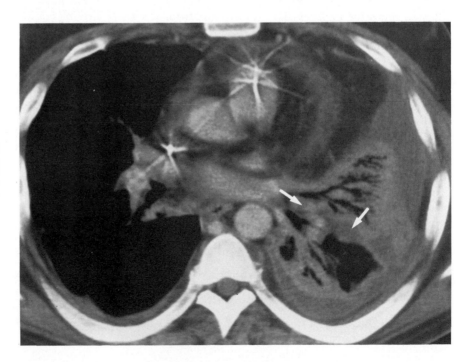

FIGURE 1–30 ■ Nonobstructive atelectasis of the left lower lobe and lingula. CT through the lower thorax demonstrates a large left pleural effusion causing compression of the left lower lobe and lingula. Fluid is visible in the lower end of the left major fissure *(arrows).*

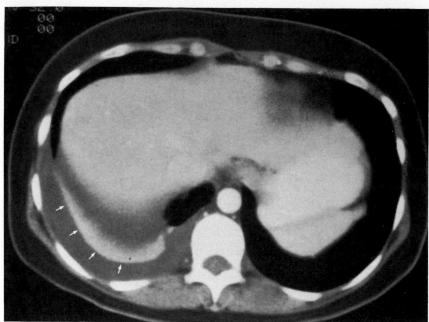

FIGURE 1–31 ■ Right lower lobe atelectasis. CT through the lower thorax demonstrates a right pleural effusion with fluid in front of and behind a collapsed lower lobe *(arrows)*, producing a pseudodiaphragm sign.

The lower lobes frequently collapse with a thin wedge of lung extending peripherally and inferiorly to approximate the diaphragm (Fig. 1–31). The collapsed lung may be misinterpreted as the diaphragm itself, with fluid in the pleural and peritoneal spaces (see also Chapter 5). Review of serial scans will demonstrate that the wedge of density is in continuity with the more cephalad collapsed lung. The central bronchi on the side of a large effusion characteristically are displaced forward.[118]

An additional advantage of CT over chest radiographs described by Naidich and co-workers[118] is that CT can usually differentiate between a malignant and benign effusion by demonstrating focal tumor deposits on the visceral or parietal pleural surfaces. This appearance of irregular, nodular pleural thickening can be seen with metastases, extension of a bronchogenic carcinoma to the pleural surface, and with mesothelioma. We have not encountered visible pleural deposits with the frequency that they describe. Although rare, tuberculous empyema may have similar CT findings of fluid and pleural masses. In the instances when cytologic examination of the pleural fluid is unrevealing, CT can also be used to guide the biopsy of focal pleural masses.

Rarely, with atelectasis from a large effusion, air-bronchograms may be absent. It has been proposed that this may be explained by the central bronchi's undergoing an element of torsion with obstruction.[119] CT cannot then distinguish between obstructive and nonobstructive atelectasis. Fortunately, this finding occurs so infrequently as not to be of practical concern.

BRONCHIAL ADENOMA AND BENIGN TUMORS

The most frequent benign neoplasms of the central bronchi are hamartomas, lipomas, and fibromas.[47, 48]

Granular cell myoblastoma, leiomyoma, chondroma, neurogenic tumors, papilloma, and bronchogenic cysts also can occur within or adjacent to the central bronchi.[47, 120, 121] Bronchial adenomas are often considered with the benign bronchial tumors because they frequently manifest in a similar manner but are low-grade malignancies.

Bronchial Adenomas ■ These tumors are uncommon, constituting only 0.6 to 1.2 per cent of tracheobronchial neoplasms.[122, 123] Over 85 per cent of adenomas arising within the bronchial tree are of the carcinoid variety.[123, 124] Cylindromas (adenoid cystic carcinomas) make up only 6 to 12 per cent of bronchial adenomas, but account for 95 per cent of tracheal adenomas.[123, 125] Carcinoid tumors are low-grade carcinomas and frequently are locally invasive. They can metastasize to regional lymph nodes and to distant sites. Most arise in the central bronchi and are visible on CT (Fig. 1–32). Bronchial obstruction is the most common presentation, and CT scans will reveal atelectasis and opacity in the subtended segment or lobe. Recurrent episodes of infection can lead to bronchiectasis or lung abscess. The obstructing mass as well as the frequent extension of the tumor beyond the bronchial wall can be visible on CT scans.[126] The tumor can also enhance following use of intravascular contrast material.[126a] In patients with adenoid cystic carcinoma and extrabronchial infiltration, the CT appearances are indistinguishable from bronchogenic carcinoma. Enlargement of regional lymph nodes can be from metastatic tumor or reactive hyperplasia of the nodes from concomitant infection (Fig. 1–33). Partial bronchial obstruction can result in hyperinflation, which will be evident on CT scans as an area of decreased density peripheral to the tumor. In instances of purely endobronchial adenomas, CT can assist in the planning of limited resection.

MR should be considered when an adrenocortico-trophic hormone–producing carcinoid is suspected and not found with CT. These tumors may show high signal intensity on T2-weighted images.[126b]

Chondromatous Hamartomas ■ These are the most common true benign neoplasms of the lung. Despite their bronchial origin, they usually manifest as a solitary pulmonary nodule and are rarely endobronchial.[127] Calcification occurs in about 30 per cent of all chondromatous hamartomas, and the frequency of calcification increases with tumor size. The pattern of calcification is stippled or conglomerate; conglomerate or "popcorn" calcification is rarely seen with other lesions.[128] Using CT, Siegelman and colleagues[28] found a focal collection of fat, typical calcifications, or both in 60 per cent of hamartomas. Endobronchial hamartomas can be resected bronchoscopically and do not tend to recur.[120]

Squamous Papillomas ■ Papillomatosis or juvenile laryngeal papillomatosis consists of an abnormal proliferation of airway mucosal cells that are thought to be of viral origin. Most lesions arise in the larynx. Distal spread to the trachea, bronchi, and lung parenchyma occurs in only about 5 per cent of patients (Fig. 1–34). CT scans can show the parenchymal and endobronchial masses (Fig. 1–35). Bronchoscopic excision of the central airway lesions using laser therapy is the preferred treatment, but the lesions recur in over 90 per cent of patients.[47, 120]

Other Tumors ■ All other benign tumors of the bronchi are rare and their demonstration on CT scans has infrequently been reported.[129, 130] Granular cell myoblastomas and lipomas tend to occur in the major bronchi and cause airway obstruction. About 50 per cent of leiomyomas arise within the central bronchi,

and the remainder occur in the lung parenchyma. Bronchial fibromas are only rarely endobronchial. Tumors of neurogenic origin rarely arise within the bronchi and more commonly manifest as solitary pulmonary nodules. When endobronchial, these benign tumors manifest with segmental or lobar collapse. CT scans can localize the site of the tumor and demonstrate the distal collapsed lung. The CT appearance of these tumors is usually nonspecific and does not differentiate them from other focal masses causing bronchial obstruction. The absence of extra-bronchial extension can suggest a benign tumor. Bronchoscopy and biopsy are usually required for diagnosis. In a report of an endobronchial lipoma, CT demonstrated the low CT numbers indicative of a fatty mass.[129] In a report of a calcified bronchial carcinoid, the CT appearance of the tumor simulated a broncholith but was more heterogeneous than would be anticipated for a broncholith.[131]

CENTRAL BRONCHOGENIC CARCINOMA

Over the past 50 years, in the Western Hemisphere bronchogenic carcinoma has established itself as the most common fatal malignancy in both men and women.[132] The prevalence, however, varies widely among countries and racial groups.[133, 134]

The frequency with which bronchogenic carcinoma arises in a central location varies with the histologic type of tumor.[135, 136] Squamous cell carcinoma most commonly arises centrally, predominantly in segmental bronchi and less commonly in lobar or main bronchi. Atelectasis or a hilar mass is therefore the most common presentation. Small-cell undifferentiated carcinoma also usually arises centrally as a hilar mass or an area of lung atelectasis or pneumo-

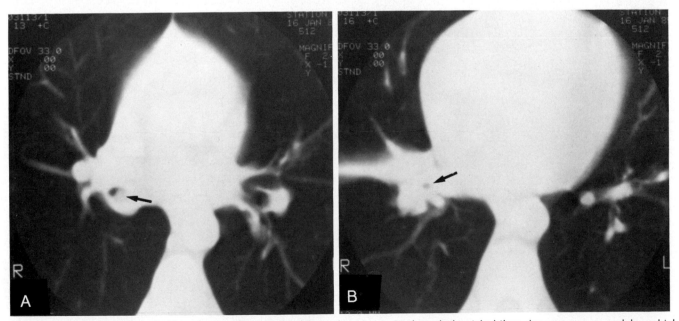

FIGURE 1–32 ■ Bronchial carcinoid producing partial middle lobe atelectasis. *A,* CT through the right hilum demonstrates an endobronchial mass *(arrow)* within the intermediate bronchus. The lung is well expanded. *B,* CT 2 cm caudad demonstrates atelectasis of the lateral segment of the right middle lobe. The lower lobe bronchus *(arrow)* is compromised, and the middle lobe bronchus is almost occluded. (Courtesy of C. Lindan, MD, San Francisco, CA.)

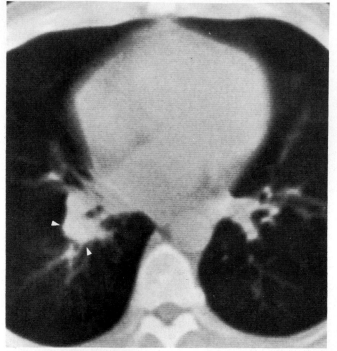

A

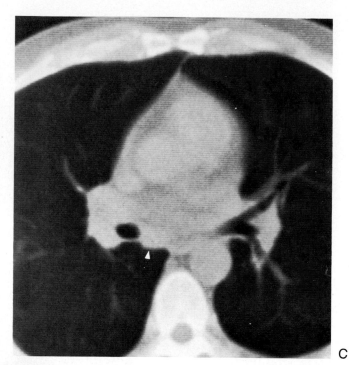

C

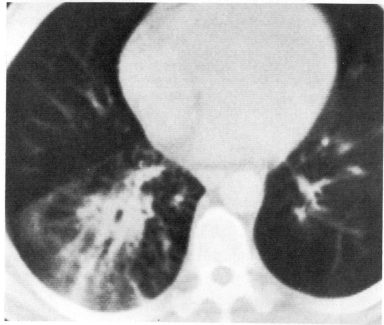

B

FIGURE 1–33 ■ Bronchial carcinoid with obstructive pneumonia. *A,* CT through the lower lobe basal segmental bronchi demonstrates a lobulated mass *(arrowheads)* compressing the bronchi. *B,* CT 2 cm caudad shows consolidation and loss of volume in the posterior and lateral basal segments of the right lower lobe. *C,* CT 4 cm cephalad shows a large azygoesophageal lymph node *(arrowhead).* At thoracotomy, a 1.3-cm × 2.0-cm carcinoid compressed the posterior and lateral basal segmental bronchi. Lymphadenopathy was found to be reactive hyperplasia without tumor.

FIGURE 1–34 ■ Pulmonary spread of laryngeal papillomatosis in a 9-year-old child with chronic laryngeal polyps. CT scans of the lower lobes demonstrate multiple nodular lesions, several with cavities. Nodules and cysts, increasing in size with time, are characteristic of parenchymal spread of papillomas.

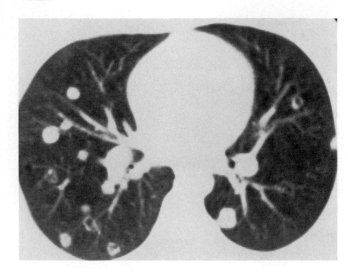

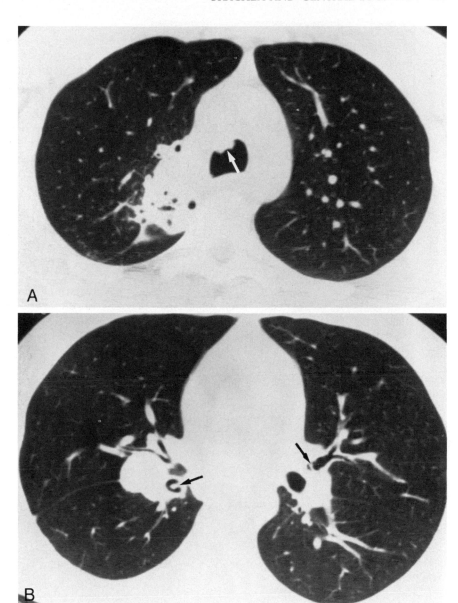

FIGURE 1–35 ■ Laryngopapillomatosis. CT scans through the mid trachea *(A)* and the lower lobe bronchi *(B)* demonstrate multiple endotracheal and endobronchial masses *(arrows),* of laryngeal papillomatosis. The right upper lobe shows atelectasis and chronic infection following occlusion of the draining bronchus. (Courtesy of David Naditch, MD, New York, NY)

nitis. Large-cell undifferentiated carcinoma infrequently has a central origin, and adenocarcinoma arises both in the lung parenchyma away from the central bronchi and centrally.

The radiographic and CT features of bronchogenic carcinoma are determined by the site of origin of the tumor and its size, growth pattern, and dissemination. At the time of presentation, the majority of central bronchogenic carcinomas are no longer amenable to surgical cure.[137] The appearance on CT scans of bronchogenic carcinoma arising in a central location has been described extensively.[138–141] The most common radiographic and CT findings are the presence of a mass causing bronchial obstruction. Atelectasis, obstructive retention of secretions, and obstructive pneumonitis can all result from bronchial obstruction. The narrowed, obstructed bronchi can routinely be demonstrated on CT scans (Figs. 1–36 and 1–37).[141a] Sites of bronchial wall thickening with-

out luminal narrowing are less common but are an important CT sign in bronchogenic carcinoma (Fig. 1–38). Thickening of the wall of a bronchus can be appreciated on CT scans at sites where lung normally makes contact with the bronchial tree. The posterior walls of the right main bronchus, right upper lobe bronchus, intermediate bronchus, distal left main bronchus, and left lower lobe bronchus are such sites. Tumor infiltration of these bronchial walls and contiguous lymphadenopathy both can cause thickening of the bronchial wall.[139] Irregularity of a thickened bronchial wall usually indicates tumor infiltration and correlates with the bronchoscopic finding of endobronchial tumor (Fig. 1–38). Bronchial narrowing may be due to mucosal tumor, submucosal infiltration by tumor, or extrinsic compression. CT cannot reliably predict mucosal involvement by bronchogenic carcinoma.[89] The presence of a mass surrounding the bronchus is, however, usually predictive of

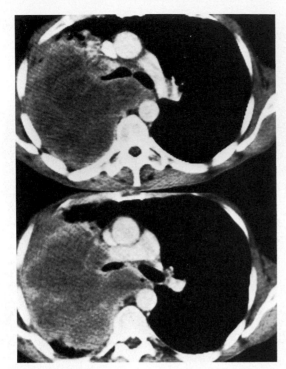

FIGURE 1–36 ■ Bronchogenic carcinoma producing bronchial obstruction and a fluid-filled lobe. Adjacent scans demonstrate inhomogeneous opacification of the right upper lobe. The right upper lobe bronchus narrows and terminates *(upper panel)*. The intermediate bronchus is compressed *(lower panel)*. The proximal tumor cannot be differentiated from the fluid-filled upper lobe on these scans. After radiation therapy to the right hilum, the right upper lobe reexpanded.

a malignant neoplasm (Fig. 1–39). Quint and co-workers[142] studied whether CT could predict the requirement for lobectomy or pneumonectomy with central bronchogenic carcinomas. They found that CT showed poor sensitivity for detecting proximal submucosal bronchial infiltration that occurs at the microscopic level. CT was also poor for determining tumor extension across fissures close to the hila, a circumstance in which pneumonectomy often becomes necessary for resection of the tumor. CT was moderately accurate in detecting tumor invasion of a central pulmonary artery or bronchus. MR may be better than CT for demonstrating angioinvasion; this technique should be considered when there is a suspicion of pulmonary artery or vein invasion.

Previously, tumor within 2 cm of the tracheal carina was considered nonresectable. Improvements in surgical techniques now allow for resection of the proximal main bronchi. Precise localization of the tumor, even when close to the tracheal carina, is thus of extreme importance.

Bronchial occlusion is most often seen with segmental bronchial tumors (see Fig. 1–37).[139] Lung window settings (−500 to −600 H) can give a false appearance of bronchial occlusion. Patency of a bronchus can be demonstrated if soft tissue window levels (20 to 50 H) are used. The most precise window levels for measuring bronchial caliber for bronchi surrounded by a mass is a level of about −150 H and a narrow window width.[27]

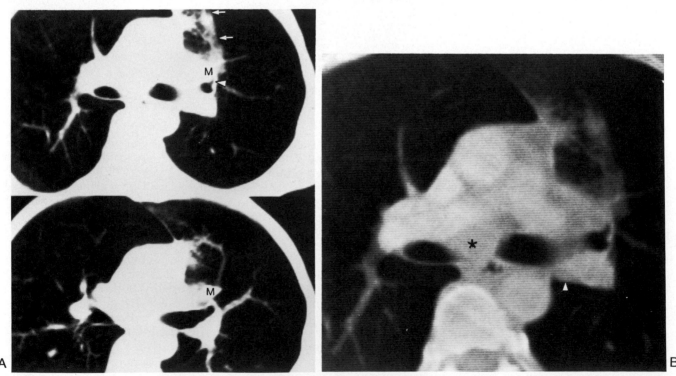

FIGURE 1–37 ■ Bronchogenic carcinoma with segmental atelectasis. *A,* Adjacent scans through the left main and upper lobe bronchi demonstrate a left anterior hilar mass (M), narrowing of the anterior segmental bronchus *(arrowhead),* and atelectasis of the anterior segment *(arrows). B,* CT at extended window settings confirms the mass and bronchial obstruction. A retrobronchial lymph node medial to the left pulmonary artery *(arrowhead)* and a subcarinal lymph node *(asterisk)* are seen.

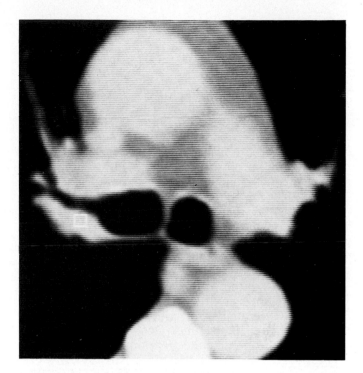

FIGURE 1–38 ■ Endobronchial bronchogenic carcinoma causing irregular narrowing of the right upper lobe bronchus. CT shows narrowing of the right upper lobe bronchus. The bronchial wall is thickened and irregular *(cursor)*. Tumor was confirmed by bronchoscopy and biopsy.

Twelve to 35 per cent of bronchogenic carcinomas manifest as an enlargement of one hilum on chest radiographs.[143, 144] The hilar enlargement can be from tumor arising in a hilar bronchus or from hilar adenopathy metastatic from a peripheral tumor. In most instances of a central tumor or hilar adenopathy, CT scans can show the abnormal enlargement and abnormal contours of the hilum. Both of these findings are most easily appreciated lateral and posterior to the hilar vessels. If interpretation of the CT scans is equivocal, a bolus injection of intravenous contrast material during rapid sequential (dynamic) scanning can separate the tumor mass from the hilar vessels (see Fig. 1–39). Bronchial obstruction predisposes to infection in the subtended lung segment. Obstructive pneumonitis or abscess formation can result. Consolidated or collapsed lung in continuity with the hilum is also most readily demonstrated after contrast material infusion.

Bronchogenic carcinoma rarely produces air-trap-

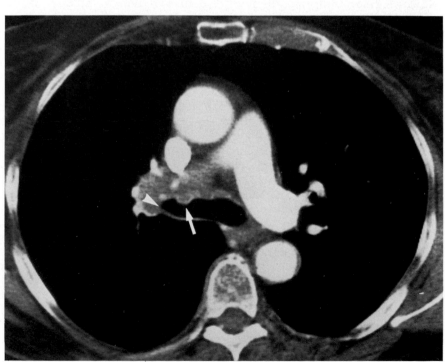

FIGURE 1–39 ■ Bronchogenic carcinoma invading the right upper bronchus lobe. CT scan at the level of the tracheal carina demonstrates a large mass arising in the right hilum, occluding the right upper lobe bronchus *(arrowhead)*, and extending into the mediastinum. The mass invades the anterior wall of the right upper lobe bronchus *(arrow)*. Tumor extension across the midline indicates the tumor is not resectable.

ping and hyperinflation of the lung subtended by a partially obstructed bronchus. Hyperlucency, when it occurs, is readily demonstrated on CT scans at appropriate window settings. The proximal bronchial tumor can also be demonstrated.

Sputum cytologic screening of people at high risk for development of bronchogenic carcinoma reveals individuals with malignant cells in their sputum, and a normal chest radiograph.[145, 146] In most of these patients, the tumor arises from a central bronchus. Painstaking fibrobronchoscopy can reveal the neoplasm in more than half of the patients.[147] CT scanning with 5-mm collimation through the central bronchi can localize the tumor in some of these cases and direct bronchoscopy to areas of special concern.[147a]

Of importance in CT of the thorax in bronchogenic carcinoma is the demonstration of intrathoracic metastases and local spread of the tumor. Lymphatic spread is usually to the hilar, mediastinal, or supraclavicular lymph nodes. Central bronchogenic carcinoma also frequently invades the mediastinum by direct growth of the tumor (see Chapters 2 and 3). Spread of bronchogenic carcinoma by way of the lymphatic system and the blood stream can be to either or both lungs or to either or both sides of the mediastinum. HRCT can accurately demonstrate lymphangitic carcinomatosis and should be considered in selected cases.[148] CT is also more sensitive than chest radiographs in detection of pulmonary nodules. In patients with suspected bronchogenic carcinoma, the entire thorax and upper abdomen should be scanned and special attention should be directed to sites of potential metastasis.

Pleural effusion is present at the time of diagnosis in 2 to 5 per cent of patients with bronchogenic carcinoma.[143] Most patients with pleural effusion have nonresectable tumor. Serous effusion usually indicates hilar lymph node involvement and lymphatic blockage. Pleural deposits from bronchogenic carcinoma causing pleural effusion may be detected with CT[118] but in our experience are uncommon.

Indications for and Therapeutic Considerations of CT and MR of the Trachea and Bronchi

The results of CT of the trachea and bronchi may have important and direct impact on the medical and surgical treatment of patients. For appropriate interpretation of CT scans, the current therapy for the diseases being imaged must be understood. For instance, surgical resection of up to 5 or 6 cm of the trachea is now feasible. CT determination of the length of a tracheal tumor and any extrinsic extension of a tumor is thus important.

The use of lasers for resection of benign lesions of the trachea and central airways is becoming widely available.[149, 150] CT can frequently determine whether a lesion is confined to the tracheal wall and amenable to this form of resection. Pearlberg and colleagues[151]

and Zwirewich and co-workers[152] have studied the role of CT in evaluating patients with cancer of the central airway for photoresection. Pearlberg showed that CT was particularly useful for defining the relationship of the sites for planned laser resection to adjacent vascular structures that could be damaged during surgery. Zwirewich and his colleagues studied patients with malignant occlusion of central bronchi. In those patients with predominantly intrinsic masses and no surrounding mass on CT that could be compressing the airway, laser resection frequently achieved patency. In those patients with masses surrounding the site of occlusion on CT, the response was less favorable.

In those centers in which experience has been obtained with CT assessment of bronchiectasis, surgeons operate without bronchoscopic confirmation.[153] This has obviated the need for bronchography in many instances and has made evaluation of the patient with suspected bronchiectasis considerably easier. In our experience, areas of focal bronchiectasis limited to one or two segments and not evident on chest radiographs are more common than is described in the literature. HRCT has become useful for evaluation of patients with unexplained chronic cough or sputum production.

The indications for CT scanning in imaging suspected abnormalities of the trachea and bronchi have largely been defined. Oblique and coned-down radiographs demonstrate most lesions protruding into the trachea and bronchi. CT can more precisely define the extrinsic extent of tracheal and bronchial lesions and their relationship to adjacent structures. The role of MR remains limited by the length of time required to obtain images and its generally poorer spatial resolution.

When the patient's symptoms, pulmonary function studies, or chest radiographs suggest compression or displacement of the trachea by an extrinsic mass, both CT and MR are likely to demonstrate the cause. A dilated or aberrant vessel or mediastinal extension of a goiter is the most common cause and both can be readily diagnosed with CT or MR. Extrinsic compression of the bronchi within a hilum is usually due to lymphadenopathy or a bronchogenic carcinoma.

CT scanning is probably indicated in all patients with masses that appear to be arising within the tracheal wall. In most of these, CT demonstrates the position and extent of the abnormality. If the mass contains calcium deposits, a benign tumor of cartilaginous origin should be considered. Rarely, a chondrosarcoma will show this finding. Extension of the mass beyond the confines of the tracheal wall is extremely suggestive of a malignant neoplasm. Unless disease in other organs or parts of the respiratory tract make the diagnosis obvious, endoscopy and biopsy invariably are necessary for diagnosis.

The use of CT for tracheal stenosis from tracheal injury requires further clarification. In our experience, CT may have a role in selecting patients for laser resection of benign strictures. If the stricture is short and high-resolution scans show that the cartilages are intact, the lesion may be suitable for this form of treatment.

CT of the entire thorax and upper abdomen is indicated in patients with endobronchial lesions suspected of being malignant neoplasms. CT can demonstrate sites suggestive of spread of the malignancy to the mediastinum, bony thorax, lung parenchyma, adrenal glands, and liver. CT can also be used to guide the bronchoscopist in performing a biopsy of abnormal bronchial sites beyond the range of direct endoscopic visibility. CT scans are also excellent for demonstrating suspected areas of atelectasis and obstructive pneumonitis. In instances of a central mass without bronchial mucosal involvement, CT-guided percutaneous biopsy can be undertaken when bronchoscopy is unrevealing.[154]

References

1. Kittredge RD: Computed tomography of the trachea: a review. Comput Tomogr 5:44, 1981.
2. Gamsu G, Webb WR: Computed tomography of the trachea: normal and abnormal. AJR 139:321, 1982.
3. Naidich DP, Terry PB, Stitik FP, Siegelman SS: Computed tomography of the bronchi. 1. Normal anatomy. J Comput Assist Tomogr 4:746, 1980.
4. Webb WR, Glazer G, Gamsu G: Computed tomography of the normal pulmonary hilum. J Comput Assist Tomogr 5:476, 1981.
5. Osborne D, Vock P, Godwin JD, Silverman PM: CT identification of bronchopulmonary segments: 50 normal subjects. AJR 142:47, 1984.
6. Jardin M, Remy J: Segmental bronchovascular anatomy of the lower lobes: CT analysis. AJR 147:457, 1986.
7. Naidich DP, Zinn WL, Ettenger NA, McCauley DI, Garay SM: Basilar segmental bronchi: thin-section CT evaluation. Radiology 169:11, 1988.
8. Gray H: Trachea. In Goss CM (ed): Gray's Anatomy of the Human Body, 28th Am ed. Philadelphia, Lea & Febiger, 1966, pp 1137–1139.
9. Fraser RG, Paré JAP, Paré PD, Fraser RS, Genereux GP: Diagnosis of Diseases of the Chest, 3d ed, Vol 1. Philadelphia, WB Saunders Company, 1988, p 37.
10. Breatnach E, Abbott GC, Fraser RG: Dimensions of the normal human trachea. AJR 141:903, 1984.
11. Griscom NT: Computed tomographic determination of tracheal dimensions in children and adolescents. Radiology 145:361, 1982.
12. Effmann EL, Fram EK, Vock P, Kirks DR: Tracheal cross-sectional area in children: CT determination. Radiology 149:137, 1983.
13. Jesseph JE, Merendino KA: The dimensional interrelationships of the major components of the human tracheobronchial tree. Surg Gynecol Obstet 105:210, 1957.
14. Fraser RG: Measurements of the caliber of human bronchi in three phases of respiration by cinebronchography. J Can Assoc Radiol 12:102, 1961.
15. Webb WR, Hirji M, Gamsu G: Posterior wall of the bronchus intermedius: Radiographic-CT correlation. AJR 141:907, 1984.
16. Boyden EA, Hartmann JF: An analysis of variations in the bronchopulmonary segments of the left upper lobes of fifty lungs. Am J Anat 79:321, 1946.
17. Griscom NT: Cross-sectional shape of the child's trachea by computed tomography. AJR 140:1103, 1983.
18. Westra D, Verbeeten B Jr: Some anatomical variants and pitfalls in computed tomography of the trachea and mainstem bronchi. I. Mucoid pseudotumors. Diagn Imag Clin Med 54:229, 1985.
19. Kormano M, Yrjana J: The posterior tracheal band: correlation between computed tomography and chest radiography. Radiology 136:689, 1980.
20. Cimmino CV: The esophageal-pleural stripe: an update. Radiology 140:609, 1981.
21. Speckman JM, Gamsu G, Webb WR: Alterations in CT mediastinal anatomy produced by an azygos lobe. AJR 137:47, 1981.
22. Westra D, Verbeeten B Jr: Some anatomical variants and pitfalls in computed tomography of the trachea and mainstem bronchi. II. Compression or anatomical variants? Diagn Imag Clin Med 54:285, 1985.
23. Schnyder PA, Gamsu G: CT of the paratracheal retrocaval space. AJR 136:303, 1981.
24. Shipley RT, McLoud TC, Dedrick CG, Shepard JA: Computed tomography of the tracheal bronchus. J Comput Assist Tomogr 9:53, 1985.
25. Morrison SC: Demonstration of a tracheal bronchus by computed tomography. Clin Radiol 39:208, 1988.
26. Webb WR, Gamsu G: Computed tomography of the left retrobronchial stripe. J Comput Assist Tomogr 7:65, 1983.
27. Webb WR, Gamsu G, Wall SD, Cann CE, Proctor E: CT of a bronchial phantom: factors affecting appearance and size measurements. Invest Radiol 19:394, 1984.
28. Himalstein MR, Gallagher JC: Tracheobronchomegaly. Ann Otol Rhinol Laryngol 82:223, 1973.
29. Bateson EM, Woo-Ming M: Tracheobronchomegaly. Clin Radiol 24:354, 1978.
30. Aaby GV, Blake HA: Tracheobronchomegaly. Ann Thorac Surg 2:64, 1966.
31. Shin MS, Jackson RM, Ho K-J: Tracheobronchomegaly (Mounier-Kuhn syndrome): CT diagnosis. AJR 150:777, 1988.
32. Williams H, Campbell P: Generalized bronchiectasis associated with deficiency of cartilage in the bronchial tree. Arch Dis Child 35:182, 1960.
33. Greene R: Saber-sheath trachea: relation to chronic obstructive pulmonary disease. AJR 130:441, 1978.
34. Rubenstein J, Weisbrod G, Steinhardt MI: Atypical appearances of saber-sheath trachea. Radiology 127:41, 1978.
35. Wilson SR, Sanders DE, Delarue NC: Intrathoracic manifestations of amyloid disease. Radiology 120:283, 1976.
36. Cook AJ, Weinstein M, Powell RD: Diffuse amyloidosis of the tracheobronchial tree: bronchographic manifestations. Radiology 107:303, 1973.
37. Kilman WJ: Narrowing of the airway in relapsing polychondritis. Radiology 126:373, 1978.
38. Hughes RAC, Berry CL, Seifert M, Lessof MH: Relapsing polychondritis. QJ Med 41:363, 1978.
39. Dolan DL, Lemmon GB Jr, Teitelbaum SL: Relapsing polychondritis. Analytical literature review and studies on pathogenesis. Am J Med 41:285, 1966.
40. Mendelson DS, Som PM, Crane R, Cohen BA, Spiera H: Relapsing polychondritis studied by computed tomography. Radiology 157:489, 1985.
41. Gibson GJ, Davis P: Respiratory complications of relapsing polychondritis. Thorax 29:726, 1974.
42. Howland WJ Jr, Good CA: The radiographic features of tracheopathia osteoplastica. Radiology 71:847, 1958.
43. Secrest PG, Kendig TA, Beland AJ: Tracheobronchopathia osteochondroplastica. Am J Med 36:815, 1964.
44. Bergeron D, Cormier Y, Desmeules M: Tracheobronchopathia osteochondroplastica. Am Rev Respir Dis 114:803, 1976.
45. Baird RB, McCartney JN: Tracheopathia osteoplastica. Thorax 21:321, 1966.
46. Massoud GE, Awwad HK: Scleroma of the upper air passages. J Faculty Radiol 10:44, 1959.
47. Caldarola VT, Harrison EG Jr, Clagett OT, Schmidt HW: Benign tumors and tumorlike conditions of the trachea and bronchi. Ann Otol Rhinol Laryngol 73:1042, 1964.
48. Gilbert JG, Mazzarella LA, Feit LJ: Primary tracheal tumors in the infant and adult. Arch Otolaryngol 58:1, 1953.
49. Weber AL, Shortsleeve M, Goodman M, Montgomery W, Grillo HC: Cartilaginous tumors of the larynx and trachea. Radiol Clin North Am 16:261, 1978.
50. Renault P: Tracheal chondroma. J Fr Med Chir Thorac 25:481, 1971.

51. Rishovits G: Tracheobronchial chondroma. Tuberkulozis 14:182, 1961.
52. Weber AL, Grillo HC: Tracheal tumors. A radiological, clinical, and pathological evaluation of 84 cases. Radiol Clin North Am 16:227, 1978.
53. Houston HE, Payne WS, Harrison EG Jr, Olsen AM: Primary cancers of the trachea. Arch Surg 99:132, 1969.
54. Ranke EJ, Presley SS, Holinger PH: Tracheogenic carcinoma. JAMA 182:519, 1962.
55. Hajdu SI, Huvos AG, Goodner JT, Foote FW Jr, Beattie EJ Jr: Carcinoma of the trachea. Clinicopathologic study of 41 cases. Cancer 25:1448, 1970.
56. Karlan MS, Livingston PA, Baker DC Jr: Diagnosis of tracheal tumors. Ann Otol Rhinol Laryngol 82:790, 1973.
57. Gamsu G, Borson DB, Webb WR: Structure and function in tracheal stenosis. Am Rev Respir Dis 121:519, 1980.
58. Fleming RJ, Medina J, Seaman WB: Roentgenographic aspects of tracheal tumors. Radiology 79:628, 1962.
59. Janower ML, Grillo HC, MacMillan AS Jr, James AE Jr: The radiological appearance of carcinoma of the trachea. Radiology 96:39, 1970.
60. Muhm JR, Crowe JK: The evaluation of tracheal abnormalities by tomography. Radiol Clin North Am 14:95, 1976.
61. Gamsu G, Nadal JA: New technique for roentgenographic study of airways and lungs using powdered tantalum. Cancer 30:1353, 1972.
62. Momose KJ, Macmillan AS Jr: Roentgenologic investigations of the larynx and trachea. Radiol Clin North Am 16:321, 1978.
63. Naidich DP, McCauley DI, Siegelman SS: Computed tomography of bronchial adenomas. J Comput Assist Tomogr 6:725, 1982.
64. Spizarny DL, Shepard J-AO, McLoud TC, Grillo HC, Dedrick CG: CT of adenoid cystic carcinoma of the trachea. AJR 146:1129, 1986.
65. Glazer GM, Axel L, Moss AA: CT diagnosis of mediastinal thyroid. AJR 138:495, 1982.
66. Kirks DR, Fram EK, Vock P, Effmann EL: Tracheal compression by mediastinal masses in children: CT evaluation. AJR 141:647, 1983.
67. Moncada R, Demos TC, Churchill R, Reynes C: Chronic stridor in a child: CT diagnosis of pulmonary vascular sling. J Comput Assist Tomogr 7:713, 1983.
68. Bisset GS III, Strife JL, Kirks DR, Bailey WW: Vascular rings: MR imaging. AJR 149:251, 1987.
69. Djalilian M, Beahrs OH, Devine KD, Weiland LH, DeSanto LW: Intraluminal involvement of the larynx and trachea by thyroid cancer. Am J Surg 128:500, 1974.
70. Daffner RH, Halber MD, Postlethwait RW, Korobkin M, Thompson WM: CT of the esophagus: II. Carcinoma. AJR 133:1051, 1979.
71. Gamsu G, Webb WR, Shallit JB, Moss AA: CT in carcinoma of the larynx and pyriform sinus: value of phonation scans. AJR 136:577, 1981.
72. Calem WS, Freund HR: Subglottic carcinoma with extensive tracheal involvement. Surgery 50:894, 1961.
73. Moss AA, Schnyder P, Thoeni RF, Margulis AR: Esophageal carcinoma: pretherapy staging by computed tomography. AJR 136:1051, 1981.
74. MacMillan AS, James AE Jr, Stitik FP, Grillo HC: Radiological evaluation of post-tracheostomy lesions. Thorax 26:696, 1971.
75. Harley HRS: Laryngotracheal obstruction complicating tracheostomy or endotracheal intubation with assisted respiration. Thorax 26:493, 1971.
76. Dunn CR, Dunn DL, Moser KM: Determinants of tracheal injury by cuffed tracheostomy tubes. Chest 65:128, 1974.
77. Grillo HC: Surgical treatment of post-intubation tracheal injuries. J Thorac Cardiovasc Surg 78:860, 1979.
78. Ross JAT: Techniques in the surgical repair of tracheal stenosis. Otolaryngol Clin North Am 12:893, 1979.
79. Toty L, Personne C, Colchen A, Leroy M, Vourc'h G: Laser treatment of postintubation lesions. In Grillo HC, Eschapasse H (eds): International Trends in General Thoracic Surgery, vol 2. Philadelphia, WB Saunders Company, 1987, p 31.
80. Martini N, Beattie EJ Jr: Less common tumors of the lung. In Shields TW (ed). General Thoracic Surgery, 2nd ed. Philadelphia, Lea & Fibiger, 1983, p 780.
81. Donoghue FE, Anderson HA, McDonald JR: Unusual bronchial tumors. Ann Otol Rhinol Laryngol 65:820, 1956.
82. Weber AL, Bird TK, Janower ML: Primary tuberculosis in childhood with particular emphasis on changes affecting the tracheobronchial tree. AJR 103:123, 1968.
83. Daly JF: Endoscopic aspects of primary tuberculosis in children. Ann Otol Rhinol Laryngol 67:1089, 1958.
83a. Choe KO, Jeong HJ, Sohn HY: Tuberculous bronchial stenosis: CT findings in 28 cases. AJR 155:971, 1990.
84. Meighan JW: Pulmonary cryptococcosis mimicking carcinoma of the lung. Radiology 103:61, 1972.
85. Citron KM, Scadding JG: Stenosing non-caseating tuberculosis (sarcoidosis) of the bronchi. Thorax 12:10, 1957.
86. Goldenberg GJ, Greenspan RH: Middle-lobe atelectasis due to endobronchial sarcoidosis, with hypercalcemia and renal impairment. N Engl J Med 262:1112, 1960.
87. Olsson T, Bjornstad-Pettersen H, Stjernberg NL: Bronchostenosis due to sarcoidosis: a cause of atelectasis and airway obstruction simulating pulmonary neoplasm and chronic obstructive pulmonary disease. Chest 75:663, 1979.
88. Henschke CI, Davis SD, Auh Y, Romano P, Westcott J, Berkmen YM, et al: Detection of bronchial abnormalities: comparison of CT and bronchoscopy. J Comput Assist Tomogr 11:432, 1987.
89. Naidich DP, Lee J-J, Garay SM, McCauley DI, Aranda CP, et al: Comparison of CT and fiberoptic bronchoscopy in the evaluation of bronchial disease. AJR 148:1, 1987.
90. Crofton J: Diagnosis and treatment of bronchiectasis: I. Diagnosis. II. Treatment and prevention. Br Med J 1:721, 1966.
91. Watanabe Y, Nishiyama Y, Kanayama H, Enomoto K, Kato K, et al: Congenital bronchiectasis due to cartilage deficiency: CT demonstration. J Comput Assist Tomogr 11:701, 1987.
92. Eliasson R, Mossberg B, Camner P, Afzelius BA: The immotile-cilia syndrome: a congenital ciliary abnormality as an etiologic factor in chronic airway infections and male sterility. N Engl J Med 297:1, 1977.
93. Wood RF, Boat TF, Doershuk CF: Cystic fibrosis. Am Rev Respir Dis 113:833, 1976.
93a. Neeld DA, Goodman LR, Gurney JW, Greenberger PA, Fink JN: Computerized tomography in the evaluation of allergic bronchopulmonary aspergillosis. Am Rev Respir Dis 142:1200, 1990.
94. Gudbjerg CE: Roentgenologic diagnosis of bronchiectasis: an analysis of 112 cases. Acta Radiol 43:209, 1955.
95. Naidich DP, McCauley DI, Khouri NF, Stitik FP, Siegelman SS: Computed tomography of bronchiectasis. J Comput Assist Tomogr 6:437, 1982.
96. Tarver RD, Conces DJ, Godwin JD: Motion artifacts on CT simulate bronchiectasis. AJR 151:1117, 1988.
97. Grenier P, Maurice F, Musset D, Menu Y, Nahum H: Bronchiectasis: assessment by thin-section CT. Radiology 161:95, 1986.
98. Phillips MS, Williams MP, Flower CDR: How useful is computed tomography in the diagnosis and assessment of bronchiectasis? Clin Radiol 37:321, 1986.
99. Joharjy IA, Bashi SA, Abdullah AK: Value of medium-thickness CT in the diagnosis of bronchiectasis. AJR 149:1133, 1987.
100. Pang JA, Hamilton-Wood C, Metreweli C: The value of computed tomography in the diagnosis and management of bronchiectasis. Clin Radiol 40:42, 1989.
101. Libshitz HI, Shuman LS: Radiation-induced pulmonary change: CT findings. J Comput Assist Tomogr 8:15, 1984.
102. Mead J, Takashima T, Leith D: Stress distribution in lungs: a model of pulmonary elasticity. J Appl Physiol 28:596, 1970.
103. Menkes H, Gamsu G, Schroter R, Macklem PT: Interdependence of lung units in isolated dog lungs. J Appl Physiol 32:675, 1972.
104. Gamsu G, Singer MM, Vincent HH, Berry S, Nadel JA: Postoperative impairment of mucus transport in the lung. Am Rev Respir Dis 114:673, 1976.
105. Robbins LL, Hale CH: The roentgen appearance of lobar and segmental collapse of the lung. III. Collapse of an entire lung or the major part thereof. Radiology 45:23, 1945.

106. Lubert M, Krause GR: Patterns of lobar collapse as observed radiologically. Radiology 56:165, 1951.

107. Krause GR, Lubert M: Gross anatomic spatial changes occurring in lobar collapse. A demonstration by means of three-dimensional plastic models. AJR 79:258, 1958.

108. Proto AV, Tocino I: Radiographic manifestations of lobar collapse. Semin Roentgenol 15:117, 1980.

109. Naidich DP, McCauley DI, Khouri NF, Leitman BS, Hulnick DH, et al: Computed tomography of lobar collapse: 1. Endobronchial obstruction. J Comput Assist Tomogr 7:745, 1983.

110. Raasch BN, Heitzman ER, Carsky EW, Lane EJ, Berlow ME, et al: A computed tomographic study of bronchopulmonary collapse. Radiographics 4:195, 1984.

111. Naidich DP, Ettinger N, Leitman BS, McCauley DI: CT of lobar collapse. Semin Roentgenol 19:222, 1984.

112. Khoury MB, Godwin JD, Halvorsen RA, Putman CE: CT of obstructive lobar collapse. Invest Radiol 20:708, 1985.

113. Woodring JH: Determining the cause of pulmonary atelectasis: a comparison of plain radiography and CT. AJR 150:757, 1988.

114. Mayr B, Ingrisch H, Haussinger K, Huber RM, Sunder-Plassmann L: Tumors of the bronchi: role of evaluation with CT. Radiology 172:647, 1989.

115. Glazer HS, Anderson DJ, Sagel SS: Bronchial impaction in lobar collapse: CT demonstration and pathologic correlation. AJR 153:485, 1989.

116. Mayr B, Heywang SH, Ingrisch H, Huber RM, Haussinger K, et al: Comparison of CT with MR imaging of endobronchial tumors. J Comput Assist Tomogr 11:43, 1987.

117. Tobler J, Levitt RG, Glazer HS, Moran J, Crouch E, et al: Differentiation of proximal bronchogenic carcinoma from postobstructive lobar collapse by magnetic resonance imaging: comparison with computed tomography. Invest Radiol 22:538, 1987.

117a. Herold CJ, Kuhlman JE, Zerhouni EA: Pulmonary atelectasis: signal patterns with MR imaging. Radiology 178:715, 1991.

118. Naidich DP, McCauley DI, Khouri NF, Leitman BS, Hulnick DH, et al: Computed tomography of lobar collapse. 2. Collapse in the absence of endobronchial obstruction. J Comput Assist Tomogr 7:758, 1983.

119. Proto AV, Merhar GL: Central bronchial displacement with large posterior pleural collections. Findings on the lateral chest radiograph and CT scans. J Can Assoc Radiol 35:128, 1984.

120. Miller DR: Benign tumors of lung and tracheobronchial tree. Ann Thorac Surg 8:542, 1969.

121. Peleg H, Pauzner Y: Benign tumors of the lung. Dis Chest 47:179, 1965.

122. Burcharth F, Axelsson C: Bronchial adenomas. Thorax 27:442, 1972.

123. Marks C, Marks M: Bronchial adenoma: a clinicopathologic study. Chest 71:376, 1977.

124. Bower G: Bronchial adenoma: a review of twenty-eight cases. Am Rev Respir Dis 92:558, 1965.

125. Giustra PE, Stassa G: The multiple presentation of bronchial adenomas. Radiology 93:1013, 1969.

126. Aronchick JM, Wexler BC, Wallace M, Epstein D, Gefter WB: Computed tomography of bronchial carcinoid. J Comput Assist Tomogr 10:71, 1986.

126a. Davis SD, Zirn JR, Govoni AF, Yankelevitz DF: Peripheral carcinoid tumor of the lung: CT diagnosis. AJR 155:1185, 1990.

126b. Doppman JL, Pass HI, Nieman LK, Findling JW, Dwyer AJ, et al: Detection of ACTH-producing bronchial tumors: MR imaging vs CT. AJR 158:39, 1991.

127. Bateson EM, Abbott EK: Mixed tumors of the lung, or hamartochondroma: a review of the radiological appearances of cases published in the literature and a report of fifteen new cases. Clin Radiol 11:232, 1960.

128. Siegelman SS, Khouri NF, Scott WW Jr, Leo FP, Hamper UM, et al: Pulmonary hamartoma: CT findings. Radiology 160:313, 1986.

129. Mendelsohn SL, Fagelman D, Zwanger-Mendelsohn S: Endobronchial lipoma demonstrated by CT. Radiology 148:790, 1983.

130. Ikezoe J, Sone S, Higashihara T, Morimoto S, Arisawa J, et al: Schwannoma of the trachea. Eur J Radiol 6:65, 1986.

131. Shin MS, Berland LL, Myers JL, Clary G, Zorn GL: CT demonstration of an ossifying bronchial carcinoid simulating broncholithiasis. AJR 153:51, 1989.

132. Silverberg E: Cancer statistics, 1987. CA 37:2, 1987.

133. Hammond EC: Lung cancer death rates in England and Wales compared with those in the U.S.A. Br Med J 2:649, 1958.

134. Korpela A, Magnus K: The incidence of lung cancer in Finland and Norway. Br J Cancer 15:393, 1961.

135. Cohen S, Hossain MS: Primary carcinoma of the lung: a review of 417 histologically proved cases. Dis Chest 49:67, 1966.

136. Kreyberg L, Liebow AA, Uehlinger EA: Histological Typing of Lung Tumors. Geneva, World Health Organization, 1967.

137. Mountain CF: Surgical prospects and priorities for clinical research. Cancer Chemother Rep 4:19, 1973.

138. Naidich DP, Stitik FP, Khouri NF, Terry PB, Siegelman SS: Computed tomography of the bronchi. 2. Pathology. J Comput Assist Tomogr 4:754, 1980.

139. Webb WR, Gamsu G, Speckman JM: Computed tomography of the pulmonary hilum in patients with bronchogenic carcinoma. J Comput Assist Tomogr 7:219, 1983.

140. Webb WR, Jensen BG, Sollitto R, de Geer G, McCowin M, et al: Bronchogenic carcinoma: staging with MR compared with staging with CT and surgery. Radiology 156:117, 1985.

141. Webb WR: Plain radiography and computed tomography in the staging of bronchogenic carcinoma: a practical approach. J Thorac Imag 2:57, 1987.

141a. Naidich DP, Funt S, Ettenger NA, Arranda C: Hemoptysis: CT-bronchoscopic correlations in 58 cases. Radiology 177:357, 1990.

142. Quint LE, Glazer GM, Orringer MB: Central lung masses: prediction with CT of need for pneumonectomy versus lobectomy. Radiology 165:735, 1987.

143. Byrd RB, Carr DT, Miller WE, Payne WS, Woolner LB: Radiographic abnormalities in carcinoma of the lung as related to histological cell type. Thorax 24:573, 1969.

144. Lehar TJ, Carr DT, Miller WE, Payne WS, Woolner LB: Roentgenographic appearance of bronchogenic adenocarcinoma. Am Rev Respir Dis 96:245, 1967.

145. Pearson FG, Thompson DW, Delarue NC: Experience with the cytologic detection, localization, and treatment of radiographically undemonstrable bronchial carcinoma. J Thorac Cardiovasc Surg 54:371, 1967.

146. Grzybowski S, Coy P: Early diagnosis of carcinoma of the lung. Cancer 25:113, 1970.

147. Marsh BR, Frost JK, Erozan YS, Carter D: Occult bronchogenic carcinoma: endoscopic localization and television documentation. Cancer 30:1347, 1972.

147a. Foster WL Jr, Roberts L Jr, McLendon RE, Hill RC: Localized peribronchial thickening: a CT sign of occult bronchogenic carcinoma. AJR 144:906, 1985.

148. Stein MG, Mayo J, Mueller N, Aberle DR, Webb WR, et al: Pulmonary lymphangitic spread of carcinoma: appearance on CT scans. Radiology 162:371, 1987.

149. Wolfe WG, Sabiston DC Jr: Management of benign and malignant lesions of the trachea and bronchi with the neodymiumyttrium-aluminum-garnet laser. J Thorac Cardiovasc Surg 91:40, 1986.

150. Brutinel WM, Cortese DA, McDougall JC, Gillo RG, Bergstralh EJ: A two-year experience with the neodymium-YAG laser in endobronchial obstruction. Chest 91:159, 1987.

151. Pearlberg JL, Sandler MA, Kvale P, Beute GH, Madrazo BL: Computed-tomographic and conventional linear-tomographic evaluation of tracheobronchial lesions for laser photoresection. Radiology 154:759, 1985.

152. Zwirewich CV, Mueller NL, Lam SC-T: Photodynamic laser therapy to alleviate complete bronchial obstruction: comparison of CT and bronchoscopy to predict outcome. AJR 151:897, 1988.

153. McLoud TC: Personal communication. 1990.

154. Sider L, David TM Jr: Hilar masses: evaluation with CT-guided biopsy after negative bronchoscopic examination. Radiology 164:107, 1987.

THE MEDIASTINUM

GORDON GAMSU

Anatomy

Cross-sectional imaging allows detailed evaluation of the mediastinum from a perspective totally different from that obtained with conventional radiographs.[1] Individual mediastinal structures and their relationships are readily visualized. Interpretation of computed tomography (CT) or magnetic resonance (MR) scans of the mediastinum necessitates a thorough knowledge of both conventional and cross-sectional anatomy. The recognition of normal mediastinal structures also requires an appreciation of the anatomic variations in individuals of different ages and physiques. Familiarity with the variations in density of mediastinal tissue and in the caliber of the mediastinal vessels is also important for diagnosing abnormality. Distortions of the mediastinal structures produced by musculoskeletal, pleural, and pulmonary disease, as well as surgery, must also be understood.

In this chapter, unless otherwise stated, we assume that the CT or MR scans are transverse and that the patient is supine. Anatomic orientation is conventional, with *anterior*, *ventral*, and *in front of* meaning toward the patient's front; *posterior, dorsal, behind* meaning toward the patient's back; *superior, cephalad,* and *above* meaning toward the patient's head; and *inferior, caudad,* and *below* meaning toward the patient's feet.

The mediastinum extends from the sternum anteriorly to the vertebral bodies posteriorly. It is bounded laterally by the parietal mediastinal pleura of each lung. Below the thoracic inlet, the mediastinum is dominated by its vascular structures, the trachea, and the esophagus. The heart and pericardium are discussed in Chapter 6.

Vascular Structures

UPPER MEDIASTINUM

Above the aortic arch and below the thoracic inlet, at a distance of 2 to 4 cm, the great arteries (arch vessels) and veins are uniformly positioned within the mediastinum (Figs. 2–1 to 2–3).[2-4] They are always visible on CT or MR scans in the transverse plane. Intravenous administration of contrast material renders them more easily identifiable on CT.

The innominate artery is the first branch of the aorta above the coronary arteries and varies only slightly in its position within the mediastinum. In about half of normal individuals, it is midline, directly anterior to the trachea. In the remainder, it is either slightly to the right or left of the midline but still anterior to the trachea. The left common carotid artery is the next branch and lies to the left of the intrathoracic trachea. At its origin, it is distinctly anterior to the trachea, and superiorly it moves to the left of the anterior half of the trachea. The left common carotid artery is usually surrounded by mediastinal fat and only rarely is in contact with the left lung. In most individuals, the left subclavian artery is the third major branch and lies to the left of the anterior two thirds of the trachea. About 10 per cent of the time, it is lateral to the posterior third of the trachea. The amount of mediastinal fat surrounding the left subclavian artery varies among individuals, and in most the artery is separated from the left lung.

The venous structures in the upper mediastinum are the right and left brachiocephalic veins, both of which are in front of the arch vessels (see Fig. 2–1). The left brachiocephalic vein courses anterior to the root of the arch vessels or aortic arch and joins the right brachiocephalic vein to form the superior vena cava (SVC) (Fig. 2–4). The right brachiocephalic vein is well forward and to the right of the trachea. Only near the thoracic inlet does it assume a position lateral to the trachea.

Below the great vessels, the aortic arch is visible for a vertical distance of 1 to 3 cm (Fig. 2–4). As the arch courses posteriorly and to the left, it often causes slight flattening of the left anterolateral wall of the trachea, with which it is in contact (Fig. 2–4). The anterior portion of the aortic arch has the SVC on its right side and the left lung on its left side. The midportion of the aortic arch is to the left of the trachea. The posterior arch lies near the left wall of the esophagus.

The SVC is in front of the trachea, separated from

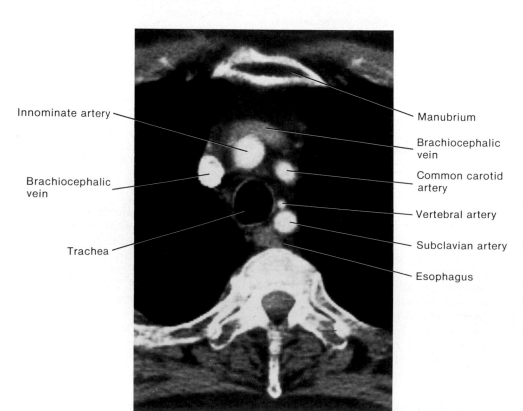

Innominate artery

Brachiocephalic vein

Trachea

Manubrium

Brachiocephalic vein

Common carotid artery

Vertebral artery

Subclavian artery

Esophagus

FIGURE 2–1 ■ Normal upper mediastinal anatomy in an adult male. CT scan is at the level of the manubrium. Contrast medium has been injected.

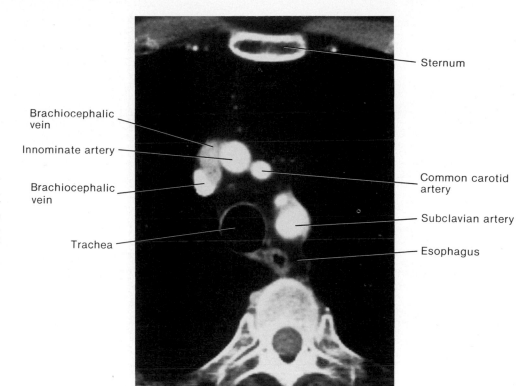

Sternum

Brachiocephalic vein

Innominate artery

Brachiocephalic vein

Common carotid artery

Subclavian artery

Trachea

Esophagus

FIGURE 2–2 ■ Normal upper mediastinal anatomy in an adult male. CT scan is at the level of the upper sternum and great vessels (1 cm caudad to the level shown in Fig. 2–1). Contrast medium has been injected.

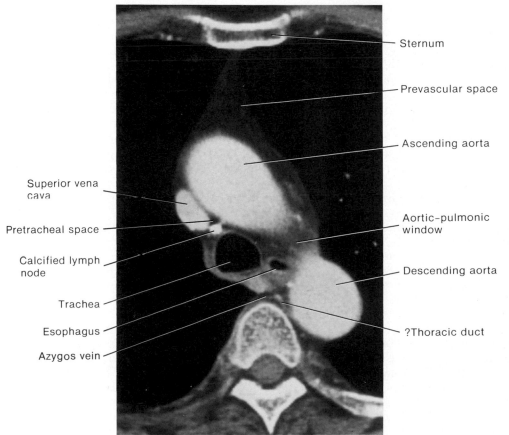

Sternum

Prevascular space

Ascending aorta

Superior vena cava

Pretracheal space

Aortic-pulmonic window

Calcified lymph node

Descending aorta

Trachea

Esophagus

?Thoracic duct

Azygos vein

FIGURE 2–3 ■ Normal mediastinal anatomy in an adult male. CT scan is at the level of the aortic-pulmonic window, above the tracheal bifurcation (1 cm caudad to the level shown in Fig. 2–4). Contrast material has been injected.

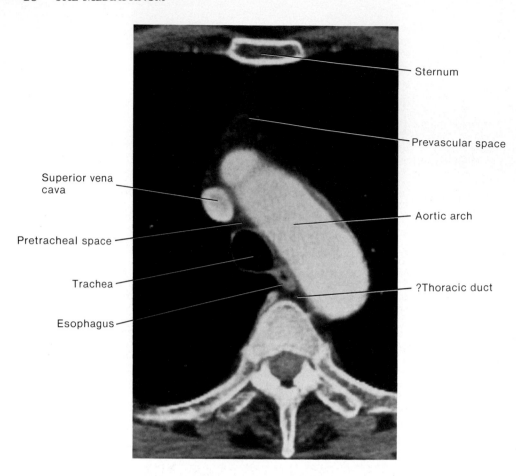

Sternum

Prevascular space

Superior vena cava

Aortic arch

Pretracheal space

Trachea

?Thoracic duct

Esophagus

FIGURE 2–4 ■ Normal mediastinal anatomy in an adult male. CT scan is at the level of the aortic arch (1 cm caudad to the level shown in Fig. 2–2). Contrast medium has been injected.

it by the pretracheal space (Fig. 2–5; see also Figs. 2–3 and 2–4). It is most often elliptic, with its long axis oriented toward the right; less commonly its orientation is anteroposterior.[5] The SVC varies considerably in size but is normally about half the size of the ascending aorta. At times, it is much smaller and may even appear as a thin crescent.

The ascending aorta lies midway between the sternum and spine (Fig. 2–5; see also Fig. 2–3). It extends vertically for 3 to 4 cm. In about two thirds of individuals, the ascending aorta directly contacts the left lung. In the remainder, it is separated from the left lung by mediastinal fat. The upper ascending aorta is separated from the lower trachea by fat within the pretracheal space (Fig. 2–5B), whereas the lower portion of the ascending aorta is immediately anterior to the right pulmonary artery (Fig. 2–6B). The main pulmonary artery is interposed between the lower ascending aorta and the left lung (Fig. 2–6B). To the right of the lower ascending aorta and slightly posterior lie the SVC and the top of the right atrium (Fig. 2–7).

The position of the SVC in relationship to the ascending aorta is variable, depending on patient habitus. The positional relationship of the descending aorta to the spinal column and esophagus varies with age, physique, and disease. In most individuals, the descending aorta is contiguous with the left anterolateral aspect of the spine (Fig. 2–7; see also Fig. 2–3). It can, however, be in the midline, or if excessively tortuous, situated directly lateral to the spine. Except in older or obese patients, the left lung inserts between the descending aorta and the left pulmonary artery, an area well shown by CT. Soft tissue that is not of fatty density, between the descending aorta and the descending left pulmonary artery and behind the left main bronchus, is usually indicative of enlarged lymph nodes or a mass.

The only consistent vascular structure to the right of the intrathoracic trachea is the arch of the azygos vein (see Fig. 2–3). The ascending azygos vein is usually in the midline or slightly to the right, in front of the spinal column (Fig. 2–7). At the level of the tracheal carina, or 1 to 2 cm above it, the azygos vein arches around the right wall of the trachea to enter the posterior wall of the SVC.

MIDDLE MEDIASTINUM

The vascular structures of the middle mediastinum are the pulmonary arteries and veins, the aorta, the azygos and hemiazygos veins, and the SVC (see Figs. 2–3 and 2–5 to 2–7).

The main pulmonary artery is visible over a vertical distance of 1 to 3 cm. Its transverse diameter measures 24.2 ± 2.2 mm (standard deviation [SD]) with an upper limit of 28.4 mm.[6] It lies to the left of the ascending aorta and is flanked by the left lung anteriorly and laterally. The right pulmonary artery courses posterolaterally to the right and slightly inferiorly. It is situated behind the root of the aorta

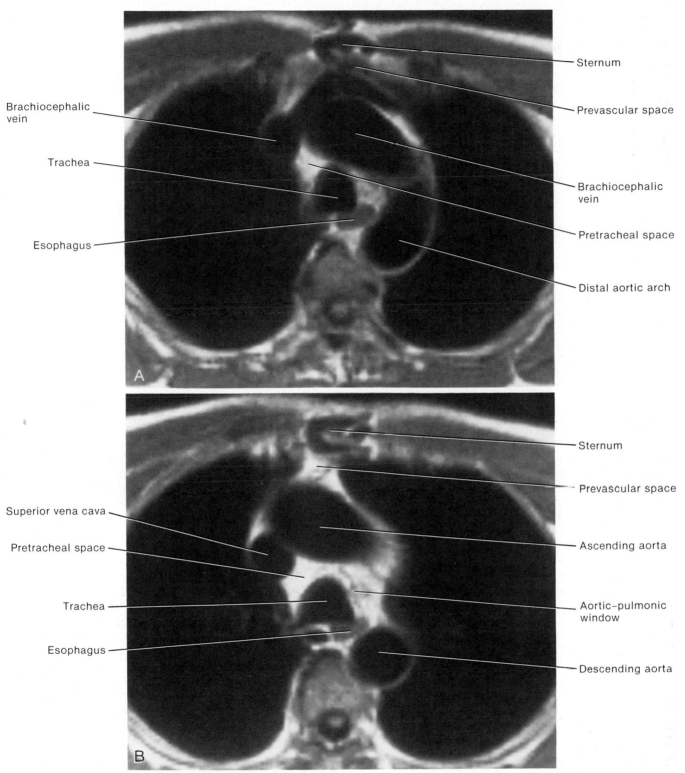

Brachiocephalic vein

Trachea

Esophagus

Sternum

Prevascular space

Brachiocephalic vein

Pretracheal space

Distal aortic arch

A

Superior vena cava

Pretracheal space

Trachea

Esophagus

Sternum

Prevascular space

Ascending aorta

Aortic–pulmonic window

Descending aorta

B

FIGURE 2–5 ■ Normal mediastinal anatomy in an adult male demonstrated on a spin–echo cardiac-gated image. *A* is at the level of the lower aortic arch; *B* is at the level of the aortic-pulmonic window.

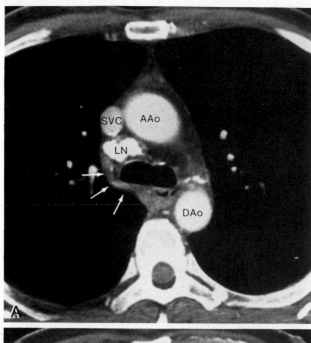

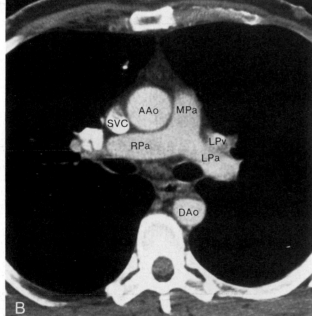

FIGURE 2–6 ■ Normal anatomy of the mid-mediastinum in an older man. Contrast material has been injected. *A*, CT scan at the level of the azygos arch *(arrows)* and tracheal bifurcation. Calcified lymph nodes are present in the pretracheal space. *B*, CT scan 2 cm caudad is at the level of the main and right pulmonary arteries. AAo = ascending aorta; MPa = main pulmonary artery; RPa = right pulmonary artery; SVC = superior vena cava; LPv = left pulmonary vein; LN = lymph node; LPa = left pulmonary artery; DAo = descending aorta.

uation of the main pulmonary artery as it arches over the left main bronchus forming the left pulmonary hilum. Occasionally, the normal main and left pulmonary arteries have a high position and lie lateral to the aortic arch.[7] Under these circumstances, these unopacified vessels may simulate a mediastinal mass on CT. On MR the structure is easily recognized as the pulmonary artery.

The upper division or anterior trunk of the right pulmonary artery arises within the mediastinum. It is evident on CT or MR, immediately behind the SVC and in front of the right main bronchus, above the right pulmonary artery (Fig. 2–8).

The left superior pulmonary vein enters the mediastinum immediately in front of the left main bronchus (Fig. 2–9). Its direction is inferior and medial, as it enters the upper posterior aspect of the left atrium. The right superior pulmonary vein enters the mediastinum 1 to 3 cm lower than the left. It is behind and to the right of the SVC and in front of the proximal right interlobular pulmonary artery (Fig. 2–10; see also Fig. 2–7). It then passes inferiorly and medially under the right pulmonary artery to enter the right upper posterior aspect of the left atrium.

LOWER MEDIASTINUM

The vascular structures contained in the lower mediastinum are the heart (see Chapter 6), the descending aorta, the azygos vein, and the hemiazygos vein (Fig. 2–11; see also Figs. 2–7 and 2–10).

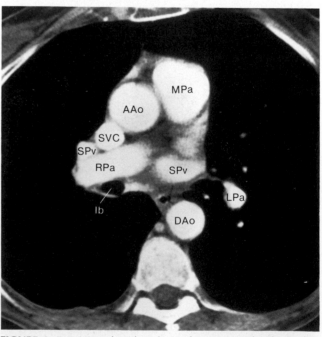

FIGURE 2–7 ■ Normal mid-mediastinal anatomy. The descending left pulmonary artery (LPa) is posterolateral to the basal bronchus, and the right pulmonary artery (RPa) is in front of the intermediate bronchus (Ib). The superior vena cava (SVC) and right superior pulmonary vein (SPv) are in front of the right pulmonary artery. The main pulmonary artery (MPa) is to the left of the ascending aorta (AAo).

and the SVC and in front of the right main and intermediate bronchi. The diameter of the right pulmonary artery at the SVC is 15.3 ± 2.9 mm.[6] The left pulmonary artery runs in a transverse plane 1 to 2 cm cephalad to the right pulmonary artery, at about the level of the tracheal carina (Fig. 2–8). Its diameter is 21.0 ± 3.5 mm. It appears as a contin-

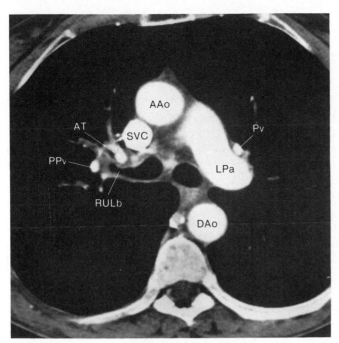

FIGURE 2–8 ■ Mid-mediastinal anatomy at the level of the tracheal bifurcation in an elderly man. Contrast material has been injected. The anterior trunk (AT) is anterior to the right upper lobe bronchus (RULb) and posterolateral to the superior vena cava (SVC). The left pulmonary artery (LPa) is above the left main bronchus. The right posterior pulmonary vein (PPv) is lateral to the upper lobe bronchus. AAo = ascending aorta; DAo = descending aorta; PV = pulmonary vein.

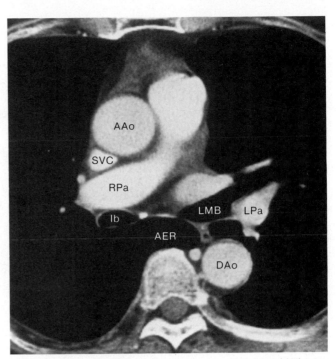

FIGURE 2–9 ■ Normal mid-mediastinal anatomy in an elderly man with a deep azygoesophageal recess (AER). The esophagus is to the left of the midline. The right lung invaginates behind the intermediate bronchus (Ib) and subcarinal space to contact the left main bronchus (LMB). The left lung protrudes between the descending aorta (DAo) and left pulmonary artery (LPa) to contact the posterior wall of the left main bronchus. The superior vena cava (SVC) is compressed between the slightly dilated ascending aorta (AAo) and right pulmonary artery (RPa).

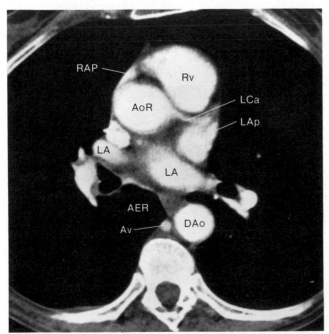

FIGURE 2–10 ■ Normal mediastinal anatomy at the level of the aortic root. Anteriorly, the outflow tract of the right ventricle (Rv) and the aortic root (AoR) are seen. The left and right atrial appendices (LAp and RAP) are indicated. The superior pulmonary veins have entered the posterior aspect of the left atrium (LA). The left coronary artery (LCa) is visible. The descending aorta (DAo) and azygos vein (Av) are anterior to the spine. AER = azygoesophageal recess.

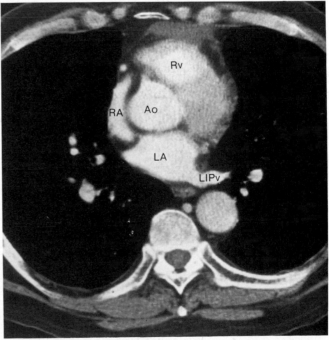

FIGURE 2–11 ■ Normal mediastinal anatomy at the level of the base of the heart in an adult male. The left and right atria (LA and RA) are demonstrated. The aorta has assumed a triangular shape, as seen at the level of the aortic valve (Ao). The right ventricle (Rv) is anterior. The left inferior pulmonary vein (LIPv) is seen entering the left atrium.

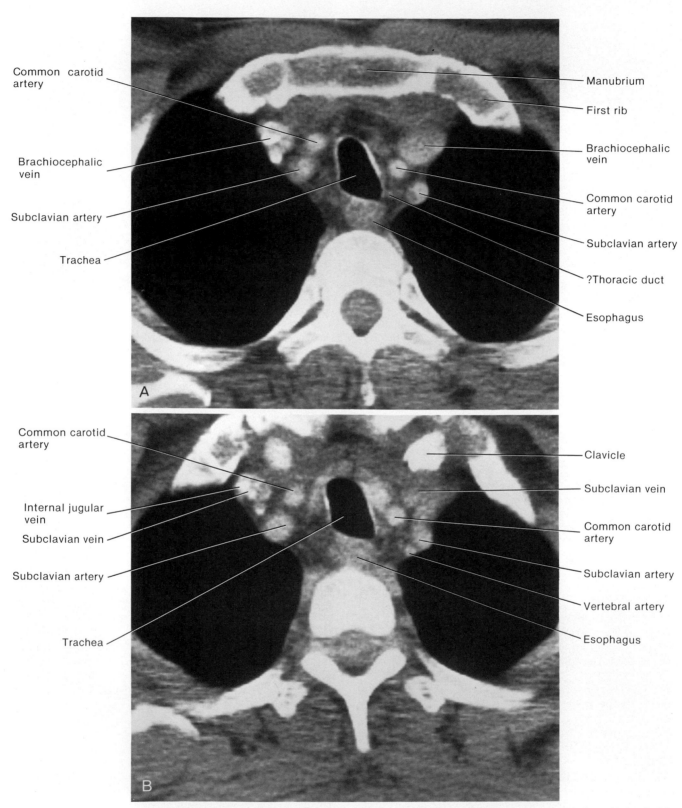

FIGURE 2–12 ■ Normal mediastinal anatomy toward the thoracic inlet. *A, B,* and *C,* Progress cephalad at 1-cm intervals from the level of the manubrium.

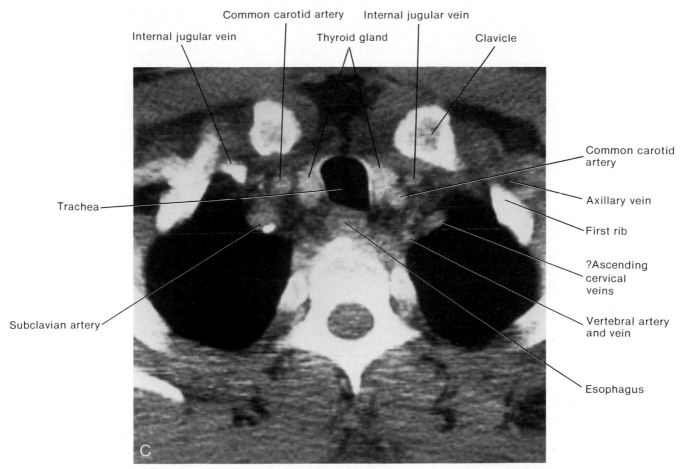

FIGURE 2–12 *Continued*

Before it enters the abdomen through the diaphragmatic retrocrural space, the descending aorta assumes a near-midline position. The caliber and the degree of tortuosity of the descending aorta vary, depending on age, physique, and the presence of vascular disease. The normal ascending aorta has a diameter of about 1.5 times that of the descending aorta. It measures 3.0 to 4.0 cm, being wider toward its base. In most individuals, the ascending azygos vein is close to the midline, to the right of the descending aorta, whereas the hemiazygos vein is posterior to the aorta. Occasionally, the thoracic duct is visible between the azygos vein and the aorta in the lower mediastinum (see Fig. 2–6B).[8] At higher levels, in the upper mediastinum, the thoracic duct assumes a position to the left of the anterior border of the spine.

THORACIC INLET

At the level of the thoracic inlet, 1 to 3 cm above the suprasternal notch, the vascular structures of the mediastinum undergo an abrupt reorientation (Fig. 2–12A to C). The innominate artery is positioned to the right of the anterior third of the trachea; it then divides into the right common carotid artery and the right subclavian artery. The right common carotid artery remains close to the right side of the trachea, whereas the right subclavian artery courses laterally toward the first rib (Fig. 2–12B, C). The right brachiocephalic vein is to the right of the posterior third of the trachea, where it receives its tributaries, the right internal jugular vein and the right subclavian vein. On the left side, the left common carotid artery is opposite the middle or posterior third of the left side of the trachea (Fig. 2–12). At the same level, the left subclavian artery moves anteriorly toward the left first rib (Fig. 2–12C). The left brachiocephalic vein maintains its anterolateral position, receiving the left internal jugular and left subclavian veins. The thoracic duct may be visible between the left common carotid and subclavian arteries.

Mediastinal Spaces

The vessels, heart, trachea, mediastinal pleura, and bony structures that border the mediastinum create real or potential spaces.[9–11] Sone and colleagues[10, 11] have outlined the potential mediastinal spaces by infusing oxygen into the mediastinum. They were able to describe the boundaries of these spaces and the anatomic communications between them.

RETROSTERNAL SPACE

The parietal mediastinal pleura becomes adherent to the inner thoracic cage lateral to the sternum.[11, 12] The retrosternal space is immediately behind and to either side of the sternum for a distance of about the width of the sternum (see Figs. 2–1 to 2–6). It is limited anteriorly by the transverse thoracic muscle.[13] Posteriorly, it is continuous with the prevascular space. This space contains fat and connective tissue and varies markedly in size among individuals. The anterior margins of the two lungs may be apposed and separated only by their pleural surfaces (see Fig. 2–6). In obese individuals, up to 2 cm of mediastinal tissue can separate the lungs, and the sternum then abuts low-density mediastinal fat.

The inner margin of the thoracic cage lateral to the sternum has a predictable contour on CT. When viewed at mediastinal window settings, it is slightly concave about half the time, whereas in the remaining individuals, it appears straight. In about 10 per cent of people, the costochondral junctions cause a slight indentation into the lungs or parasternal soft tissue. At the level of the anterior ends of the first ribs, a prominent indentation into the subapex of the lung is common.

Small lymph nodes are normally present along the internal mammary vascular bundle, but they are not visible on CT or MR. The internal mammary arteries and veins are frequently evident but may not be discernible without intravenously administered contrast material. After contrast infusion, one to three, but usually two, vessels are visible on each side of the sternum (see Fig. 2–2).[13a] They are immediately extrapleural and 2 to 5 cm from the midline (i.e., lateral to the sternum by one third to one half of its width). The artery is usually lateral, and the vein medial.[14]

PREVASCULAR SPACE

The anterior mediastinum contains a potential space known as the prevascular space (see Figs. 2–1 to 2–10). It is continuous with the retrosternal space in front and is bordered laterally by the lungs. Posteriorly, it is limited by the heart, SVC, main pulmonary artery, ascending aorta, and arch vessels. On the left side, the prevascular space extends lateral to the ascending aorta and is continuous with the aortic-pulmonic window (see Figs. 2–5A and 2–6B). The size of the prevascular space depends on the patient's adiposity and physique. The density of the fat in the prevascular space also varies in normal people. Less than half of the time it is low density typical of fat, while about one third of the time its density is that of soft tissue; and in the remainder, the density is irregular and inhomogeneous. Ill-defined bands of higher density are frequently visible crossing the prevascular space.

The normal contents of the prevascular space are the left and right brachiocephalic veins and the thymus gland. At the level of the origin of the arch vessels, or the upper ascending aorta, the left brachiocephalic vein crosses from upper left to lower right. If unopacified with contrast, the left brachiocephalic vein may be mistaken for an anterior mediastinal mass (see Fig. 2–1).[15]

The normal thymus lies within the prevascular mediastinal fat over a vertical distance of 5 to 7 cm. Arising from the third pharyngeal pouches, the thymus is distinctly bilobed. In the infant and young child, this feature cannot be appreciated on CT or MR, and the thymus fills the mediastinum between the great vessels and ascending aorta, and the sternum (Fig. 2–13). In the young, the anterior aspect of the thymus is against the anterior chest wall, and the lateral margins are convex, impinging on the medial aspects of the lungs.[16] The CT density of thymus is distinctly greater than that of mediastinal fat (Fig. 2–14), and its MR intensity is homogeneous, less than fat, and slightly higher than that of muscle on T1-weighted images.[17] The thymus is visible in all individuals under the age of 30.[18, 19] The normal thymus increases in size until about puberty but does not increase relative to the mediastinum after age 3; this is explained by the more rapid growth of the thorax than of the thymus gland.

With increasing age, through adolescence and young adulthood, the thymus gland assumes its adult shape. Its shape becomes bilobed or triangular in cross section. When bilobed, each lobe may be oval, elliptic, or semilunar and measures 1 to 4 cm in length and 0.5 to 1.5 cm in thickness.[18] The thymus appears slightly larger on MR than on CT, probably because of motion during imaging. The left lobe is usually dominant and more frequently visible than the right on both CT and MR.

With increasing age, the thymus gland undergoes fatty involution, decreasing in size and conspicuousness. In individuals who are age 50, it may be visible

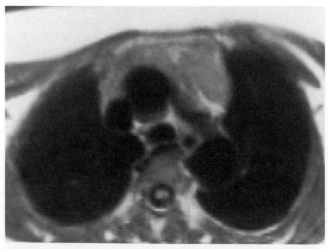

FIGURE 2–13 ■ Normal thymus in a 9-year-old child. T1-weighted spin-echo image shows the normal thymus filling the anterior mediastinum. The intensity of the thymus is slightly greater than that of normal muscle.

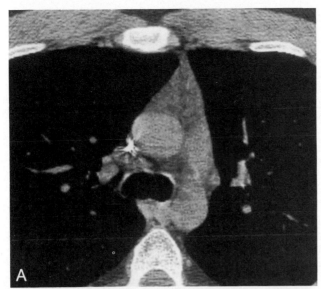

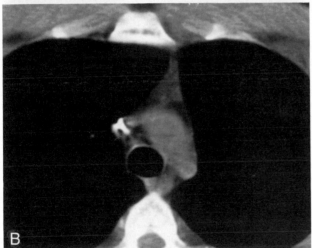

FIGURE 2–14 ■ Normal thymus in the adult. *A*, High-resolution (HR) CT scan in an 18-year-old male shows normal thymic tissue anterior to the ascending aorta and main pulmonary artery. *B*, CT scan in a 35-year-old male shows partial involution of the normal thymus, which is anterior to the ascending aorta.

on CT or MR as a distinct entity or only as an inhomogeneity of the prevascular mediastinal fat (see Fig. 2–6A).[18–21] MR can discriminate more clearly than CT between the involuted thymus and mediastinal fat.

Not uncommonly the right lobe of the thymus extends between the superior vena cava and ascending aorta into the pretracheal space. Enlargement of this variant lobe, whether due to mass or cyst, can present as a pretracheal, middle mediastinal mass.

Normal lymph nodes can be visible in the prevascular space, and in patients who have had granulomatous disease small, noncalcified nodes are common. In about 10 per cent of people, a tubular structure runs superoinferiorly, lateral to the aortic arch. This structure is probably a mediastinal vein or the phrenic nerve, but its nature is not certain.

PRETRACHEAL SPACE

The pretracheal space has particular significance in CT or MR of the mediastinum. It contains many lymph nodes draining both lungs and the mediastinal organs. In addition, it is the space through which transcervical mediastinoscopy is performed. The pretracheal space does not border the lungs, and on radiographs masses or lymph nodes in this space must be of considerable size before becoming visible. CT and MR can demonstrate subtle enlargement of pretracheal lymph nodes.

The pretracheal space extends vertically from the thoracic inlet to the tracheal carina (see Figs. 2–1 to 2–6). The structures bordering the space depend on the level in the mediastinum. At lower levels, the space is bounded by the anterior convexity of the trachea, the medial wall of the azygos arch, the posteromedial wall of the superior vena cava, and the posterior wall of the ascending aorta (see Fig. 2–6A).[22] On the left side, it is limited by the aortic arch or is continuous with the aortic-pulmonic window. Above the aortic arch, the pretracheal space is between the anterior arch of the trachea and the innominate artery in front and the left common carotid and left subclavian arteries to the left. The superior vena cava and right brachiocephalic vein border the pretracheal space on the right. Above the thoracic inlet the space continues into the deep fascial spaces of the neck.

The size of the pretracheal spaces varies widely among individuals. It increases with increasing mediastinal fat, age, and aortic unfolding. The CT density of the space is usually uniform and of fatty density. As with mediastinal "fat" in general, the density varies among individuals. In one study,[22] the mean density of inferior pretracheal space in normal individuals was found to range from -107 H to $+48$ H.

Around the trachea, within the fat and fibrous connective tissue, are numerous lymph nodes. In about 90 per cent of normal individuals, one or more lymph nodes are visible medial to the azygos arch (Fig. 2–6A). (See also the section on mediastinal lymph nodes.)

The pretracheal space also contains the superior retroaortic recess of the pericardium, visible on CT or MR in 50 to 65 per cent of normal individuals. It appears as a low-density or low-intensity, well-defined oval or crescentic structure behind the aortic root, at about the level of the tracheal carina (Fig. 2–15).[23, 24]

AORTIC-PULMONIC WINDOW

The aortic-pulmonic window is situated beneath the aortic arch and above the left pulmonary artery.[25] This space is bounded medially by the lower trachea and esophagus and laterally by the left lung. It is continuous with the inferior pretracheal space medially and the prevascular space to the left of the ascending aorta (see Figs. 2–5B and 2–6A).

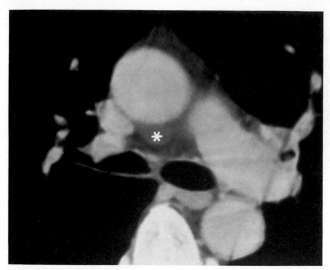

FIGURE 2–15 ■ Superior recess of the pericardium. The low-density ovoid superior retroaortic recess of the pericardium (asterisk) is within the precarinal space behind the aortic root.

On chest radiographs, the aortic-pulmonic window has a height of 1 to 3 cm. On scans obtained with the patient supine, the window may span less than a single 1-cm scan and is then obscured by volume-averaging from the undersurface of the aortic arch and the superior surface of the left pulmonary artery.[26] On supine CT or MR scans, the left lung rarely penetrates this space, although it does appear to do so on erect chest radiographs. The aortic-pulmonic window is usually inhomogeneous, with high-density bands coursing through it. Lying between two pulsatile vascular structures, it is also prone to distortion by motion artifacts.

The aortic-pulmonic window contains fat, lymph nodes (including the ductus node), the ligamentum arteriosum, and the recurrent laryngeal nerve.[27] Occasionally on CT a tubular structure appears to course across it that may be the ligamentum arteriosum, although this is speculative (Fig. 2–6A).

SUBCARINAL SPACE

Extending inferiorly from the pretracheal space is the subcarinal space. This is one of the more difficult areas of the mediastinum to assess with radiographs.[28] The height of the subcarinal space is approximately 2 cm. Its upper portion is bounded anteriorly by the right pulmonary artery and the mediastinal portion of the left superior pulmonary vein (see Figs. 2–6B, 2–7, and 2–8). The right and left main bronchi flank this space on either side. The esophagus, which is posterior and usually to the left of the midline, runs through the subcarinal space. The azygos vein, anterior to the spine, is posterior within the space. The right lung contacts the mediastinum behind the right main bronchus and intermediate bronchus and bounds the subcarinal space posterolaterally. In its lower portion, the space is limited on the right by the intermediate bronchus and inferiorly by the left atrium. In asthenic individ-

uals and in patients with emphysema, the aorta may be in the midline and may form the posterior border of the subcarinal space.

A distinctive pad of mediastinal fat is seen on CT and MR above the left atrium and beneath the tracheal carina, and its CT density is moderately inhomogeneous. Three to five lymph nodes normally occupy the subcarinal space.

RETROTRACHEAL SPACE AND POSTERIOR MEDIASTINUM

The mediastinum posterior to the trachea and heart is elegantly displayed by CT.[29, 30] Between the thoracic inlet and the azygos arch, the appearance of the retrotracheal region is determined by the relative positions of the esophagus and aorta and by the degree of contact of the right lung with the mediastinum. In about 50 per cent of individuals, the right lung contacts one quarter to one half of the posterior wall of the trachea (see Figs. 2–1 to 2–4). In the other 50 per cent, the right lung penetrates the retrotracheal mediastinum to a lesser extent, and the retrotracheal space is filled with mediastinal fat and connective tissue. When the trachea lies close to the spinal column, the retrotracheal space is small, and the right lung is precluded from entering it. In the supine patient, the midesophagus often is slightly to the left of the midline, and about one third of the time, the center of the esophagus is completely to the left of the lower trachea.

Variations in size, shape, and configuration of the posterior mediastinum are evident in the retrocardiac region. The position of the descending aorta varies with age, physique, and degree of lung inflation. It may be distinctly to the left of the spinal column, or it may approach the midline. Toward the diaphragmatic crura, the descending aorta invariably is in the midline. The esophagus likewise varies in position until it approaches the diaphragm. The ascending azygos vein maintains a fairly constant position in the midline or slightly to the right of the midline, anterior to the spinal column.

The lower posterior mediastinum is in direct continuity with the subcarinal space (see Figs. 2–7 and 2–10). The right lung always contacts the posterior wall of the right main and intermediate bronchi, although in about 10 per cent of normal individuals, the azygos arch abuts the medial posterior wall of the right main bronchus.[31] Posteromedial to the bronchial tree, the right lung may intrude deeply into the posterior mediastinum and contact the esophagus, aorta, and azygos vein. Alternatively, the lower posterior mediastinum may be filled with mediastinal fat, preventing the lung from contact with these structures. In the latter instance, the right border of the posterior mediastinum is a straight line from the intermediate bronchus, pulmonary vein, or left atrium to the spine. In about 20 per cent of individuals, the anteroposterior dimension of the mediastinum is small. The bronchial tree, right pulmonary vein, and the heart are all close to the spine. In

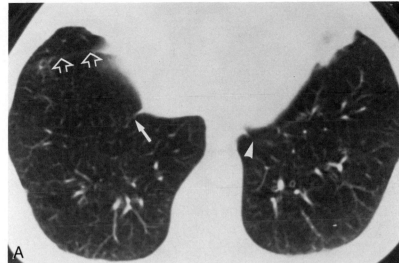

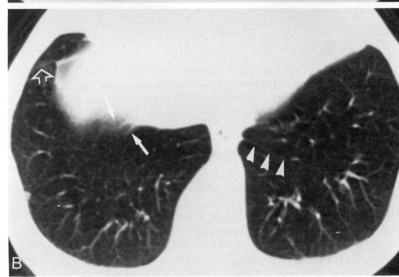

FIGURE 2–16 ■ Normal inferior pulmonary ligament, phrenic nerve, and major fissure. *A* and *B,* On the left side, the four pleural layers of the inferior pulmonary ligament *(arrowheads)* are seen. On the right, the pleura investing the right phrenic nerve *(arrows)* is shown. The lower end of the right major fissure *(open arrows)* is farther anterior on the right.

normal adults, the contour of the right posteroinferior mediastinum is more commonly concave or straight. Occasionally, the esophagus bulges to the right in this area and can be mistaken for a mass or adenopathy. In children and infants, as well as about 30 per cent of young adults, the mediastinum itself may bulge to the right, producing a right posterior mediastinal convexity.[32]

In our experience, normal lymph nodes are not visible on CT scans of the posterior mediastinum. The azygos vein is seen in most individuals, and in more than 50 per cent, the hemiazygos or accessory hemiazygos vein is also visible on the left side, immediately behind the descending aorta. The hemiazygos vein crosses behind the aorta to join the azygos vein between the eighth and tenth dorsal vertebrae, whereas the accessory hemiazygos crosses one or two vertebral bodies higher.[33] These anastomoses are infrequently opacified with contrast material and should not be mistaken on CT for enlarged posterior mediastinal lymph nodes.

The inferior pulmonary ligament is a double layer of pleura that extends inferiorly from the inferior pulmonary veins on each side to anchor the lower lobes to the mediastinum and medial diaphragm. The space between these pleural layers of the ligament is a potential site for accumulation of mediastinal air, and the ligament can be a natural barrier to the distribution of pleural fluid. The ligament can be seen on CT as a slightly posteriorly directed thin line, extending laterally from the region of the lower esophagus variably as far as the mid-hemidiaphragm. It is seen on at least one side in about 60 per cent of normal individuals (Fig. 2–16A, B).[34, 35] A second single or double line anterior to the inferior pulmonary ligament, extending laterally from the inferior vena cava (IVC) on the right and the left atrium on the left, is formed by the phrenic nerve, pericardiophrenic vessels, and their investing pleura (Fig. 2–16A).[36] The early CT descriptions of the normal inferior pulmonary ligament mistakenly included the phrenic nerve and overestimated the frequency with which the ligament is demonstrated. Anterior to both the inferior pulmonary ligaments and the phrenic

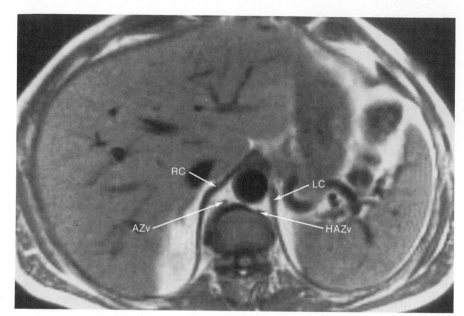

FIGURE 2–17 ■ Normal anatomy of the retrocrural space. MR demonstrates the right and left diaphragmatic crura (LC and RC). The retrocrural space contains high-intensity fat outlining the azygos vein (AZv) and hemiazygos vein (HAZv).

nerves, the medial extent of the lower major fissure may be evident as it contacts the heart and may be low in density or high in MR intensity from contained mediastinal fat.

RETROCRURAL SPACE

The retrocrural space is the inferior extension of the posterior mediastinum.[37, 38] The diaphragmatic crura originate as muscle bundles caudad to the esophageal hiatus and anterior to the aortic hiatus. The bundles join across the midline and then separate into right and left components at the level of the celiac artery. Inferiorly, the two crura become fibrous tendons that blend with the anterior longitudinal ligament of the second and third lumbar vertebrae (Figs. 2–17 and 2–18) (see Chapter 5). The two arching crura form the lateral and anterior boundaries of the aortic hiatus. The right crus is noticeably larger and longer than the left. Each crus passes from one side of the vertebral body to the anterior wall of the aorta. Several structures in addition to the aorta traverse the retrocrural space (or aortic hiatus). The thoracic duct and azygos vein lie to the right of the aorta; the hemiazygos vein is to the left. Intercostal arteries and splanchnic nerves also course through this space. The density of this space is uniform and low, equivalent to that of retroperitoneal fat. Except for the aorta, the normal structures within the retrocrural space do not measure more than 6 mm in transverse diameter when viewed at a window width of 200 H and a level of 10 to 30 H. Some of the structures seen on CT opacify with intravenous contrast material. Normal lymph nodes are either too small to be visible or are less than 6 mm in diameter.

Mediastinal Lines

Mediastinal lines observed on chest radiographs are either interfaces between the lung and mediastinal soft tissues or viscera or sites where the two lungs contact each other.

ANTERIOR JUNCTION LINE

The anterior junction line lies anterior to the aorta and heart, where the anteromedial portion of each lung approaches the midline. It is seen on 20 to 25 per cent of normal anteroposterior chest radiographs, commencing at the manubrium and extending inferiorly and slightly to the left for several centimeters.[39, 40] The line represents the visceral and parietal pleurae of each lung and a small quantity of mediastinal fat between them. In the 20 to 25 per cent of instances when the anterior junction line is visible on chest radiographs, the lungs have approximated anteriorly, producing a thin line in an anteroposterior plane (Fig. 2–19). In the other 75 to 80 per

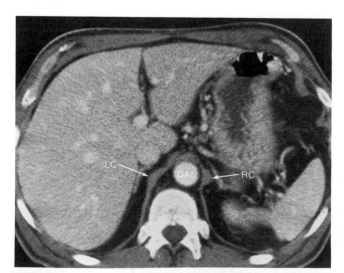

FIGURE 2–18 ■ Normal anatomy of the retrocrural space. The larger right diaphragmatic crus (RC) meets the left crus (LC) anterior to the descending aorta (DAo). The retrocrural space contains several small structures, none larger than 6 mm in diameter.

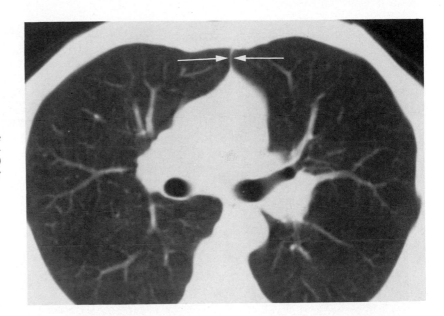

FIGURE 2–19 ■ Normal anterior junction line. The two lungs approach the midline anterior to the ascending aorta. The anterior junction line *(arrows)* consists of four layers of pleura and a varying quantity of mediastinal fat.

cent, the lungs are either separated by mediastinal fat or the line lies in an oblique plane and is not visible on radiographs. CT can demonstrate the causes of obliteration of the anterior junction line, the commonest of which are an ascending aortic aneurysm, lymphadenopathy, or an anterior mediastinal tumor.[41]

POSTERIOR JUNCTION LINE

The two lungs approximate behind the esophagus and in front of the spine above the aortic arch. On chest radiographs of the erect patient, the posterior junction line projects vertically as a stripe of variable thickness, visible through the tracheal air column. It invariably extends above the suprasternal notch, which distinguishes it from the anterior junction line. Variations in the normal thickness of the posterior junction line limit its use in defining mediastinal disease. On CT in the supine patient, mediastinal structures tend to lie against the spine, so it is unusual for the lungs to appose posteriorly (Fig. 2–20). In the prone patient, the posterior junction line is seen more frequently.

When air is present in the esophagus, a soft tissue stripe may appear on frontal radiographs and on CT, separating air in the lungs from air within the esophagus (Fig. 2–20). This is the esophageal-pleural stripe and may be present on either side or both sides of the esophagus.[42, 43] The stripe comprises visceral and parietal pleurae, mediastinal fat, and the esophageal wall. Thickening of the esophageal-pleural stripe can be from disease affecting the pleura, mediastinal contents, or the esophageal wall, and CT will usually demonstrate the precise cause.

RIGHT PARATRACHEAL STRIPE

The right paratracheal stripe is an important and sensitive indicator of disease on chest radiographs. In most adults, this stripe or line is up to 4 mm thick, when measured between air in the right lung and air in the trachea.[44] The stripe comprises pleura, mediastinal fat, connective tissue, and the wall of the trachea. On CT, the right wall of the trachea is demonstrated in all individuals (see Figs. 2–1 to 2–5). The extent of contact of the right lung with the right wall of the trachea varies, but in most instances the posterior one half to two thirds of the trachea contacts the right lung. Absence of the right paratracheal stripe on radiographs is usually from excessive mediastinal fat separating the trachea from the right lung. Abnormal thickening of the stripe can be caused by tracheal, mediastinal, or pleural disease. The most common cause is enlarged pretracheal lymph nodes, extending to the right of the trachea. CT can invariably explain the cause of an abnormally wide right paratracheal stripe.

POSTERIOR TRACHEAL BAND OR STRIPE

On about 80 per cent of well-penetrated lateral chest radiographs, a line up to 5 mm wide can be seen posterior to the tracheal air column.[29, 30, 45] This posterior tracheal stripe consists of tracheal wall, mediastinal tissues, and pleura, between air in the trachea and air in the right lung (see Figs. 2–2 and 2–4). The stripe is the posterior continuation of the right paratracheal stripe. It will not be visible on chest radiographs when the right lung does not enter the retrotracheal mediastinum sufficiently to produce a tangential interface. On CT in the supine patient, the right lung normally contacts less than 50 per cent of the posterior tracheal wall. This stripe is also absent on chest radiographs when there is a small tracheoesophageal recess or a fat-filled retrotracheal space. The width of the posterior tracheal stripe can vary over its length with differing amounts of retrotracheal tissue.

The posterior stripe may appear thickened on chest radiographs when the esophagus contains air and is in midline because the anterior esophageal wall then contributes to the thickness of the stripe. CT can

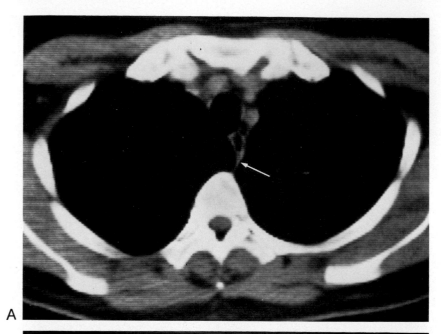

A

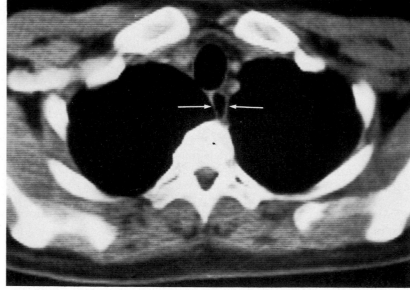

B

FIGURE 2–20 ■ Normal anatomy of the posterior junction line in a 39-year-old man. *A*, The two lungs appose behind the esophagus to produce a single line *(arrow)*. *B*, Two cm cephalad, air in the esophagus produces right and left esophageal-pleural stripes *(arrows)*.

distinguish between thickening of the stripe due to disease and thickening due to variation in the position of the esophagus.

Abnormal thickening of the stripe is most commonly caused by primary or recurrent carcinoma of the esophagus.[45, 46] Thickening may also result from esophageal dilatation, tracheal tumors, and mediastinal lymphadenopathy.

LEFT PARATRACHEAL REFLECTION

On the left side, above the aortic arch, the lung is precluded from contacting the left tracheal wall in all but an occasional individual (see Figs. 2–1 and 2–2).[47] On frontal chest radiographs, an interface between the left lung and left subclavian artery is evident about 75 per cent of the time, and a more medial interface is seen in about 30 per cent of chest

radiographs. CT shows that this medial interface is usually between the left upper lobe and left upper mediastinum, lateral to the trachea and in front of the left subclavian artery. A third interface, which can be confusing, occurs between the left lung and the left upper mediastinum, behind the left subclavian artery. Abnormalities that can cause lateral displacement of the left paratracheal reflection or interface are most commonly vascular variants such as a persistent left SVC, or cardinal vein. Adenopathy can also occur in this region but is difficult to detect on chest radiographs and is usually found with CT or MR.

Mediastinal Lymph Nodes

Since the original report by Schnyder and Gamsu[22] of the number and size of the pretracheal lymph nodes at the level of the azygos vein, several investigators have described the number, frequency, and appearance of normal mediastinal lymph nodes on CT.[48–53] Important for CT and MR are the size and number of normal lymph nodes at different sites within the mediastinum. In general, mediastinal lymph nodes lie with their long axis in a craniocaudal direction,[54] and CT or MR images the nodes in the transverse, or shorter, axis. Most lymph nodes appear round or oval on transverse mediastinal images. They are usually contained within mediastinal fat and are clearly visible as discrete structures. Opacification of mediastinal vessels can, on occasion, assist in differentiating a node from a tortuous or aberrant vessel.[55] Lymph nodes are scattered throughout the mediastinum, and normally there are over 100 nodes within the mediastinum. Under normal circumstances, only a small percentage is visible.

Certain lymph node groups are not routinely imaged on CT or MR. At these sites, any visible lymph node should be viewed with suspicion of being abnormally enlarged. The nodes that are not imaged are the internal mammary nodal chains; the circumcardiac nodes around the base of the heart; the lymph nodes around the lower esophagus and in the inferior pulmonary ligaments; and the posterior pre- and paraspinal nodes.

The sites at which normal lymph nodes are routinely imaged are around the trachea, in the subcarinal space, in the aortic-pulmonic window, and in the prevascular space. Even within these sites, the number and size of visible lymph nodes vary. Table 2–1 summarizes the usual number and size, as well as the approximate maximum number and size of nodes at each site, displayed on CT.[48–52] It should be remembered that in about 1 per cent of individuals, normal nodes greater than 15 mm in transverse diameter will be imaged, and in about 5 per cent, nodes between 10 and 15 mm can be found. The common sites for these large but normal nodes are the lower pretracheal and subcarinal spaces. Mediastinal lymph nodes may also be nonspecifically large owing to distant inactive granulomatous diseases or reactive hyperplasia, especially with centrally obstructing tumors. Unopacified vessels that cross the mediastinum may also be mistaken for enlarged lymph nodes.[55] The CT and MR imaging characteristics of mediastinal nodes do not enable the differentiation between malignant and benign nodes. Occasionally, lymph nodes enhance on CT with intravascular contrast material and show unopacified centers. This finding has been described in tuberculous adenopathy but is unusual. We have seen it in other conditions, including metastases from intrathoracic and extrathoracic sources. At present, the sole criterion for abnormality of mediastinal nodes is nodal size. The routine clinical use of a diameter of 10 mm as the upper limit for normal nodes is convenient but must be recognized as a simplification.

Quint and colleagues[50] have described the sites at which CT has difficulty in showing normal lymph nodes. The left paratracheal and left tracheobronchial nodes may be difficult to demonstrate because of overlapping pulsatile vessels at these sites. The relative effectiveness of CT and MR in detecting abnormal lymph nodes has been studied in patients with bronchogenic carcinoma. CT has better spatial resolution, whereas MR has better contrast resolution, especially with cardiac-gated images. The results are that CT and MR show comparable detection rates. However, some studies indicate that both may not detect nodes even up to 40 mm in diameter.[56]

Techniques of Examination

The techniques for performing CT or MR of the mediastinum differ among institutions.[57, 58] A routine format can be established that will be suitable for most clinical circumstances. Occasionally, the examination must be modified to obtain the images most appropriate to the problem being investigated. The dose of contrast material and timing of contrast infusion for CT have been investigated,[59–61] and the results of these studies can be exploited to obtain optimum intravascular opacification.

Respiration

Most patients are able to suspend respiration long enough to complete at least one scan if not multiple scans. If possible, CT scans should always be obtained with the patient breath holding. If breath holding is not possible, the patient should mouth-breathe quietly to minimize motion artifacts.

The optimum lung volume is deep inspiration (near total lung capacity), which is reproducible and provides the best demonstration of the lungs and mediastinum. Most patients achieve full inspiration more comfortably and are able to sustain this lung volume after taking a few deep breaths. This may be a useful routine to adopt, especially for older patients.

For MR of the mediastinum, T1- and T2-weighted spin-echo imaging is generally favored.[58] Although rapid scanning techniques are being developed, routine spin-echo imaging precludes breath holding. Patients are instructed to breathe quietly without stopping.

TABLE 2–1 ■ Normal Lymph Node Number and Size at Various Sites

SITE	NUMBER Usual	NUMBER Maximum	SIZE (mm) Usual	SIZE (mm) Maximum	SIZE (mm) Unusual
Upper trachea (L or R)	0-3	5-8	3-5	7	—
Lower trachea (L or R)	2-4	3-6	5-10	10	15
Aortic-pulmonic window	0-3	3-6	5-7	9	12
Subcarinal space	0-3	2-3	6-10	11	16
Prevascular space	0-2	5-10	3-6	8	—

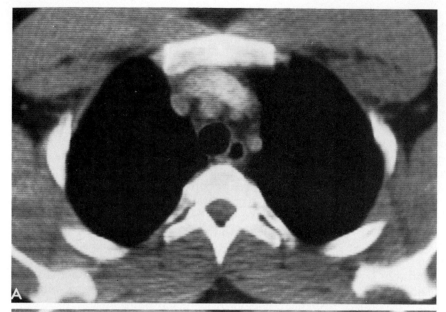

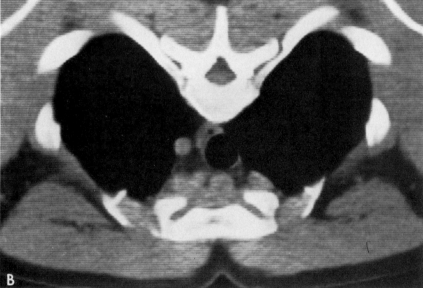

FIGURE 2–21 ■ Normal upper mediastinal anatomy, demonstrating differences between supine (A) and prone (B) scans. On the prone scan, the arch vessels are displaced forward against the sternum. The left brachiocephalic vein is compressed and is no longer seen. The esophagus assumes a near-midline position.

Position

Most CT imaging of the thorax is performed with the patient supine. In adults, the patient's arms are placed above the head to reduce scan artifacts. On scans obtained with the patient prone, the heart and mediastinum tend to fall forward toward the sternum (Fig. 2–21).[62] For the evaluation of posterior mediastinal masses or structures such as the esophagus, prone scans may be more appropriate, although this has not become standard practice. For patients unable to lie supine or prone, scans can also be obtained in the decubitus position, although this position does not have any specific advantage in the mediastinum. Scanners with a wide aperture allow the examination to be performed with the patient seated; direct coronal scans are then possible.[63] This orientation has not demonstrated advantages over the routine supine position.

Most MR scans are now obtained with the patient supine, but with their arms by their sides. Streak artifacts from the shoulder girdle are not a consideration with MR imaging. For patients who experience claustrophobia in the magnet, the prone position may be more comfortable, even though this position makes cardiac-gating more difficult.

Contrast Material

Intravenous infusion of contrast material greatly facilitates the interpretation of CT scans of the mediastinum but is not necessary in all instances. Intravascular contrast material outlines normal vascular landmarks, facilitates the detection of vessel enlargement and abnormal vessels, and by enhancement can show highly vascular masses. The accepted precautions with intravenous iodinated contrast agents must be observed. In many institutions, non-ionic contrast agents are routinely used. The usual adult dose is 150 to 200 mL of contrast (300 to 350 mg of iodine/mL) administered with a power injector.

The protocol that we use in adults for a GE 9800 scanner consists of three bolus injections of 60 mL each, administered at a rate of 2 mL/sec. Scanning commences 35 to 45 sec after initiation of the injection. The first bolus is for a series of contiguous 10-mm collimated scans from above the lung apices to a level through the aortic arch. Scans are in pairs, with a 12- to 15-sec delay between each pair to allow the patient to take a single breath. The second bolus is for about 16 scans, using 5-mm collimation through the pulmonary hila. The scan sequences are similar to the first series. The third bolus is for a series of 10-mm collimated scans through the lower thorax and upper abdomen to include the liver and adrenal glands.

Precise timing and contrast volumes must be modified for different scanners, patients of different weight, and for specialized studies such as investigations of suspected aortic dissection or arteriovenous anomalies. For these situations, a bolus of contrast should be injected at predetermined levels, usually at a rate of 2 mL/sec, followed by rapid sequential scanning without movement of the CT table.

Intravascular contrast material for MR of the thorax has received limited investigation.[64] At present, only gadolinium-DTPA (Gd-DTPA) is available for commercial use. In general, Gd-DTPA is an extracellular marker that shortens relaxation times by its paramagnetic effect. Preliminary investigations have shown that Gd-DTPA causes enhancement of many masses.[65] It has not been demonstrated that paramagnetic contrast agents assist in separating malignant from benign masses or sufficiently increase the intensity of small mediastinal masses so as to make them more conspicuous. For the present, Gd-DTPA is still experimental for mediastinal imaging.

Technical Considerations

The major cause of degradation of CT images of the mediastinum is the presence of streak artifacts from the edges of contrast-enhanced, pulsatile vascular structures and from the shoulder girdle. These artifacts can be diminished by using the shortest possible scan times. Attention also should be given to patient positioning, and use of the appropriate scan-file for the size of the patient. In general, for thoracic imaging a high-resolution reconstruction algorithm is used.[66] This is mainly for the smaller structures in the lungs but does not detract from images of the mediastinum.

A projection radiograph (e.g., scout view) is routine in planning mediastinal CT. For focal lesions, the projection radiograph can be correlated with the conventional chest radiographs to determine the number of CT scans needed to demonstrate the area of interest. A projection radiograph is especially useful in planning CT of vascular lesions such as aortic dissections, for which specific levels are to be studied with rapid sequential scans.

The most appropriate window levels and window widths for viewing the mediastinum are determined by the equipment and the eye of the beholder. Generally, for the mediastinum, a window width between 300 and 500 H and a window level between 0 and 60 H are used.

The technical factors for MR of the mediastinum can be varied widely, depending on the information required. For most applications, spin-echo imaging with the occasional addition of limited flip-angle imaging for vascular anatomy is used.[67] The precise details of sequences vary with the scanner and its field strength. The technique that we use for a high field strength magnet consists of T1- and T2-weighted transaxial sequences through the thorax and upper abdomen. T1 weighting is achieved by cardiac-gating to every heart beat for 1024 beats. For the T1 sequence, a 256 × 256 matrix is used with 2 averages and an echo time (TE) of 20 ms. For T2 weighting, cardiac-gating is to every other beat, with a 128 × 256 matrix and a TE of 20/80. Coronal or orthogonal images are optional.

For an intermediate field strength magnet (0.35 T), T1 and T2 weighting are again achieved by cardiac-gating to every heart beat and every other heart beat, respectively. Usually, four averages are used instead of two. Coronal imaging is again optional. With new equipment, different forms of respiratory and flow compensation are available and should be used.[68] For a suspected lesion of the brachial plexus or chest wall, surface coils can be used for transaxial, coronal, or sagittal imaging. More detailed anatomy of a smaller field-of-view can be obtained.

Pathology

Vascular Anomalies

ARTERIAL ANOMALIES

The paired aortic arches found in the embryo may develop anomalously and may result in malformations of the thoracic aorta and great vessels (Fig. 2–22 and Table 2–2). The majority of patients with aortic arch anomalies are asymptomatic. When a complete vascular ring is present, symptoms can result from airway or esophageal compression. Most patients with arch malformations have a mediastinal abnormality on a chest radiograph that can be mistaken for a mass or can be suggestive of the anomaly. In patients with aortic arch anomalies, CT or MR is often obtained to investigate the mediastinal mass or mediastinal widening. Baron and co-workers[69] found 5 of 71 mediastinal masses evaluated with CT to be arch anomalies. Arch anomalies can also be incidental and can present potentially confusing findings in a patient undergoing CT or MR for other reasons.

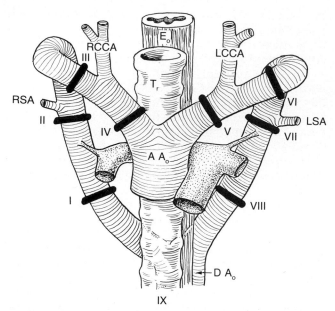

FIGURE 2–22 ■ Schematic representation of the embryonic development of the paired aortic arches with sites of potential interruption. The ascending aorta (AAo) divides into a right and left arch. The right arch gives rise to the common carotid artery (RCCA) and right subclavian artery (RSA), whereas the left arch branches off the left common carotid artery (LCCA) and left subclavian artery (LSA). The aortic arches unite behind the trachea (Tr) and esophagus (Eo) to form the descending aorta (DAo). I = normal; II = left aortic arch with aortic diverticulum; III = left aortic arch with an aberrant right subclavian artery; IV = left aortic arch with an aberrant right innominate artery; V = right aortic arch with an aberrant left innominate artery; VI = right aortic arch with an aberrant left subclavian artery; VII = right aortic arch with mirror-image branching (rare); VIII = right aortic arch with mirror-image branching (common); IX = double aortic arch (no interruption).

Webb[70] and McLoughlin[71] and their colleagues showed that if an aortic anomaly is suspected, computed tomography is a simple, noninvasive method for accurately determining the abnormality. Only the more common arterial anomalies are discussed.

Coarctation of the Aorta ■ This localized deformity of the media of the artery, resulting in an infolding of the aortic wall, accounts for about 7 per cent of congenital heart diseases.[72] An eccentric narrowing of the aortic lumen results. Coarctation most often occurs distal to the left subclavian artery. Usually the segment of aorta between the left subclavian artery

TABLE 2–2 ■ Aortic Arch Anomalies

Left aortic arch with aberrant right subclavian artery
Left aortic arch with aberrant right innominate artery
Left aortic arch with right descending aorta
Right aortic arch with mirror-image branching
Right aortic arch with aberrant left subclavian artery
Right aortic arch with aberrant left innominate artery
Right aortic arch with isolation of the left subclavian artery
Double aortic arch with both arches patent
Double aortic arch with partial atresia of one
Cervical aortic arch
Atresia of the aortic arch
Coarctation of the aorta
Aortic valve atresia
Supravalvular aortic stenosis

and the coarctation is also hypoplastic and slightly narrowed.

CT in patients with coarctation of the aorta can demonstrate a narrow, deformed aortic isthumus—the segment of aorta between the left subclavian artery and the ligamentum arteriosum.[5, 73–75] The coarctation itself is probably not seen, and CT cannot image webs or short strictures in such vessels as the aorta. CT in two cases of pseudocoarctation of the aorta showed the high, anteriorly situated distal arch and the buckled proximal descending aorta.[76] A portion of the left lung was seen indenting the mediastinum between the redundant aortic arch and the spine. The latter finding is occasionally seen in normal individuals and may not be specific for pseudocoarctation. It is unlikely that these CT features can allow the diagnosis of pseudocoarctation of the aorta to be made with accuracy.

MR imaging is particularly well suited to imaging the aorta and its developmental anomalies.[77–80] If the patient (or the magnetic gradient angle) is rotated about 30° into the left antero-oblique position, sagittal MR images will generally pass through both the ascending and descending aortas (Fig. 2–23).[81] MR also can be obtained in children as young as newborns, with high accuracy for aortic lesions.

In coarctation of the aorta, the site, severity, and length of the stenotic segment can be defined. Additional important information that can be obtained from MR images includes the relationship of the coarctation to the great vessels, and the size of ascending and descending aortas. Von Schulthess and colleagues[78] studied 13 patients with coarctation of the thoracic aorta, demonstrating a discrete or diffuse stenotic segment in 12 of them. The cardiac-gated, spin-echo MR images also showed postste-

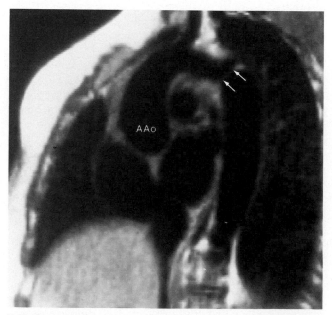

FIGURE 2–23 ■ Aortic coarctation. Left anterior oblique cardiac-gated MR image demonstrates a moderately dilated ascending aorta (AAo) with an aortic coarctation (*arrows*) in the typical location.

notic dilatation and sites of dilated collateral vessels. Following surgical repair of the stenosis, complications such as restenosis, aneurysms, and hematoma were well displayed with MR. At present, MR is the favored technique for confirming the suspected diagnosis of aortic coarctation and may obviate the need for angiograms in some cases.

Aberrant Subclavian Artery ■ An aberrant right subclavian artery in the presence of an otherwise normal aorta is the most common anomaly of aortic arch development, occurring in approximately 1 in 200 people.[82] The anomalous subclavian artery arises from the distal aortic arch as its last major vessel. The aberrant artery crosses the posterior mediastinum obliquely upward from left to right. Symptoms are uncommon, but widening of the superior mediastinum and bowing of the trachea anteriorly are not infrequently seen on chest radiographs. Several

CT findings reflect the aortic maldevelopment. The aortic arch, higher than normal with a more directly anteroposterior orientation, is visible, as is the aberrant right subclavian artery arising from the medial wall of the posterior portion of the arch or from the beginning of the descending aorta (Fig. 2–24). Dilatation of the origin of the aberrant right subclavian artery is common and if excessive is called a diverticulum of the aorta. Unless it is recognized as the dilated segment of an anomalous artery, it can be misdiagnosed as an aortic aneurysm.[82] An actual aneurysm of an aberrant subclavian artery is rare but does occur.

An aberrant left subclavian artery arises from a right aortic arch and is less common than an aberrant right subclavian artery, occurring in approximately 1 in 1000 people.[83] About 10 per cent of patients with this anomaly also have congenital heart disease. The

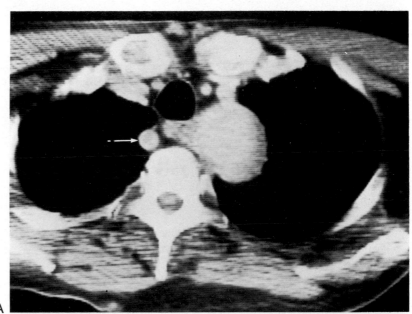

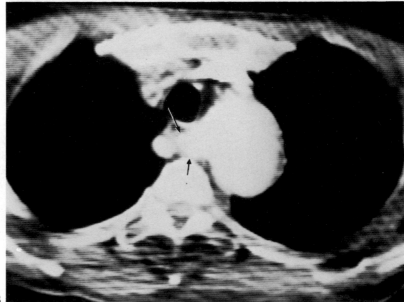

FIGURE 2–24 ■ Aberrant right subclavian artery in an asymptomatic older male. *A,* CT scan shows an abnormally situated right subclavian artery *(arrow).* *B,* Ten mm caudad, the dilated proximal segment of the anomalous right subclavian artery *(arrows)* is seen.

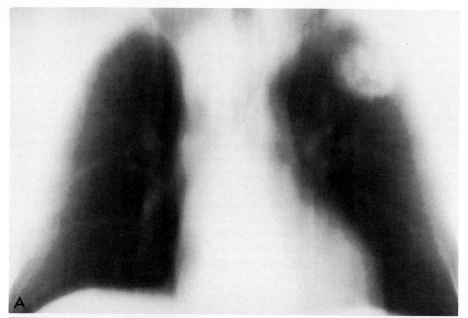

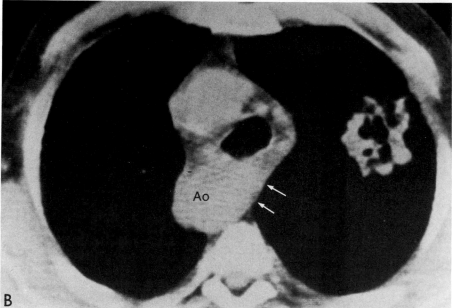

FIGURE 2–25 ■ Right aortic arch with aberrant left subclavian artery in a 68-year-old man. *A*, A conventional tomogram shows a left upper lobe bronchogenic carcinoma and a right mediastinal mass. *B*, CT scan shows that the right mediastinal mass is a right aortic arch (Ao). The dilated proximal segment of an anomalous left subclavian artery *(arrows)* is also demonstrated.

FIGURE 2–26 ■ Azygos lobe. The right lung within the azygos lobe protrudes into the mediastinum behind the superior vena cava *(upper arrow)* and the trachea *(lower arrow).*

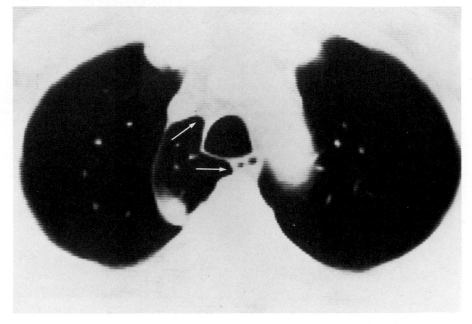

CT appearances of the malformed aorta and aberrant left subclavian artery are similar to those seen with an aberrant right subclavian artery, although the posterior portion of the aortic arch is often more midline than normal, assuming a position behind the trachea and displacing the esophagus to the left.

MR is equal to CT for displaying aberrant subclavian vessels.[79, 84] MR can demonstrate the relationship of these vessels to the trachea and esophagus and can show compression caused by vascular rings.

Right Aortic Arch Malformation ■ By definition, a right aortic arch is to the right of the trachea and esophagus. The normal arrangement of the arch vessels is determined by the site at which the left aortic arch is embryonically interrupted.

With a right aortic arch and aberrant left subclavian artery, embryonic interruption is between the left common carotid artery and the left subclavian artery (Fig. 2–25). This form of arch malformation has been detailed earlier in the chapter.

Two kinds of aberrant left subclavian artery with a right aortic arch can occur. In one, the descending aorta descends on the left of the spine. In the other, it descends on the right. With both variations, a vascular ring is present, although tracheoesophageal compression is rare.

An additional very rare anomaly of the right aortic arch, which can be diagnosed from CT or MR, is the aberrant left innominate artery. The branching order of the arch vessels can usually be ascertained, and in the case of an aberrant left innominate artery, the origin of the right common carotid artery is before the right subclavian artery. The anomalous aberrant left innominate artery arises from the medial aspect of the distal right arch and produces a symptomatic vascular ring.

When embryonic aortic interruption is distal to the left subclavian artery, mirror-image branching is produced.[85] Two types are found; the commoner occurs when interruption is distal to the left ductus arteriosus and a vascular ring is not produced. Virtually all patients with this type of branching have congenital heart disease, usually tetralogy of Fallot or truncus arteriosus. A rare form of mirror-image right aortic arch occurs when the left arch is interrupted proximal to the left ductus arteriosus.[86]

The CT or MR findings in some of these rare forms of right aortic arch malformations have been described, and the diagnoses can readily be made.[79] For example, if a right aortic arch with mirror-image branching of the arch vessels is shown and if a dilated retrotracheal aorta is seen, the rarer form of mirror-image branching should be suggested.

Double Aortic Arch ■ Double aortic arch is the most important of the arch anomalies producing a vascular ring.[87] It is rarely associated with congenital heart disease, but symptoms of tracheoesophageal compression are common. Two broad groups of double aortic arch are found. In the first, both arches are patent and functional; in the second group, a portion of the left arch is atretic.

The CT and MR findings in double aortic arch have been described in several reports.[70, 71, 79] They accurately reflect the anatomic position of the aortic arches and arch vessels. The right arch is usually the larger and higher, and it courses behind the esophagus to join the left arch. The aorta usually descends on the left. Images near the thoracic inlet demonstrate the four arch vessels, situated symmetrically around the trachea and each arising independently from the two aortic arches.

VENOUS ANOMALIES

Anomalies of the great thoracic veins rarely result in symptoms but can cause confusing mediastinal contours on chest radiographs that call for further evaluation using CT or MR. They may also produce unusual vascular structures that can be seen incidentally on CT or MR obtained for other reasons. It is important, therefore, to recognize them and to know their appearances.

Anomalous development may involve the vena caval systems or the azygos systems. Only the more common anomalies, for which the findings have been reported, are discussed. The principles apply to other venous anomalies, and they all can be defined accurately.

Azygos Lobe ■ The most common maldevelopment of the thoracic veins is lateral displacement of the arch of the azygos vein. This anomaly occurs in 0.4 to 1.0 per cent of the population and is referred to as an "azygos lobe," because the medial portion of the right upper lobe is trapped by the abnormally positioned azygos fissure and vein. The abnormal position of the azygos veins derives from the premature descent of the right posterior cardinal vein. A portion of the right upper lobe lung bud becomes trapped between the azygos fissure and the mediastinum.

CT has been instrumental in defining the spectrum of alterations in mediastinal anatomy found with an azygos lobe.[5, 88] The azygos vein is displaced cephalad and joins either the SVC, in an abnormal position near the junction of the left and right brachiocephalic veins, or the right brachiocephalic vein. The superior 2 to 3 cm of the ascending azygos vein is displaced to the right of the spine and, as it leaves the spine, may resemble a lung nodule when viewed on a single CT scan. Frequently, the axis of the SVC is abnormally oriented toward the left. The contact between the right upper lobe and the mediastinum also differs from normal when an azygos lobe is present. The lung often excessively intrudes between the SVC and the trachea and contacts their medioposterior and anterior walls, respectively (Fig. 2–26). This intrusion can often be seen on lateral chest radiographs as a lucency behind the SVC. Also, the lung within the azygos lobe often intrudes into the retrotracheal space, displacing the esophagus to the left and outlining the posterior wall of the trachea.

Left Superior Vena Cava ■ Persistence of the embryonic left anterior cardinal vein results in a left SVC.

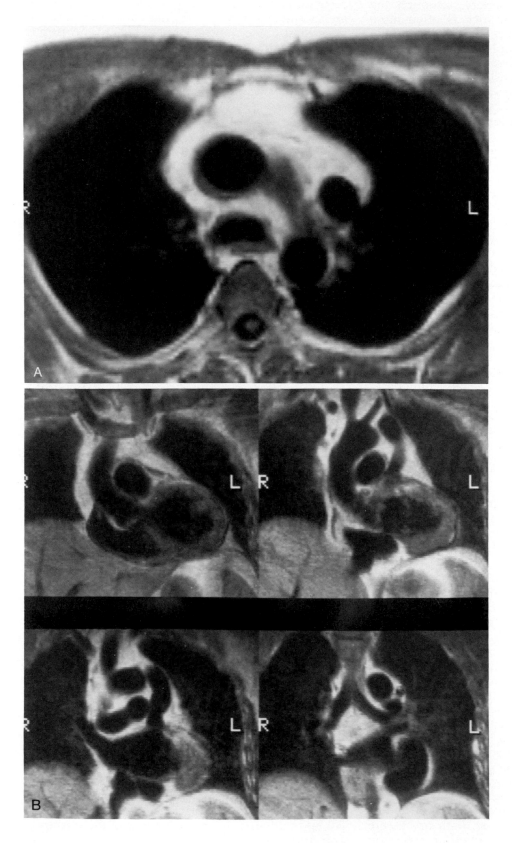

FIGURE 2–27 ■ Persistent left superior vena cava. *A,* Cardiac-gated MR image demonstrates a large anomalous vessel to the left of the aortic-pulmonic window. The right superior vena cava is absent. *B,* Cardiac-gated coronal MR image confirms the persistent left superior vena cava coursing lateral to the main pulmonary artery and posterior to the left atrium to join the coronary venous system.

This relatively common anomaly is present in 0.3 per cent of normal individuals and about 5 per cent of patients with congenital heart disease.[89] Eighty to ninety per cent of people with a left SVC also have a right SVC.[90] In two thirds of these, the left brachiocephalic vein is small or absent. The left SVC may be smaller than its counterpart on the right, or the two may be equal in size. Communication of the left SVC with the hemiazygos system may be present. In patients with a left SVC, an additional contour to the left superior mediastinum is frequently visible on frontal radiographs. CT or MR may be obtained to investigate this abnormal contour, or, alternatively, a left SVC may be an incidental finding on scans obtained for other reasons.

The CT or MR findings of a left SVC are readily apparent.[90–93] Within the upper mediastinum, the left SVC is positioned lateral to the left common carotid artery and anterior to the left subclavian artery. (Fig. 2–27). As it descends, the vein is visible to the left of the aortic arch and main pulmonary artery (Fig. 2–27). It then passes in front of the left hilum and enters the oblique coronary veins and coronary sinus, posterior to the left atrium and ventricle. In the upper mediastinum, the position of the left SVC resembles that of its counterpart on the right, whereas at lower levels, it is more posterior.

A rare similar anomaly is a left brachiocephalic vein that descends along the left upper mediastinum, in a position similar to a persistent left SVC.[90] The anomalous vein then crosses the mediastinum through the aortic-pulmonic window, posterior to the ascending aorta and anterior to the lower trachea. It joins the right brachiocephalic vein to form a shortened right superior vena cava.

Azygos and Hemiazygos Continuation of the Inferior Vena Cava (IVC) ■ The IVC is derived from three sets of paired veins: supracardinal, subcardinal, and postcardinal.[92, 94] If the infrahepatic segment of the IVC, derived from subcardinal veins, fails to achieve patency, the intermediate segments of the supracardinal veins join the IVC to the azygos or hemiazygos system. This anomaly can be associated with congenital heart disease and polysplenia or, less commonly, asplenia.[95, 96]

Berdon and Baker[97] have shown that azygos continuation of the IVC can be suspected from the radiographic appearances of an enlarged azygos system. However, an enlarged azygos system has frequently been mistaken for a mediastinal mass or posterior mediastinal lymphadenopathy. With hemiazygos continuation of the IVC, the dilated hemiazygos vein may not communicate with the azygos system and courses up the left side of the mediastinum to produce a retroaortic mass and sometimes a mass around the aortic arch. The suprahepatic portion of the IVC is derived from hepatic sinusoids, and the intrathoracic IVC is usually present with azygos continuation. Therefore, the finding of an IVC on chest radiographs does not exclude the diagnosis of azygos or hemiazygos continuation.

The CT or MR findings of azygos continuation of the IVC, or of hemiazygos continuation of the IVC with connection to the azygos system, are definitive enough to preclude a venogram for diagnosis.[96, 98, 99] In patients with azygos continuation of the IVC or with hemiazygos continuation of the IVC with connection to the azygos vein, findings in the upper thorax are the same. The ascending azygos vein, the azygos arch, and the distal SVC are dilated from increased blood flow. In azygos continuation, the dilated azygos vein exits the abdomen through the retrocrural space (Fig. 2–28 A to D). Without infusion of contrast medium, the dilated azygos vein can be mistaken for a retrocrural mass. The vein ascends in a normal position in front of the spine, along or slightly right of the midline. The dilated azygos is often equal to the aorta in diameter (Fig. 2–29 A and B). With hemiazygos continuation of the IVC having an azygos connection, the dilated hemiazygos vein lies posterior to the aorta and to the left of the spine.[100] It then crosses the posterior mediastinum to join the azygos system. In hemiazygos continuation of the IVC without azygos connection, the dilated hemiazygos vein stays on the left and drains into a dilated left superior intercostal vein or persistent left SVC.[101]

Several anomalies associated with azygos and hemiazygos continuation of the IVC can occur and should be sought on CT or MR scans. Among these are a left IVC, duplication of the IVC, polysplenia, and congenital heart disease.

Disease of the Thoracic Aorta

AORTIC ANEURYSMS

By definition, an aneurysm of the thoracic aorta is a dilatation of all the components of the vessel wall. The morphologic types of aortic aneurysms are saccular, fusiform, dissecting, false, and sinus of Valsalva. This section deals only with saccular and fusiform aneurysms. Acquired aortic aneurysms are arteriosclerotic, luetic, mycotic, traumatic, or from medial necrosis; both saccular and fusiform aneurysms are most commonly arteriosclerotic. The diameter of a fusiform aortic aneurysm is by definition greater than 4 cm.[102] A saccular aneurysm can be smaller than 4 cm and still be considered an aneurysm. Fomon and colleagues[103] have shown that the potential for rupture of an aortic aneurysm is directly related to its wall tension and thus to the size of the aneurysm. Aneurysms less than 5 cm in diameter have a negligible incidence of rupture; those that are 5 to 10 cm in diameter, if untreated, have approximately a 10 per cent chance of rupturing; and those more than 10 cm have a 50 per cent chance of rupturing.

The majority of thoracic aortic aneurysms can be suspected from chest radiographs.[104, 105] The most common radiographic findings are a mediastinal mass or an enlarged segment of the aorta that often contains wall calcification. Displacement and, less frequently, compression of the esophagus or of the trachea and bronchi may be visible on radiographs.

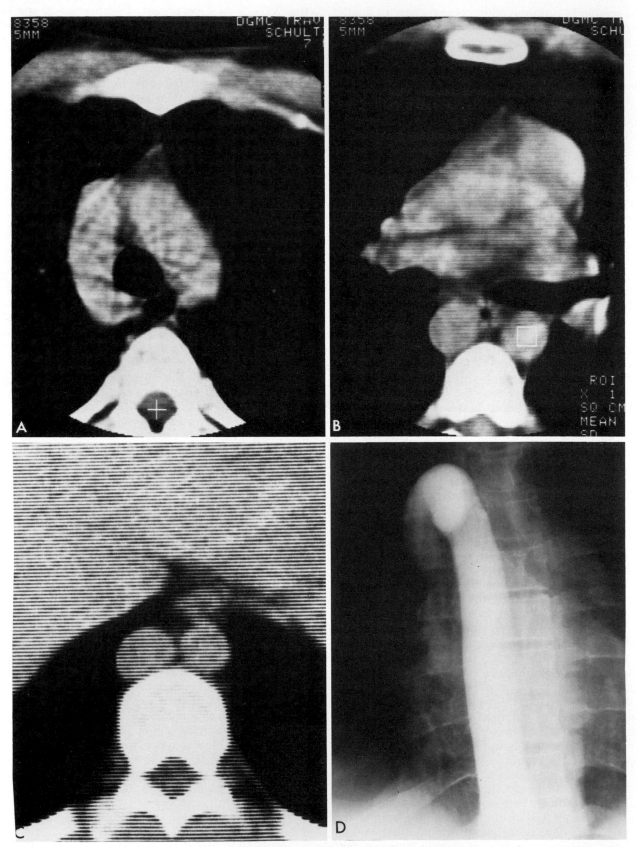

FIGURE 2–28 ■ Azygos continuation of the inferior vena cava in a 29-year-old woman with a right upper mediastinal mass. *A*, CT scan at the level of the aortic arch demonstrates an enlarged azygos arch to the right of the trachea. *B* and *C*, At the level of the tracheal carina and diaphragm, the ascending azygos vein is equal in size to the descending aorta. *D*, The thoracic portion of an inferior venacavogram shows the dilated azygos vein. The inferior vena cava did not communicate with the right atrium.

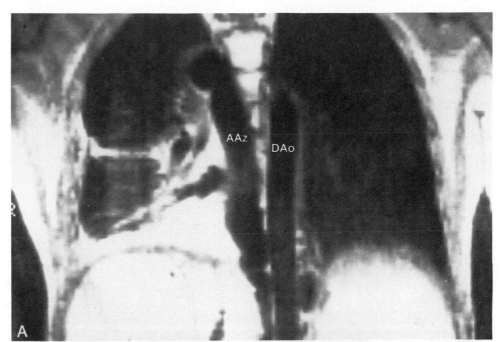

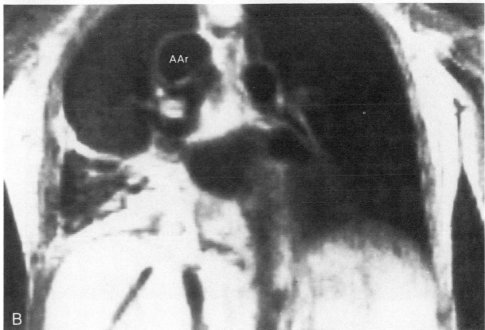

FIGURE 2–29 ■ Azygos continuation due to an inferior vena caval stricture in a young female with right lower lobe pneumonia and a right mediastinal mass. *A,* Coronal MR image demonstrates a massive dilated ascending azygos vein (AAz) equal in size to the descending aorta (DAo). *B,* Two cm anteriorly, the massive dilated azygos arch (AAr) is demonstrated. The infrahepatic portion of the inferior vena cava is also seen.

Erosion of thoracic vertebrae and posterior ribs can also occur but is uncommon.

CT can delineate a mediastinal mass as an aneurysm, characterize it, and show its exact location. Fusiform thoracic aortic aneurysms have characteristic appearances, and in most patients, the diagnosis is readily apparent (Fig. 2–30).[74, 106, 107] They can show the following CT characteristics: dilatation of the aorta, usually greater than 4 cm in diameter; curvilinear or plaquelike calcification; intraluminal thrombus; contrast enhancement of the patent portion of the lumen; displacement of mediastinal structures; and bone erosion of vertebral bodies.

Thrombus within thoracic aortic aneurysms is seen on CT in 86 to 100 per cent of patients (Fig. 2–31).[106, 107] These figures apply to arteriosclerotic aneurysms but are probably similar for those aneurysms from other causes. Machida and Tasaka[107] have shown that the most common configuration is a complete ring of thrombus surrounding the aortic lumen. In our experience, rings of thrombi occur mainly in large fusiform aneurysms. Smaller thrombi tend to form crescents, involving from one quarter to more than two thirds the circumference of the aneurysm.[106]

Calcification in the wall of aortic aneurysms is visible on CT scans in 83 to 100 per cent of patients (Fig. 2–31).[106, 107] It tends to appear as discontinuous

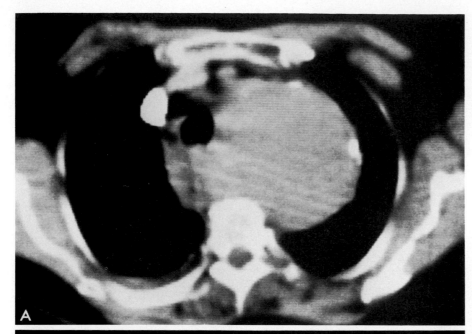

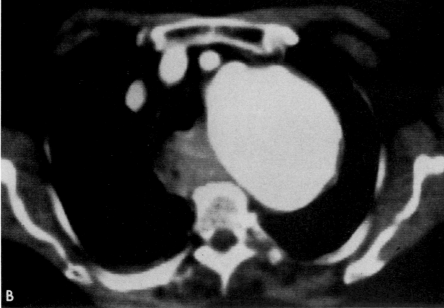

FIGURE 2–30 ■ Ruptured aortic aneurysm in a 68-year-old woman with a clinical finding of aortic dissection. *A*, Dynamic CT scan during contrast material injection demonstrates a large aneurysm of the aortic arch with rim calcification. *B*, Later in the same sequence, the aortic aneurysm has opacified with contrast material. The retrotracheal mass is from mediastinal hematoma.

plaques and curvilinear segments. Machida and Tasaka[107] reported calcification within the mural thrombus of aortic aneurysms in 17 per cent of patients.

The most common site of thoracic aneurysms is the descending aorta.[105] The esophagus is displaced to the right, whereas the trachea and bronchi are displaced anteriorly. The arch of the aorta is the next most common site, and the ascending aorta is the least common. Aneurysms of the arch and ascending aorta produce displacement and compression of mediastinal structures. Fusiform aneurysms rarely involve the entire aorta.

A leaking or ruptured thoracic aortic aneurysm shows extensive tissue density from mediastinal hematoma. A left pleural effusion may be evident. With a bolus injection of contrast medium, rarely the material can be seen escaping beyond the confines of the aorta (see Fig. 2–30). Following blunt thoracic trauma, CT may help in determining a need for arteriography when the chest radiograph is normal.[107a] A mediastinal hematoma or contour abnormality of a great vessel probably indicates a need for an arteriogram.

Thoracic aortic aneurysms can undoubtedly be diagnosed with a high degree of accuracy using CT and injected contrast material. Bolus injections of contrast medium with rapid sequential scans can assist in detailing the aneurysm. However, for CT to replace aortography in the preoperative assessment of patients with intrathoracic aneurysms, it must procure all the information required to determine the appropriate surgical approach to the lesion.[108] The size of the aneurysm and whether the arch vessels

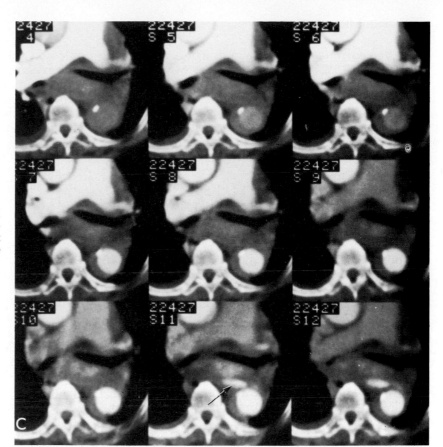

FIGURE 2–30 *Continued* ■ *C,* Sequential scans at a lower level demonstrate opacification of a descending aorta of normal caliber and escape of contrast material *(arrow)* into the mediastinum. Extensive mediastinal hematoma is present.

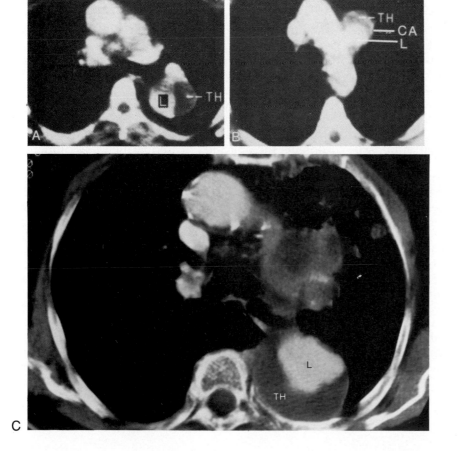

FIGURE 2–31 ■ Aortic aneurysm in three patients. The differing configuration of the lumen and mural thrombus is typical. The left hilar mass in C is a bronchogenic carcinoma. CA = calcium, L = lumen, TH = thrombus.

are affected must be ascertained. The status of the remainder of the aorta also must be evaluated and thus the CT examination must image the entire aorta.

MR can demonstrate fusiform and saccular aneurysms of the ascending aorta, aortic arch, and descending aorta.[77, 109] The relationship of the aneurysm to the arch vessels can be defined on sagittal images or images obtained in the oblique sagittal plane. This oblique image can be obtained by elevating the patient's right shoulder about 30° and imaging in the sagittal plane, or by using electronic angulation of the slice-selective gradient along a line parallel to the aortic arch.

The precise diameter of thoracic aortic aneurysms can be measured from MR images, and the maximum diameter can be monitored over time. In the patient with a thoracic aortic aneurysm and chest pain, MR is ideal for detecting mediastinal hematoma, which suggests rupture of the aneurysm. MR is also effective in demonstrating the presence of a thrombus within a thoracic aortic aneurysm. On gated spin-echo images, the lumen of the aneurysm shows a signal void, whereas the thrombus demonstrates variable signal intensity, depending on the age and composition of the thrombus. The distinction between increased signal due to thrombus and slow signal in an aneurysm can be achieved by using phase-shift technique or gradient-echo images.[110, 111]

AORTIC DISSECTIONS

Aortic dissection is the most common acute emergency involving the aorta.[112] Dissection results from a tear in the vessel wall with penetration of blood into the media to create a false channel, or false lumen. The false channel is usually between the inner one third and outer two thirds of the media. In most instances, a predisposing weakness of the media is present in the form of Erdheim's cystic medial necrosis, Marfan's syndrome, Ehler-Danlos syndrome, or arteritis.[112, 113] Arteriosclerosis and syphilis account for less than 5 per cent of the cases.

The classification of aortic dissection into two types[113] has become generally accepted, and the type is directly related to prognosis and therapy. Type A dissection, affecting the ascending aorta or the ascending and descending aorta, accounts for 60 to 70 per cent of dissections. Involvement of the aortic valve ring and ostia of the coronary arteries can produce aortic incompetence and left heart failure. Type B dissection extends distally from the aortic isthmus, near the aortic insertion of the ligamentum arteriosum. The chest radiograph in aortic dissection is frequently abnormal, but the findings are not specific.[114] Widening of the aorta or a progressive change in its configuration on sequential radiographs is highly suspicious, and the site of mediastinal widening may suggest the type of dissection. An unexplained discrepancy between the sizes of the ascending and descending aorta can also suggest dissection. The esophagus and trachea may be displaced, although this can also be seen with aortic aneurysms. A left pleural effusion, an apical pleural cap, or paraspinous widening may each indicate leakage from an aortic dissection. Enlargement of the cardiac silhouette or evidence of acute left heart failure may be due to an aortic insufficiency or hemopericardium. The most specific radiographic sign of aortic dissection is the displacement of intimal calcification away from the outer margin of the aorta by at least 4 to 5 mm, even though this sign is found only in a small minority of patients. CT scans obtained without intravascular contrast material can show, in half of the patients, a difference in CT density between the true and false lumens of the dissection. Displacement of intimal calcification away from the apparent wall of the aorta is also more apparent before than after contrast material infusion. Nevertheless, CT studies before contrast infusion are not advocated (Fig. 2–32).

CT scans are generally more revealing after infusion of contrast material. High concentrations of intravascular contrast material are desirable. Rapid sequential scanning after injection of 100 mL of contrast material at 2 mL/sec is most helpful. A series of seven to nine rapid sequential scans is obtained initially at each of three levels: through the aortic arch, at the tracheal bifurcation, and above the diaphragm.[106, 115] A frontal CT projection radiograph is used to determine the correct levels for the sequential scans. If a dissection involving the descending aorta (type A or type B) is shown, scanning should be continued to determine the inferior extent of the dissection and the status of the aorta's abdominal branches. The entire thoracic aorta and arch vessels should then be scanned, with an additional infusion of contrast material if necessary.

When a dissection is present, the outer diameter of the aorta is invariably larger than 5 cm but usually less than 10 cm.[116] The diameter of the opacified true lumen is usually smaller than normal and often appears flattened or distorted. The space between the opacified true lumen and the outer aortic margin contains the opacified or unopacified false lumen. A discrepancy in the size of the ascending and descending aorta is only a confirmatory sign of aortic dissection.

The definitive CT finding for acute aortic dissection is the presence of two opacified channels with an intimal flap between them (Fig. 2–33).[106, 116–118] The two channels are visible in at least 75 per cent of symptomatic patients with acute aortic dissection. In the ascending aorta, the false lumen is usually anterior, whereas in the descending aorta, it is usually posterolateral. The CT density of contrast within the true lumen is often different from that of the false lumen, reflecting a difference in the flow rate of contrast material in each channel. The slower flow is usually in the false lumen, and this can be demonstrated with rapid sequential scanning. CT is more sensitive than angiography in demonstrating any difference in opacification between the two channels.

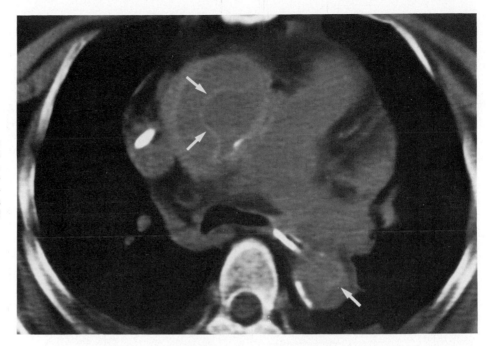

FIGURE 2–32 ■ Type A aortic dissection in a cadaver. The blood within the aorta is of lower density than the aortic wall. Intimal flaps *(arrows)* divide both the descending and ascending aorta. Calcification is visible in the aortic wall. Catheters are present in the superior vena cava and esophagus.

Calcified, atheromatous plaques occur in the intima of the aortic wall and are particularly well displayed on CT scans. In 25 to 56 per cent of patients with aortic dissection, these plaques become displaced along with the intima, away from the rest of the aortic wall.[106, 116–118] Intimal calcification, displaced inward from the aortic contour, however, is not pathognomonic of aortic dissection. In several conditions, soft tissue density between a calcified plaque and the apparent aortic contour can produce the same appearance.[115] For example, calcification within a mural thrombus of an aortic aneurysm can appear displaced from the aortic wall. A periaortic hematoma or incidental soft tissue mass surrounding the aorta

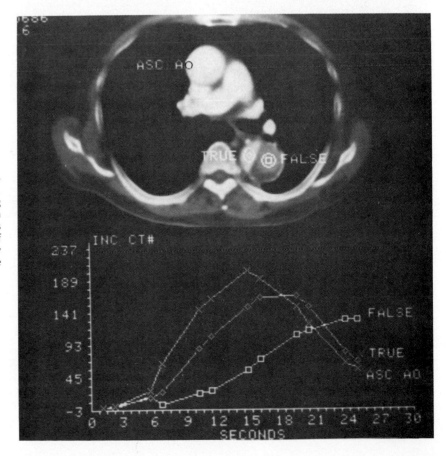

FIGURE 2–33 ■ Type B aortic dissection with time-density plot from multiple sequential CT scans. Fields-of-interest are plotted from the ascending aorta (ASC AO), true lumen (TRUE), and false lumen (FALSE). The relative increase in attenuation values *(vertical axis)* reflects the passage of a bolus of contrast material through the areas of interest. Flow through the false lumen is slower than through the true lumen or ascending aorta.

likewise can simulate a calcified plaque displayed from the apparent outer contour of the aorta. Occasionally, a saccular aneurysm contiguous to the calcified aortic wall or a tortuous descending aorta gives the appearance of displaced calcification. Therefore, aortic dissection should not be diagnosed from the appearance of "displaced" calcification alone. All the scans should be examined before the final diagnosis is considered.

CT is highly accurate for the diagnosis of aortic dissection. Thorsen and colleagues[119] and Oudkerk and co-investigators[120] both found no false-negative diagnoses and only one false-positive diagnosis in their studies. In perhaps as many as 25 per cent of patients with acute aortic dissections, the false channel is thrombosed and does not opacify. It remains controversial whether some of these instances could represent bleeding into the wall of the aorta from rupture of the vasa vasorum, without an intimal tear, as proposed by Yamada and co-workers.[121] The false channel is thrombosed more frequently with subacute and chronic aortic dissection. If seen on only a few scans, a thrombosed false lumen without displaced intimal calcification may be confused with a fusiform aortic aneurysm containing a crescentic thrombus. The site and length of an aortic dissection, together with its other features, should make the differentiation possible in most cases.

MR can generally provide a definite diagnosis of aortic dissection by demonstrating the two channels

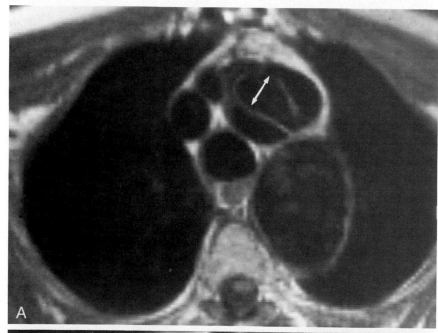

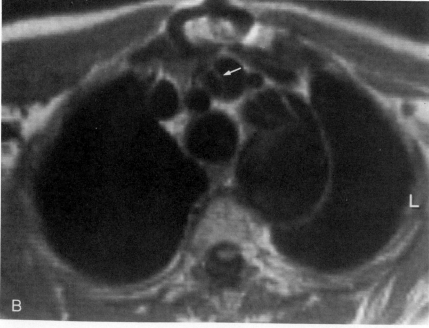

FIGURE 2–34 ■ Type A aortic dissection. *A,* Cardiac-gated MR image demonstrates a distinct flap *(arrows)* within the ascending aorta. The descending aorta is markedly dilated. *B,* Three cm superiorly the dissection is seen extending into the right common carotid with the flap *(arrow)* visible.

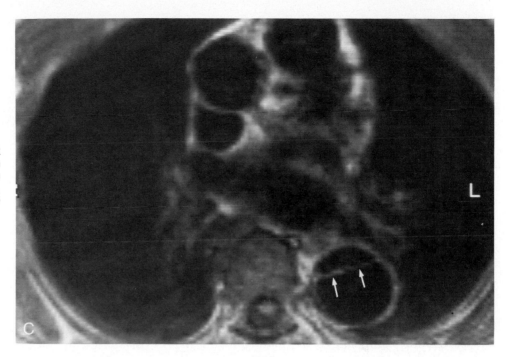

FIGURE 2–34 *Continued* ■ *C*, MR image 9 cm inferiorly. The dissection involves the descending aorta, with the flap *(arrows)* crossing the aorta, dividing the descending aorta into two distinct channels.

and the intimal flap between them (Fig. 2–34).[77, 122–124] The true and false channels can frequently be distinguished because of the presence of signal within the false channel, owing to either slow blood flow or thrombus. Even when the false channel contains thrombus, it is frequently possible to differentiate the signal intensity of thrombus from that of the intimal flap. Blood within the mediastinum can be recognized, thereby demonstrating the presence of periaortic hematoma. Likewise, blood within the pericardial sac can be recognized, indicating leakage from the false channel.

The accuracy of MR for the diagnosis of aortic dissection has been assessed. Radiologists with MR experience have about a 95 per cent sensitivity and 90 per cent specificity for detection of aortic dissection.[125] Fluid in the superior pericardial recesses around the aortic root, however, can be misinterpreted on MR as an aortic dissection.[126] Other pitfalls in interpretation are not uncommon and include unusual origins of the arch vessels; an unusual position of the left brachiocephalic vein; aortic plaque; and motion artifacts.[126a]

CT and MR can evaluate the results of repair of thoracic aortic dissection.[122, 127] In many cases, two channels persist, and the intimal flap is visible distal to the site of insertion of the aortic graft. The flow in the two channels produces a signal void rendering the intimal flap evident. MR also can monitor the size of the false channel and provide early detection of an aneurysm of the false channel.

In general, patients with type A dissections are surgical candidates, whereas those with type B are treated medically.[128–130] Regardless of therapy, the presence and type of dissection should be ascertained promptly once the patient's condition has stabilized. CT or MR should be performed within hours of the patient's admission to the hospital. Definitive therapy for type A dissections is based on the site of the intimal tear; the extent of dissecting hematoma; the degree of involvement of aortic branches; the presence of an associated aneurysm or pseudoaneurysm; and patency of the false channel.[129, 130] Surgery in type A dissection usually consists of insertion of an ascending aortic graft and an aortic valve prosthesis when incompetence is present, and of ensuring that the patency of the coronary arteries is maintained.

As in the case of aortic aneurysm, if CT or MR provides all the required information, aortography can be obviated. Patients in whom the false channel is thrombosed are usually excluded from surgical therapy and further angiographic studies are not warranted. Also, if a definite diagnosis of a type B dissection without an aneurysm can be made, surgery is usually not indicated and aortography is unnecessary.

CT, or preferably MR, should be the initial examination for patients suspected of having subacute or chronic aortic dissection. The majority of these patients are treated medically, and both these techniques are appropriate, noninvasive methods of confirming the diagnosis and type of dissection.

Patients treated either surgically or medically for aortic dissection are prone to serious immediate and long-term complications.[127, 131, 132] Complications consist of an extension of the dissecting hematoma; aneurysm formation, which occurs in 15 to 25 per cent of patients; aortic valvular insufficiency; and aortic rupture. Turley and colleagues[133] showed a remarkably high incidence of persistent patency of the false channel after surgery. Radiographic and angiographic monitoring of patients with a persistent false channel has been advocated,[134] but CT and MR are more convenient and rapid methods of repeatedly evaluating the aorta.[135, 136] After surgery, CT or MR should be performed in a manner similar to that previously described. The examination should be directed toward the detection of potential complications. Teflon grafts, often inserted at the site of the intimal tear, are radiodense and visible on CT scans.[135, 137] Dacron grafts are usually not dense enough to be visible with CT. After many years, Dacron grafts may calcify and can be seen radiographically and with CT.

Venous Occlusion

Obstruction of the SVC and other superior mediastinal veins is not as uncommon as formerly thought.[138, 139] The symptoms and signs that result from SVC or thoracic inlet venous obstruction are known as the SVC syndrome. Most patients with SVC syndrome have a malignant tumor involving the mediastinum. In over 80 per cent of these cases, the responsible tumor is a bronchogenic carcinoma, commonly arising in the right upper lobe.[140] Other causes include malignancies originating in the thymus or thyroid, lymphomas, or metastases to the mediastinal lymph nodes. Benign causes of the syndrome are fibrosing mediastinitis, granulomatous mediastinitis (especially histoplasmosis), multinodular goiter, aortic aneurysm, trauma, irradiation, thrombosis from indwelling intravascular devices,

and primary thrombosis of the SVC.[141] In a minority of patients, no cause can be found.

SVC obstruction produces a distinct constellation of clinical findings.[139–141] Suffusion and cyanosis of the face may be accompanied by edema of the head, neck, and arms. The veins of the head and neck are prominently distended. Dilated collateral veins of the chest wall are often visible. Venous pressure in the upper extremities can be elevated to above 20 mm Hg.

Radiographs of the chest frequently reveal a mediastinal mass.[138, 142] The mass may be the compressing tumor, but it may also be composed of dilated mediastinal and azygos veins.[142, 143, 143a] CT and MR can usually confirm the diagnosis and define the site of venous obstruction (Fig. 2–35).[93, 144–147] Occasionally, the SVC is intact, and a bilateral occlusion of the brachiocephalic veins will be found. Dilated collateral venous channels, involving the azygos system, or passing through the chest wall, are also often visible on CT or MR. With neoplasms, CT or MR can determine the extent of the tumor mass and the presence of additional mediastinal abnormalities.[93, 145–147]

The thoracic veins are normally well defined on contrast-enhanced CT. Intravascular filling defects can be readily demonstrated (Fig. 2–36.) Engel and colleagues[144] used CT to study 50 patients with SVC syndrome, which was due to malignancy in 36 pa-

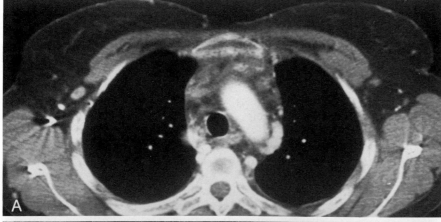
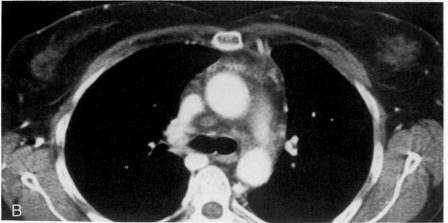

FIGURE 2–35 ■ Sclerosing mediastinitis with obliteration of the superior vena cava above the azygos arch. *A* and *B*, CT scan through the upper mediastinum demonstrates absence of upper superior vena cava and brachiocephalic veins. Dilated collateral veins involve the chest wall, accessory azygos, and accessory hemiazygos systems. The superior vena cava is reconstituted from the azygos arch.

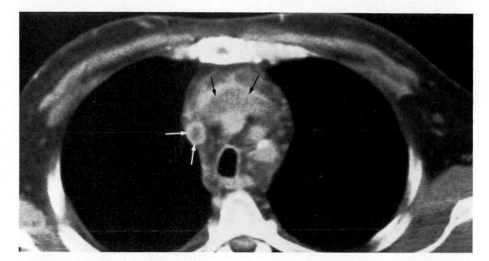

FIGURE 2–36 ■ Venous thrombosis in a man with right upper lobe squamous cell carcinoma and superior vena cava syndrome. Thrombus, outlined by contrast material, is seen within the right *(white arrows)* and left *(black arrows)* brachiocephalic veins. Opacified collateral veins are seen in the anterior chest wall. The superior vena cava is occluded by tumor inferior to the plane of the scan.

tients and benign causes in 14. In about half of these 50, the SVC was the site of obstruction, whereas in the other half, other upper thoracic veins were involved. Engel and co-workers proposed two criteria for a diagnosis of venous obstruction: nonopacification of veins downstream from the site of obstruction and opacification of collateral veins. In about a third of their patients, when no soft tissue mass was identified, the obstruction was attributed to thrombosis, or radiation mediastinitis and fibrosis.

Contrast material–related flow patterns, especially with a bolus injection, can simulate venous thrombosis. Therefore, care should be taken in interpreting these examinations.[148] As a general rule, in patients with suspected venous thrombosis, contrast material should be infused simultaneously into both the upper extremities.

Weinreb and co-workers[147] and McMurdo and colleagues[93] used MR to evaluate mediastinal and thoracic inlet venous obstructions. They found that MR could demonstrate the site of obstruction and the presence of a mass equally well as CT. On spin-echo MR, thrombi composed of blood elements and thrombi composed of tumor have similar imaging characteristics. Both can have signal intensity that varies from high to low on T2- as well as T1-weighted images. Gradient-echo images may in some instances make this distinction in the following way. Tumor is usually of intermediate signal intensity, whereas blood-containing thrombus is very low in signal intensity on cine-MR. The reason for this is that the magnetic susceptibility effects of blood elements within a thrombus composed of blood can cause the thrombus to have very low signal intensity on gradient-echo images (which are sensitive to magnetic susceptibility).

MR signal from slowly flowing blood and on occasion from normally flowing blood in mediastinal veins must be distinguished from a thrombus.[67, 149, 150] With slow flow there is usually a rim of low signal intensity between the thrombus and the wall of the vein. When first and second echo images are available, the signal intensity of slowly flowing blood usually increases in the second echo image. With gradient-echo images, the high signal from flowing blood is readily distinguished from a thrombus.[150a] A third method for distinguishing flow signal from an intravascular thrombus is with phase-encoded images in which only moving protons are imaged.[151]

Lymphadenopathy

The detection of mediastinal lymph node enlargement is an important function of pulmonary radiology. CT and MR can detect mediastinal and hilar lymphadenopathy not otherwise apparent on chest radiographs and can confirm suspicious adenopathy. The frequency and size of normal mediastinal lymph nodes were detailed earlier in this chapter. In general, mediastinal lymph nodes appear as discrete, nonenhanced, round or slightly irregular densities of various sizes. On CT, mediastinal lymph nodes are of soft tissue density, which usually distinguishes them easily from the background of mediastinal fat and connective tissue. On T1-weighted spin-echo sequences, lymph nodes are intermediate in signal intensity and conspicuous against the high signal intensity of fat.[146, 152] On T2 weighting, lymph nodes have an intensity similar to that of fat, and therefore blend with mediastinal fat.

Mediastinal lymph nodes do not frequently show some of the imaging characteristics of lymph nodes in the neck. For instance, they uncommonly enhance on CT after intravascular contrast material and infrequently show low-density necrosis. Im and colleagues[153] have described rim enhancement of mediastinal lymph nodes in tuberculous adenopathy. This is a finding we have also seen in adenopathy from metastases.[154] At this time, there are no distinguishing features between normal and abnormal nodes with CT, except for size.

Several groups[53, 152, 155] have attempted to identify MR characteristics that could distinguish between benign and malignant lymph nodes. In general, both malignant and benign nodes demonstrate wide variations in their measured T1 and T2 relaxation values.

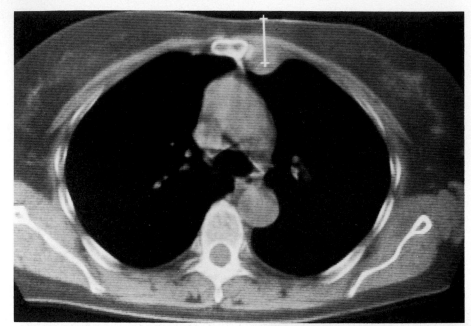

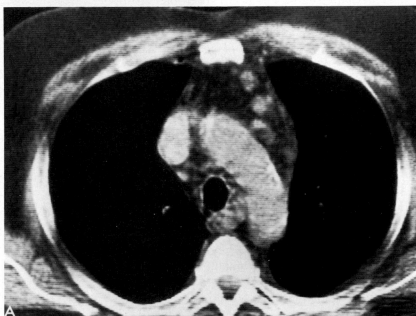

FIGURE 2–37 ■ Enlarged internal mammary lymph node in a 64-year-old asymptomatic woman with a retrosternal density on a routine lateral chest radiograph. The mass on the left *(bottom of marker)* represents an enlarged internal mammary lymph node. Other scans showed a breast mass on the left that had not been palpable but was subsequently found to be carcinoma.

FIGURE 2–38 ■ Enlarged lymph nodes in the prevascular space and aortic-pulmonic window, in an elderly patient with poorly differentiated carcinoma of the left lung. *A,* CT scan shows enlarged nodes in the prevascular space anterior to the aortic arch. *B,* CT scan 2 cm caudad demonstrates massively enlarged nodes in front of the ascending aorta, in the aortic-pulmonic window, and to the left of the trachea. (Nodes of this size in a patient with bronchogenic carcinoma have a high probability of being malignant. Only the paratracheal node could be reached by cervical mediastinoscopy. The calcified azygos node behind the superior vena cava is due to previous granulomatous disease.)

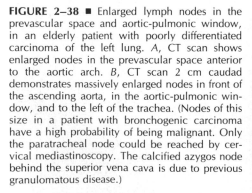

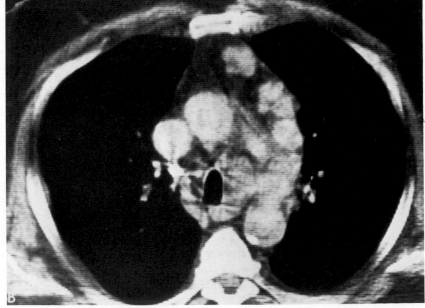

With grouped data, malignant nodes tend to have shorter T1 and T2 values than do benign causes of mediastinal adenopathy. In practical terms, this is not sufficient to be of diagnostic value. Whether MR spectroscopy or MR imaging with new pulse sequences or special MR contrast materials will be able to improve our ability to discriminate between benign and malignant lymphadenopathy remains speculative.

The main lymph node groups of the mediastinum are the internal mammary, prevascular, pretracheal, aortic-pulmonic, subcarinal, posterior mediastinal, and circumcardiac nodes.

INTERNAL MAMMARY LYMPH NODES

Normal internal mammary lymph nodes are not demonstrated on CT or MR scans. After injection of contrast material, two or three small internal mammary vessels may be visible on CT. Enlarged internal mammary nodes exhibit a characteristic focal soft tissue convexity protruding into the lung, lateral to the sternum (Fig. 2–37).[155a] Ege[156] and Rose and colleagues[157] have shown that the position of the internal mammary nodes varies from midline to 5.3 cm from the midline. Costal cartilages can also produce a convexity lateral to the sternum; but by observation of contiguous scans, this potential pitfall in diagnosis can be avoided. Internal mammary lymph node enlargement is rare in granulomatous diseases or metastatic bronchogenic carcinoma.

Internal mammary lymph node enlargement is common in patients with metastatic breast carcinoma. CT, in conjunction with other imaging studies, can assist in the staging of breast cancer and in the

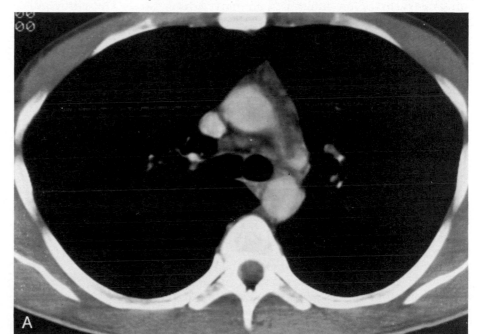

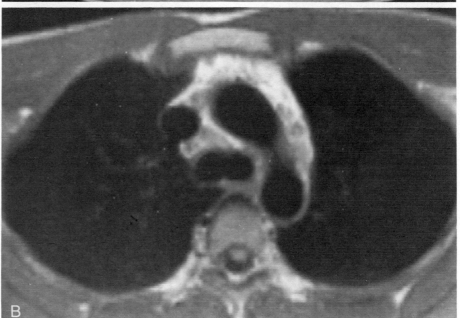

FIGURE 2–39 ■ Mediastinal adenopathy in a patient with AIDS and Kaposi's sarcoma. *A,* CT scan shows prevascular aortic-pulmonic window and pretracheal lymphadenopathy. *B,* T1-weighted MR image shows the nodes more clearly than CT scan because of better contrast between nodes and mediastinal fat.

detection of nodal recurrence.[158, 159, 160] Scatarige and colleagues[160] used CT to study 219 women with breast cancer at various stages of their disease. They found enlarged nodes, ranging in size from 6 mm to 6 cm, in 20.5 per cent of patients. Lymphadenopathy was most common at only one intercostal space—usually the second—but occurred in as many as four spaces.

The only other condition in which internal mammary adenopathy is seen with any frequency is lymphoma. Hopper and colleagues[161] studied over 100 patients with Hodgkin's disease. They found internal mammary adenopathy, unsuspected from chest radiographs, in 34.6 per cent of patients, whereas the chest radiograph was abnormal at this site in only 4 of 107 patients. CT is thus considerably more sensitive than lateral radiographs in demonstrating internal mammary adenopathy. Very rarely an aneurysm of an internal mammary artery can produce a mass in this location.[161a]

PREVASCULAR LYMPH NODES

One to six normal nodes are seen at this site on CT or MR in about 75 per cent of patients. They are not larger than about 8 mm and appear as discrete, round densities. Nodes of this size can be from prior granulomatous disease or may be normal. Enlarged prevascular lymph nodes are commonly due to bronchogenic carcinoma, lymphoma, sarcoidosis, metastasis, and many other conditions that can affect thoracic lymph nodes. The CT appearance of prevascular adenopathy varies from discrete, round or slightly irregular densities to large, lobulated conglomerate masses (Figs. 2–38 and 2–39). Lymphoma characteristically produces lobulated masses of matted nodes. CT and MR are considerably more sensitive than chest radiographs in the detection and identification of prevascular lymphadenopathy.

PRETRACHEAL LYMPH NODES

The pretracheal space, between the anterior trachea and the ascending aorta and arch vessels, contains numerous lymph nodes. The azygos lymph nodes in the right tracheobronchial angle are the most frequently imaged of the pretracheal nodes. They are present in over 95 per cent of normal people and are about 4 to 8 mm in transverse diameter. An occasional normal azygos node can be 10 or 11 mm in diameter. Lymph nodes at other sites in the pretracheal space are usually smaller and less frequently visible on CT or MR. The pretracheal lymph nodes are the mediastinal nodes most commonly involved in thoracic diseases (Figs. 2–40 and 2–41). Only when considerably enlarged do they distort the contour of the right mediastinum and become visible on chest radiographs as widening of the right paratracheal stripe. The pretracheal lymph nodes are thus often not detected from chest radiographs and are detected only on transaxial CT or MR images. Muller and colleagues[162] correlated the radiographic signs of right paratracheal adenopathy with the CT findings in 98 patients. In those patients with nodes larger than 15 mm in diameter, the right paratracheal stripe was widened in only 31 per cent. This is partially explained by the fact that these nodes are anterolateral to the trachea, and the distance between the tracheal lumen and right lung with large nodes may not be increased. In only 42 per cent of patients with adenopathy was the azygos vein–node complex enlarged on chest radiographs. Similarly, convexity of the SVC was seen in only about one half of patients with lymphadenopathy.

AORTIC-PULMONIC LYMPH NODES

The region of the aortic-pulmonic window often suffers from partial volume-averaging with the superior surface of the left pulmonary artery or the undersurface of the aortic arch on both CT and MR.[163] The aortic-pulmonic window can be demonstrated better with 5-mm than 10-mm CT collimation. Usually, two to four—but up to eight or ten—normal lymph nodes are visible in the aortic-pulmonic window, in about 80 per cent of individuals. They measure about 4 to 8 mm in diameter, and a normal node of up to 10 mm can occasionally be found. The aortic-pulmonic window also contains an irregular tubular density, presumably the ligamentum arteriosum, that should not be mistaken for an enlarged lymph node. Enlarged lymph nodes in the aortic-pulmonic window typically appear as round or slightly irregular, non-enhanced densities (Fig. 2–42; see also Fig. 2–41A). Chest radiographs are less sensitive in detecting aortic-pulmonic window ade-

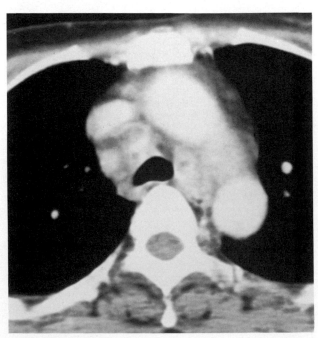

FIGURE 2–40 ■ Tuberculous lymphadenopathy. CT scan, following contrast material injection, demonstrates edge-enhancement of pretracheal and left paratracheal enlarged lymph nodes, proved to be tuberculosis. (Courtesy of J-G Im, MD, Seoul, Korea.)

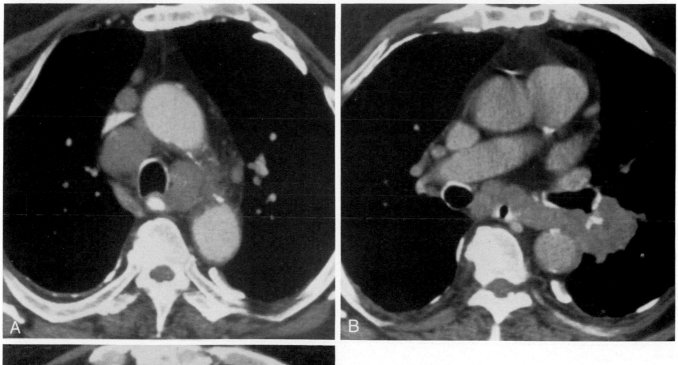

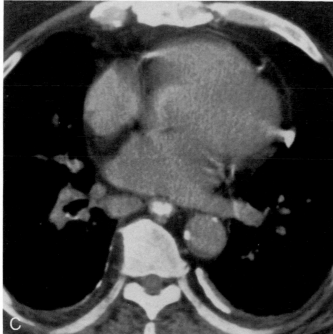

FIGURE 2–41 ■ Metastatic bronchogenic carcinoma in a patient with asbestos exposure. *A,* CT scan through the mid-mediastinum demonstrates enlarged lymph nodes in the pretracheal space, aortic-pulmonic window, and prevascular space. Oral contrast material is visible in the esophagus, and intravascular contrast in the superior vena cava. *B,* Four cm inferiorly, extensive hilar and subcoronal adenopathy is present. Adenopathy is seen behind the left main stem bronchus, obliterating the space between the descending aorta and the descending left pulmonary artery. *C,* Three cm inferior to *B,* paraesophageal lymph nodes are seen on the right, in the region of the inferior pulmonary ligament. Multiple calcified, asbestos-related pleural plaques are visible bilaterally on all three scans.

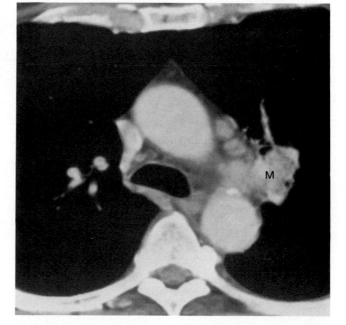

FIGURE 2–42 ■ Bronchogenic carcinoma arising in the left hilum with aortic-pulmonic window invasion and adenopathy. CT scan shows a left hilar mass (M) with direct invasion into the aortic-pulmonic window and also separate lymphadenopathy. The lymph nodes show mild edge-enhancement following contrast material injection.

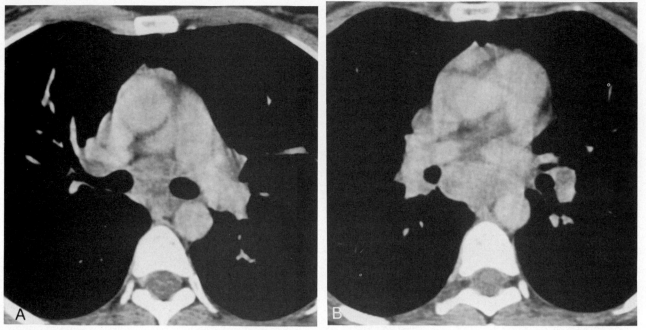

FIGURE 2–43 ■ Sarcoidosis with subcarinal and hilar adenopathy. *A* and *B*, CT scans show extensive subcarinal and bilateral hilar adenopathy. The nodes in the azygoesophageal recess and right hilum separate the intermediate bronchus and right lung. The esophagus is displaced posteriorly and to the left.

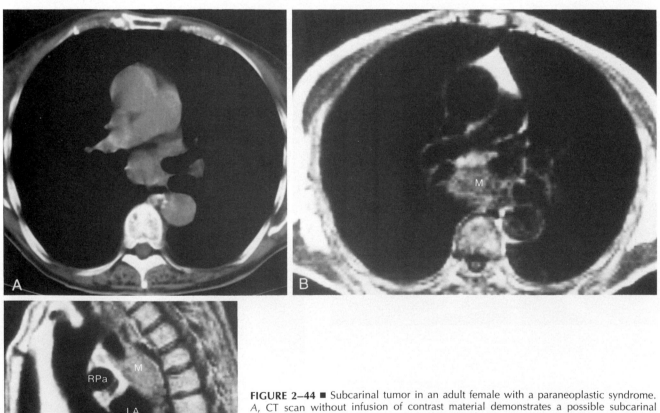

FIGURE 2–44 ■ Subcarinal tumor in an adult female with a paraneoplastic syndrome. *A*, CT scan without infusion of contrast material demonstrates a possible subcarinal density suggestive of a mass. *B*, T1-weighted MR image at the same level as *A* shows a mass (M) with lower signal intensity than mediastinal fat. *C*, Sagittal MR demonstrates the mass (M) above the left atrium (LA) and behind the right pulmonary artery (RPa). Biopsy of the mass showed a small-cell bronchogenic carcinoma.

nopathy than previously thought. Lymphadenopathy that can be demonstrated with CT in the aortic-pulmonic window is visible on chest radiographs only about half the time.[27]

SUBCARINAL LYMPH NODES

In about 90 per cent of individuals, one to three normal lymph nodes are visible on CT in the subcarinal region. The subcarinal region can contain the largest normal nodes in the mediastinum—up to 15 mm in diameter. It also frequently is the site of calcified nodes from prior granulomatous disease. Lymphatic pathways from both lungs pass through the subcarinal space, and subcarinal lymph nodes are almost as commonly enlarged as the azygos nodes in a variety of diseases (Fig. 2–43; see also Fig. 2–41).

Subcarinal lymph nodes can be markedly enlarged without being visible on chest radiographs, and CT is considerably more sensitive than chest radiographs in detecting subcarinal lymphadenopathy (Fig. 2–

44). Muller and colleagues[28] studied the subcarinal region in 90 patients using chest radiographs and CT. In patients with subcarinal adenopathy, only 23 per cent showed an abnormal azygoesophageal recess interface, and 40 per cent an increase in subcarinal density on chest radiographs.

POSTERIOR MEDIASTINAL LYMPH NODES

Although normal lymph nodes are present along the spinal vertebral bodies, they are not demonstrated on CT or MR. Focal lateral displacement of one or both paraspinal interfaces, detected from chest radiographs, can be due to posterior mediastinal adenopathy but also to several other causes.[164, 165] Inflammatory, traumatic, or neoplastic disease extending from the spine, as well as dilated vessels, may cause widening of the paraspinous line (Fig. 2–45). When spinal abnormalities are not evident, lymph node enlargement becomes a common cause of paraspinal line displacement (see Fig. 2–41C). Enlarged lymph nodes may be due to lymphoma,

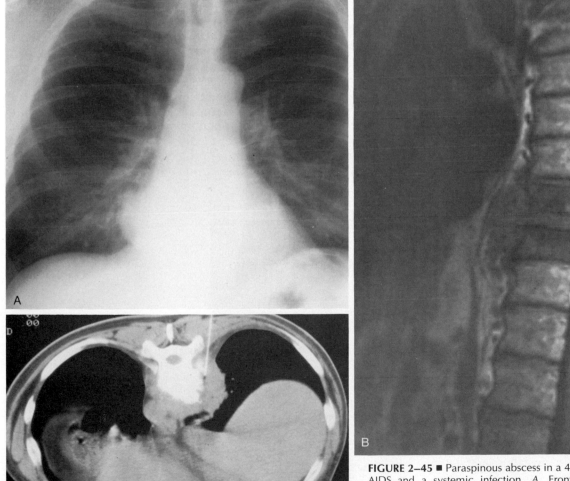

FIGURE 2–45 ■ Paraspinous abscess in a 45-year-old male with AIDS and a systemic infection. *A,* Frontal chest radiograph demonstrates a mass behind the right side of the heart. *B,* Spinal MR image demonstrates reduced intensity in two vertebral bodies with posterior and anterior masses. *C,* CT-guided aspiration of the mass demonstrated a paraspinous *Staphylococcus aureus* infection.

metastasis, or inflammation. Efremidis and co-workers[164] showed that CT is an excellent method for investigating paraspinous widening; they were able to confirm radiographic findings and determine the extent of disease in 11 patients with paraspinal widening. Enlarged paravertebral lymph nodes appear as discrete, nonenhanced densities, often displacing normal mediastinal structures. CT is more sensitive than lymphangiography in detecting and identifying posterior mediastinal adenopathy.[165] Occasionally, steroid-induced lipomatosis causes paraspinal widening, and CT can readily diagnose this abnormality.[166]

CIRCUMCARDIAC LYMPH NODES

Lymph nodes form a chain around the pericardial attachment to the diaphragm, but normal circumcardiac nodes cannot be shown on CT or MR. Circumcardiac nodes are not commonly involved in most diseases affecting the thorax or in diseases metastatic to the mediastinum. The exception to this general rule is mediastinal lymphoma, which, when it recurs, classically affects the circumcardiac nodes (Fig. 2–46).[167–169] On CT or MR, circumcardiac lymph node enlargement can be detected with greater sensitivity than from chest radiographs and can be distinguished from benign causes of a mass at this site, especially an epicardial fat pad or a pleuropericardial cyst.[168, 169]

Benign Lesions

CT is currently used to detect mediastinal abnormalities not visible on chest radiographs and to characterize, localize, and determine the anatomic relationships of lesions detected from radiographs.

Often the results of CT profoundly influence the patient's care. This is especially true when lesions can be diagnosed as benign from CT, obviating further investigation. When CT is able to identify a mediastinal mass as a vessel, fatty mass, or thin-walled cyst, benignity is usually assumed. The CT or MR findings characterizing as benign many homogeneous solid, soft tissue masses have not been established, and further investigation is necessary in this area.[44, 170] Areas of high attenuation can be found in mediastinal masses owing to calcium deposition, high iodine content, or acute hemorrhage.[170a] Although diffuse high attenuation suggests benignity, this finding may be misleading.

For mediastinal masses, spin-echo MR and CT provide similar morphologic information. Although the spatial resolution of MR in the mediastinum, even with cardiac-gating, does not equal that of CT, contrast resolution between most masses and the surrounding mediastinal vessels and fat is excellent provided that the appropriate imaging sequence is used. Thus the conspicuousness of most mediastinal masses is equal for MR and CT. In general, MR is better than CT for demonstrating the relationship of a mediastinal mass to the surrounding vessels.[171] MR can also demonstrate vascular invasion or compression by a mediastinal mass. Flow signal from a compressed vessel must however be differentiated from vascular invasion by the compressing neoplasm. Cine-MR is useful for making this distinction. Partial volume-averaging of high signal intensity from mediastinal fat and signal void from vessels can produce the intermediate signal of most mediastinal masses.[113] This phenomenon occasionally can be seen in the aortic-pulmonic window region but is not usually a practical problem. The same broad categorization of masses into fatty, cystic, vascular, or solid

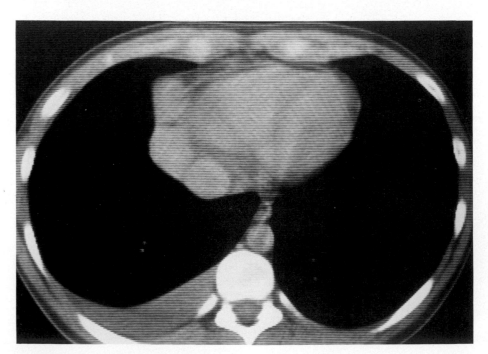

FIGURE 2–46 ■ Circumcardiac lymph nodes from recurrent lymphoma. CT scan shows several large lymph nodes to the right of the heart within the circumcardiac lymph node chain. A free-flowing right pleural effusion is present.

that can be achieved with CT can be obtained with MR.

FATTY MASSES

With the advent of CT, the frequent deposition of fat within the mediastinum has become apparent.[172, 173] Fat is easily identified by its low density (−20 H to −100 H). In the study by Pugatch and colleagues,[174] almost half of 39 benign mediastinal abnormalities investigated with CT were composed of fat. Fatty lesions occurred in the superior, anterior, and posterior mediastinum, although the superior mediastinum was the most common site of mediastinal adiposity or lipomatosis. Paraspinous deposition of fat in steroid-induced thoracic lipomatosis can also produce smooth symmetric widening of the paraspinous lines.[166] In two other studies, fat-containing masses constituted 3 to 10 per cent of all mediastinal lesions evaluated using CT.[175, 176] The usual clinical circumstances leading to investigation with CT occur when a superior mediastinal mass or diffuse mediastinal widening is seen on chest radiographs. The patient is often obese or may be receiving steroids. On CT, mediastinal fat in obese or cushingoid patients is low in density and of uniform consistency.

Like CT, MR can demonstrate diffuse mediastinal lipomatosis. T1-weighted images distinguish between mediastinal fat, with a T1 value of 300 to 400 ms, and most soft tissue masses with T1 values between 1200 and 1600 ms.[146] Localized fatty masses visible on CT can derive from a number of causes. A prominent epicardial fat pad is the most common fatty mass in the thorax and is easily recognized on CT or MR. Paling and Williamson[177] have described the variations on chest radiographs and CT scans of the left epicardial fat pad. They showed that a moderately large fat pad could be present on CT without being radiographically evident, and also that cardiomegaly or a levoposition of the heart could artificially simulate the radiographic appearance of a fat pad.

Lipomas can manifest in the anterior mediastinum, but they also occur in the middle and posterior mediastinum and adjacent to the diaphragm.[178] Thymolipomas are anterior mediastinal benign tumors and frequently reach a large size and bulge to both sides of the mediastinum (Fig. 2–47). On CT they may be indistinguishable from a lipoma but may have fibrous bands passing through them, as well as large vascular channels. Occasionally, a chyle-containing lymphangioma in the anterior mediastinum shows low density on CT or high signal intensity on MR and could be mistaken for a mediastinal lipoma or thymolipoma. Differentiation between benign and malignant fatty mediastinal masses can be difficult. The diagnosis of benignity of fatty mediastinal masses often is presumptive, because liposarcoma and fibroliposarcoma are rare mediastinal tumors, occurring most commonly in the posterior mediastinum and only occasionally in the anterior mediastinum. Liposarcoma also should have more high-density elements than benign fat, should be more

inhomogeneous, and can show features of diffuse mediastinal invasion.

Extraperitoneal or omental fat can herniate through the foramen of Morgagni or of Bochdalek or through the esophageal hiatus. These fatty masses manifest as low-density mediastinal lesions and can be difficult to distinguish from a primary mediastinal lesion. Careful scrutiny of multiple images can frequently demonstrate the extrathoracic origin of the mass.

CYSTIC MASSES

Cysts constitute 15 to 20 per cent of all mediastinal masses.[179] The most common are bronchogenic, enterogenous, pleuropericardial, and thymic. Most benign mediastinal cysts do not produce symptoms and can become large before they are discovered. They are usually found incidentally on chest radiographs. In addition to these congenital cysts, many predominantly solid tissue masses may have cystic components or may develop areas of lower CT attenuation secondary to necrosis, liquefied hemorrhage, or cystic degeneration.[180, 181] Included among the former are dermoids, teratomas, and lymphangiomas and among the latter thymic Hodgkin's disease, metastases, neurofibromas, and intrathoracic goiters.

Most congenital mediastinal cysts have a density of 0 H to 20 H, which is less than that of muscle but greater than that of fat. Some benign cysts have viscous fluid with a density in the range of 20 H to 50 H or, uncommonly, up to 100 H, equivalent to that of solid tumors.[182–184] Cysts containing serous fluid, such as pericardial cysts, typically have long T1 and T2 relaxation values producing low signal intensity on T1-weighted images.[170, 185] On T2 weighting they can increase in relative signal intensity because of their water content, which has a long T2 value. Bronchogenic and degenerative cysts may contain a high concentration of mucin or protein, may have a short T1 relaxation value, and may appear intense on both T1- and T2-weighted images.

The CT features of a congenital mediastinal cyst that suggest benignity are (1) homogeneous attenuation, usually in the range of 0 to 20 H; (2) a smooth, well-defined, thin wall that usually enhances with intravascular contrast material; (3) a regular shape—round, oval, or tubular; (4) no enhancement of the cystic content; (5) no infiltration of surrounding structures; and (6) a typical location within 5 cm of the tracheal carina. Masses that show most or all of the features are invariably benign.[186] Confirmation of the diagnosis can be made by transbronchial or transtracheal aspiration.

Bronchogenic and enterogenous cysts arise from the airway and esophagus, respectively, most commonly near the tracheal carina. They frequently protrude into the posterior mediastinum and may be extremely large when first discovered.[187, 188] An abrupt increase in size can be caused by hemorrhage into the cyst. On CT scans, bronchogenic cysts appear unilocular with uniform density (Fig. 2–48). Their attenuation value depends on the content of the cyst and can vary from 0 to over 100 H. On spin-

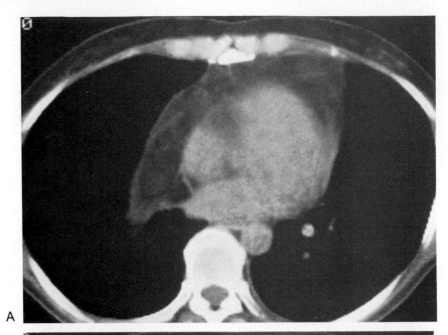

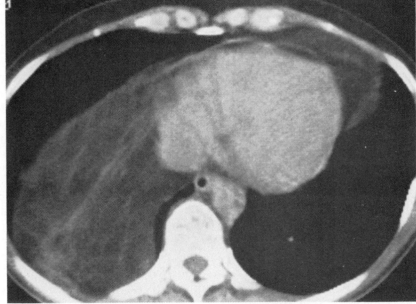

FIGURE 2–47 ■ Mediastinal thymolipoma. *A* and *B*, CT scans through the lower thorax show a low-density mass in the anterior mediastinum, in front of the heart and on the right extending to the posterior chest wall. Strands of fibrous tissue course through the mass. At thoracotomy, a 10-kg thymolipoma was removed.

echo MR images, they are usually bright on T1- and T2-weighted images. The wall of the cyst is usually thin and the inner margin smooth. Although bronchogenic cysts displace adjacent structures, they are usually clearly demarcated from the surrounding mediastinal organs.

Pleuropericardial cysts are congenital, smooth, round-to-oval lesions that are invariably connected to the pericardium. In about two thirds of instances, they arise from the right cardiophrenic angle. Other sites of origin are the left cardiophrenic angle, the anterior and superior mediastinum, and, rarely, the pericardium posterior to the heart.[187] Occasionally, pleuropericardial cysts are pedunculated, and on CT scans, the connection of the cysts to the pericardium is not evident. They appear smooth and thin-walled, and their contents are homogeneous, with a density

usually ranging from 0 H to 20 H but sometimes higher (Fig. 2–49).[188] On MR the cystic fluid is usually intermediate to high in intensity on T1-weighted images, increasing on T2-weighted images. These lesions are malleable, and as Pugatch and colleagues[188] showed, they can change shape on CT when the patient is in the prone or decubitus position.

True congenital thymic cysts are rare and originate from the thymopharyngeal duct.[189] They can occur anywhere along the course of the embryonic thymus gland from the angle of the mandible to the manubrium. Most do not cause symptoms, but if large, they can produce tracheal or cardiac compression.[190, 191] Mediastinal thymic cysts are usually round and frequently are multiloculated. Hemorrhage into the cyst is common, and the cyst cavity often contains

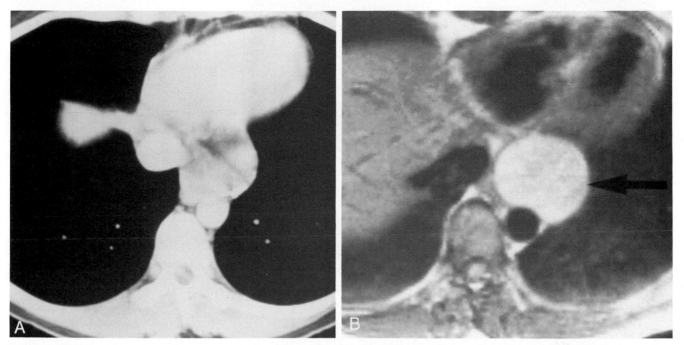

FIGURE 2–48 ■ Bronchogenic cyst in an asymptomatic young adult male with an abnormal chest radiograph. *A*, CT scan demonstrates a mass behind the heart and in front of the descending aorta. *B*, Cardiac-gated, T1-weighted MR image more clearly defines the mass *(arrow)*, which is homogeneous and high in intensity. At surgery, a bronchogenic cyst was removed.

old blood, necrotic material, and cholesterol crystals. It can thus be anticipated that the CT attenuation values of the cystic fluid may vary considerably from those of water.

Thymomas often undergo cystic degeneration. If degeneration is extensive, the CT and gross appearance of the lesion is indistinguishable from that of a thymic cyst.[189] Cystic degeneration can also occur in Hodgkin's disease and germ cell tumors around the thymus and can produce a similar appearance. An anterior or superior mediastinal cyst is seldom a congenital thymic cyst, and the commoner, more ominous alternative lesions should be considered first.

Pancreatic pseudocysts can manifest as a mass in the posterior or inferior mediastinum. CT can then demonstrate their cystic nature and their extension through the retrocrural portion of the diaphragm (Fig. 2–50).[192, 193] We have seen one pancreatic pseudocyst in which the cystic mass appeared thick on CT. CT is probably the most precise method of determining the thoracic and abdominal extent of a pancreatic pseudocyst.

Cystic teratomas can be benign or malignant, cystic or solid, although the cystic lesions tend to be benign. One reported benign cystic teratoma[194] demonstrated CT findings of a well-circumscribed anterior mediastinal mass composed of fat and soft tissue density. Subsequent studies have shown marked variability in the thickness of the wall and the CT density of the contents of benign cystic teratomas (Fig. 2–51).[195, 196]

Other lesions that can undergo cystic degeneration and show mixed solid and cystic elements on CT or MR include mediastinal carcinomas; metastases to lymph nodes, especially from thyroid, testes, and melanoma of the skin; and nerve root tumors, especially schwannomas and neurofibromas. Cystic degeneration of a solid mass is more likely to occur following radiation or chemotherapy but can be seen prior to treatment.

VASCULAR MASSES

As described earlier in this chapter, a dilated or aberrant vessel is a common cause of a mediastinal mass. CT and MR can readily identify these masses. In most circumstances, a structure that enhances on CT after intravascular contrast material to the same extent as the great vessels is a dilated vessel. Some solid tumors can enhance markedly with contrast but should not be mistaken for a vessel. Mediastinal masses that usually enhance following administration of intravascular contrast material include intrathoracic extension of a goiter, paragangliomas, benign lymphoid hyperplasia (Castleman's disease), carcinoids, parathyroid adenomas, and, occasionally, highly malignant tumors.[197–199]

SOLID MASSES

Mediastinal masses of relatively uniform soft tissue density constitute a varied group. A circumscribed solid mediastinal mass can be inflammation, a primary benign neoplasm, or a primary malignant neoplasm. Large single lymph nodes or conglomerate nodes can also appear masslike on CT. With MR, a group of small discrete lymph nodes may appear to coalesce into a single large node or mass, although

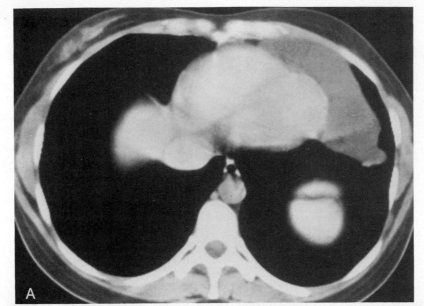

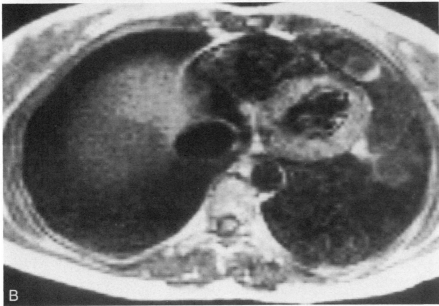

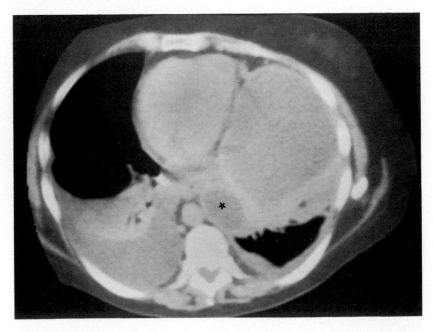

FIGURE 2–49 ■ Compound pericardial cyst in an asymptomatic young male. *A,* CT scan through the apex of the heart demonstrates a large paracardiac mass on the left side with a density that is higher than fat but lower than muscle. *B,* Gated MR shows that the mass is multiloculated and low in intensity on T1 weighting.

FIGURE 2–50 ■ Mediastinal extension of pancreatic pseudocyst in a 41-year-old patient with pancreatitis. CT shows a thick wall cyst *(asterisk)* to the left of the descending aorta, which has entered the posterior mediastinum through the aortic hiatus. Bilateral pleural effusions are present. Air in the left pleural space is from a previous thoracentesis.

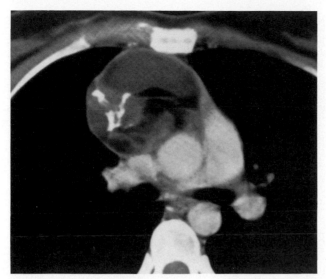

FIGURE 2–51 ■ Benign cystic teratoma in a young female with an asymptomatic mediastinal mass. CT shows a 7-cm anterior mediastinal mass with a thin, well-defined capsule. The mass contains low-density fat, soft tissue density, and bony components. A fat–soft tissue level is present in the center of the mass.

this is not frequently a problem with newer MR scanners. Lymphoma, granulomatous disease, and metastases can all appear as solid masses. A mass is considered solid if most of its density on CT is greater than that of fat or of water (Fig. 2–52).[200] Attenuation values can be quite imprecise in the mediastinum, and solid soft tissue masses can range from 15 H to 50 H. Calcification can occur in mediastinal masses and, if diffuse, usually indicates benignity. However, teratocarcinomas and thymomas can be heavily calcified. Calcification within a mass or within lymph nodes usually cannot be demonstrated on MR. Occasionally, large calcified deposits produce a striking area of signal void.[170]

The appearance of the boundary between a mass and the surrounding mediastinum has been extensively discussed. If a distinct plane of cleavage is visible around the mass and the mediastinal fat planes are preserved, the mass is often considered benign; but this is not a reliable sign of benignity, especially in cases of thymoma.[201] Small sites of mediastinal infiltration by malignant neoplasms may not be demonstrated on CT or MR.

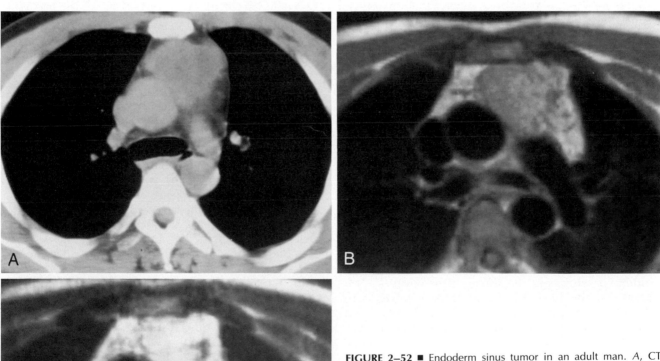

FIGURE 2–52 ■ Endoderm sinus tumor in an adult man. *A,* CT scan shows an anterior mediastinal mass displacing the aorta and the main pulmonary artery posteriorly. The mass is of uniform soft tissue density. *B,* T1-weighted MR image demonstrates the mass contiguous with the aorta and main pulmonary artery. The mass is moderately inhomogeneous. *C,* On T2 weighting, the mass is equal to mediastinal fat in signal intensity and is poorly imaged. At thoracotomy, an anterior mediastinal tumor was readily resected.

When CT or MR shows that the mediastinum is widely infiltrated and mediastinal structures are encased, the mass is usually malignant.[202] Benign masses such as granulomatous disease can however elicit an inflammatory response and demonstrate an ill-defined margin, simulating malignancy. Many mediastinal masses do not have clear-cut CT or MR features of either benignity or malignancy; therefore, a qualified interpretation is warranted. With MR, benign neoplasms do not differ significantly from malignant neoplasms either in intensity or relaxation values.[170, 203]

Thymic Abnormalities

THYMIC HYPERPLASIA

Thymic hyperplasia, also known as thymic lymphoid follicular hyperplasia, is characterized by an enlargement of the thymus with preservation of the gland's general architecture. The lymphoid follicles are hyperplastic, and the thymic medulla is diffusely infiltrated with lymphocytes and plasma cells. The association of thymic hyperplasia with myasthenia gravis and thyrotoxicosis is well known.[204, 205]

In about 50 per cent of patients with thymic hyperplasia, the gland is sufficiently enlarged to produce an anterior mediastinal mass on chest radiographs that can be detected readily with CT. On CT the axes of each lobe are increased compared with those of normal individuals of the same age.[206, 207] The greater than normal thickness of at least one lobe is most striking. In an occasional patient, thymic hyperplasia appears as a rounded mass on CT (Fig. 2–53). The CT density of thymic hyperplasia is similar to that of the normal young thymus and higher than that of the involuting thymus of adults. In some patients, small calcifications are evident on high-resolution CT images, and in others, cystic degeneration of the germinal centers may produce an inhomogeneous appearance to the hyperplastic thymus. In 30 to 50 per cent of patients with proven thymic hyperplasia, CT shows a normal-sized thymus.[208, 209]

The MR spin-echo appearance of thymic hyperplasia has been described, and the resolution of MR scanners is sufficient to image this entity.[208] MR intensity of the hyperplastic thymus is lower than that of surrounding mediastinal fat on T1-weighted images and should be easily visible in the anterior mediastinum. Whether MR will be able to discriminate between thymic hyperplasia and malignant processes on the basis of relaxation times is not known and appears doubtful.

THYMOMA

The role of imaging in patients with a suspected thymoma is complex. In patients with myasthenia gravis, the CT or MR demonstration of an otherwise occult mass can indicate the necessity for thymectomy. Also, CT and MR may demonstrate extension of an invasive thymoma to the mediastinum or pleura and thus may change the therapeutic approach. One

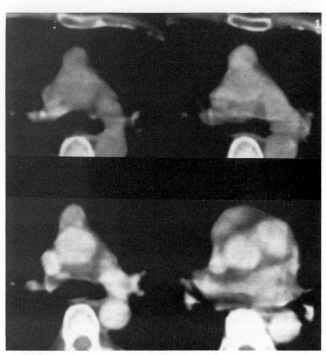

FIGURE 2–53 ■ Hyperplasia of the thymus. Serial CT scans demonstrate a round mass in the right lobe of the thymus. The mass enhances following administration of intravascular contrast material. At surgery, the thymus was resected and contained areas of thymic hyperplasia. (Courtesy of Pierre Schnyder, MD, Lausanne, Switzerland.)

third to one half of thymomas are malignant.[201, 210–212] The distinction between benign and malignant thymoma may be difficult even from histologic sections. Thus, the prognosis and therapeutic approach is frequently determined by whether the tumor has invaded beyond its capsule. The concept of invasion of the thymus through its fibrous capsule is of major importance. CT and MR have become the most precise modalities for the presurgical determination of the extent of a thymoma.

Noninvasive Thymoma ■ Most noninvasive thymomas appear on transaxial images as round or oval, well circumscribed, and between 1 and 10 cm in diameter, replacing the normal thymus. Thymomas less than 2 cm in diameter may appear as no more than a focal bulge on the contour of the normal thymus. The CT density of a thymoma is similar to that of normal young thymus and is usually only slightly affected by the administration of intravenous contrast material. Intratumoral calcifications are found in about one quarter of noninvasive thymomas.[207, 210, 213] Their presence however is not indicative of benignity. Areas of cystic degeneration are also found within noninvasive thymoma and appear on CT as areas of lower density, similar to the degenerative changes seen with thymic hyperplasia.

Thymomas occur along the thymolymphatic duct and are not limited to the prevascular space. They are most commonly found in an inverted U shape around the base of the heart but can arise anywhere between the lower pole of the thyroid gland and the anterior surface of the pericardium.[207] They may even

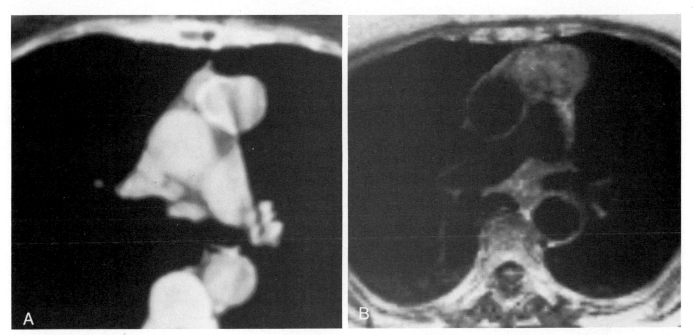

FIGURE 2–54 ■ Benign spindle cell thymoma in an asymptomatic female. *A*, CT scan demonstrates an anterior mediastinal mass in the left lobe of the thymus with a well-defined capsule. *B*, T1-weighted MR image demonstrates the mass, which appears more inhomogeneous than on CT scan. The capsule is not as well demonstrated with MR as with CT.

arise in the middle mediastinum. Thus imaging for detection of thymoma must encompass the entire mediastinum.

Administration of intravenous contrast material only slightly enhances the CT density of the tumor, but when combined with 3 to 5 mm scans, it can help to distinguish the capsule of the tumor from the pericardium, pleura, and mediastinal contents. Demonstration that a thymoma is noninvasive is important, as less than 2 per cent of encapsulated thymomas will recur after surgery (Fig. 2–54).[214]

Information on the MR of thymoma is limited. In the published cases, the lesion was well demarcated within the anterior mediastinum.[170, 208, 215] Thymomas have a short T1 relaxation time but still show good contrast from mediastinal fat on T1-weighted images. Whether MR is better than CT for defining capsular invasion by thymomas is not known.

Invasive Thymoma ■ CT is the most precise method for detecting local and regional spread of invasive thymoma. Invasive thymoma appears on CT as an irregular, ill-defined mass, usually within the prevascular mediastinal space. The main feature of mediastinal invasion is the obliteration of the tissue planes defined by mediastinal fat.[208, 210] This may be difficult to detect, however, and false-positive and false-negative results on CT are not uncommon. Close attention must therefore be paid to the mediastinal recesses that surround the aorta, pulmonary arteries, and SVC.

The mediastinal organs most likely to be invaded by a thymoma are the trachea, the great arteries and veins, the mediastinal pleura, and the pericardium (Fig. 2–55). Once the tumor reaches the pleural surface, it can extend anteriorly around the chest

wall or posteriorly along the mediastinal pleura.[216] Pleural extension across the pleura by droplet spread, without continuity with the primary tumor, is seen in about 15 per cent of advanced malignant thymomas.[217] CT is the best method of detecting extension of the pleura and transpleural droplet spread (Fig. 2–56). In patients with suspected invasive thymoma, CT or MR examination of the thorax should thus always encompass the entire thorax, to the most inferior extent of the posterior costophrenic sulci.

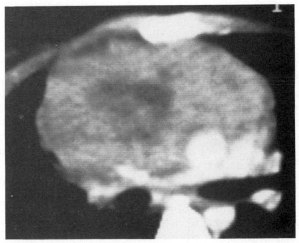

FIGURE 2–55 ■ Invasive thymoma in a patient with myasthenia gravis. CT scan, following injection of intravenous contrast material, demonstrates a large anterior mediastinal mass without a defined capsule. The mass is inhomogeneous with enhancing portions. The great vessels are displaced posteriorly. Regions of necrosis with low intensity are present within the mass. (Courtesy of Pierre Schnyder, MD, Lausanne, Switzerland.)

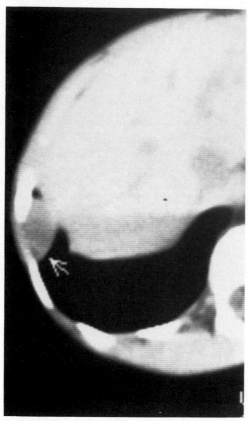

FIGURE 2–56 ■ Transpleural spread of malignant thymoma. CT of the right lower thorax demonstrates a pleural base mass in the right lateral costophrenic angle *(arrow)*, representing transpleural droplet metastases from a malignant thymoma.

Invasive thymoma can spread directly across the pleura into the lung parenchyma, although this is less common than the mediastinal or pleural route. Extrathoracic extension of invasive thymoma is not uncommon, and direct invasion of the diaphragm, or through the aortic or esophageal hiatuses has been reported.[218, 219] When diaphragmatic deposits of tumor are found with CT or MR, the examination should be extended to include the abdomen.

Invasive thymoma is usually more heterogeneous than noninvasive thymoma on CT, although this finding is not by itself indicative of a malignant neoplasm. Areas of tumor necrosis are usually more clearly demonstrated after intravenous administration of contrast material. The tumor usually becomes denser as it enhances, whereas the necrotic areas are lower in density and do not change their density. The contrast between the tumor and mediastinal fat and vessels may also increase with intravascular contrast.

On CT, intratumoral calcifications and areas of cystic degeneration are equally common in invasive and noninvasive thymoma. The only definitive findings of invasion are detection of regional or distant metastases.[146, 210, 220] In two cases of invasive thymoma that we have observed, MR showed the tumor readily delineated from mediastinal fat. Neither of our cases, however, had the short T1 relaxation time reported by Ross and colleagues.[215]

THYMOLIPOMA

Thymolipoma (lipothymoma) is a benign, anterior mediastinal mass arising from the thymus. It has a well-formed fibrous capsule that surrounds mature fat, containing thymic rests (see Fig. 2–47). This lesion produces few symptoms and 50 per cent of thymolipomas are first detected from chest radiographs as an asymptomatic mediastinal mass.[221, 222] They can, however, reach a large size and compress adjacent structures, and even the heart.[223] When both the fatty and thymic portions of the tumor are demonstrated on CT or MR, the correct diagnosis can be strongly suspected. When the tumor appears to be only fat and the solid thymic components are not evident, only its position within the mediastinum can suggest the diagnosis. As with thymomas, tumoral calcification can be found.[207, 221, 222]

On MR, the tumor has the imaging characteristics of a fatty mass and is intense on T1- and T2-weighted images. In one case that we observed, large vascular channels and linear strands of lower signal intensity coursed through the tumor.

MYASTHENIA GRAVIS

The roles of CT and MR in the evaluation of patients with myasthenia gravis depend on the clinical approach to the problem in any given institution. A thymoma or thymic hyperplasia is found in 10 to 20 per cent of patients with myasthenia gravis, and one third to one half of these thymomas are malignant.[189, 212, 220, 224–226] When chest radiographs demonstrate an anterior mass, CT or MR should be obtained to determine the extent of the lesion and detect possible occult metastases. If no mass is evident on chest radiographs and thymectomy is routinely performed, CT or MR is probably not indicated. CT or MR can detect small thymomas that could be malignant and are not evident radiographically. CT or MR should therefore be obtained when surgery is to be undertaken if a thymoma can be demonstrated. In the clinical context of myasthenia gravis, CT is highly sensitive and relatively specific in detecting occult thymomas, especially in patients over the age of 40.[201, 208, 220, 225, 226] Contiguous thin sections should be obtained to help differentiate thymic hyperplasia and thymoma. In most circumstances, detection of a thymoma indicates the need for thymectomy, even though the prognosis for patients affected by myasthenia gravis is much worse with a thymoma than without one.[170] Removal of the tumor does not improve the prognosis.

LYMPHOMA

Thymic involvement in patients with mediastinal Hodgkin's disease occurs in about one third of cases, both at the initial presentation stage and during relapse. The CT and MR features have both been reported.[155, 180, 206, 207, 227] The more common CT finding is that of a well-defined mass in the anterior mediastinum that enhances slightly after intravenous injection of contrast material. Regional lymphadenopathy may be evident on CT. Especially following radiation, the tumor can undergo cystic degeneration, producing a large multicystic mediastinal mass without other specific findings.[180, 228] CT can usually differentiate between lymphadenopathy and an enlarged thymus. CT is obtained to display the extent and stage of the lesion. In most instances, lymphoma is not restricted to the thymus, and CT is the most precise method of defining lymphadenopathy at other sites within the mediastinum and thoracic cage. In the absence of lymphadenopathy, the solitary thymic mass is unlikely to be lymphoma.[227]

Although the MR imaging characteristics of isolated or primary thymic lymphoma have not been described, several studies have investigated mediastinal lymphoma in general.[155, 229] Mediastinal Hodgkin's disease has a relatively low signal intensity on T1-weighted images, similar to that of muscle, and readily contrasts with mediastinal fat. In most cases, mediastinal Hodgkin's disease also has a high signal intensity on T2-weighted images. The occasional mass that remains low in signal intensity on T2-weighted images is less likely to involute following therapy, possibly reflecting a large amount of fibrous stroma within the tumor.[230]

OTHER NEOPLASMS

Several other tumors can arise within or around the thymus. The commonest of these are germ cell and carcinoid tumors.[202, 231, 233] Germ cell tumors arise from malignant transformation of germinal elements.[233a] In adults the incidence of benign germ cell tumors is equal in men and women, whereas the malignant varieties have a strong male predominance. The benign is teratoma, and the malignant are teratocarcinomas, embryonal carcinomas, seminomas, endodermal sinus tumors, and choriocarcinomas (Fig. 2–57). Sixty per cent of all germ cell tumors are benign teratomas. Their cystic and fatty components are readily identified on CT and MR, but these features are not specific for benignity. Thin-walled cystic teratomas are usually benign and do not invade adjacent structures, but when large they may compress adjacent organs.

The more malignant of these germ cell tumors have CT and MR features similar to those of invasive thymomas. They can have low-density or low-intensity necrotic areas, areas of cystic degeneration, and even intratumoral calcifications. They can invade the mediastinum, pleura, and pericardium and produce a CT or MR appearance indistinguishable from invasive thymoma. The only clearly differentiating feature is that they do not have the propensity for transpleural droplet spread. Seminomas are similar in imaging characteristics to the other germ cell tumors.[207, 234, 235] They can be inhomogeneous and may contain cystic areas, and calcifications within the tumor are frequent. Enhancement of the solid portions of the tumor after administration of intravascular contrast material is common but is not diagnostically specific. Invasion of the mediastinum

is diagnosed from CT and MR images by obliteration of tissue planes and replacement of mediastinal fat by tumor. Vascular compression and invasion may be detected with CT after infusion of contrast material, but are more readily seen with MR.

Carcinoid tumors arising in the thymus are rare and are associated with Cushing's syndrome or the multiple endocrine neoplasia syndrome.[189, 225, 232] About 40 per cent of thymic carcinoids have Cushing's syndrome, but, unlike foregut carcinoid tumors, do not produce the carcinoid syndrome. Thymic carcinoid tumors can be small and not visible on CT or MR, or large, aggressive, and metastatic to distant sites. Their CT findings are similar to those of invasive thymoma, with superior vena caval obstruction an unusually common finding. The conventional chest radiograph can be normal, and the thymus should be evaluated with CT or MR in all patients with unexplained Cushing's syndrome.

THYMIC CYSTS

True or congenital thymic cysts are exceedingly rare, and most cysts within the thymus are degenerative within tumors such as thymomas, or they occur after radiation therapy for Hodgkin's disease.[228, 236]

Congenital thymic cysts are usually within the thymus but can occur anywhere along the thymolymphatic duct. Most patients are asymptomatic, and the cyst is found on a chest radiograph or CT as an unexpected finding. Their CT density is usually in the range of water, but may be higher or lower.[207, 218] CT density up to 50 H represents hemorrhage or cellular debris within the cyst, whereas low values down to −30 H may indicate cholesterol deposits within the cyst. Thymic cysts should appear intense on T2-weighted images, as seen in one case we have observed (Fig. 2–58).

On CT, the wall of a thymic cyst is invariably thin (1 to 2 mm thick) and sharply defined. It can enhance following a bolus of intravenous contrast material. Most cysts are unilocular, but multilocular cysts have also been described.[237] Thymic cysts are not uncommonly surrounded by a small amount of thymic tissue.

REBOUND THYMIC HYPERPLASIA

The thymus involutes and diminishes in size in response to systemic stress, such as chemotherapy, burns, surgery, or high glucocorticoid levels in Cushing's syndrome.[238, 243] Rebound hyperplasia with enlargement to greater than normal size can occur in children and adults following removal of the stress, or discontinuation of chemotherapy.[239–242] Choyke and colleagues[244] found regrowth of the involuted thymus in all young patients following chemotherapy and a rebound increase, to a volume 50 per cent greater than baseline, in about 20 per cent of their patients. Kissin and co-workers[245] found a similar occurrence in 11.6 per cent of patients studied by CT, 3 to 14 months after initiation of chemotherapy.

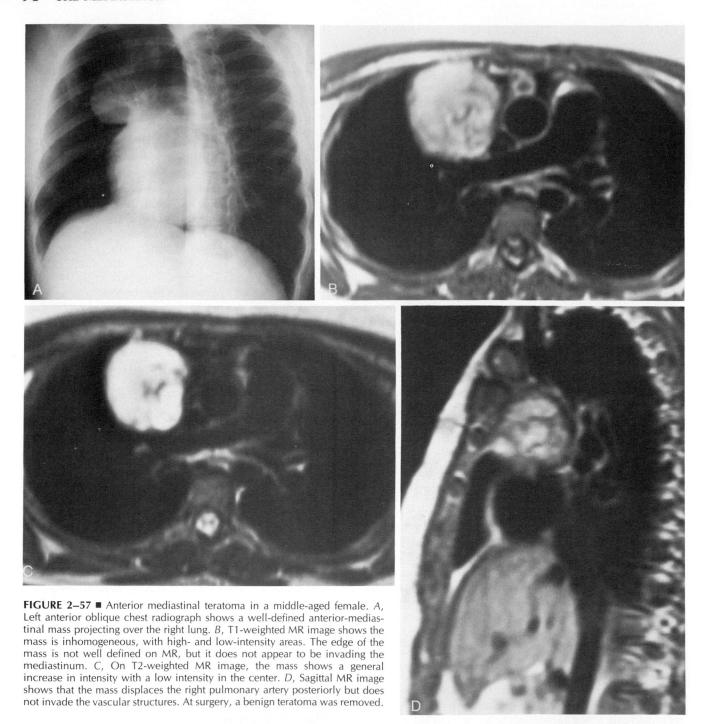

FIGURE 2–57 ■ Anterior mediastinal teratoma in a middle-aged female. *A,* Left anterior oblique chest radiograph shows a well-defined anterior-mediastinal mass projecting over the right lung. *B,* T1-weighted MR image shows the mass is inhomogeneous, with high- and low-intensity areas. The edge of the mass is not well defined on MR, but it does not appear to be invading the mediastinum. *C,* On T2-weighted MR image, the mass shows a general increase in intensity with a low intensity in the center. *D,* Sagittal MR image shows that the mass displaces the right pulmonary artery posteriorly but does not invade the vascular structures. At surgery, a benign teratoma was removed.

The CT appearance of the enlarged thymus is similar to that of other causes of thymic hyperplasia, usually with preservation of the bilobed shape of the thymus. The importance of this finding is to distinguish rebound thymic hyperplasia from metastases to the anterior mediastinum, or lymphomatous involvement of the mediastinal nodes and thymus.

Mediastinal Abnormalities

MEDIASTINAL GOITER

Mediastinal goiters constitute 5 to 10 per cent of all resected mediastinal masses.[237, 246] They are most commonly found in the pretracheal space but can occur anywhere in the mediastinum.[247] In most patients, aberrant thyroid tissue is biologically active and will concentrate radioiodine.[248] In practice, however, nuclear imaging can detect less than 50 per cent of mediastinal goiters, and routine nuclear scanning of mediastinal masses has not become accepted. Most patients with a mediastinal goiter have CT as part of their evaluation for a mediastinal mass. If the diagnosis of goiter can be made, surgery is often obviated.

The thyroid gland is readily evaluated by CT.[247, 249–252] The attenuation values of thyroid tissue are usually greater than those of soft tissue, ranging intravenous contrast material; and the typical location in the pretracheal space (Fig. 2–59).

Multinodular goiters are usually equal to or lower in intensity than the normal thyroid on T1-weighted images and high in intensity on T2-weighted images.[170, 253] The high intensity on T2 weighting is due to adenomatous hyperplasia within the goiter. High intensity on T1-weighted images can be from subacute hemorrhage or proteinaceous fluid within a colloid cyst (Fig. 2–60).[254, 255] In most circumstances, mediastinal goiters are inhomogeneous on T2-weighted images and less so on T1 weighting. Coronal images are useful for displaying mediastinal goiters because they can demonstrate both the cervical and thoracic components of the goiter.[256] A disadvantage of MR is its inability to display calcification within a goiter. However, displacement of

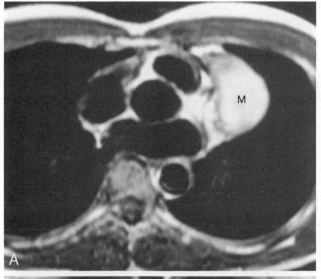

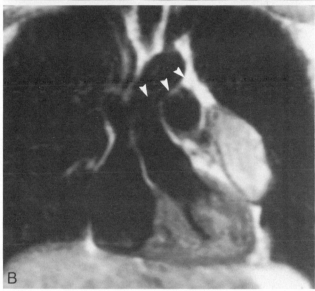

FIGURE 2–58 ■ Congenital thymic cyst in an asymptomatic adult male. *A*, Cardiac-gated MR image demonstrates a mass to the left of the base of the heart. The mass (M) is homogeneous and appears not to be infiltrating the mediastinum. *B*, Coronal MR image shows a plane of cleavage *(arrowheads)* between the mass and the heart, probably representing the pericardium. (Courtesy of Clark Carrol, MD, Houston, TX.)

from 57 ± 11 H in patients having chronic thyroiditis to 112 ± 10 H in normal individuals. As Kaneko and colleagues[249] have shown, only in patients with hypothyroidism does the density of the thyroid approach that of normal soft tissue.

Aberrant thyroid tissue, in either the neck or the mediastinum, can be diagnosed with CT because of the initial high CT density of the mass.[247, 253] In virtually all patients, mediastinal goiters are extensions from a cervical multinodular goiter into the pretracheal space.[250, 251] Additional features that suggest the diagnosis include well-defined borders of the mass; punctate, coarse, or ring calcifications; inhomogeneity with nonenhancing, low-density sites; marked, rapid, and prolonged enhancement of the mass by at least 25 H following administration of

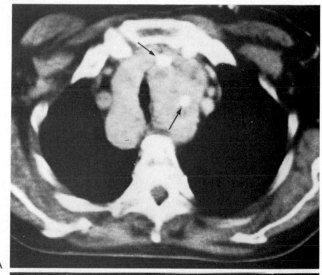

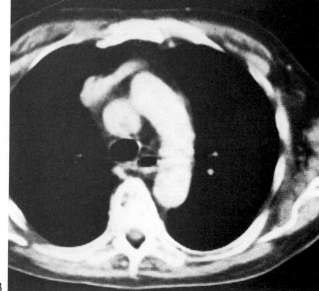

FIGURE 2–59 ■ Mediastinal extension of a goiter discovered incidentally on a chest radiograph. *A*, CT scan shows the goiter surrounding and compressing the upper intrathoracic trachea. Focal calcifications *(arrows)* were not apparent on chest radiographs. *B*, During infusion of contrast material, the mass (lower in the pretracheal space) demonstrates pronounced, immediate contrast enhancement.

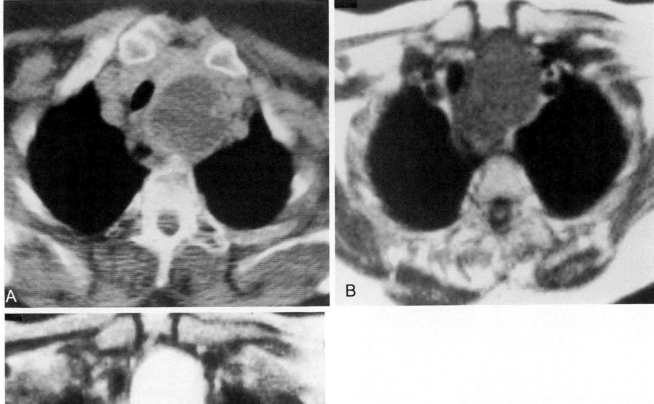

FIGURE 2–60 ■ Mediastinal extension of a goiter. *A*, CT scan shows an inhomogeneous mass with a lower-density center in the upper mediastinum, displacing the trachea and esophagus from left to right. *B*, T1-weighted MR image shows the mass as inhomogeneous. The great vessels displaced toward the left are better seen than on CT scan. *C*, On T2 weighting, the mass shows a marked increase in signal intensity, greater than that of fat, owing to a colloid cyst within the goiter.

mediastinal vessels, the trachea, and the esophagus is clearly depicted with MR.

Most patients with an intrathoracic goiter are asymptomatic, and the abnormality is detected on a routine chest radiograph. Occasionally, symptoms of airway or esophageal compression are experienced. The combination of findings on CT or MR is sufficiently characteristic for the diagnosis to be made in most instances.

MEDIASTINAL PARATHYROID ABNORMALITIES

Accessory parathyroid tissue may be present anywhere between the cricoid cartilage and the root of the aorta. In fact, 2 per cent of normal parathyroid glands are in the mediastinum. Most are in the upper prevascular space, but occasionally they can be in the middle or posterior mediastinum.[257, 258] Normal

mediastinal parathyroid glands are too small to be recognized on CT.

Neck exploration with resection of parathyroid tissue usually cures primary hyperparathyroidism, and the incidence of persistent hyperparathyroidism after surgery is only 1.4 to 5.4 per cent.[259] Persistent hyperparathyroidism can be due to parathyroid hyperplasia with insufficient tissue having been removed, or to failure to remove a functioning parathyroid adenoma. Determining the site of abnormal parathyroid hormone production in patients with persistent hyperparathyroidism is often difficult. Many imaging techniques have been advocated, including selective arteriography, venous sampling, ultrasound, CT, MR, and technetium/thallium scintigraphy.[260, 261]

A small percentage of parathyroid adenomas occupy the mediastinum, and the majority of these are less than 2 cm in diameter. CT can demonstrate mediastinal adenomas in 29 to 80 per cent of cases (Fig. 2–61).[257, 258, 260, 262] This wide range in the detection rate probably reflects differences in scanner capabilities. Mediastinal parathyroid adenomas tend to be extremely vascular, and enhancement with an intravenous bolus of contrast material probably occurs in the majority of them.

On MR most parathyroid adenomas are low in signal intensity on T1-weighted images (Fig. 2–61) and markedly increase in intensity on T2-weighted images.[263] About 10 per cent of adenomas are of low intensity on both T1- and T2-weighted images, and occasionally an adenoma is intense with both se-quences. The mediastinal adenoma appears as a well-circumscribed mass, usually in the anterior medias-tinum near the thoracic inlet in close proximity to the great vessels or in front of the ascending aorta. Limited studies show that about 75 per cent of mediastinal adenomas are detected with MR.[256, 263]

In patients with persistent hyperparathyroidism following neck exploration, a combination of nonin-vasive studies is indicated.[260, 261] High-resolution ul-trasound and thallium/technetium scintigraphy de-tect most cervical adenomas. If one or both of these are negative, CT and MR should be obtained and should employ high-resolution techniques of both the neck and mediastinum. Selective venous sam-pling for parathyroid hormone assay and angiogra-

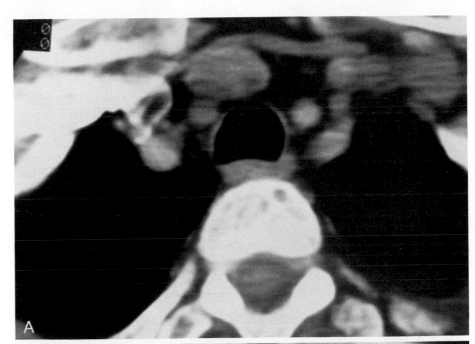

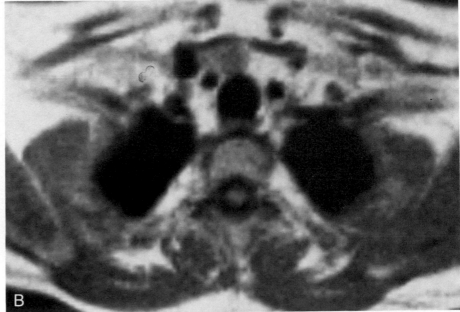

FIGURE 2–61 ■ Superior mediastinal para-thyroid adenoma in a patient with recurrent hyperparathyroidism following neck explo-ration. *A*, CT scan demonstrates a 2-cm mass immediately in front of the trachea. *B*, T1-weighted MR at the same level dem-onstrates the mass, which is low in signal intensity and can be readily distinguished from mediastinal fat.

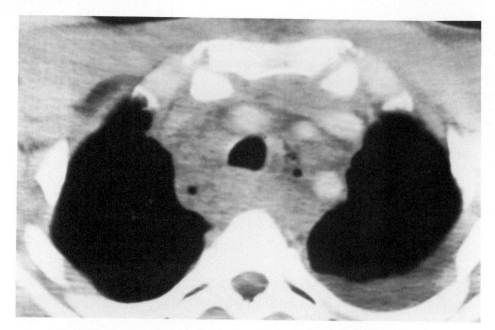

FIGURE 2–62 ■ Acute mediastinitis following cardiac surgery. CT scan through the upper mediastinum demonstrates diffuse mediastinal widening, with gas bubbles visible in the soft tissues of the mediastinum. The normal low density of fat is replaced by inhomogeneous, higher-density soft tissue. A left pleural effusion is present. Intravascular contrast material opacifies the vessels.

phy generally should be reserved for those instances when an adenoma has still not been localized.

MEDIASTINITIS AND MEDIASTINAL ABSCESS

Infections of the mediastinum are uncommon compared with those of the abdomen or of the lung. Rupture or perforation of the esophagus is the cause of acute mediastinitis in over 90 per cent of cases. The remaining 10 per cent are due to an infected median sternotomy, extension of infection from the neck, trauma to the pharynx or trachea (including tracheostomy), penetrating chest wounds, disruption of surgical anastomoses, and complication of oral surgery.[264-266] The responsible organisms are usually a mixture of pyogenic bacteria, including anaerobes, and gram-positive and gram-negative bacilli. Acute mediastinitis is often life-threatening and produces impressive clinical manifestations. Swift diagnosis and appropriate therapy, including prompt surgical drainage, are mandatory. Description of the CT findings of acute mediastinitis and of mediastinal abscess are limited.[267-269] CT usually demonstrates diffuse mediastinal widening, with obliteration of the normal fat planes or a focal mass with ill-defined edges. Low-density sites represent areas of necrosis. Gas bubbles or a gas collection strongly suggests

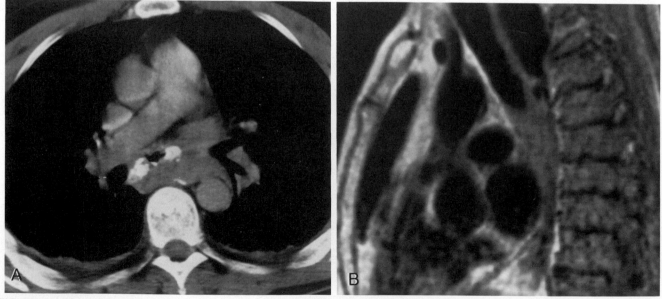

FIGURE 2–63 ■ Mediastinal abscess in a man with dysphagia. *A*, CT scan demonstrates a subcarinal mass with an irregular air-containing space. High-density areas are residual barium from a previous esophagram. *B*, Sagittal MR demonstrates the mass behind the right pulmonary artery, above the left atrium, and below the tracheal carina. At mediastinal exploration, a perforated esophagus with a mediastinal abscess, due to a fish bone, was found.

acute pyogenic mediastinitis or an abscess (Figs. 2–62 and 2–63). If an abscess contains gas, the inner margin of the wall usually is shaggy and thick. The abscess wall frequently enhances following administration of intravascular contrast material.

Fibrosing mediastinitis is characterized by an excessive fibrotic reaction within the mediastinum.[270] It is most commonly the result of infection with histoplasmosis but has been seen with tuberculosis, lymphatic obstruction, and as an autoimmune disease.[271, 272] The fibrosis can produce a solid mediastinal mass or can be progressive, with encasement, compression, and occlusion of the SVC, tracheobronchial tree, esophagus, or pulmonary vessels. Both CT and MR can provide important information as to the extent of the process and can collaborate on the diagnosis.

CT demonstrates one or more ill-defined masses, usually between 2 and 5 cm in diameter.[273] The mid-mediastinum and adjacent subcarinal space are most commonly involved. Extension into one or both hila occurs frequently. Calcification, which is stippled or dense, usually is present, scattered throughout the mass or masses. Narrowing or obstruction of mediastinal vessels and of the aerodigestive tracts can be a prominent feature. Intravascular contrast material assists in demonstrating the site of vascular narrowing and collateral venous channels (Fig. 2–64). When bronchial narrowing is present, postobstructive lung consolidation may lead to an erroneous diagnosis of a lung neoplasm with mediastinal invasion.

Rholl and colleagues[274] used MR to study seven patients with fibrosing mediastinitis. They found that

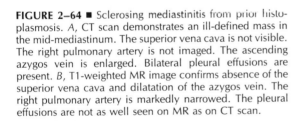

FIGURE 2–64 ■ Sclerosing mediastinitis from prior histoplasmosis. A, CT scan demonstrates an ill-defined mass in the mid-mediastinum. The superior vena cava is not visible. The right pulmonary artery is not imaged. The ascending azygos vein is enlarged. Bilateral pleural effusions are present. B, T1-weighted MR image confirms absence of the superior vena cava and dilatation of the azygos vein. The right pulmonary artery is markedly narrowed. The pleural effusions are not as well seen on MR as on CT scan.

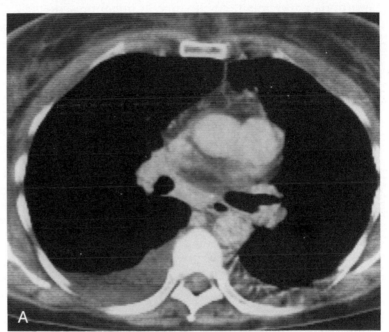
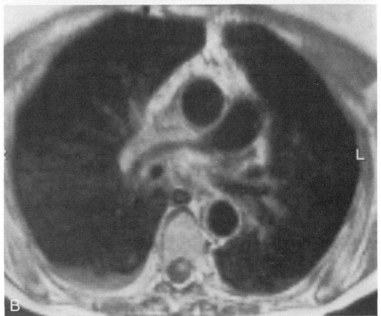

MR provided complementary information regarding vascular compromise. Although MR does not demonstrate calcification, important in the diagnosis, it does show that the masses are low in intensity on T1- and T2-weighted images, suggesting their benign nature.[275]

Bronchogenic Carcinoma

Bronchogenic carcinoma is the most common fatal malignancy in both men and women and is a leading cause of death in the industrialized world. Although the increasing incidence is tapering off in men, it continues at an alarming rate in women.[275, 276] Surgical removal of all the tumor, with or without adjuvant radiotherapy or chemotherapy, currently offers the only hope for cure. Thus, precise determination of the extent of the tumor is essential for planning appropriate treatment. At the time of initial presentation, about 60 per cent of bronchogenic carcinomas are nonresectable, judged by symptoms, clinical presentation, and investigation short of thoracotomy. Of the remainder, occult metastases can be detected in about one third with imaging studies such as CT, MR, and radionuclear scintigraphy.

Over 95 per cent of bronchogenic carcinomas arise from bronchial or bronchiolar epithelial or glandular elements. They constitute the four main types of bronchogenic carcinoma: squamous cell carcinoma, adenocarcinoma, large-cell carcinoma, and small-cell carcinoma. Alveolar-bronchiolar cell carcinoma is a variant of adenocarcinoma. Poorly differentiated or undifferentiated forms of the listed types compose about 20 per cent of bronchogenic carcinomas. Small-cell bronchogenic carcinoma (SCBC) frequently is disseminated at the time of presentation and is generally not considered with the others, which are grouped together as non–small-cell bronchogenic carcinoma (NSCBC). New, aggressive, combined surgical and chemotherapeutic approaches to SCBC show some promise for localized disease but are mainly experimental.[277, 278] In general, discussion of imaging, staging, and therapy is limited to NSCBC. Imaging of bronchogenic carcinoma requires evaluation of the lungs, mediastinum, pleura, chest wall, and upper abdomen. The CT and MR imaging of bronchogenic cancer is also discussed in Chapters 1, 3, and 4.

STAGING CLASSIFICATIONS

Imaging of NSCBC requires a precise delineation of the extent of the tumor. The American Joint Committee for Cancer Staging and End-Results Reporting (AJC) has developed a system for classifying the anatomic extent of cancer, including NSCBC.[279] The staging system was revised for bronchogenic carcinoma in 1986 to reflect the changing surgical approaches to advanced local disease.[280] The staging classification has several purposes. It allows uniform description of the extent of the tumor; comparison of various modes of therapy; prediction of prognosis; and increasingly, decisions on suitability of treatment including thoracotomy.

The AJC classification uses the well-known tumor-nodal involvement metastasis (TNM) method of staging. Imaging techniques are incorporated primarily into the initial clinical-diagnostic portion of the system. T describes the extent of the primary tumor, N the presence of regional lymph node metastasis, and M the presence of extrathoracic metastases (Table 2–3). The system does not consider the histologic type of NSCBC, even though it is known to affect the outcome. Tumors are divided into four stages, based on their anatomic extent (Table 2–3). The changes in the 1986 AJC revision for NSCBC mainly separate advanced local disease amenable to surgical resection from those carcinomas that are nonresectable.[280] The previous three stages are replaced by four. Also, stage III is divided into IIIA, which designates carcinomas that are potentially resectable, and IIIB, which describes carcinomas that are generally considered nonresectable (Table 2–3). When the TNM classification is used for NSCBC, the 5-year survival rate decreases as the stage increases, from about 65 per cent for stage I to less than 10 per cent for stage IV.[281, 282]

The role of CT and MR in evaluating patients with bronchogenic carcinoma is multifaceted and complex. In most circumstances, patients with NSCBC have one of these two studies performed. A comparison of the two procedures is considered later in this section. A survey of thoracic surgeons has shown wide variation in the circumstances in which they order CT and use the results.[283] This reflects marked differences in (1) the surgical approach to NSCBC; (2) differences in sampling tumor at various sites such as the mediastinal nodes; and (3) the reliability with which the results of CT and MR are considered by surgeons.

MEDIASTINAL INVASION

NSCBC arising near the mediastinum can invade directly into the mediastinum by contiguous spread across the pleura. Tumor that involves the parietal mediastinal pleura or pericardium without invasion of the aerodigestive organs, mediastinal vessels, or heart is classified as T3 and is considered by many surgeons to be resectable (Fig. 2–65). Invasion of these mediastinal organs by the carcinoma is classified as T4, and the carcinoma is generally nonresectable (Fig. 2–66A and B). Both CT and MR can sometimes demonstrate the extent of mediastinal invasion by a tumor. This distinction between T3 and T4 mediastinal tumor invasion is of critical importance in the decision whether to perform a thoracotomy. In many instances of T4 tumors CT and MR demonstrate encasement, narrowing, or obstruction of mediastinal organs or tumor crossing the midline and can therefore reliably indicate that the tumor is nonresectable. For instance, a carcinoma causing SVC obstruction, whether clinically evident or not, is nonresectable. Direct tumor involvement

TABLE 2–3 ■ TNM Staging of Lung Cancer

T (PRIMARY TUMOR)

T0	No evidence of primary tumor
T1	Tumor 3 cm or less in greatest diameter, limited to lung, with no invasion proximal to lobar bronchus
T2	Tumor > 3 cm, invades visceral pleura or produces collapse or consolidation of less than entire lung, must be > 2 cm distal to the carina
T3	Tumor focally invading parietal pleura, chest wall, diaphragm, or mediastinal pleura or pericardium; < 2 cm from the carina or producing collapse on consolidation of entire lung
T4	Tumor of any size involving heart, great vessels, trachea, esophagus, vertebral body, or carina, or producing malignant pleural effusion

N (NODAL INVOLVEMENT)

N0	No nodal metastases
N1	Metastases to ipsilateral hilar nodes
N2	Metastases to ipsilateral mediastinal nodes or subcarinal nodes
N3	Metastases to contralateral hilar or mediastinal lymph nodes or scalene or supraclavicular lymph nodes

M (DISTANT METASTASES)

M0	Metastases absent
M1	Metastases present

RESECTABLE STAGES				UNRESECTABLE STAGES			
Stage I	T1	N0	M0	Stage IIIB	Any T	N3	M0
	T2	N0	M0		T4	Any N	M0
Stage II	T1	N1	M0	Stage IV	Any T	Any N	M1
	T2	N1	M0				
Stage IIIA	T3	N0	M0				
	T3	N1	M0				
	T1	N2	M0				
	T2	N2	M0				
	T3	N2	M0				

of the aortic-pulmonic window may be surgically removed if the recurrent laryngeal nerve is not involved; tumor at this site indicates the need for careful laryngoscopic evaluation of the vocal cords.

Local mediastinal invasion by a T3 carcinoma causing obliteration of fat planes can sometimes be difficult to detect with CT. The CT density of a bronchogenic carcinoma may be similar to that of mediastinal fat, and the accuracy of CT in showing this type of spread has been only moderate. T1-weighted MR images show better contrast between tumor and fat

and can probably distinguish between T3 and T4 tumors more easily than CT scans, although this is difficult to prove statistically.[283a]

Several groups have investigated the ability of CT and MR to predict mediastinal invasion by a contiguous carcinoma and thus its resectability.[284–289] Scott and co-investigators[288] found that CT predicted pericardial invasion in only one of three cases and all three were resected at surgery. Glazer and colleagues[289] used the following as their CT criteria for resectability of paramediastinal tumor otherwise in-

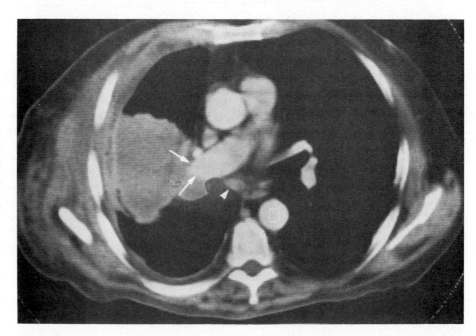

FIGURE 2–65 ■ Locally advanced T3 bronchogenic carcinoma. CT scan shows a large right lung mass contiguous with the right pulmonary artery (arrows), causing blurring of the margin of the arterial wall. An enlarged lymph node (arrowhead) is visible in the subcarinal space. At surgery, the tumor could be peeled off the pulmonary artery. The lymph node showed reactive hyperplasia.

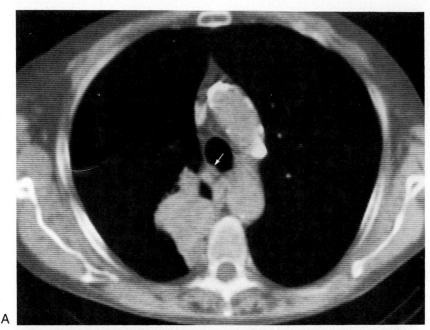

A

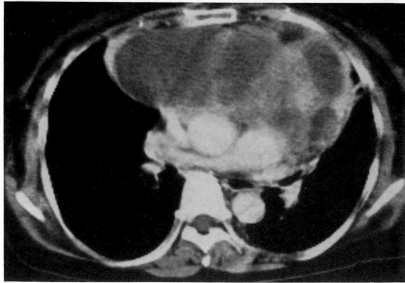

B

FIGURE 2–66 ■ Nonresectable T4 bronchogenic carcinoma in two patients. *A*, Right upper lobe carcinoma invades the mediastinum and produces thickening of the tracheal wall *(arrow)*. At bronchoscopy, biopsy of the tracheal wall at this site revealed invasion by the tumor. *B*, Massive necrotic anterior mediastinal squamous carcinoma that arose in the left lung. The vascular structures of the mediastinum are displaced posteriorly. Low-density areas represent sites of necrosis. (*B* courtesy of S. Landon, MD, Oakland, CA.)

determinate for invasion: (1) 3 cm or less contact between the tumor and the mediastinum, (2) less than a 90° circumferential contact between the tumor and the aorta, and (3) the presence of a clear plane of mediastinal fat between the tumor mass and mediastinal structures. Ninety-seven per cent of masses with one or more of these criteria were resectable; three fourths did not in fact invade the mediastinum, and the others had limited invasion. In general, the accuracy of CT for mediastinal invasion has only been between 50 and 70 per cent.[284–289] Even though from our experience MR appears better than this, it gives only marginally better results than CT, even for tumor invasion of vascular structures.[283a, 284, 285, 290]

BRONCHIAL TUMOR

CT detection of endobronchial tumor and sites of bronchial obstruction or narrowing is highly accurate

and can assist the bronchoscopist in selecting sites for bronchial biopsy. CT has higher spatial resolution than MR and is better for diagnosing endobronchial tumor. Bronchogenic carcinoma more than 2 cm distal to the tracheal carina is classified as T2 and can usually be resected by pneumectomy. Quint and colleagues,[291] in using CT to predict whether lobectomy or pneumectomy would be required for resection of a central NSCBC, found that CT frequently could not predict proximal submuscular extension of tumor. This is an important observation that should not be overlooked in interpreting CT scans of endobronchial tumor. Carcinomas close to the tracheal carina (classified as T3) can be resected. In fact, they can be resected even if the lower ipsilateral trachea is involved. Improved surgical techniques allow for reimplantation of the contralateral main bronchus into the resected lower trachea. Tumor crossing the midline to involve the tracheal carina and contralateral main stem bronchus, is classified as T4 and is nonresectable. The ability of CT or MR to accurately predict proximal bronchial extension of bronchogenic carcinoma is not known. Visible tumor is evident at bronchoscopy or surgery and should be assessed during those procedures. The endoscopist should always be made aware of the precise location of extratracheal or extrabronchial masses that could be biopsied by a transbronchial approach.[292]

MEDIASTINAL LYMPH NODE METASTASES

The size, distribution, and CT and MR appearance of normal lymph nodes in the mediastinum have been discussed earlier in this chapter. For practical purposes, lymph nodes that measure more than 10 mm in transverse diameter on CT or MR are considered abnormal. In about 5 per cent of normal individuals, however, a normal node is found that measures up to 15 mm and occasionally a normal node up to 20 mm is found. It is often assumed that all lymph nodes larger than 10 mm in diameter can be demonstrated with CT or MR. This is incorrect. In a study presented by Webb and colleagues,[56] involving about 160 patients with NSCBC, nodes up to 25 mm in diameter were missed by either CT or MR, or both. The likelihood of metastases in mediastinal lymph nodes in patients with bronchogenic carcinoma, the so-called "prior probability of disease being present," is important. In patients selected for CT or MR investigation, the incidence of nodal metastases is probably 20 to 40 per cent.[293–295] Patient selection may greatly affect this incidence. Nevertheless, studies with markedly different incidences should be viewed with suspicion as containing a skewed population. In patients with clinically resectable bronchogenic carcinoma, the incidence of normal-sized nodes containing tumor shown on CT or MR is difficult to determine, but probably ranges between 5 and 15 per cent.[56, 276, 296]

Mediastinal lymph nodes are less intense than mediastinal fat on T1-weighted spin-echo images because of their considerably longer T1 relaxation values. T1-weighted images are thus the most useful for detecting lymph nodes. The ability of MR potentially to discriminate between enlarged nodes containing tumor and benign enlarged nodes has been investigated.[53, 297] The T1 relaxation times of malignant nodes average out to be longer than those of benign nodes, both in vivo and in vitro. The overlap between benign and malignant nodes however precludes this finding from being of clinical value. The addition of gadolinium-DTPA as an intravascular contrast does not assist in separating benign from malignant nodes.

The lobe of origin of an NSCBC will partially determine the mediastinal nodal groups to which the tumor will metastasize.[298–330] Right upper lobe carcinomas tend to metastasize to the ipsilateral, right paratracheal, azygos, and precarinal nodes, usually after involving the upper and midhilar nodes. Only about 10 per cent cross the midline to the left pretra-

cheal nodes or prevascular anterior mediastinal nodes. Right lower lobe carcinomas metastasize more widely to the right hilar, pretracheal, subcarinal, precarinal, and inferior ligament nodes. Left upper lobe NSCBC with mediastinal involvement spreads to both left and right sides of the mediastinum in about 35 per cent of instances. Left lower lobe carcinomas metastasize most widely, to almost all nodal groups.

Detection of enlarged mediastinal nodes can have significant impact on the subsequent handling of the patient with suspected NSCBC. There are three commonly used methods for sampling mediastinal lymph nodes: cervical mediastinoscopy for pretracheal and paratracheal nodes; parasternal mediastinotomy for aortic-pulmonic and preaortic nodes; and transbronchial bronchoscopic needle biopsy.[292, 301, 302] The accuracy of these techniques is only about 80 per cent, because most surgeons sample only enlarged nodes, thus missing intracapsular metastases. Also each approach is capable of sampling only a small percentage of mediastinal nodes. The decisions to sample mediastinal nodes and the approach are often based on the results of CT and MR.[283] If no enlarged nodes are present, most thoracic surgeons forego a sampling procedure prior to thoracotomy. With the revised AJC classification, tumor within nodes ipsilateral to the carcinoma itself or in the subcarinal region is designated N2 (stage IIIA) and does not preclude curative resection. Several studies have shown 30 to 45 per cent 5-year survival rates for patients with N2 nodes, treated by resection and mediastinal stripping, and usually adjuvant radiotherapy.[303, 304] The presence of enlarged contralateral N3 nodes (stage IIIB) thus is of critical importance. N3 NSCBC is considered by virtually all thoracic surgeons to constitute nonresectable disease (Figs. 2–67 and 2–68). It is thus essential to detect and make known to the surgeon the presence of contralateral adenopathy that should be sampled by the most appropriate method.

COMPARISON OF IMAGING MODALITIES

Chest radiographs and conventional tomograms have a sensitivity of only about 50 per cent for detecting mediastinal lymph node metastases from bronchogenic carcinoma. Their specificity however is high, and most patients have nonresectable N3 disease when mediastinal widening is present on a chest radiograph (Fig. 2–69). CT should nevertheless be obtained to exclude benign causes for the mediastinal widening and to demonstrate possible diffuse infiltration of the mediastinum by tumor. Tumor diffusely infiltrating the mediastinum shows replacement of mediastinal fat by tumor and encasement of vessels and airways. Although extracapsular (i.e., extranodal) mediastinal tumor is well known, it has received scant description in the radiology literature. CT and MR can detect this entity and obviate further unnecessary investigation. CT in this circumstance can also aid in the planning of radiation therapy.

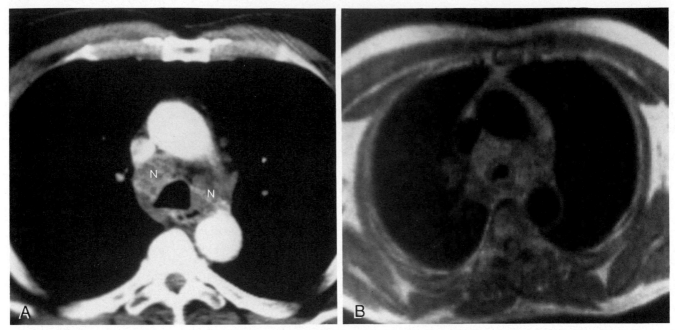

FIGURE 2–67 ■ N3 contralateral mediastinal lymph nodes from a left lower lobe bronchogenic carcinoma. *A*, CT scan following contrast material injection demonstrates enlarged lymph nodes (N) in the aortic-pulmonic window and in the pretracheal space, on the right side. *B*, T1-weighted MR shows replacement of mediastinal fat by enlarged lymph nodes on both sides of the mediastinum. Biopsy of these nodes at mediastinoscopy revealed metastatic adenocarcinoma.

Both CT and MR are capable of showing enlarged lymph nodes within the mediastinum. Neither, though, can distinguish between metastasis and benign reactive hyperplastic nodal enlargement. CT can demonstrate benign calcification within nodes enlarged from prior granulomatous disease, a finding not seen with MR. The sensitivity, specificity, and accuracy of CT and MR for the detection of medias-

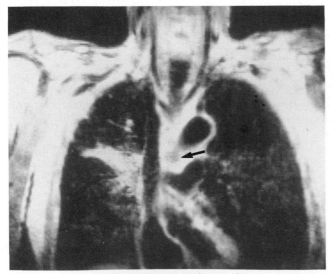

FIGURE 2–68 ■ Contralateral N3 nodes in the aortic-pulmonic window. Coronal MR demonstrates atelectasis of the anterior segment of the right upper lobe due to an endobronchial tumor. A contralateral N3 node *(arrow)* is visible deep in the aortic-pulmonic window. Biopsy of this node demonstrated metastatic tumor, making the tumor nonresectable.

tinal nodal metastases from NSCBCs have been extensively investigated.[56, 91, 284–286, 305–329] The results of early CT studies (1978–1985) are in general at variance with the results of later ones (1986–1990). Most of the early studies showed a sensitivity and specificity of 0.75 to 0.95 and an accuracy of 0.80 to 0.90. These optimistic results reflect early studies with biased patient selection, small sample sizes, and enthusiastic investigators. Later studies have been much less encouraging and have shown considerably less promising results. Most later studies have larger study populations, better control of their results, and more precise definitions of abnormality. The general results for the later studies give sensitivities and specificities of 0.50 to 0.65 and accuracy of about 0.60. MR studies have given very similar results.[283a] The interpretation of a patient's scan regarding the likelihood of mediastinal lymph node metastases must thus be extremely circumspect. Even nodes up to 4 cm in diameter can be benign or missed with CT and MR, and nodes of normal size can contain tumor.[296] Emphasis should be on those nodes that are likely to contain tumor and should be biopsied. It is clear that additional research should be undertaken to better characterize mediastinal lymph nodes.

RESECTABILITY OF BRONCHOGENIC CARCINOMA

The staging of bronchogenic carcinoma cannot be directly translated into surgical resectability. For the individual patient with bronchogenic carcinoma, the physician's decision as to whether resection should be attempted is complex.[330] The aggressive attitudes of surgeons toward such an operation varies widely, and the presence of tumor in low or high mediastinal

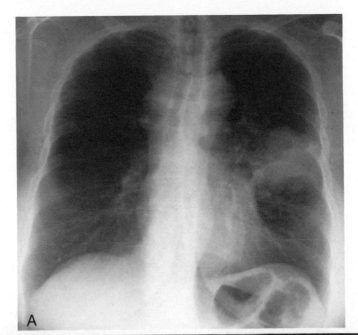

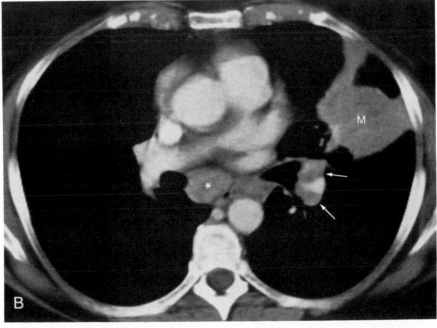

FIGURE 2–69 ■ Nonresectable bronchogenic carcinoma with contralateral mediastinal adenopathy. *A,* Chest radiograph shows a large mass in the left midlung. Widening of the right paratracheal stripe is seen. *B,* CT scan through the midthorax, following intravenous contrast material injection, demonstrates the left lung mass (M) and left hilar adenopathy. Lymph nodes are seen in the subcarinal space *(asterisk)* and behind the left main bronchus. Other scans demonstrated the right paratracheal adenopathy. In the presence of bronchogenic carcinoma, the large size and distribution of these lymph nodes make the likelihood of metastases high.

lymph nodes remains controversial. Mountain[331] has summarized the current variations in the approach to advanced local disease. Concomitant disease, age, symptoms, and the presence of distant metastases must all be taken into consideration. An excellent review of the problem by Mittman and Bruderman[330] is available. Recommendations based solely on CT or MR findings therefore are inadequate. CT and MR have a role in the evaluation of bronchogenic carcinoma, although the limitations and pitfalls in interpretation of both types of images must be fully appreciated.

Whether well-differentiated squamous cell carcinomas or adenocarcinomas that manifest as peripheral nodules should be studied with CT or MR is also controversial. When the chest radiograph shows a normal mediastinum, the incidence of spread of these tumors in mediastinal nodes is low. The probability that small mediastinal lymph nodes detected only by CT contain tumor is also low, and many surgeons resect regional nodes in these patients. One study,[332] however, showed significant findings with CT in 5 of 31 patients, whereas another study[333] showed significant mediastinal lymphadenopathy in only 1 of 23 patients.

Lymphoma

The malignant lymphomas are part of a spectrum of lymphoproliferative disorders, all of which can involve the thorax. A histologic classification (Table 2–4) is most widely used but should be replaced

TABLE 2–4 ■ Classification of Malignant Lymphomas

RYE CLASSIFICATION OF HODGKIN'S DISEASE

Histologic Findings	Prevalence (%)	
	Adults	Children
Lymphocytic predominance	5-10	11
Nodular sclerosis	50-80	65
Mixed cellularity	15-40	18
Lymphocytic depletion	5-10	1
Unclassified	<5	5

NCI CLASSIFICATION OF NON-HODGKIN'S LYMPHOMAS

Histologic Findings	Prevalence (%)
Low-grade malignant lymphomas	
Small lymphocytic consistent with chronic lymphocytic leukemia, plasmacytoid	3.6
Follicular, small cleaved cell	22.5
Follicular, mixed cell	7.7
Intermediate-grade malignant lymphoma	
Follicular, large cell	3.8
Diffuse, small cleaved cell	6.9
Diffuse, mixed cell (small), and large cell	6.9
Diffuse, large cell (cleaved/noncleaved)	19.7
High-grade malignant lymphoma	
Immunoblastic, large cell	7.9
Lymphoblastic, large cell	4.2
Small noncleaved cell (Burkitt's/non-Burkitt's)	5.0
Miscellaneous	
Mycosis fungoides, histiocytic, extramedullary, unclassifiable, others	11.2

when lymphoid function is better understood.[334, 335] At the time of presentation, 65 to 70 per cent of patients with Hodgkin's lymphoma have intrathoracic disease, the mediastinum being involved in 90 per cent.[336, 337] The mediastinum is the only site of Hodgkin's lymphoma in about 25 per cent of all patients. Non-Hodgkin's lymphoma is usually a more widespread disease at presentation, with thoracic involvement in only 40 per cent of patients and isolated mediastinal disease in less than 10 per cent. Hodgkin's disease is staged according to the extent of disease and whether symptoms are present (Table 2–5).[334, 335] Hodgkin's disease has a 75 to 80 per cent cure rate for all stages,[338] and there is a closer correlation between the stage and prognosis for Hodgkin's lymphoma than for non-Hodgkin's lymphoma. Patients with stages I and II Hodgkin's disease have a 98 per cent 5-year survival rate (disease-free, 78 per cent) without mediastinal disease and an 88 per cent 5-year survival rate (disease-free, 66 per cent) with it. Patients with stage III Hodgkin's disease, on the other hand, have only a 75 per cent 5-year survival rate.[337]

Survival, especially in Hodgkin's lymphoma, is directly related to early and adequate treatment.[338, 339] In most instances, treatment is with radiation alone for local disease, and chemotherapy and radiation for disseminated disease.[161, 338] New protocols for treating patients with malignant lymphoma are being developed continually. For the

therapy to be appropriate, extensive evaluation of lymph nodes and potentially affected organs must be undertaken. Among the nonradiologic investigations are hematologic and bone marrow studies and sampling of tissues from abdominal organs, lymph nodes at multiple sites, and the spleen. Radiologic studies include chest radiographs, isotope studies, lung and mediastinal CT or MR, and lymphangiography.

Hodgkin's disease is more predictable in its behavior than non-Hodgkin's lymphoma, because it tends to spread to contiguous nodal chains.[339a] This pattern is reflected in the chest radiograph. The most common finding in intrathoracic lymphoma is mediastinal lymph node enlargement. Filly, Blank, and Castellino,[336] in a study of 300 patients with untreated malignant lymphoma, found radiographically demonstrated intrathoracic disease in 67 per cent of the patients with Hodgkin's disease and in 43 per cent of patients with non-Hodgkin's lymphoma. In 90 per cent of those with Hodgkin's disease and in only 46 per cent of those with non-Hodgkin's lymphoma, lymph nodes involved the prevascular and pretracheal compartments alone, or in combination with other nodal groups. Internal mammary lymph node enlargement was much more frequent in Hodgkin's disease, whereas isolated posterior mediastinal and paracardiac nodal enlargement was reported only in non-Hodgkin's lymphoma. Hilar lymphadenopathy was found in about 20 per cent of patients with mediastinal Hodgkin's disease and correlated closely with lung involvement.

Several studies have used CT to better define the distribution of intrathoracic involvement in Hodgkin's and non-Hodgkin's lymphoma.[161, 169, 340–344] The nodal groups most commonly involved are the anterior mediastinal, paratracheal, aortic-pulmonic window, hilar, subcarinal, and internal mammary groups (Fig. 2–70). Nodal sites of disease most likely to be detected by CT and not shown on chest radiographs are the subcarinal, internal mammary, and hilar nodes. Both Hodgkin's and non-Hodgkin's lym-

TABLE 2–5 ■ Ann Arbor Staging of Hodgkin's Disease

STAGE	DEFINITION
I	Involvement of a single lymph node region (I) or of a single extralymphatic organ or site (I$_E$)
II	Involvement of two or more lymph node regions on the same side of the diaphragm (II) or localized involvement of an extralymphatic organ or site and of one or more lymph node regions on the same side of the diaphgram (II$_E$)
III	Involvement of lymph node regions on both sides of the diaphragm (III), which may also be accompanied by involvement of the spleen (III$_S$), by localized involvement of an extralymphatic organ or site (III$_E$), or both (III$_{SE}$)
IV	Diffuse or disseminated involvement of one or more extralymphatic organs or tissues with or without associated lymph node involvement

The absence or presence of fever, night sweats, and/or unexplained loss of 10% or more of body weight in the 6 months preceding admission are to be denoted in all cases by the suffix letters A or B, respectively.

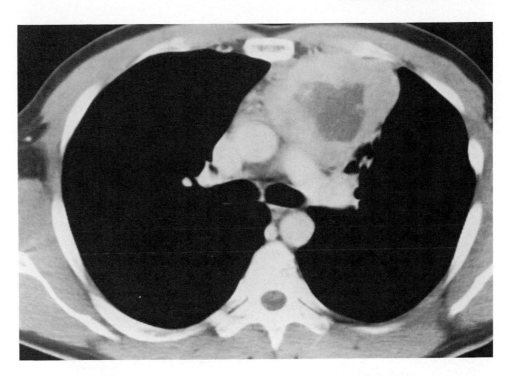

FIGURE 2–70 ■ Non-Hodgkin's lymphoma in a young male with a mediastinal mass. CT scan following injection of contrast material demonstrates a large anterior mediastinal mass. The mass shows enhancement with contrast material, with a low-density center representing necrosis within the tumor. The lymphoma was thought to have arisen within the left lobe of the thymus.

phoma have two main pathways of extranodal extension from the mediastinum. Tumor can spread from the anterior and posterior mediastinum to involve the extrapleural soft tissues of chest wall and pericardium. Pilepich and colleagues[345] found this form of spread in over 50 per cent of patients with mediastinal lymphoma. Tumor can also extend directly from the mediastinum and hila to the lymphoid tissue around the bronchi. Detection of tumor at these sites often causes the radiation ports to be changed to include the newly discovered tumor.

Heron and co-workers[227] used CT to study the size of the thymus in patients with Hodgkin's disease. The thymus was enlarged in 30 per cent of patients at initial presentation and could readily be distinguished from enlarged anterior mediastinal lymph nodes. In 50 episodes of suspected relapse of Hodgkin's lymphoma, thymic enlargement was found in 38 per cent, always in combination with enlarged mediastinal nodes. The authors emphasized that after treatment, thymic enlargement could be due to rebound hyperplasia.

The appearance on CT of nodal involvement with Hodgkin's lymphoma is distinctive. The nodes can be enlarged and discrete or form conglomerate masses. In most instances, the nodes or masses will not enhance with intravascular contrast material. Calcification within nodes containing Hodgkin's lymphoma can occur following radiation or chemotherapy. About 20 per cent of patients with Hodgkin's disease will show sites of lower CT density within their nodal masses.[345a] These patients do not have a different response rate or course compared with patients without nodal necrosis.

In general, all patients with Hodgkin's lymphoma undergo CT of the thorax, whether or not the chest radiograph is normal. Additional sites of involvement are found in up to 40 per cent, staging is changed in up to 20 per cent, and therapy is altered in up to 25 per cent.[161, 337, 342, 346]

Non-Hodgkin's lymphoma is a more diffuse and less predictable disease than Hodgkin's lymphoma. Nevertheless, Khoury and colleagues[343] found that CT showed disease not suspected from chest radiographs in 28 per cent and added significant information for all patients with suspected abnormalities. They concluded that CT was useful in untreated patients with stage I and II disease and in treated patients with radiographs suggestive of relapse.

MR has been used to study mediastinal lymphoma, both before and after treatment.[229, 230, 347] Although it was originally thought that MR may demonstrate intensity difference between lymphoma-containing nodes and normal nodes, this has not proved to be true. Several authors have shown that the intensity and T1 and T2 relaxation times for lymphoma are similar to those for other malignant diseases.[152, 155, 202] von Schulthess and colleagues[203] showed that lymphomas are usually lower than fat on T1- and T2-weighted images but occasionally show high intensity on T2 weighting (Fig. 2–71). Images obtained with fat saturation techniques can however assist in defining the extent of the adenopathy and the extranodal extension from the mediastinum extrapleurally to the chest wall (Fig. 2–72). Occasionally, high-grade malignant non-Hodgkin's lymphoma shows inhomogeneous areas of high and low intensity reflecting foci of fibrosis or necrosis.[230] On the other hand, most low-grade non-Hodgkin's lymphomas have a homogeneous signal intensity pattern.[347a] Others have found no differences in MR imaging characteristics between high- and low-grade lymphomas.[347b]

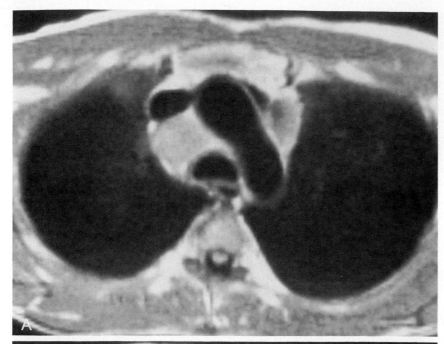

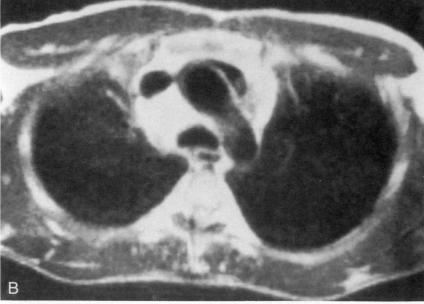

FIGURE 2–71 ■ Hodgkin's disease with mediastinal adenopathy. *A*, T1-weighted spin-echo image demonstrates enlarged lymph nodes in the pretracheal space displacing the superior vena cava forward. Enlarged lymph nodes are also seen lateral to the aortic arch. *B*, T2-weighted image shows the lymph nodes have increased in intensity and now equal the intensity of mediastinal fat.

Recurrent intrathoracic Hodgkin's disease does not commonly involve previously irradiated areas. In two studies, the incidence of in-field recurrence was only between 5 and 20 per cent, and invariably the original tumor mass was very large.[348, 349] A problem in the imaging of patients following treatment for Hodgkin's disease is the involution of the mediastinal nodal masses after treatment. Residual masses are detected in up to 50 per cent of patients. Most of these masses do not contain viable malignant cells. The incidence of recurrence, however, is twice as high when patients have a residual mass than when no mass can be imaged.[348] Nyman and co-workers[230] have found that large masses with a low tumor:fat or tumor:muscle intensity ratio on pretreatment T2-weighted images involuted poorly (Fig. 2–73). After treatment, all lymphomas showed a significant decrease in T2 values and signal intensity ratios. Following chemotherapy or radiation therapy, the successfully treated lymphoma masses should reach a stable size in two to three months.[350, 351] Any subsequent increase in size should be highly suggestive of probable recurrence of the lymphoma. Zerhouni and colleagues[229] have suggested that, following treatment, persistence of high signal intensity or an increase in signal intensity on T2-weighted images may also suggest in-field recurrence in Hodgkin's disease. This interesting finding still needs confirmation.

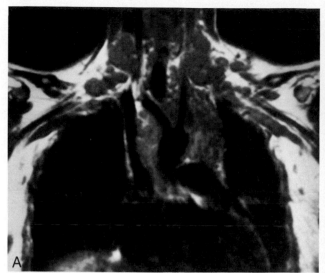
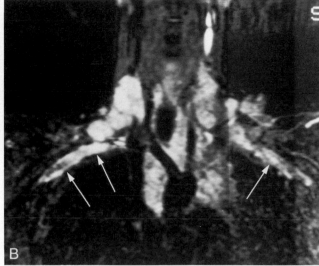

FIGURE 2–72 ■ Distribution of mediastinal and neck lymph nodes in Hodgkin's lymphoma. *A,* Coronal T1-weighted image demonstrates low-intensity lymph nodes in the neck and upper mediastinum. *B,* Using a fat-suppression (STIR) imaging sequence, the tumor containing lymph nodes has markedly increased in relative signal intensity. Extrapleural extension of the tumor to the chest wall, over the apices of the lungs *(arrows),* is now better appreciated. (Courtesy of Colleen Bergen, MD, Palo Alto, CA.)

Indications for CT and MR Scans of the Mediastinum

CT and to a much lesser extent MR have become firmly established as primary modalities for imaging morphology of the mediastinum. It is generally accepted that CT is the more sensitive and more specific of the two. Virtually all mediastinal abnormalities detected on chest radiographs, or suspected from clinical examination, are confirmed with CT. As yet, MR is not a routine imaging study for noncardiac mediastinal diseases apart from suspected disease of the aorta and major mediastinal arteries and veins.

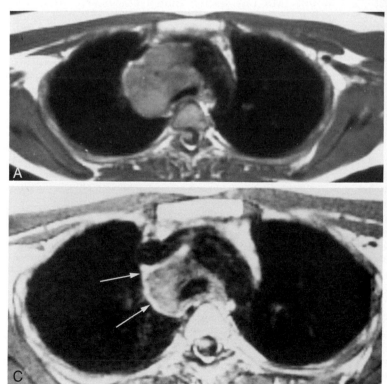
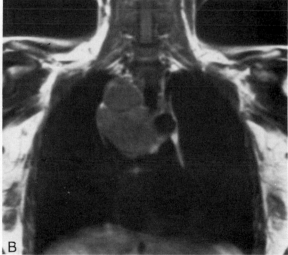

FIGURE 2–73 ■ Lymphoma with persistent low intensity on T2 weighting. *A,* T1-weighted spin-echo MR image demonstrates a moderately low-intensity mass of lymph nodes displacing the trachea posteriorly. The intensity of the lymph nodes is slightly higher than that of muscle. *B,* Coronal T1-weighted MR image confirms the presence of the lymph nodes involving the pretracheal space and extending into the aortic-pulmonic window. *C,* T2-weighted spin-echo MR image shows that the lymph nodes have remained relatively low in signal intensity. The peripheral high intensity *(arrows)* is probably due to slow-flowing blood in the displaced azygos arch.

Detection of Disease

The detection of abnormalities in the mediastinum is clearly better with CT than with chest radiographs or conventional tomograms. In fact, CT has completely replaced conventional tomography for thoracic imaging in general and imaging of the mediastinum in particular. Whenever the detection of mediastinal disease can affect patient care, CT is the imaging modality of choice. This is most apparent for the detection of lymphadenopathy, whether benign or malignant. CT is now routine for patients with suspected bronchogenic carcinoma, lymphoma, or extrathoracic malignancy, when detection of lymph nodes could alter therapy. When the CT examination is conducted for detection of lymphadenopathy, most radiologists use intravascular contrast material to obtain opacification of the mediastinal vessels. Detection of mediastinal adenopathy in patients with non–small-cell bronchogenic carcinoma requires careful reevaluation in the light of recent studies. The sensitivity, specificity, and accuracy of these studies are less than earlier studies showed and are quite disappointing. They indicate that carcinoma within normal-sized nodes, substantially enlarged hyperplastic nodes without tumor, and undetected enlarged nodes (both by CT and MR) are all significant problems. The inability of CT to detect subtle mediastinal invasion and submucosal mediastinal bronchial extension by bronchogenic carcinoma is also a problem. Most studies have shown comparable results for CT and MR in detecting enlarged mediastinal lymph nodes. Our impression is that this is true in most instances if studies of equal quality are compared. The major difference is that good quality CT is routine, whereas poor quality MR of the thorax is still not uncommon. MR of the thorax can show major degradation of the images in an unpredictable and frustrating manner. The role of CT and MR for following the course of patients treated for lymphoma remains unclear. MR studies that claim the modality can predict response to therapy or detect early recurrence may be important but are still provisional. The entire clinical problem needs to be kept in appropriate prospective.

Both MR and CT can screen patients with suspected congenital vascular abnormalities and disease of the great vessels and aorta. MR is more accurate than CT in defining the presence and extent of aortic dissections; this therefore is one area in which MR routinely should be favored over CT. Another important potential application for MR is the detection and mapping of sites of venous obstruction in the thorax. This area requires additional study, especially with flow-sensitive MR techniques such as gradient-echo sequences.

In patients with myasthenia gravis, CT or MR can detect thymic masses not evident on chest radiographs. When the presence of a mass will influence the decision to remove the thymus, one of these studies should be obtained. Similarly, in the patient with persistent hyperparathyroidism following neck dissection, CT or MR should be undertaken to include the entire thorax to search for an aberrantly situated parathyroid adenoma.

Characterization of Disease

The attenuation coefficients of biologic tissues as measured by the Hounsfield number (H) have a reasonably linear relationship to the physical density of the tissue. Density in the mediastinum is sufficiently precise in most cases to differentiate fat, cyst fluid, and soft tissue. The cystic component of some mediastinal masses can however approach soft tissue density. Infusion of intravascular contrast material frequently demonstrates the enhancing wall of a cystic mediastinal mass. MR can similarly discriminate among those tissues within the mediastinum. MR is insensitive for detecting calcium within nodes and masses, which is a distinct disadvantage. Virtually all mediastinal masses or suspected masses can be imaged with CT to determine the mass constituents, relationships to surrounding structures, and extensions within the mediastinum. Both CT and MR readily define the cause of a diffusely widened mediastinum and anomalies of the veins and arteries.

CT has been a revolutionary advance in mediastinal imaging. Its ability to exclude significant abnormality and to detect subtle morphologic derangement is remarkable. It is now so established as to be almost routine for imaging most patients with thoracic disease. However, its limitations must clearly be appreciated, especially its specificity for enlarged lymph nodes. MR has shown that it can nearly equal the resolution of CT in the mediastinum when good quality studies are obtained. The hope that MR would have higher specificity for characterizing mediastinal disease has not been realized. The future challenge for CT and MR of the mediastinum is to improve their discriminatory power for malignant and nonmalignant tissues.

References

1. Heitzman ER, Goldwin RL, Proto AV: Radiologic analysis of the mediastinum utilizing computed tomography. Radiol Clin North Am 15:309, 1977.
2. Kolbenstvedt A, Kolmannskof F, Aakhus T: Arterial structures of the chest and abdomen at computer tomography. Acta Radiol (Diagn) 20:703, 1979.
3. Goldwin RL, Heitzman ER, Proto AV: Computed tomography of the mediastinum: normal anatomy and indication for the use of CT. Radiology 124:235, 1977.
4. Zylak CJ, Pallie W, Jackson R: Correlative anatomy and computed tomography: a nodule on the mediastinum. Radiographics 2:555, 1982.
5. Speckman JM, Gamsu G, Webb WR: Alterations in CT mediastinal anatomy produced by an azygos lobe. AJR 137:47, 1981.
6. Kuriyama K, Gamsu G, Stern RG, Cann CE, Herfkens RJ, et al: CT-determined pulmonary artery diameters in predicting pulmonary hypertension. Invest Radiol 19:16, 1984.

7. Mencini RA, Proto AV: The high left and main pulmonary arteries: a CT pitfall. J Comput Assist Tomogr 6:452, 1982.

8. Schnyder PA, Hauser H, Moss A, Gamsu G, Brasch R, et al: CT of the thoracic duct. Eur J Radiol 3:18, 1983.

9. Hyson EA, Ravin CE: Radiographic features of mediastinal anatomy. Chest 75:609, 1979.

10. Sone S, Higashihara T, Morimoto S, Yokota K, Ikezoe J, et al: Normal anatomy of thymus and anterior mediastinum by pneumomediastinography. AJR 134:81, 1980.

11. Sone S, Higashihara T, Morimoto S, Yokota K, Ikezoe J, et al: Potential spaces of the mediastinum: CT pneumomediastinography. AJR 138:1051, 1982.

12. Mitsuoka A, Kitano M, Ishii S: Gas-contrasted computed tomography of the mediastinum. J Comput Assist Tomogr 5:588, 1981.

13. Clemente CD (ed): Gray's Anatomy, 30th ed. Philadelphia, Lea & Febiger, 1984.

13a. Glassberg RM, Sussman SK, Glickstein MF: CT anatomy of the internal mammary vessels: importance in planning percutaneous transthoracic procedures. AJR 155:397, 1990.

14. Glassberg RM, Sussman SK: Life-threatening hemorrhage due to percutaneous transthoracic intervention: importance of the internal mammary artery. AJR 154:47, 1990.

15. Taber P, Chang LWM, Campion GM: The left brachiocephalic vein simulating aortic dissection on computed tomography. J Comput Assist Tomogr 3:360, 1979.

16. Heiberg E, Wolverson MK, Sundaram M, Nouri S: Normal thymus: CT characteristics in subjects under age 20. AJR 138:491, 1982.

17. Siegel MJ, Glazer HS, Wiener JI, Molina PL: Normal and abnormal thymus in childhood: MR imaging. Radiology 172:367, 1989.

18. Baron RL, Lee JKT, Sagel SS, Peterson RR: Computed tomography of the normal thymus. Radiology 142:121, 1982.

19. de Geer G, Webb WR, Gamsu G: Normal thymus: Assessment with MR and CT. Radiology 158:313, 1986.

20. Dixon AK, Hilton CJ, Williams GT: Computed tomography and histological correlation of the thymic remnant. Clin Radiol 32:225, 1981.

21. Francis IR, Glazer GM, Bookstein FL, Gross BH: The thymus: re-examination of age-related changes in size and shape. AJR 145:249, 1985.

22. Schnyder PA, Gamsu G: CT of the pretracheal retrocaval space. AJR 136:303, 1981.

23. Levy-Ravetch M, Auh YH, Rubenstein WA, Whalen JP, Kazam E: CT of the pericardial recesses. AJR 144:707, 1985.

24. McMurdo KK, Webb WR, von Schulthess GK, Gamsu G: Magnetic resonance imaging of the superior pericardial recesses. AJR 145:985, 1985.

25. Heitzman ER, Lane EJ, Hammack DB, Rimmler LJ: Radiological evaluation of the aortic-pulmonic window. Radiology 116:513, 1975.

26. Webb WR, Moore EH: Differentiation of volume averaging and mass on magnetic resonance images of the mediastinum. Radiology 155:413, 1985.

27. Jolles PR, Shin MS, Jones WP: Aortopulmonary window lesions: detection with chest radiography. Radiology 159:647, 1986.

28. Muller NL, Webb WR, Gamsu G: Subcarinal lymph node enlargement: Radiographic findings and CT correlation. AJR 145:15, 1985.

29. Kormano M, Yrjana J: The posterior tracheal band: Correlation between computed tomography and chest radiography. Radiology 136:689, 1980.

30. Cimmino CV: The esophageal-pleural stripe: an update. Radiology 140:609, 1981.

31. Landay MJ: Azygos vein abutting the posterior wall of the right main and upper lobe bronchi: a normal CT variant. AJR 140:461, 1983.

32. Onitsuka H, Kuhns LR: Dextroconvexity of the mediastinum in the azygoesophagus recess: a normal variant in young adults. Radiology 135:126, 1980.

33. Takesugi JE, Godwin JD: CT appearance of the retroaortic anastomoses of the azygos system. AJR 154:41, 1990.

34. Cooper C, Moss AA, Buy J-N, Stark DD: CT appearance of the normal inferior pulmonary ligament. AJR 141:237, 1983.

35. Rost RC, Proto AV: Inferior pulmonary ligament: computed tomographic appearance. Radiology 148:479, 1983.

36. Berkemen YM, Davis SD, Kazam E, Auh YH, Yankelevitz D, et al: Right phrenic nerve: anatomy, CT appearance, and differentiation from the pulmonary ligament. Radiology 173:43, 1989.

37. Callen PW, Korobkin M, Isherwood I: Computed tomographic evaluation of the retrocrural prevertebral space. AJR 129:907, 1977.

38. Shin MS, Berland LL: Computed tomography of retrocrural spaces: normal, anatomic variants, and pathologic conditions. AJR 145:81, 1985.

39. Cimmino CV: The anterior mediastinal line on chest roentgenogram. Radiology 82:459, 1964.

40. Berne AS, Gerle RD, Mitchel GE: The mediastinum: normal roentgen anatomy and radiologic techniques. Semin Roentgenol 4:3, 1969.

41. Figley MM: Mediastinal minutiae. Semin Roentgenol 4:22, 1969.

42. Proto AV, Lane EJ: Air in the esophagus: a frequent radiographic finding. AJR 129:433, 1977.

43. DeGinder WL: Pleuro-esophageal line in normal chest roentgenogram. JAMA 167:437, 1958.

44. Savoca CJ, Austin JHM, Goldberg HI: The right paratracheal stripe. Radiology 122:295, 1977.

45. Putman CE, Curtis AM, Westfriend M, McLoud TC: Thickening of the posterior tracheal stripe: a sign of squamous cell carcinoma of the esophagus. Radiology 121:533, 1976.

46. Yrjiana J: The posterior tracheal band and recurrent esophageal carcinoma. Radiology 126:615, 1980.

47. Proto AV, Corcoran HL, Ball JB Jr: The left paratracheal reflection. Radiology 171:625, 1989.

48. Genereux GP, Howie JL: Normal mediastinal lymph node size and number: CT and anatomic study. AJR 142:1095, 1984.

49. Glazer GM, Gross BH, Quint LR, Francis IR, Bookstein FL, et al: Normal mediastinal lymph nodes: number and size according to American Thoracic Society mapping. AJR 144:261, 1985.

50. Quint LE, Glazer GM, Orringer MB, Francis IR, Bookstein FL: Mediastinal lymph node detection and sizing at CT and autopsy. AJR 147:469, 1986.

51. Kiyono K, Sone S, Sakai F, Imai Y, Watanabe T, et al: The number and size of normal mediastinal lymph nodes: a postmortem study. AJR 150:771, 1988.

52. Ingram CE, Belli AM, Lewars MD, Reznek RH, Husband JE: Normal lymph node size in the mediastinum: a retrospective study in two patient groups. Clin Radiol 40:35, 1989.

53. Dooms GC, Hricak H, Crooks LE, Higgins CB: Magnetic resonance imaging of the lymph nodes: comparison with CT. Radiology 153:719, 1984.

54. Beck E, Beattie EJ Jr: The lymph nodes in the mediastinum. J Int Coll Surg 29:247, 1958.

55. Glazer HS, Aronberg DJ, Sagel SS: Pictorial essay. AJR 144:267, 1985.

56. Webb WR, Gatsonis CA, Zerhouni EA, Heelan RT, Glazer GM, et al: Comparison of CT and MR imaging in lung cancer staging: preliminary results of the RDOG imaging study. Presented at the Annual Meeting of the Radiological Society of North America. Chicago, November 1989.

57. Heitzman ER: Computed tomography of the thorax: current perspectives. AJR 136:2, 1981.

58. Gamsu G, Sostman D: Magnetic resonance imaging of the thorax. Am Rev Respir Dis 139:254, 1989.

59. Newhouse JH, Murphy RX Jr: Tissue distribution of soluble contrast: effect of dose variation and changes with time. AJR 136:463, 1981.

60. Burgener FA, Hamlin DJ: Contrast enhancement in abdominal CT: bolus vs. infusion. AJR 137:351, 1981.

61. Young SW, Noon MA, Nassi M, Castellino RA: Dynamic computed tomography body scanning. J Comput Assist Tomogr 4:168, 1980.

62. Ball WS, Wicks JD, Mettler FA Jr: Prone-supine change in organ position: CT demonstration. AJR 135:815, 1980.

63. van Waes PFGM, Zonneveld FW: Patient positioning for direct coronal computed tomography of the entire body. Radiology 142:531, 1982.

64. Wolf G: Current status of MR imaging contrast agents: special report. Radiology 172:709, 1989.

65. Wikstroem MG, Moseley ME, White DL, Dupon JW, Winkelhake JL, et al: Contrast-enhanced MRI of tumors: comparison of Gd-DTPA and a macromolecular agent. Invest Radiol 24:609, 1989.

66. Zwirewich CV, Terriff B, Muller NL: High spatial-frequency (bone) algorithm improves quality of standard CT of the thorax. AJR 153:169, 1989.

67. Spritzer C, Gamsu G, Sostman HD: Magnetic resonance imaging of the thorax: techniques, current applications, and future directions. J Thorac Imag 4:1, 1989.

68. Haacke EM, Lenz GW: Improving image quality in the presence of motion by using rephasing gradients. AJR 148:1251, 1987.

69. Baron RL, Levitt RG, Sagell SS, Stanley RJ: Computed tomography in the evaluation of mediastinal widening. Radiology 138:107, 1981.

70. Webb WR, Gamsu G, Speckman JM, Kaiser JA, Federle MP, et al: CT demonstration of mediastinal aortic arch anomalies. J Comput Assist Tomogr 6:445, 1982.

71. McLoughlin MJ, Weisbrod G, Wise DJ, Yeung HPH: Computed tomography in congenital anomalies of the aortic arch and great vessels. Radiology 138:399, 1981.

72. Friedman WF: Congenital heart disease. In Petersdorf RG, Adams RD, Braunwald E, Isselbacher KJ, Martin JB, et al (eds): Principles of Internal Medicine. New York, McGraw-Hill Book Company, 1983, p 1392.

73. Godwin JD, Herfkens RJ, Brundage BH, Lipton MJ: Evaluation of coarctation of the aorta by computed tomography. J Comput Assist Tomogr 5:153, 1981.

74. White RD, Lipton MJ, Higgins CB, Federle MP, Pogany AC, et al: Non-invasive evaluation of suspected thoracic aortic disease by contrast-enhanced computed tomography. Am J Cardiol 57:282, 1986.

75. White RD, Dooms GC, Higgins CB: Advances in imaging thoracic arotic disease. Invest Radiol 21:761, 1986.

76. Gaupp RJ, Fagan CJ, Davis M, Epstein NE: Pseudo-coarctation of the aorta. J Comput Assist Tomogr 5:571, 1981.

77. Glazer HS, Gutierrez FR, Levitt RG, Lee JKT, Murphy WA: The thoracic aorta studies by MR imaging. Radiology 157:149, 1985.

78. von Schulthess GK, Higashino SM, Higgins SS, Didier D, Fisher MR, et al: Coarctation of the aorta: MR imaging. Radiology 158:469, 1986.

79. Kersting-Sommerhoff BA, Sechtem UP, Fisher MR, Higgins CB: MR imaging of congenital anomalies of the aortic arch. AJR 149:8, 1987.

80. Rees S, Somerville J, Ward C, Martinez J, Mohiaddin RH, et al: Coarctation of the aorta: MR imaging in late postoperative assessment. Radiology 173:499, 1989.

81. Feiglin DH, George CR, MacIntyre WJ, O'Donnell JK, Go RT: Gated cardiac magnetic resonance structural imaging: Optimization by electronic axial rotation. Radiology 154:129, 1985.

82. Klinkhamer AC: Aberrant right subclavian artery. Clinical and roentgenologic aspects. AJR 97:438, 1966.

83. Baron MG: Right aortic arch. Circulation 44:1137, 1971.

84. Didier D, Higgins CB, Fisher MR, Osaki L, Silverman NH, Ceitlin MD: Congenital heart disease: gated MR imaging in 72 patients. Radiology 158:227, 1986.

85. Shuford WH, Sybers RG, Edwards FK: The three types of right aortic arch. AJR 109:67, 1970.

86. Taber P, Chang LWM, Campion GM: Diagnosis of retroesophageal right aortic arch by computed tomography. J Comput Assist Tomogr 3:684, 1979.

87. Shuford WH, Sybers RG, Weens HS: The angiographic feature of double aortic arch. AJR 116:125, 1972.

88. Smathers RL, Buschi AJ, Pope TL, Brenbridge AN, Williamson BR: The azygous arch: normal and pathologic CT appearance. AJR 139:477, 1982.

89. Cha EM, Khoury GH: Persistent left superior vena cava: radiologic and clinical significance. Radiology 103:375, 1972.

90. Webb WR, Gamsu G, Speckman JM, Kaiser JA, Federle MP, et al: Computed tomographic demonstration of mediastinal venous anomalies. AJR 139:157, 1982.

91. Huggins TJ, Lesar ML, Friedman AC, Puatt RS, Thane TT: CT appearance of persistent left superior vena cava. J Comput Assist Tomogr 6:294, 1982.

92. Kellman GM, Alpern MB, Sandler MA, Craig BM: Computed tomography of vena caval anomalies with embryologic correlation. Radiographics 8:533, 1988.

93. McMurdo KK, de Geer G, Webb WR, Gamsu G: Normal and occluded mediastinal veins: MR imaging. Radiology 159:33, 1986.

94. Chuang VP, Mena CE, Hoskins PA: Congenital anomalies of the inferior vena cava. Review of embryogenesis and presentation of a simplified classification. Br J Radiol 47:206, 1974.

95. Royal SA, Callen PW: Congenital anomalies of the inferior vena cava. Review of embryogenesis and presentation of a simplified classification. Br J Radiol 47:206, 1974.

96. Churchill RJ, Wesby G III, Marsan RE, Moncada R, Reynes CJ, et al: Computed tomographic demonstration of anomalous inferior vena cava with azygos continuation. J Comput Assist Tomogr 4:398, 1980.

97. Berdon WE, Baker DH: Plain film findings in azygos continuation of the inferior vena cava. AJR 104:452, 1968.

98. Ginaldi S, Chuang VP, Wallace S: Absence of the hepatic segment of the inferior vena cava with azygos continuation. J Comput Assist Tomogr 4:112, 1980.

99. Mayo J, Gray R, St. Louis E, Grossman H, Mc Laughlin M, et al: Anomalies of the inferior vena cava. AJR 140:339, 1983.

100. Floyd GD, Nelson WP: Developmental interruption of the inferior vena cava with azygos and hemiazygos substitution. Unusual radiographic features. Radiology 119:55, 1976.

101. Haswell DM, Berrigan TJ Jr: Anomalous inferior vena cava with accessory hemiazygos continuation. Radiology 119:51, 1976.

102. Cooley RN, Schreiber MH: Radiology of the heart and great vessels. In Cooley RN, Schreiber MH (eds): Golden's Diagnostic Radiology, 3rd ed. Baltimore: Williams & Wilkins, 1978, pp 603–604.

103. Fomon JJ, Kurzweg FT, Broadway RK: Aneurysms of the aorta: a review. Ann Surg 165:557, 1967.

104. Higgins CB, Silverman NR, Harris RD, Albertson KW: Localized aneurysms of the descending thoracic aorta. Clin Radiol 26:474, 1975.

105. Joyce JW, Fairbairn JF II, Kincaid OW, Juergens JL: Aneurysms of the thoracic aorta: a clinical study with special reference to prognosis. Circulation 29:176, 1964.

106. Godwin JD, Herfkens RL, Skioeldebrand CG, Federle MP, Lipton MJ: Evaluation of dissections and aneurysms of the thoracic aorta by conventional and dynamic CT scanning. Radiology 126:125, 1980.

107. Machida K, Tasaka A: CT patterns of mural thrombus in aortic aneurysms. J Comput Assist Tomogr 4:840, 1980.

107a. Richardson P, Mirvis SE, Scorpio R, Dunham CM: Value of CT in determining the need for angiography when findings of mediastinal hemorrhage on chest radiographs are equivocal. AJR 156:273, 1991.

108. Cooley DA, DeBakey ME: Surgical considerations of intrathoracic aneurysms of the aorta and great vessels. Ann Surg 135:660, 1952.

109. Zeitler E, Kaiser W, Schuierer G, Stetter E, Oppelt A, et al: Magnetic resonance imaging of clots in the heart and vascular system. Ann Radiol (Paris) 28:105, 1985.

110. White EM, Edelman RR, Wedeen VJ, Brady TJ: Intravascular signal in MR imaging: use of phase display for differentiation of blood flow signal from intraluminal disease. Radiology 161:245, 1986.

111. Laub GA, Kaiser WA: MR angiography with gradient motion rephasing. J Comput Assist Tomogr 12:377, 1988.

112. Doroghazi RM, Slater EE, eds. Aortic dissection. New York, McGraw-Hill Book Company, 1983.

113. Robert WC: Aortic dissection: anatomy, consequences, and causes. Am Heart J 101:195, 1981.

114. Itzchak Y, Rosenthal T, Adar R, Rubinstein ZJ, Lieberman V, Deutsch V: Dissecting aneurysm of the thoracic aorta: reappraisal of radiologic diagnosis. AJR 125:559, 1975.

115. Godwin JD, Breiman RS, Speckan JM: Problems and pitfalls on the evaluation of thoracic aortic dissection by computed tomography. J Comput Assist Tomogr 6:750, 1982.

116. Gross SC, Barr I, Eyler WR, Khaja F, Goldstein S: Computed tomography in dissection of the thoracic aorta. Radiology 136:135, 1980.

117. Larde D, Belloir C, Vasile N, Frija J, Ferrane J: Computed tomography of aortic dissection. Radiology 136:147, 1980.

118. Heiberg E, Wolverson M, Sundaram M, Connors J, Susman N: CT findings in thoracic aortic dissection. AJR 136:13, 1981.

119. Thorsen MK, San Dretto MA, Lawons TL, Foley WD, Smith DF, et al: Dissecting aortic aneurysms: Accuracy of computed tomography diagnosis. Radiology 148:773, 1983.

120. Oudkerk M, Overbosch E, Dee P: CT recognition of acute aortic dissection. AJR 141:671, 1983.

121. Yamada T, Tada S, Harada J: Aortic dissection without intimal rupture: Diagnosis with MR imaging and CT. Radiology 168:347, 1988.

122. Amparo EG, Higgins CB, Hricak H, Sollitto R: Aortic dissection: magnetic resonance imaging. Radiology 155:399, 1985.

123. Geisinger MA, Risius B, O'Donnell JA, Zelch MG, Moodie DS, et al: Thoracic aortic dissections: Magnetic resonance imaging. Radiology 155:407, 1985.

124. Dinsmore RE, Wedeen VJ, Miller SW, Rosen BR, Fifer M, et al: MRI of dissection of the aorta: recognition of the intimal tear and differential flow velocities. AJR 146:1286, 1986.

125. Kersting-Sommerhoff BA, Higgins CB, White RD, Sommerhoff CP, Lipton MJ: Aortic dissection: magnetic resonance imaging: sensitivity and specificity of MR imaging. Radiology 166:651, 1988.

126. Winer-Muram HT, Gold RE: Effusion in the superior pericardial recess simulating a mediastinal mass. AJR 154:69, 1990.

126a. Solomon SL, Brown JJ, Glazer HS, Mirowitz SA, Lee JKT: Thoracic aortic dissection: pitfalls and artifacts in MR imaging. Radiology 177:223, 1990.

127. Yamaguchi T, Guthaner DF, Wexler L: Natural history of the false channel of type A aortic dissection after surgical report: CT study. Radiology 170:743, 1989.

128. Dalen JE, Alpert JS, Cohn LH, Black H, Collins JJ: Dissection of the thoracic aorta—medical or surgical therapy? Am J Cardiol 34:803, 1974.

129. Strong WW, Moggio RA, Stansel HC Jr: Acute aortic dissection—twelve medical and surgical experience. J Thorac Cardiovasc Surg 68:815, 1974.

130. Miller DV, Stinson EB, Oyer PE, Rossiter SJ, Reitz BA, et al: Operative treatment of aortic dissections: experience with 125 patients over a sixteen-year period. J Thorac Cardiovasc Surg 78:365, 1979.

131. Thomas CS Jr, Alford WC Jr, Burrus GR, Frist RA, Stoney WS: The effectiveness of surgical treatment of acute aortic dissection. Ann Thorac Surg 26:42, 1978.

132. Miller DC: Surgical management of aortic dissections: Indications, preoperative management, and long-term results. In Doroghazi RM, Slater EE (eds): Aortic Dissections. New York, McGraw-Hill, 1983, pp 193–243.

133. Turley K, Ullyot DJ, Gowin JD, Wilson JM, Lipton M, et al: Repair of thoracic aorta. Evaluation of false lumen utilizing computed tomography. J Thorac Cardiovasc Surg 81:61, 1981.

134. Guthaner DF, Miller DC, Silverman JF, Stinson EB, Wexter L: Fate of the false lumen following surgical repair of aortic dissections: An angiographic study. Radiology 133:1, 1979.

135. Mathieu D, Keta K, Loisance D, Cachera JP, Rousseau M, et al: Postoperative CT follow-up of aortic dissection. J Comput Assist Tomogr 10:216, 1986.

136. McNamara MT, Higgins CB: Cardiovascular applications of magnetic resonance imaging. Magn Reson Imag 2:167, 1984.

137. Godwin JD, Turley K, Herfkens RJ, Lipton MJ: Computed tomography for follow-up of chronic aortic dissection. Radiology 139:655, 1981.

138. Parish JM, Marschke RF Jr, Dines DE, Lee RE: Etiologic consideration in superior vena cava syndrome. Mayo Clin Proc 56:407, 1981.

139. Schraufnagel DE, Hill R, Leech JA, Pare JAP: Superior vena cava obstruction. Am J Med 70:1169, 1981.

140. Gosh BC, Cliffton EE: Malignant tumors with superior vena cava obstruction. NY State J Med 73:283, 1973.

141. Mahajan V, Strimlan V, VanOrstrand HS, Loop FD: Benign superior vena cava syndrome. Chest 68:32, 1975.

142. Steinberg I: Dilatation of the hemiazygos veins in superior vena caval occlusion simulating mediastinal tumor. AJR 87:248, 1962.

143. Berk RN: Dilatation of the left superior intercostal vein in the plain-film diagnosis of chronic superior vena caval obstruction. Radiology 83:419, 1964.

143a. Dudiack CM, Olson MC, Posniak HV: CT evaluation of congenital and acquired abnormalities of the azygos system. RadioGraphics 11:259, 1991.

144. Engel IA, Auh YH, Rubenstein WA, Sniderman K, Whalen JP, et al: CT diagnosis of mediastinal and thoracic inlet venous obstruction. AJR 141:521, 1983.

145. Moncada R, Cardella R, Demos TC, Churchill RJ, Love L, et al: Evaluation of superior vena cava syndrome by axial CT and CT phlebography. AJR 143:731, 1984.

146. Gamsu G, Webb WR, Sheldon P, Kaufman L, Crooks LE, et al: Nuclear magnetic resonance imaging of the thorax. Radiology 147:473, 1983.

147. Weinreb JC, Mootz A, Cohen JM: MRI evaluation of mediastinal and thoracic inlet venous obstruction. AJR 146:679, 1986.

148. Godwin JD, Webb WR: Contrast-related flow phenomena mimicking pathology on thoracic computed tomography. J Comput Assist Tomogr 6:460, 1982.

149. Bradley WG, Waluch V: Blood flow: magnetic resonance imaging. Radiology 154:443, 1985.

150. Axel L: Blood flow effects in magnetic resonance imaging. AJR 143:1157, 1984.

150a. Hansen ME, Spritzer CE, Sostman HD: Assessing the patency of mediastinal and thoracic inlet veins: value of MR imaging. AJR 155:1177, 1990.

151. Edelman RR, Mattle HP, Atkinson DJ, Hoogewoud HM: MR angiography. AJR 154:937, 1990.

152. Dooms GC, Hricak II, Moseley ME, Bottles K, Fisher M, et al: Characterization of lymphadenopathy by magnetic resonance relaxation times: preliminary results. Radiology 155:691, 1985.

153. Im JG, Sone KS, Kang HS, Park JH, Yeon KM, et al: Mediastinal tuberculous lymphadenitis: CT manifestations. Radiology 164:115, 1987.

154. Yousem DM, Scatarige JC, Fishman EK, Siegelman SS: Low-attenuation thoracic metastases in testicular malignancy. AJR 146:291, 1986.

155. Nyman R, Rhen S, Ericsson A, Glimelius B, Hagberg H, et al: An attempt to characterize malignant lymphoma in spleen, liver and lymph nodes with magnetic resonance imaging. Acta Radiol 28:527, 1987.

155a. Scataridge JC, Boxen I, Smathers RL: Internal mammary lymphadenopathy: imaging of a vital lymphatic pathway in breast cancer. RadioGraphics 10:857, 1990.

156. Ege G: Internal mammary lymphoscintigraphy. Radiology 118:101, 1976.

157. Rose CM, Kaplan WD, Marck A: Lymphoscintigraphy of the internal mammary lymph nodes. Int J Radiat Oncol Biol Phys (Suppl 2) 2:102, 1977.

158. Meyer JE, Munzenrider JE: Computed tomographic demonstration of internal mammary lymph-node metastasis in patients with locally recurrent breast carcinoma. Radiology 139:661, 1981.

159. Lindfors KK, Meyer JE, Busse PM, Kopans DB, Munzenrider JE, et al: Evaluation of local and regional breast cancer recurrence. AJR 145:833, 1985.

160. Scatarige JC, Fishman EK, Zinreich ES, Brem RF, Almaraz R: Internal mammary lymphadenopathy in breast carcinoma: CT appraisal of anatomic distribution. Radiology 167:89, 1988.

161. Hopper KD, Diehl LF, Lesar M, Barnes M, Granger E, Baumann J: Hodgkin disease: clinical utility of CT in initial staging and treatment. Radiology 169:17, 1988.

161a. Giles JA, Sechtin AG, Waybill MM, Moser RP, Jr: Bilateral internal mammary artery aneurysms: a previously unreported cause for an anterior mediastinal mass. AJR 154:1189, 1990.

162. Muller NL, Webb WR, Gamsu G: Paratracheal lymphadenopathy: Radiographic findings and correlation with CT. Radiology 156:761, 1985.

163. Webb WR, Moore EH: Differentiation of volume averaging and mass on magnetic resonance images of the mediastinum. Radiology 155:413, 1985.

164. Efremidis SC, Dan SJ, Cohen BA, Mitty HA, Rabinowitz JG: Displaced paraspinal line: role of CT and lymphography. AJR 136:505, 1981.

165. Cohen WN, Seidelmann FE, Bryan PJ: Computed tomography of localized adipose deposits presenting as tumor masses. AJR 128:1007, 1977.

166. Streiter ML, Schneider HJ, Proto AV: Steroid-induced thoracic lipomatosis: Paraspinal involvement. AJR 139:679, 1982.

167. Jochelson MS, Balikian JP, Mauch P, Liebman H: Peri- and paracardial involvement in lymphoma: a radiographic study of 11 cases. AJR 40:483, 1983.

168. Bledin A, Bernardino ME, Libshitz HI: Cardiophrenic angle nodes: an unusual CT finding of advanced metastatic disease. Comput Tomogr 4:193, 1980.

169. Cho CS, Blank N, Castellino RA: CT evaluation of cardiophrenic angle lymph nodes in patients with malignant lymphoma. AJR 143:719, 1984.

170. Gamsu G, Stark DS, Webb WR, Moore EH, Sheldon PE: Magnetic resonance imaging of benign mediastinal masses. Radiology 151:709, 1984.

170a. Glazer HS, Molina PL, Siegel MJ, Sagel SS: High-attenuation mediastinal masses on unenhanced CT. AJR 156:45, 1991.

171. Gamsu G, Sostman D: Magnetic resonance imaging of the thorax. Am Rev Respir Dis 139:254, 1989.

172. Rohlfing BM, Korobkin M, Hall AD: Computed tomography of intrathoracic omental herniation and other mediastinal fatty masses. J Comput Assist Tomogr 1:181, 1977.

173. Bein ME, Mancuso AA, Mink JH, Hansen GC: Computed tomography in the evelution of mediastinal lipomatosis. J Comput Assist Tomogr 2:379, 1978.

174. Pugatch RD, Faling LJ, Robbins AH, Spira R: CT diagnosis of benign mediastinal abnormalities. AJR 143:685, 1980.

175. McLoud TC, Wittenberg J, Ferrucci JT Jr: Computed tomography of the thorax and standard radiographic evaluation of the chest: A comparative study. J Comput Assist Tomogr 3:170, 1979.

176. Mendez G Jr, Isikoff MB, Isikoff SK, Sinner WN: Fatty tumors of the thorax demonstrated by CT. AJR 133:207, 1979.

177. Paling MR, Williamson BRJ: Epipericardial fat pad: CT findings. Radiology 165:335, 1987.

178. Rothman SLG, Simeone JF, Allen WE, Putman CE, Redman HC: Computerized tomography in the assessment of disease of the thorax. Comput Tomogr 1:181, 1977.

179. Oldham HN Jr: Mediastinal tumors and cysts (collective review). Ann Thorac Surg 11:246, 1971.

180. Federle MP, Callen PW: Cystic Hodgkin's lymphoma of the thymus: computed tomography appearance. J Comput Assist Tomogr 3:542, 1979.

181. Glazer HS, Siegel MJ, Sagel SS: Low-attenuation mediastinal masses on CT. AJR 152:1173, 1989.

182. Marvasti MA, Mitchell GE, Burke WA, Meyer JA: Misleading density of mediastinal cysts on computerized tomography. Ann Thorac Surg 31:167, 1981.

183. Nakata H, Nakayama C, Kimoto T, Nakayama T, Tsukamoto Y, et al: Computed tomography of mediastinal bronchogenic cysts. J Comput Assist Tomogr 6:733, 1982.

184. Mendelson DS, Rose JS, Efremidis SC, Kirschner PA, Cohen BA: Bronchogenic cysts with high CT numbers. AJR 140:463, 1983.

185. Webb WR, Gamsu G, Stark DD, Moon KL, Moore EH: Evaluation of magnetic resonance sequences in imaging mediastinal tumors. AJR 143:723, 1984.

186. Kuhlman JE, Fishman EK, Wang KP, Zerhouni EA, Siegelman SS: Mediastinal cysts: diagnosis by CT and needle aspiration. AJR 150:75, 1988.

187. Rogers CI, Seymour EQ, Brock JG: Atypical pericardial cyst location: the value of computed tomography. J Comput Assist Tomogr 4:683, 1980.

188. Pugatch RD, Braver JH, Robbins AH, Faling LJ: CT diagnosis of pericardial cysts. AJR 131:515, 1978.

189. Rosai J, Levine GD: Tumors of the Thymus. Atlas of Tumor Pathology, 2nd series. Washington, DC, Armed Forces Institute of Pathology, 1976, pp 132–140.

190. Gouliamos A, Striggaris K, Lolas C, Deligeorgi-Politi H, Vlahos L: Thymic cyst. J Comput Assist Tomogr 6:172, 1982.

191. Alee G, Logue B, Mansour K: Thymic cyst simulating multiple cardiovascular abnormalities and presenting with pericarditis and pericardial tamponade. Am J Cardiol 31:377, 1973.

192. Ovens GR, Arger PH, Mulhern CB Jr, Coleman BG, Gohel V: CT evaluation of mediastinal pseudocyst. J Comput Assist Tomogr 4:256, 1980.

193. Wittich GR, Karnel F, Schurawitzki H, Jantsch H: Percutaneous drainage of mediastinal pseudocysts. Radiology 167:51, 1988.

194. Scully RE, Galdabini JJ, McNeely U: Weekly clinico-pathological exercises: case 25. N Engl J Med 296:1467, 1977.

195. Friedman AC, Pyatt RS, Harmman DS, Downey EF Jr, Olson WB: CT of benign cystic teratomas. AJR 138:659, 1982.

196. Suzuki M, Takashima T, Itoh H, Choutoh S, Kuwamura I, et al: Computed tomography of mediastinal teratomas. J Comput Assist Tomogr 7:74, 1983.

197. Onik G, Goodman PC: CT of Castleman disease. AJR 140:691, 1983.

198. Komaiko MS, Lee ME, Birnberg FA: The contrast-enhanced paravascular neoplasm: a potential CT pitfall. J Comput Assist Tomogr 4:516, 1980.

199. Spizarny DL, Rebner M, Gross BH: CT evaluation of enhancing mediastinal masses. J Comput Assist Tomogr 11:990, 1987.

200. Webb WR, Jensen BG, Sollitto R, de Geer G, McCowin M, et al: Bronchogenic carcinoma: staging with MR compared with staging with CT and surgery. Radiology 156:117, 1985.

201. Fon GT, Bein ME, Mancuso AA, Keesey JC, Lupetin AR, et al: Computed tomography of the anterior mediastinum in myasthenia gravis. Radiology 142:135, 1982.

202. Lee KS, Im JG, Han CH, Han MC, Kim CW, et al: Malignant primary germ cell tumors of the mediastinum: CT features. AJR 153:947, 1989.

203. von Schulthess GK, McMurdo K, Tscholakoff D, de Geer G, Gamsu G, et al: Mediastinal masses: MR imaging. Radiology 158:289, 1986.

204. Gunn A, Michie W, Irvine WJ: The thymus in thyroid disease. Lancet 2:776, 1964.

205. Franken EA Jr: Radiologic evidence of thymic enlargement in Graves' disease. Radiology 91:20, 1968.

206. Baron RL, Lee JK, Sagel SS, Peterson RR: Computed tomography of the normal thymus. Radiology 142:121, 1982.

207. Walter E: Computertomographische diagnostik des Thymus. In Huber H (ed): Jahrbuch 1983 der Schweizerischen Gesellschaft fuer Radiologue und Nuklearmedizin, Vol 208. 1983, pp 25–34.

208. Batra P, Herrmann C Jr, Mulder D: Mediastinal imaging in myasthenia gravis: correlation of chest radiography, CT, MR, and surgical findings. AJR 148:515, 1987.

209. Chen J, Weisbrod GL, Herman SJ: Computed tomography and pathologic correlations of thymic lesions. J Thorac Imag 3:61, 1988.

210. Baron RL, Lee JK, Sagel SS, Levitt RG: Computed tomography of the abnormal thymus. Radiology 142:127, 1982.

211. Castlemann B, Norris EH: Pathology of the thymus in myasthenia gravis: a study of 35 cases. Medicine (Baltimore) 28:27, 1949.

212. Goldman A, Cutermann J, Keeseytal JC: Myasthenia gravis and invasive thymoma: a 20-year experience. Neurology 25:1021, 1975.

213. Harper RAK, Guyer PB: The radiological features of thymic tumors: a review of 65 cases. Clin Radiol 16:97, 1965.

214. Fechner RE: Recurrence of non-invasive thymomas. Report of four cases and review of the literature. Cancer 23:1423, 1969.

215. Ross JS, O'Donovan PB, Novoa R, Mehta A, Buonocore E, et al: Magnetic resonance of the chest: initial experience with imaging and in vivo T1 and T2 calculations. Radiology 152:95, 1984.

216. Zerhouni EA, Scott WW Jr, Baker RR, Wharam MD, Siegelmann SS: Invasive thymomas: diagnosis and evaluation by computed tomography. J Comput Assist Tomogr 6:92, 1982.

217. McCrea ES, Maslar JA: Thymoma with distant intrathoracic implants, with CT confirmation. Cancer 50:1612, 1982.

218. Siegelman SS, Scott WW Jr, Baker RR, Fishman EK: CT of the thymus. In Siegelmann SS (ed): Computed Tomography of the Chest. New York, Churchill Livingstone, 1984, pp 233–271.

219. Scatarige JC, Fishman EK, Zerhouni EA, Siegelman SS: Transdiaphragmatic extension of invasive thymoma. AJR 144:31, 1985.

220. Moore AV, Korobkin M, Olanow W, Ravin CE, Putman CE, et al: Thymoma detection by mediastinal CT: patients with myasthenia gravis. AJR 138:217, 1982.

221. Teplick JG, Nedvick A, Haskin ME: Roentgenographic features of thymolipoma. AJR 117:873, 1973.

222. Peake JB, Zeigler MG: Thymolipoma: report of three cases. Am Surg 43:477, 1977.

223. Yeh HC, Gordon A, Kirschner PA, Cohen BA: Computed tomography and sonography of thymolipoma. AJR 140:1131, 1983.

224. Batata MA, Martini N, Huvos AG, Aguilar RI, Beattie EJ: Thymomas: clinicopathologic features, therapy, and prognosis. Cancer 34:398, 1974.

225. Brown LR, Muhm JR, Sheedy PF II, Unni KK, Bernatz PE, et al: The value of computed tomography in myasthenia gravis. AJR 140:31, 1983.

226. Ellis K, Austin JHM, Jaretzki A III: Radiologic detection of thymoma in patients with myasthenia gravis. AJR 151:873, 1988.

227. Heron CW, Husband JE, Williams MP: Hodgkin disease: CT of the thymus. Radiology 167:647, 1988.

228. Lindfors KK, Meyer JE, Dedrick CG, Hassell LA, Harris NL: Thymic cysts in mediastinal Hodgkin disease. Radiology 156:37, 1985.

229. Zerhouni EA, Fishman EK, Jones R, Siegelman SS, Soulen RL: MR imaging of "sterilized" lymphoma (abstr). Radiology 161:207, 1986.

230. Nyman RS, Rehn SM, Glimelius BLG, Hagberg HE, Hemmingsson AL, et al: Residual mediastinal masses in Hodgkin disease: prediction of size with MR imaging. Radiology 170:435, 1989.

231. Brown LR, Aughnbaugh GL, Wick MR, Baker BA, Salassa RM: Roentgenologic diagnosis of primary corticotropin-producing carcinoid tumors of the mediastinum. Radiology 142:143, 1982.

232. Birnberg FA, Webb WR, Selch MT, Gamsu G, Goodman PC: Thymic carcinoid tumors with hyperparathyroidism. AJR 139:1001, 1982.

233. Levitt RG, Husband JE, Glazer HS: CT of primary germ-cell tumors of the mediastinum. AJR 142:73, 1984.

233a. Nichols CR: Mediastinal germ cell tumors—clinical features and biologic correlates. Chest 99:472, 1991.

234. Livesay JJ, Mink JH, Fee HJ, Bein ME, Sample WF, et al: The use of computed tomography to evaluate suspected mediastinal tumors. Ann Thorac Surg 27:305, 1979.

235. Shin MS, Ho KJ: Computed tomography of primary mediastinal seminomas. J Comput Assist Tomogr 7:990, 1983.

236. Baron RL, Sagel SS, Baglan RJ: Thymic cysts following radiation therapy of Hodgkin disease. Radiology 141:593, 1981.

237. Wychilis AR, Payne WSA, Clagett OT, Woolner LB: Surgical treatment of mediastinal tumors. J Thorac Cardiovasc Surg 62:379, 1971.

238. Gelfand DW, Goldman AS, Law AJ: Thymic hyperplasia in children recovering from thermal burns. J Trauma 12:813, 1972.

239. Rizk G, Cuteo L, Amplatz K: Rebound enlargement of the thymus after successful corrective surgery for transformation of the great vessels. AJR 116:528, 1972.

240. Cohen M, Hill CA, Cangir A, Sullivan MP: Thymic rebound after treatment of childhood tumors. AJR 135:151, 1980.

241. Shin MS, Ho KJ: Diffuse thymic hyperplasia following chemotherapy for nodular sclerosing Hodgkin's disease. An immunologic rebound phenomenon? Cancer 51:30, 1983.

242. Levine GD, Rosai J: Thymic hyperplasia and neoplasia: a review of current concepts. Hum Pathol 9:495, 1978.

243. Doppman JL, Oldfield EH, Chrousos GP, Nieman L, Udelsman R, et al: Rebound thymic hyperplasia after treatment of Cushing's syndrome. AJR 147:1145, 1986.

244. Choyke PL, Zeman RK, Gootenberg JE, Hoffer F, Frank JA: Thymic atrophy and regrowth in response to chemotherapy: CT evaluation. AJR 149:269, 1987.

245. Kissin CM, Husband JE, Nicholas D, Eversman W: Benign thymic enlargement in adults after chemotherapy: CT demonstration. Radiology 163:67, 1987.

246. Benjamin SP, McCormack IJ, Effler DB, Groves LK: Primary tumors of the mediastinum. Chest 62:297, 1972.

247. Binder RE, Pugatch RD, Faling LJ, Kanter RA, Sawin CT: Diagnosis of posterior mediastinal goiter by computed tomography. J Comput Assist Tomogr 4:5552, 1980.

248. Irwin RS, Braman SS, Arvanitidis AN, Hamolsky MW: [131]I thyroid scanning in preoperative diagnosis of mediastinal goiter. Ann Intern Med 89:73, 1978.

249. Kaneko T, Matsumoto M, Fukui K, Hori T, Katayama K: Clinical evaluation of thyroid CT values in various thyroid conditions. Comput Tomogr 3:1, 1979.

250. Morris UL, Colletti PM, Ralls PW, Boswell WD, Lapin SA, et al: CT demonstration of intrathoracic thyroid tissue. J Comput Assist Tomogr 6:821, 1982.

251. Bashist B, Ellis K, Gold RP: Computed tomography of intrathoracic goiters. AJR 140:455, 1983.

252. Glazer GM, Axel L, Moss AA: CT diagnosis of mediastinal thyroid. AJR 138:495, 1982.

253. Higgins CB, McNamara MT, Fisher MR, Clark OH: MR imaging of the thyroid. AJR 147:1255, 1985.

254. Gefter WB, Spritzer CE, Eisenberg B, Livolsi VA, Axel L, et al: Thyroid imaging with high field strength surface-coil MR. Radiology 164:483, 1987.

255. Noma S, Nishimura K, Togashi K, Itoh K, Fujisawa I, et al: Thyroid gland: MR imaging. Radiology 164:495, 1987.

256. Higgins CB, Auffermann W: MR imaging of thyroid and parathyroid glands: a review of current status. AJR 151:1095, 1988.

257. Krudy AG, Doppman JL, Brennan MF: The detection of mediastinal parathyroid glands by computed tomography, selective arteriography, and venous sampling. Radiology 140:739, 1981.

258. Doppman JL, Krudy AG, Brennan MF, Schneider P, Lasker RD, et al: CT appearance of enlarged parathyroid glands in the posterior superior mediastinum. J Comput Assist Tomogr 6:1099, 1982.

259. Brennan MF, Doppman JL, Marx SJ, Spiegel AM, Brown EM, et al: Reoperative parathyroid surgery for persistent hyperparathyroidism. Surgery 83:669, 1978.

260. Miller DL, Doppman JL, Shawker TH, Krudy AG, Norton JA, et al: Localization of parathyroid adenomas in patients who have undergone surgery. Part 1. Noninvasive imaging methods. Radiology 162:133, 1987.

261. Levin KE, Gooding GAW, Okerlund M, Higgins CB, Norman D, et al: Localizing studies in patients with persistent or recurrent hyperparathyroidism. Surgery 102:917, 1987.

262. Sommer B, Welter HF, Spelsberg F, Schrer U, Lissner J: Computed tomography for localizing enlarged parathyroid

glands in primary hyperparathyroidism. J Comput Assist Tomogr 6:521, 1982.

263. Auffermann W, Guis M, Tavares NJ, Clark OH, Higgins CB: MR signal intensity of parathyroid adenomas: correlation with histopathology. AJR 153:873, 1989.

264. Payne WS, Larson RH: Acute mediastinitis. Surg Clin North Am 49:999, 1969.

265. Enquist RW, Blanek RR, Butler RH: Nontraumatic mediastinitis. JAMA 236:1048, 1976.

266. Starr MG, Gott VL, Towsend TR: Mediastinal infection after cardiac surgery. Ann Thorac Surg 38:414, 1984.

267. de Graaff CS, Falke TH, Bakker W: Computerized tomography in acute mediastinitis. Europ J Radiol 1:180, 1981.

268. Goodman LG, Kay HR, Teplick SK, Mundth ED: Complications of median sternotomy: computed tomographic evaluation. AJR 141:225, 1983.

269. Carrol CL, Jeffrey RB Jr, Federle MP, Vernacchia FS: CT evaluation of mediastinal infections. J Comput Assist Tomogr 11:449, 1987.

270. Light AM: Idiopathic fibrosis of mediastinum: a discussion of three cases and review of the literature. J Clin Pathol 31:78, 1978.

271. Goodwin RA, Nickell JA, Des Pres RM: Mediastinal fibrosis complicating healed primary histoplasmosis and tuberculosis. Medicine 51:227, 1972.

272. Morgan AD, Loughridge LW, Calne RY: Combined mediastinal and retroperitoneal fibrosis. Lancet 1:67, 1966.

273. Weistein JB, Aronberg DJ, Sagel SS: CT of fibrosing mediastinitis: findings and their utility. AJR 141:247, 1983.

274. Rholl KS, Levitt RG, Glazer HS: Magnetic resonance imaging of fibrosing mediastinitis. AJR 145:255, 1985.

275. Farmer DW, Moore E, Amparo E, Webb WR, Gamsu G, et al: Calcific fibrosing mediastinitis: demonstration of pulmonary vascular obstruction by magnetic resonance imaging. AJR 143:1189, 1984.

275a. Silverberg E: Cancer statistics. CA 37:2, 1987.

276. Blot WJ, Fraumeni JF: Changing patterns of lung cancer in the United States. Am J Epidemiol 115:664, 1982.

277. Evans WK, Murray N, Feld R, Coy P, Clarke D, et al: Canadian multicentre randomized trial comparing standard and alternating combination chemotherapy in extensive small cell lung cancer (abstr). Fourth World Lung Cancer Conference, Toronto, 1985, No. 560:77.

278. Messeih AA, Schweitzer JM, Lipton A, Harvey HA, Simmonds MA, et al: Addition of etoposide to cyclophosphamide, doxorubicin, and vincristine for remission induction and survival in patients with small cell lung cancer. Cancer Treat Rep 71:61, 1987.

279. Beahrs OH, Henson DE, Hutter RV, Myers MH (eds): Manual for Staging of Cancer, 3rd ed. Philadelphia, JB Lippincott Company, 1988, pp 115–121.

280. Mountain CF: A new international staging system for lung cancer. Chest (suppl) 89:225S, 1986.

281. Tisi GM, Friedman PJ, Peters RM, Pearson G, Carr D, et al: Clinical staging of primary lung cancer. Am Rev Respir Dis 127:659, 1983.

282. Roeslin N, Chalkadakis G, Dumont P, Witz JP: A better prognostic value from a modification of lung cancer staging. J Thorac Cardiovasc Surg 94:504, 1987.

283. Epstein DM, Stephenson LW, Gefter WB, van der Voorde F, Aronchik JM, et al: Value of CT in the preoperative assessment of lung cancer: a survey of thoracic surgeons. Radiology 161:423, 1986.

283a. Webb WR, Gatsonis C, Zerhouni EA, Heelan RT, Glazer GM, et al: CT and MR imaging in staging non-small cell bronchogenic carcinoma: Report of the Radiologic Diagnostic Oncology Group. Radiology 178:705, 1991.

284. Martini N, Heelan R, Westcott J, Bains MS, McCormack P, et al: Comparative merits of conventional, computed tomographic, and magnetic resonance imaging in assessing mediastinal involvement in surgically confirmed lung carcinoma. J Thorac Cardiovasc Surg 90:639, 1985.

285. Webb WR, Jensen BG, Sollitto R, de Geer G, McCowin M, et al: Bronchogenic carcinoma: staging with MR compared with staging with CT and surgery. Radiology 156:117, 1985.

286. Rendina ES, Bognolo DA, Mineo TC, Gualdi GF, Caterino M, et al: Computed tomography for the evaluation of intrathoracic invasion by lung cancer. J Thorac Cardiovasc Surg 94:57, 1987.

287. Wursten HU, Vock P: Mediastinal infiltration of lung carcinoma (T4No-1): the positive predictive value of computed tomography. J Thorac Cardiovasc Surg 35:355, 1987.

288. Scott IR, Muller NL, Miller RR, Evans KG, Nelems B: Resectable stage III lung cancer: CT, surgical, and pathologic correlation. Radiology 166:75, 1988.

289. Glazer HS, Kaiser LR, Anderson DJ, Molina PL, Emami B, et al: Indeterminate mediastinal invasion in bronchogenic carcinoma: CT evaluation. Radiology 173:37, 1989.

290. Kameda K, Adachi S, Kono M: Detection of T-factor in lung cancer using magnetic resonance imaging and computed tomography. J Thorac Imag 3:73, 1988.

291. Quint LE, Glazer GM, Orringer MB: Central lung masses: prediction with CT of need for pneumonectomy versus lobectomy. Radiology 165:735, 1987.

292. Schenk DA, Strollo PJ, Pickard JS, Santiago RM, Weber CA, et al: Utility of the Wang 18-gauge transbronchial histology needle in the staging of bronchogenic carcinoma. Chest 96:272, 1989.

293. Acosta JL, Manfredi F: Selective mediastinoscopy. Chest 71:150, 1977.

294. Naruke T, Suemasu K, Ishikawa S: Lymph node mapping and curability at various levels of metastasis in resected lung cancer. J Thorac Cardiovasc Surg 76:832, 1978.

295. Ashraf MH, Milsom PL, Walesby RK: Selection by mediastinoscopy and long-term survival in bronchial carcinoma. Ann Thorac Surg 30:208, 1980.

296. Gross BH, Glazer GM, Orringer MB, Spizarny DL, Flint A: Bronchogenic carcinoma metastatic to normal-sized lymph nodes: Frequency and significance. Radiology 166:71, 1988.

297. de Geer G, Webb WR, Sollitto R, Golden J: MR characteristics of benign lymph node enlargement in sarcoidosis and Castleman's disease. Europ J Radiol 6:145, 1986.

298. Borrie J: Primary carcinoma of the bronchus: prognosis following surgical resection. Ann R Coll Surg 10:165, 1952.

299. Nohl-Oser HC: An investigation into the lymphatic and vascular spread of carcinoma of the bronchus. Thorax 11:172, 1956.

300. Watanabe Y, Shimizu J, Tsubota M, Takashi I: Mediastinal spread of metastatic lymph nodes in bronchogenic carcinoma: mediastinal nodal metastases in lung cancer. Chest 97:1059, 1990.

301. Graves WG, Martinez MJ, Carter PL, Barry MJ, Clarke JS: The value of computed tomography in staging bronchogenic carcinoma: a changing role for mediastinoscopy. Ann Thorac Surg 40:57, 1985.

302. Staples CA, Muller NL, Miller RR, Evans KG, Nelems B: Mediastinal nodes in bronchogenic carcinoma: comparison between CT and mediastinoscopy. Radiology 167:367, 1988.

303. Holmes EC: Surgical adjuvant therapy of non–small-cell lung cancer. J Surg Oncol (suppl) 1:16, 1989.

304. Kris MG, Gralla RJ, Martini N, Stampleman LV, Burhe MT: Preoperative and adjuvant chemotherapy in locally advanced non–small cell lung cancer. Surg Clin North Am 67:1051, 1987.

305. Underwood GH Jr, Hooper RG, Axelbaum SP, Goodwin DW: Computed tomographic scanning of the thorax in the staging of bronchogenic carcinoma. N Engl J Med 300:777, 1979.

306. Shevland JE, Chiu LC, Schapiro RL, Young JA, Rossi NP: The role of conventional tomography and computed tomography in assessing the resectability of primary lung cancer: a preliminary report. J Comput Tomogr 2:1, 1978.

307. Chang AE, Schaner EG, Conkle DM, Doppman JL, Rosenberg SA: Evaluation of computed tomography in the detection of pulmonary metastases: a prospective study. Cancer 43:913, 1979.

308. Ekholm S, Albrechtsson U, Kugelberg J, Tylen U: Computed tomography in preoperative staging of bronchogenic carcinoma. J Comput Assist Tomogr 4:763, 1980.

309. Faling LJ, Pugatch RD, Jung-Legg Y, Daly BDT Jr, Hong WK, et al: Computed tomographic scanning of the mediastinum in the staging of bronchogenic carcinoma. Am Rev Respir Dis 124:690, 1981.

310. Osborne DR, Korobkin M, Ravin CE, Putman CE, Wolfe WG, et al: Comparison of plain radiography, conventional tomography, and computed tomography in detecting intrathoracic lymph node metastases from lung carcinoma. Radiology 142:157, 1982.

311. Rea HH, Shevland JE, House AJS: Accuracy of computed tomographic scanning in assessment of the mediastinum in bronchial carcinoma. J Thorac Cardiovasc Surg 81:825, 1981.

312. Baron RL, Levitt RG, Sagel SS, White MJ, Roper CL, et al: Computed tomography in the preoperative evaluation of bronchogenic carcinoma. Radiology 145:727, 1982.

313. Lewis JW, Madrazo BL, Gross SC, Eyler WR, Magilligan DJ Jr, et al: The value of radiographic and computed tomography in the staging of lung carcinoma. Ann Thorac Surg 34:553, 1982.

314. Richey HM, Matthews JI, Helsel RA, Cable H: Thoracic CT scanning in the staging of bronchogenic carcinoma. Chest 85:218, 1984.

315. Glazer GM, Orringer MB, Gross BH, Quint LE: The mediastinum in non–small cell lung cancer: CT-surgical correlation. AJR 142:1101, 1984.

316. Frederick HM, Bernardino ME, Baron M, Colvin R, Mansour K, et al: Accuracy of chest computerized tomography in detecting malignant hilar and mediastinal involvement by squamous cell carcinoma of the lung. Cancer 54:2390, 1984.

317. Heelan RT, Martini N, Westcott JW, Bains MS, Watson RC, et al: Carcinoma involvement of the hilum and mediastinum: computed tomographic and magnetic resonance evaluation. Radiology 156:111, 1985.

318. Coulomb M, Escolano E, Rose-Pittet L, Blanc-Jouvan F, Lebas JF, et al: L'extension ganglionnaire médiastinale dans le cancer primitif des bronches: corrélations entre la tomodensitométrie, l'imagerie par résonance magnétique et la médiastinoscopie. A propos de 50 observations. J Radiol 68:549, 1987.

319. Musset D, Grenier P, Carette MF, Frija G, Hauuy MP: Primary lung cancer staging: prospective comparative study of MR imaging with CT. Radiology 160:607, 1986.

320. Daly BDT, Faling LJ, Bite G, Gale ME, Bankoff MS, et al: Mediastinal lymph node evaluation by computed tomography in lung cancer. J Thorac Cardiovasc Surg 94:664, 1987.

321. Patterson GA, Ginsberg RJ, Poon PY, Cooper JD, Goldberg M: A prospective evaluation of magnetic resonance imaging, computed tomography, and mediastinoscopy in the preoperative assessment of mediastinal node status in bronchogenic carcinoma. J Thorac Cardiovasc Surg 94:679, 1987.

321. Patterson GA, Ginsberg RJ, Poon PY, Cooper JD, Goldberg M: A prospective evaluation of magnetic resonance imaging, computed tomography, and mediastinoscopy in the preoperative assessment of mediastinal node status in bronchogenic carcinoma. J Thorac Cardiovasc Surg 94:679, 1987.

322. Osada H, Nakajima Y, Taira Y, Yokote K, Noguchi T: The role of mediastinal and multi-organ CT scans in staging presumable surgical candidates with non–small-cell lung cancer. Japan J Surg 17:362, 1987.

323. Poon PY, Bronskill MJ, Henkelman RM, Rideout DF, Shulman HS, et al: Mediastinal lymph node metastases from bronchogenic carcinoma: detection with MR imaging and CT. Radiology 162:651, 1987.

324. Buy JN, Ghossain MA, Poirson F, Bazot M, Meary E, et al: Computed tomography of mediastinal lymph nodes in non–small cell lung cancer: a new approach based on the lymphatic pathway of tumor spread. J Comput Assist Tomogr 12:545, 1988.

325. Batra P, Brown K, Collins JD, Ovenfors CO, Steckel RJ: Evaluation of intrathoracic extent of lung cancer by plain chest radiography, computed tomography, and magnetic resonance imaging. Am Rev Respir Dis 137:1456, 1988.

326. Ratto GB, Mereu C, Motta G: The prognostic significance of mediastinal lymph nodes in patients with lung cancer. Chest 93:807, 1988.

327. Whittlesey D: Prospective computed tomographic scanning in the staging of bronchogenic cancer. J Thorac Cardiovasc Surg 95:876, 1988.

328. Grenier PH, Dubray B, Carett MF, Frijia G, Musset D, et al: Preopeative thoracic staging of lung cancer: CT and MR evaluation. Diagn Interv Radiol 1:23, 1989.

329. McLoud TC, Kosiuk JP, Templeton PA, Shepard JAO, Moore EH, et al: CT in the staging of bronchogenic carcinoma: update of analysis by correlative lymph node mapping and sampling. Presented at the Annual Meeting of Radiological Society of North America, November 1989.

330. Mittman C, Bruderman I: Lung cancer: to operate or not? Am Rev Respir Dis 116:477, 1977.

331. Mountain CF: Expanded possibilities for surgical treatment of lung cancer: survival in stage IIIa disease. Chest 95:1045, 1990.

332. Heavey LR, Glazer GM, Gross BH, Francis IR, Orringe MB: The role of CT in staging radiographic $T_1N_0M_0$ lung cancer. AJR 146:285, 1986.

333. Pearlberg JL, Sandler MA, Beute GH, Madrazo BL: $T_1N_0M_0$ bronchogenic carcinoma: assessment by CT. Radiology 157:187, 1985.

334. Castellino RA: Hodgkin disease: practical concepts for the diagnostic radiologist. Radiology 159:305, 1986.

335. Wang Y: Classification of non-Hodgkin's lymphoma. AJR 147:205, 1986.

336. Filly R, Blank N, Castellino RA: Radiographic distribution of intrathoracic disease in previously untreated patients with Hodgkin's disease and non-Hodgkin's lymphoma. Radiology 120:277, 1976.

337. North LB, Fuller LM, Hagegeister FB, Rodgers RW, Butler JJ, et al: Importance of initial mediastinal adenopathy in Hodgkin disease. AJR 138:229, 1982.

338. Hoppe RT: The contemporary management of Hodgkin disease. Radiology 169:297, 1988.

339. Henry L: Long survival in Hodgkin's disease. Clin Radiol 21:203, 1970.

339a. Rosenberg SA, Kaplan HS: Evidence for an orderly progression in the spread of Hodgkin's disease. Cancer Res 26:1225, 1966.

340. Rostock RA, Stanley SS, Lenhard RE, Wharam MD, Order SE: Thoracic CT scanning for mediastinal Hodgkin's disease: results and therapeutic implications. Int J Radiat Oncol Biol Phys 9:1451, 1983.

341. Glazer HS, Lee JKT, Balfe DM, Mauro MA, Griffith R, Sagel SS: Non-Hodgkin lymphoma: computed tomographic demonstration of unusual extranodal involvement. Radiology 149:211, 1983.

342. Castellino RA, Blank N, Hoppe RT, Cho C: Hodgkin disease: contributions of chest CT in the initial staging evaluation. Radiology 160:603, 1986.

343. Khoury MB, Godwin JD, Halvorsen R, Hanun Y, Putman CE: Role of chest CT in non-Hodgkin lymphoma. Radiology 158:659, 1986.

344. Jochelson MS, Balikian JP, Mauch P, Liebman H: Peri- and paracardial involvement in lymphoma: a radiographic study of 11 cases. AJR 140:483, 1983.

345. Pilepich MV, Rene JB, Munzenrider JE, Carter BL: Contributions of computed tomography to the treatment of lymphomas. AJR 131:69, 1978.

345a. Hopper KD, Diehl LF, Cole BA, Lynch JC, Meilstrup JW, McCauslin MA: The significance of necrotic mediastinal lymph nodes on CT in patients with newly diagnosed Hodgkin disease. AJR 155:267, 1990.

346. Salonen O, Kivisaari L, Standertskjold-Nordernstam CG, Oksanen K, Lappalainen K: Chest radiography and computed tomography in the evaluation of mediastinal adenopathy in lymphoma. Acta Radiol 28:747, 1987.

347. Nyman R, Rehn S, Glimelius B, Hagberg H, Hemmingsson A, et al: Magnetic resonance imaging, chest radiography, computed tomography and ultrasonography in malignant lymphoma. Acta Radiol 28:253, 1987.

347a. Rehn SM, Nyman RS, Glimelius BLG, Hagberg HE, Sundstrom JC: Non-Hodgkin lymphoma: predicting prognostic grade with MR imaging. Radiology 176:249, 1990.

347b. Negendank WG, Al-Katib AM, Karanes C, Smith MR: Lymphomas: MR imaging contrast characteristics with clinical-pathologic correlations. Radiology 177:209, 1990.

348. North LB, Fuller LM, Sullivan-Halley JA, Hagemeister FB: Regression of mediastinal Hodgkin disease after therapy: evaluation of time interval. Radiology 164:599, 1987.

349. Mauch P, Goodman R, Hellman S: The significance of mediastinal involvement in early stage Hodgkin's disease. Cancer 42:1039, 1978.

350. Chen JL, Osborne BM, Butler JJ: Residual fibrous masses in treated Hodgkin's disease. Cancer 60:407, 1987.

351. Cosset FT, Cherel P, Renaudy N, Carde P, Piekarski JD: Thoracic CT-scanning follow-up of residual mediastinal masses after treatment of Hodgkin's disease. Radiother Oncol 11:119, 1988.

CHAPTER 3

PULMONARY HILA

GORDON GAMSU

The transverse axial anatomy of the hila is simple when the relationships of the pulmonary arteries and veins to the bronchial tree are understood. Variations in the positions of the arteries, veins, and bronchi are small and do not produce major differences in the appearances of the hila. The normal computed tomographic (CT) and magnetic resonance (MR) anatomy of the pulmonary hila have been described in detail.[1-5]

Anatomy

The pulmonary hilum cannot be anatomically defined with precision but is generally considered to be "the depression on the mediastinal surface of the lung where the bronchus, blood vessels, and nerves enter."[6] More important than a strict anatomic definition of the hilum is an understanding of the pulmonary arteries and veins and their relationship to the bronchial tree from the site in the mediastinum where they approach the lungs to their segmental branches and tributaries (Fig. 3–1). The bronchial anatomy has been detailed in Chapter 1. The branches of the pulmonary artery accompany their respective bronchi as they pass from the medias-

tinum into each lung. In contrast, the pulmonary veins course in directions separate from the bronchi and are more variable in position.

The right pulmonary artery divides within the mediastinum into upper and lower divisional arteries. The upper division of the right pulmonary artery (anterior trunk) is immediately in front of the right main bronchus. After a short, obliquely upward course it divides, usually into three branches, each of which accompanies a right upper lobe segmental bronchus. The apical arterial branch is anteromedial to its bronchus. The anterior and posterior pulmonary arterial branches tend to be medial to their respective bronchi. The lower division of the right pulmonary artery (interlobar artery) is anterolateral to the intermediate bronchus. The first branches of the interlobar artery consist of one to three ascending branches arising from its anterolateral surface to supply a portion of the posterior segment of the right upper lobe. Next are branches accompanying the superior segmental bronchus of the right lower lobe and, at a slightly lower level, a branch accompanying the right middle lobe bronchus. The superior segmental artery and right middle lobe artery are usually lateral to their respective bronchi but vary in position. The basal branches of the lower lobe artery accom-

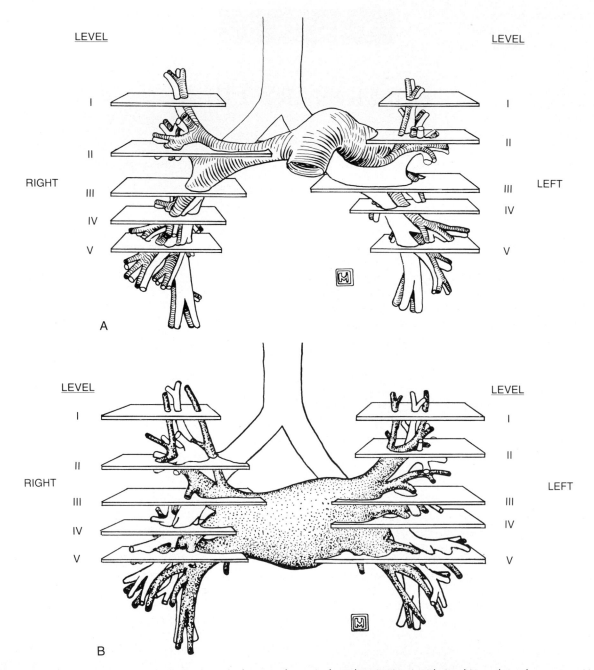

FIGURE 3–1 ■ Schema of the normal hila. The bronchial tree is shown in frontal projection in relationship to the pulmonary arteries (A) and pulmonary veins (B). Designated levels refer to levels in the text and to Figures 3–3 through 3–9.

pany the basal segmental bronchi but also vary in position.

The veins contributing to the hilar contours on the right side are the superior and inferior pulmonary veins. The right superior pulmonary vein is a constant structure with two major tributaries. In most people the right posterior pulmonary vein lies lateral to the apical bronchus and courses forward in the angle between the anterior and posterior segmental bronchi of the right upper lobe. It forms the superior pulmonary vein by joining the apical anterior pulmonary vein in front of the interlobar artery before entering the mediastinum. The middle lobe tributary

of the superior pulmonary vein primarily drains the middle lobe and passes medial to the middle lobe bronchus. It then enters the mediastinum and joins with the superior pulmonary vein. The right inferior pulmonary vein primarily drains the lower lobe. It is the only vascular structure that crosses behind the bronchial tree on the right, which it does at about the level of the basal segmental bronchi.

The top of the left hilum is about 2 cm higher than the right, and its vascular structures vary more in position than those on the right. The left pulmonary artery does not divide into distinct upper and lower divisions. Four to eight upper lobe arterial branches arise from the superior and lateral surfaces of the main trunk of the left pulmonary artery. The branch most constantly present is an apical segmental artery coursing medial to the apical posterior segmental bronchus. An anterior branch medial to the anterior segmental bronchus is also frequently present. A posterior subsegmental branch is an inconstant finding. The left pulmonary artery passes over the left main bronchus and turns rapidly caudad as the descending left pulmonary artery. A posterior branch to the superior segment of the left lower lobe and an anterior branch to the lingular segments of the upper lobe are the first two major branches of the descending segment of the left pulmonary artery as it courses lateral to the lower lobe bronchus. The pulmonary arterial branches of both the lingular and the superior segments accompany their respective bronchi. Lateral branches supplying portions of the left lower lobe are also often present. The descending left pulmonary artery then divides with the basal segmental bronchi to supply the remainder of the left lower lobe.

The left pulmonary veins are similar to those found on the right. The superior pulmonary vein has posterior and apical anterior tributaries that converge and enter the mediastinum anterior to the left main bronchus. The middle pulmonary vein tributary of the superior pulmonary vein usually drains the lingular segments of the left upper lobe and enters the mediastinum slightly caudal to the superior pulmonary vein. The inferior pulmonary vein is a posterior

hilar structure and, as on the right, passes posterior to the dividing lower lobe segmental bronchi.

Accurate assessment of the normal and abnormal hilum requires an understanding of the hilar contours. Additional information can be obtained with opacification of the hilar vessels using intravascular contrast material.[3] The hilar contours can be determined with CT window settings usually used to view the lungs (level -500 to -750 Hounsfield units [H]; width 800 to 1500 H). The intramediastinal pulmonary arteries and veins are best seen at soft tissue CT settings suitable for viewing the mediastinum (level, 0 to 60 H; width, 250 to 500 H). The frequency with which CT scans demonstrate the hilar bronchi, arteries, and veins depends on their size and orientation and on the collimation of the CT scan. The large central structures and those that are cut either transversely or longitudinally are invariably visible. The segmental bronchi and vessels that course obliquely through the plane of the image (e.g., the middle lobe segmental bronchi), are shown less frequently on 1-cm collimated CT scans. With 5-mm collimation, bronchi and vessels as far as segmental and subsegmental bronchi can be routinely imaged.[7]

On spin-echo, cardiac-gated MR images of hila, only vessel walls and bronchi as far as lobar divisions are identified. Imaging degradation and poor resolution preclude accurate visualization of more distal vessels or bronchi.[8] MR and CT scans both demonstrate normal soft tissue that is predominantly fat

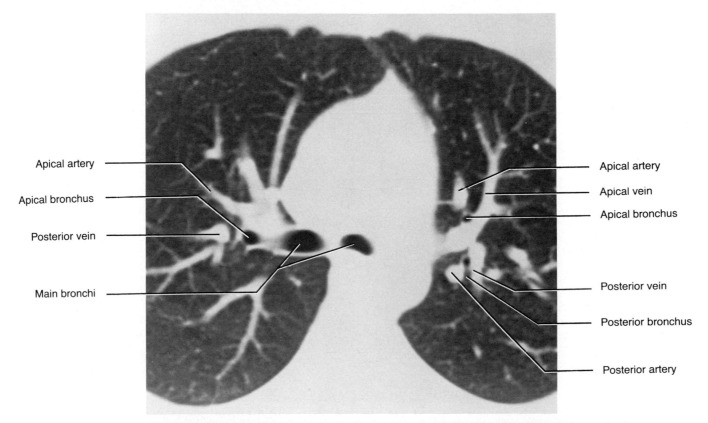

Apical artery

Apical bronchus

Posterior vein

Main bronchi

Apical artery

Apical vein

Apical bronchus

Posterior vein

Posterior bronchus

Posterior artery

FIGURE 3–2 ■ Normal superior hilar anatomy in an adult man showing the relationships of the bronchi, arteries, and veins.

and small lymph nodes within the hila.[8] Normal lymph nodes up to 1 cm in transaxial diameter can be seen within both hila.

For descriptive purposes, we will deal with CT and MR appearances of the right and left hila sepa-rately. Figures 3–2 through 3–7 are serial 6- and 10-mm CT scans through the normal hila from superior to inferior levels. Each CT image is accompanied by a labeled schema of the hilum at that level. Selected MR images are included.

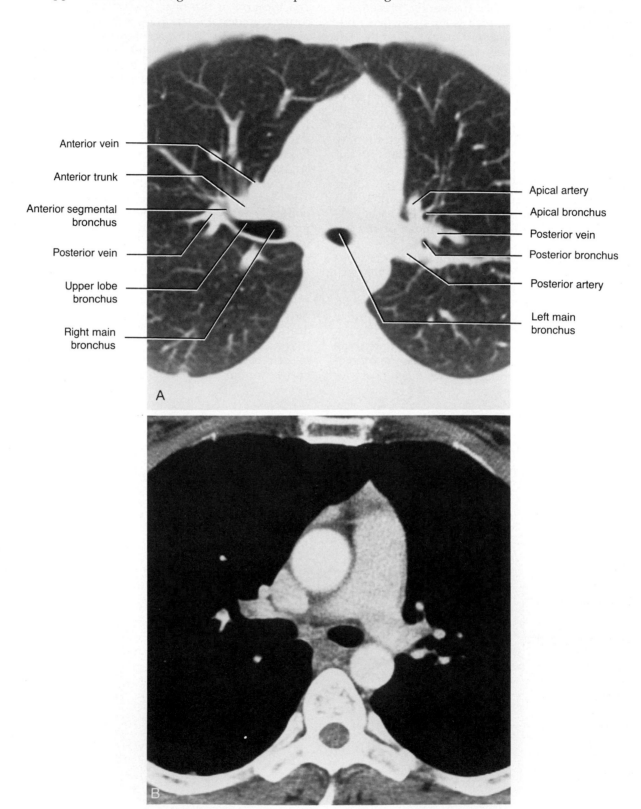

Anterior vein

Anterior trunk

Anterior segmental bronchus

Posterior vein

Upper lobe bronchus

Right main bronchus

Apical artery

Apical bronchus

Posterior vein

Posterior bronchus

Posterior artery

Left main bronchus

FIGURE 3–3 ■ Normal right upper hila and left superior hilar anatomy showing the relationships of the bronchi, arteries, and veins. *A*, CT scan at lung window settings. *B*, CT scan at soft tissue window settings.

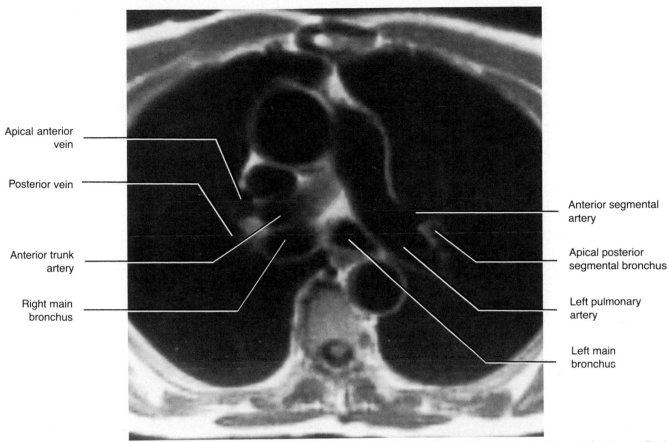

Apical anterior
vein

Posterior vein

Anterior trunk
artery

Right main
bronchus

Anterior segmental
artery

Apical posterior
segmental bronchus

Left pulmonary
artery

Left main
bronchus

FIGURE 3–4 ■ Normal right and left hilar anatomy showing the relationships of the bronchi, arteries, and veins. Cardiac-gated MR scan. Partial volume of the upper surface of the right pulmonary artery and mediastinal fat produces a masslike effect in the mid-mediastinum.

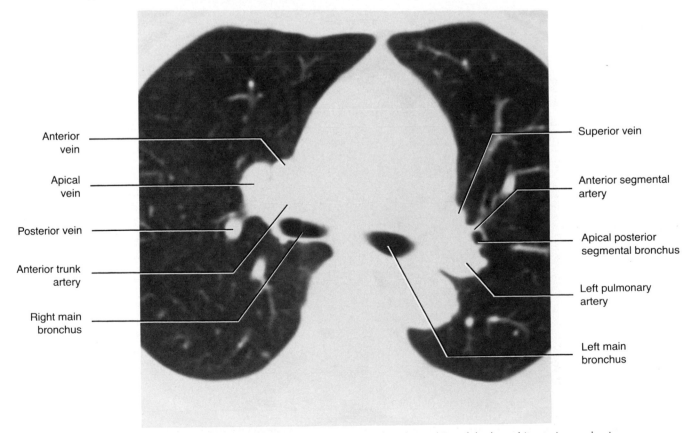

Anterior
vein

Apical
vein

Posterior vein

Anterior trunk
artery

Right main
bronchus

Superior vein

Anterior segmental
artery

Apical posterior
segmental bronchus

Left pulmonary
artery

Left main
bronchus

FIGURE 3–5 ■ Normal right and left upper hilar anatomy showing the relationships of the bronchi, arteries, and veins.

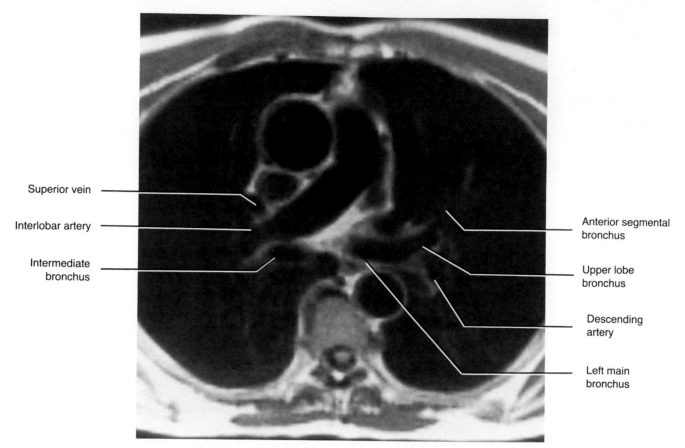

Superior vein

Interlobar artery

Intermediate bronchus

Anterior segmental bronchus

Upper lobe bronchus

Descending artery

Left main bronchus

FIGURE 3–6 ■ Normal right and left hilar anatomy showing the relationships of the bronchi, arteries, and veins. Cardiac-gated MR scan.

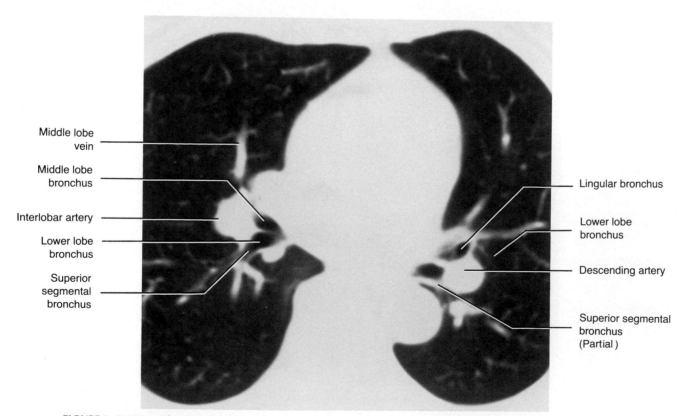

Middle lobe vein

Middle lobe bronchus

Interlobar artery

Lower lobe bronchus

Superior segmental bronchus

Lingular bronchus

Lower lobe bronchus

Descending artery

Superior segmental bronchus (Partial)

FIGURE 3–7 ■ Normal right and left midhilar anatomy showing the relationships of the bronchi, arteries, and veins.

Right Hilum

RIGHT APICAL SEGMENTAL BRONCHUS (LEVEL I)

The superior right hilum is at about the same level as the tracheal bifurcation (see Fig. 3–2). The apical segmental bronchus is seen in cross section lateral to the lower trachea or to the right main bronchus and is usually flanked on its medial side by the apical segmental pulmonary artery and on its lateral side by the posterior tributary of the superior pulmonary vein. CT scans may show branches of these vessels coursing outward from the right superior hilum, but normally any additional tissue is not visible at this level.

RIGHT MAIN BRONCHUS (LEVEL II)

The short right main bronchus bifurcates into the right upper lobe bronchus and the intermediate bronchus about 1 cm below the tracheal carina (see Fig. 3–3). The upper lobe bronchus arises from the lateral aspect of the main bronchus and courses laterally for 1 to 2 cm. It then usually trifurcates into anterior, posterior, and apical segmental bronchi. CT scans show the lobar bronchus and the anterior and posterior segmental bronchi on one image. The anterior segmental bronchus lies in a more horizontal plane than the posterior bronchus, which is directed obliquely cephalad. The anterior bronchus is thus frequently seen over a greater distance than its posterior counterpart. The apical bronchus is imaged on the immediately cephalic scan.

The upper division of the right pulmonary artery (anterior trunk) lies anterior to the right main bronchus (see Figs. 3–3B and 3–4). In the transverse axial plane it is cut obliquely and produces an oval density immediately anterior to the right main bronchus and contained within the mediastinum. The anteroposterior diameter of the anterior trunk is approximately equal to the diameter of the adjacent right main bronchus. At this level or slightly caudad, the horizontal anterior segmental pulmonary artery is medial to the anterior segmental bronchus. The posterior tributary of the superior pulmonary vein is quite constant in position; it was found in 82 per cent of 50 lungs studied by Boyden and Scannell.[9] On CT images it produces a distinctive round or oval density laterally in the angle between the anterior and posterior segmental bronchi (see Fig. 3–3). Also visible at this level, but less constant in position, is the apical anterior tributary of the superior pulmonary vein, which forms a subpleural convexity in the anterior hilum between the anterior trunk and the superior vena cava.

The posterior upper right hilum is devoid of vascular structures. The lung, with very few exceptions, is closely applied to the posterior walls of the distal right main bronchus and right upper lobe bronchus and medial to the right upper lobe posterior segmental bronchus (see Figs. 3–2 through 3–4).

On cardiac-synchronized MR images at this level, the upper lobe bronchus is visible, whereas its anterior and segmental branches are seen about half the time. The oval lucency of the anterior trunk of the right pulmonary artery is usually seen anterior to the main or right main bronchus (see Fig. 3–4). The pulmonary veins are less constantly demonstrated. A small amount of fat or soft tissue can be present lateral to the artery and anterior to the upper lobe bronchus.

RIGHT INTERMEDIATE BRONCHUS (LEVEL III)

The intermediate bronchus extends vertically for 3 to 4 cm between the origin of the right upper lobe and the right middle lobe bronchi (see Fig. 3–5). It is present in cross section on three or four adjacent 1-cm-thick images. The interlobar pulmonary artery courses laterally and inferiorly from the mediastinum, moving from a position anterior to the intermediate bronchus to a position lateral to the bronchus at its termination.

In its upper portion, the interlobar artery gives rise to two to four ascending branches that supply posterior regions of the right upper lobe. At this level, the posterior and apical anterior pulmonary veins come together in the anterior hilum (see Fig. 3–5), producing adjacent convexities on the anterior surface of the interlobar artery lateral to the superior vena cava and right upper atrium.

One to two centimeters lower, the interlobar artery takes a more lateral position in relation to the intermediate bronchus (see Fig. 3–6). One to three arterial branches course posteriorly to supply the superior segment of the right lower lobe (see Fig. 3–7). These branches, together with the interlobar artery, give the hilar contour a reverse comma or elongated S shape at this level. The two pulmonary veins of the anterior hilum combine at about this level to form the superior pulmonary vein, which then enters the mediastinum.

MR scans demonstrate the same vascular and airway structures that are seen on CT. In addition, in most subjects a collection of fat-intensity soft tissue is evident in the anterior hilum lateral to the proximal interlobar pulmonary artery. It varies between 5 and 15 mm in diameter, and about half the time it is 10 mm or more in diameter.

RIGHT MIDDLE LOBE BRONCHUS (LEVEL IV)

The right middle lobe bronchus arises from the anterolateral surface of the intermediate bronchus 4 to 5 cm below the tracheal carina. It courses anteriorly, laterally, and inferiorly for 1 to 3 cm before dividing into its segmental bronchi (Fig. 3–8). The middle lobe bronchus is visible, usually on two adjacent images, coursing in an anterolateral and inferior direction at about 45°. The medial and lateral segmental bronchi of the middle lobe cannot always be seen on the CT scan. The medial segmental bronchus lies in a more horizontal plane than the lateral segmental bronchus and is more frequently demonstrated. The bronchus to the superior segment of the right lower lobe is usually visible at the level of the orifice of the right middle lobe bronchus or 1

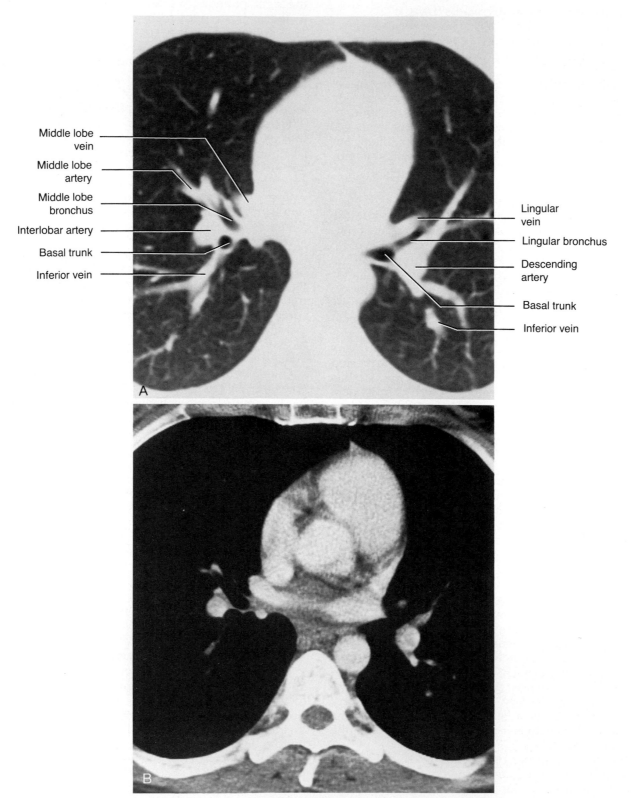

Middle lobe vein

Middle lobe artery

Middle lobe bronchus

Interlobar artery

Basal trunk

Inferior vein

Lingular vein

Lingular bronchus

Descending artery

Basal trunk

Inferior vein

FIGURE 3–8 ■ Normal right and left midhilar anatomy showing the relationships of the bronchi, pulmonary arteries, and pulmonary veins. *A,* CT scan at lung window settings. *B,* CT scan at soft tissue window settings.

cm superiorly (see Fig. 3–7). It arises from the posterolateral right lower lobe bronchus. CT scans at the level of the right middle lobe and superior segmental bronchi clearly show the descending right pulmonary artery that lies lateral to the bronchi between the right middle lobe bronchus anteriorly and the superior segmental bronchus posteriorly, forming a distinct oval density with a smooth lateral contour. As many as three branches, but usually only one, arise from its anterolateral surface, coursing forward to accompany the right middle lobe bronchi (see Fig. 3–8).[10] At about the same level, pulmonary artery branches to the superior segment of the lower lobe extend posteriorly to accompany the superior segmental bronchus on its lateral surface. The middle pulmonary vein tributary of the superior pulmonary vein can be seen between the right middle lobe bronchus and the mediastinum approximately 50 per cent of the time.

Lung tissue always outlines the posterior hilum at this level, sharply defining the posterior wall and often part of the medial wall of the intermediate bronchus and adjacent mediastinum. When the superior segmental bronchus is visible, its medial wall contacts the parenchyma of the right lower lobe.

MR images at the level of the middle lobe bronchus demonstrate the same findings seen on the CT scan, but with less frequency and clarity. The segmental bronchi are only inconsistently demonstrated, and, again, small amounts of soft tissue are evident in the lateral hilum around the bronchi and hila.

RIGHT BASAL BRONCHI (LEVEL V)

The right lower lobe bronchus divides into its four basal segmental bronchi approximately 1 cm below the level of the origin of the right middle lobe bronchus.[11] CT scans always show one or more basal segmental bronchi (Fig. 3–9). At this level, the relationship of the segmental pulmonary artery branches to the bronchial tree varies. The branching pulmonary arteries course in oblique planes. At their branch points, they often have a lobular, round, or oval appearance, usually adjacent to bronchi. Naidich and colleagues[7] have shown that all of the basal bronchi can be identified using thin-section contiguous CT scans (Fig. 3–10). The divisions into subsegmental bronchi could be seen in 56 per cent of instances in the right lower hilum. In situations in which an abnormality is suspected, 1.5- to 5-mm sections can improve detection of bronchial wall thickening or small endobronchial masses.

CT scans at about the level of the origin of the lower lobe segmental bronchi demonstrate the right inferior pulmonary vein (see Fig. 3–9). It passes behind the bronchial tree and courses medially toward the left atrium. Usually the inferior pulmonary vein is horizontal, and a 2- to 4-cm segment can be seen entering the posterolateral left atrium. This is

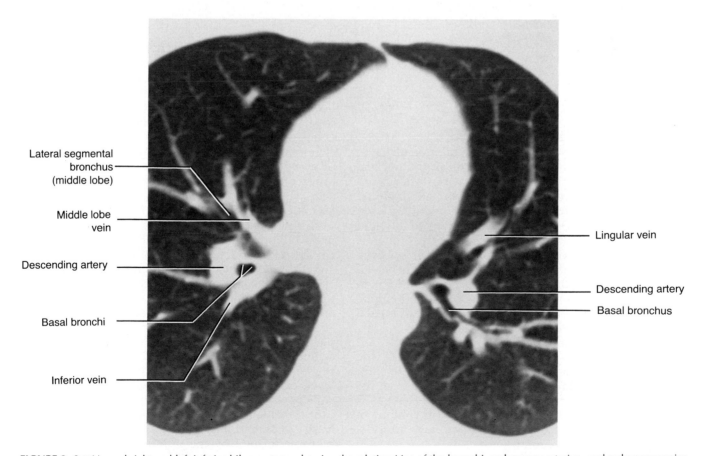

FIGURE 3–9 ■ Normal right and left inferior hilar anatomy showing the relationships of the bronchi, pulmonary arteries, and pulmonary veins.

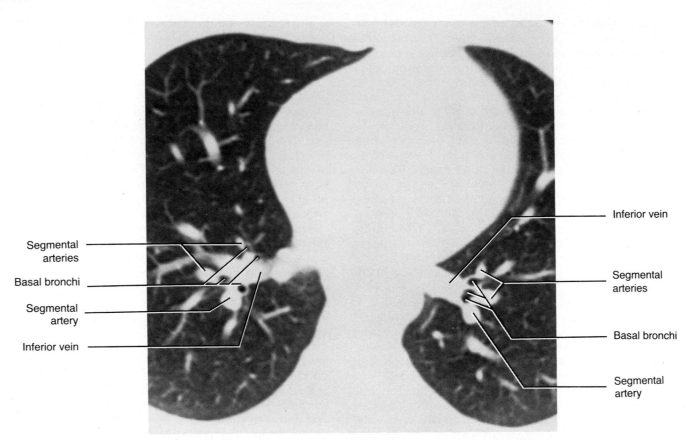

Segmental arteries

Basal bronchi

Segmental artery

Inferior vein

Inferior vein

Segmental arteries

Basal bronchi

Segmental artery

FIGURE 3–10 ■ Five-millimeter collimated CT scan through the basal segmental bronchi demonstrates segmental and subsegmental branches. The pulmonary artery branches tend to be toward the costal pleura in their relationship to the bronchi.

the only level below the azygos vein at which the lung does not contact the posterior surface of the right bronchial tree.

Left Hilum

LEFT APICAL POSTERIOR BRONCHUS (LEVEL I)

The left superior hilum is similar in appearance to the right superior hilum. At the level of the tracheal carina, or 1 cm cephalad, the apical posterior bronchus is visible in cross section. Occasionally both the apical and posterior subsegmental bronchi are seen (see Figs. 3–2 and 3–3). A vein analogous to the right posterior pulmonary vein lies lateral to the bronchus in more than half of normal subjects.[12] It is the only normal structure lateral to the bronchus at this level. Frequently an additional vein is present anterior to the apical posterior bronchus. One of the upper lobe pulmonary artery branches is usually present medial to the bronchial tree.

At a slightly caudal level, the top of the left pulmonary artery borders the medial side of the apical posterior bronchus (see Fig. 3–4). Four to eight arterial branches to the left upper lobe arise from the superior surface of the left pulmonary artery as it arches over the left main bronchus. The contour of the superior surface of the left pulmonary artery is thus variable and irregular.

Mencini and Proto[13] described a normal variation in the configuration of the main and left pulmonary arteries that may simulate a mediastinal mass. Occasionally a high-riding left pulmonary artery can occur lateral to the aortic arch and displace the left medial upper lobe away from the mediastinum. This is an isolated anomaly that can be recognized as the pulmonary artery after injection of contrast medium or by noting its continuity with the main pulmonary artery on inferior scans.

LEFT PULMONARY ARTERY (LEVEL II)

The normal hilar contour at the level of the left main pulmonary artery varies little. CT scans 1 to 2 cm below the tracheal carina pass through the horizontal portion of the left pulmonary artery, which is above the distal left main bronchus and proximal left upper lobe bronchus (see Fig. 3–5). The artery has an oval appearance in cross section and is directly lateral to the proximal left main bronchus. About 75 per cent of the time, the left upper lobe anterior segmental bronchus arises with the apical posterior segmental bronchus from a common trunk.[14] At this level, or 1 cm caudad, the anterior segmental bronchus is visible about 90 per cent of the time (see Fig. 3–5). It usually has a horizontal orientation, and at least 1 to 3 cm of its length can be seen. The posterior hilum is formed by the pulmonary artery, which is smoothly rounded and gives off one to three arterial branches. The anterior hilum, medial to the anterior segmental bronchus, is variably lobulated. The CT appearance of the anterior left hilum is formed by a composite of the superior pulmonary vein and one or more branches of the pulmonary artery to the anterior segment.

On MR scans, the left pulmonary artery, the upper lobe bronchial tree laterally, and the superior vein anteriorly are usually seen (see Fig. 3–4).[5] Soft tissue (i.e., nodes or fat) is not apparent at this level.

LEFT UPPER LOBE BRONCHUS (LEVEL III)

Two to four centimeters below the tracheal carina, the left main bronchus divides into the left upper lobe and left lower lobe bronchi. This is at the level of the midportion of the intermediate bronchus on the right side. The left upper lobe bronchus courses laterally and is visible on one or two adjacent CT images. In 75 per cent of individuals, the anterior and apical posterior segmental bronchi arise as a common trunk, directed superiorly, and the lingular bronchus appears as the continuation of the left upper lobe bronchus, coursing anteriorly, laterally, and inferiorly (see Fig. 3–6). In 25 per cent of people, the left upper lobe bronchus trifurcates into anterior, apical posterior, and lingular bronchi. The course of the proximal anterior segmental bronchus parallels the lingular bronchus, and it may be difficult to differentiate the two. The direction of the anterior segmental bronchus, however, is invariably more anterior than that of the lingular bronchus.

The contour of the left hilum at this level is relatively simple. Anterior to the left upper lobe bronchus and medial to the anterior and lingular segmental bronchi, the hilum consists of pulmonary venous structures. The superior pulmonary vein enters the mediastinum at about the level of the anterior segmental bronchus to produce a small anterior convexity (see Fig. 3–5). Depending on its size and position, the vein may extend inferiorly to lie medial to the lingular bronchus as well. Lateral to the lower lobe bronchus and behind the upper lobe bronchus, the descending left pulmonary artery forms a distinct oval density (see Figs. 3–6 through 3–8). Both anterior and posterior branches arise from the pulmonary artery at this level, producing a somewhat lobular appearance. An arterial branch to the lingula can be seen in about 50 per cent of normal persons, and a posterior branch to the superior segment of the lower lobe can be found in about 80 per cent.

Webb and Gamsu[4] have shown that on CT a small segment of the posterior wall of the left main bronchus and the medial wall of the left lower lobe bronchus are usually contacted by the superior segment of the left lower lobe that invaginates between the descending pulmonary artery and bronchus laterally and the aorta and esophagus medially, forming the retrobronchial recess (see Figs. 3–6 and 3–8). When the anteroposterior diameter of the chest is narrow or the aorta is dilated, lung is excluded from this region. The proximity of lung to the bronchial tree facilitates the recognition of nodal enlargement or bronchial abnormalities at this site.

On spin-echo MR images, the bronchi and pulmonary vessels are imaged as far as their lobar branches (see Fig. 3–6). More distal vessels and airways are inconsistently imaged. Because of the nature of MR images, the confluence of veins entering the left mediastinum is particularly well seen. Soft tissue representing fat and lymph nodes up to 5 mm in diameter is demonstrated in most normal subjects. A thin layer of fatty tissue 3 to 10 mm thick separates the posterior wall of the distal left main bronchus from the adjacent descending pulmonary artery (see Fig. 3–6).[4] A similar layer may also be present medially between the artery and superior segmental bronchus.

LEFT LOWER LOBE BRONCHUS (LEVEL IV)

Three to five centimeters below the tracheal carina and 1 cm below the origin of the left lower lobe bronchus, the superior segmental bronchus of the lower lobe is seen along its axis (see Fig. 3–7). As on the right, the proximal superior segmental bronchus is usually seen on only one image and is not seen in all instances. It extends directly posteriorly, usually flanked by a branch of the pulmonary artery on its lateral side and a tributary of the inferior pulmonary vein medially. At this level, the pulmonary artery is lateral to the lower lobe bronchus and has a bilobed or oval contour. The anterior wall of the left lower lobe bronchus is devoid of vessels and routinely is contacted by lung tissue.[14a] CT images sometimes show the middle pulmonary tributary of the superior pulmonary vein as it crosses in front of the hilum toward the left atrium (see Fig. 3–8).

LEFT BASAL BRONCHI (LEVEL V)

The left inferior hilum is very similar in appearance to the right inferior hilum and is usually seen at about the same level. CT and MR scans show the left inferior pulmonary vein as it passes behind the dividing lower lobe segmental bronchi (see Fig. 3–10). On CT scans, the segmental pulmonary arteries are visible in cross section as oval or elongated segments near the bronchi they accompany.

In the studies by Naidich and co-workers[7] using high-resolution CT (HRCT), all of the left basal segmental bronchi and 35 per cent of the subsegmental bronchi could be identified. As with the right, the branching pattern is variable, but this technique can reliably detect subtle endobronchial involvement by a mass or endobronchial obstruction.

Techniques of Examination

Computed tomography of the hila is usually performed as part of an examination of the entire thorax. The hilar images should be observed while the patient is still in the scanner, as additional images, with or without contrast and usually using 1.5- to 5-mm collimation, can better define any abnormality that is detected. The techniques used for CT of the thorax vary widely among institutions.[15] With modern equipment, the study can be modified to suit the problem under consideration. Glazer and colleagues[3] have shown that dynamic scanning during incremental movement of the scanner table during intravenous bolus injection of a contrast medium gives excellent detail of the hilar vessels—a technique that has become widely accepted. We routinely use 5-mm collimation for scans through the hila.

CT Imaging

RESPIRATION AND POSITION

CT scanning should be performed during suspended respiration at maximal inspiration. In older patients and patients who are dyspneic, a few preliminary deep breaths will make it easier to maintain full inspiration. A nose clip may also assist patients in holding their breath.

The supine position is usually used, with the patient's arms extended above the head. Because the hila have limited mobility, the prone and decubitus positions offer no advantage over the supine position.

CONTRAST MEDIUM

Contrast medium is usually administered to opacify the mediastinal vessels. The hilar vessels will necessarily be opacified, and masses can be distinguished from enlarged vessels within the hilum. The usual dose of contrast medium is 125 to 150 mL of 60 per cent contrast (35.25 to 42.3 g of organically bound iodine). The most frequent method of administered contrast is by rapid-drip infusion. Alternatively, a large bolus of contrast material (75 mL of 60 per cent contrast) can be given immediately before scanning. When higher concentrations of intravascular iodine are required, a bolus injection of 25 to 30 mL of 60 or 76 per cent contrast should be given, followed by rapid sequential scanning at a specific level.

TECHNICAL CONSIDERATIONS

Evaluating the pulmonary hila requires observation of a wide range of CT densities. The most accurate assessment of hilar contours and normal bronchi is achieved with settings used for the lungs. A window level between −500 and −750 H and a window width of 800 to 1500 H are usually used. These settings, however, obscure detail of adjacent mediastinal structures and tend to underestimate the internal diameter of the bronchi and overestimate bronchial narrowing. The hilar structures, adjacent mediastinum, and bronchi should also be observed at a window level of 0 to 60 H and a window width of 250 to 500 H. Rapid sequential scans through the hila are also viewed at these soft tissue window settings.

At a window level of about -450 H and a window width of 1000 to 1500 H, the hilar contours, struc-

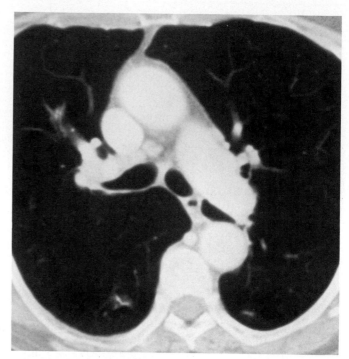

FIGURE 3–11 ■ CT scan through the midhila at extended window settings (window width 1500 H) demonstrates hilum contours, vessels, and bronchi, all on a single scan.

tures, and bronchi can be seen on a single image (Fig. 3–11). Bronchial narrowing and obstruction are more precisely delineated than at lung window levels. The relationship of hilar abnormalities to adjacent mediastinal structures can be seen more easily at these extended window settings.

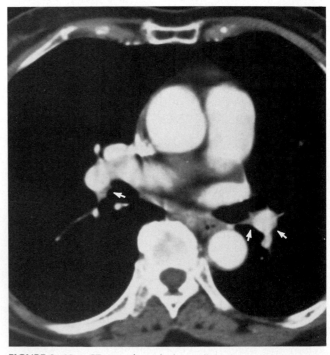

FIGURE 3–12 ■ CT scan through the midhila demonstrates bilateral deposits of normal fat *(arrows)*.

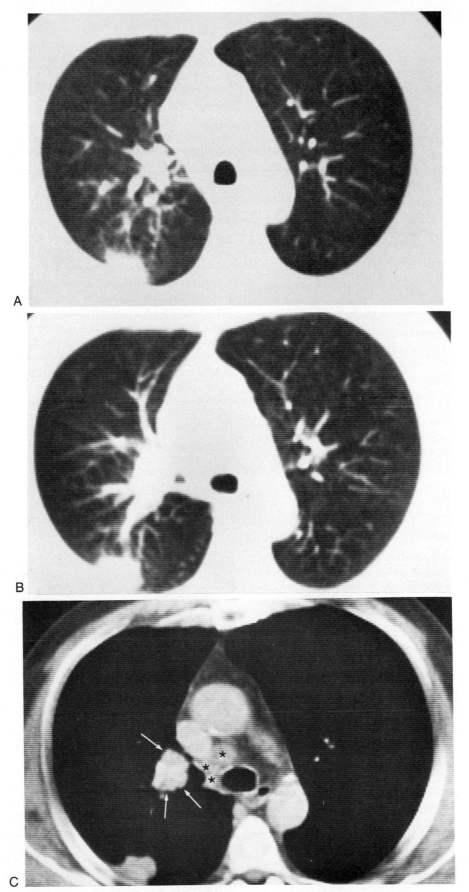

FIGURE 3–13 ■ Bronchogenic carcinoma with hilar metastases. Frontal radiograph shows a right upper lobe mass and enlargement of the superior right hilum. *A,* CT scan shows a mass larger than normal vessels involving the superior right hilum. Posteriorly the primary tumor is visible. *B,* CT scan 1 cm caudal to the level seen in *A* shows the hilar mass obliterating the apical segmental bronchus. *C,* CT scan at the same level but at soft tissue window settings shows multiple nodes in the superior hilum *(arrows)*. Pretracheal lymphadenopathy is also present *(asterisks).*

131

MR Imaging

MR imaging of the hila has been predominantly with spin-echo techniques in the transaxial plane.[16, 17] MR scanners have used field strengths between 0.35 and 1.5 tesla (T). Various pulse sequences have been employed. The repetition time (TR) can be varied between 300 and 1800 ms and the echo delay time (TE) between 30 and 90 ms. Since becoming available, electrocardiogram (ECG) gating has become routine and greatly improves imaging of the mediastinum and hila. With ECG gating, the effective TR is about 700 ms, and the images are T1 weighted. ECG, or cardiac, gating is usually selected for systole so that vessels appear void of signal with only the vessel wall demonstrated. In addition to axial images, some authors have used coronal plane imaging, although it is not generally part of the routine for hilar or mediastinal imaging.

Low flip angle imaging of the hila has been reported for specific circumstances. Posteraro and colleagues[18] used gradient-recalled acquisition in the steady state (GRASS) imaging to identify intravascular emboli within proximal pulmonary arteries. At present, these sequences are not of general application. Limited experience with ultrashort TE sequences of less than 1 ms show promise for imaging the pulmonary and hilar vessels, although these techniques are still experimental and not commercially available.

Pathology

CT Signs of Hilar Abnormalities

To identify an abnormal hilum requires detailed knowledge of the normal variations in hilar contours and bronchial appearances at each level. This understanding can only be achieved by careful observation of many normal cases. CT of the hila uses as a basis the bronchial anatomy and the relationship of the vascular hilar structures to the bronchial tree. Normal hila are composed predominantly of bronchi and vessels. At extended window settings and with HRCT scans, small quantities of fat and small lymph nodes may be demonstrated at the sites previously described; any other tissue is abnormal (Fig. 3–12). The objective findings of an abnormal hilum are found posteriorly, where lung normally contacts the bronchial tree. The finding of endobronchial abnormalities in conjunction with an adjacent mass also helps to identify an abnormal hilum. Local or generalized alteration or irregularity in hilar contours is at least partially subjective and is more difficult to define precisely. Because hilar abnormalities are frequently focal, involving only one or two levels, a systematic evaluation of each level on both sides is essential.

ABNORMAL RIGHT HILUM

Abnormalities of the superior right hilum are easily detected. The apical segmental bronchus is invariably present in cross section, and the vessels accompanying the bronchus are only slightly bigger than the bronchus. Any larger density should raise suspicion of an abnormality (Fig. 3–13). Obliteration or narrowing of the bronchus is usually accompanied by an extrinsic mass.

At the level of the right upper lobe bronchus, the presence of tissue in the posterior hilum greater than the anticipated thickness of the bronchial wall is abnormal (Fig. 3–14). Rarely, a posterior or superior pulmonary vein passes behind the right main bronchus. Laterally, the posterior pulmonary vein is usually present between the anterior and posterior segmental bronchi and is about one half to three fourths the size of the right main bronchus. Any additional density lateral to the bronchial bifurcation indicates lymphadenopathy or a mass. Anteriorly, the anterior pulmonary artery trunk should not be larger than about one-and-one-half times the size of the adjacent right main bronchus. The anterior trunk has multiple branches that course anteriorly and laterally, but the main artery should not extend lateral to a vertical plane through the posterior pulmonary vein.

At the level of the intermediate bronchus, the posterior right hilum is also relatively easy to evaluate. The right lung routinely contacts the posterior bronchial tree for the full length of the intermediate bronchus. The anterior hilum at this level is the most difficult area in which to detect subtle abnormalities. The interlobar pulmonary artery lies partially in front of and partially lateral to the intermediate bronchus. Its branches extend laterally, superiorly, and posteriorly and course in oblique planes to the transverse

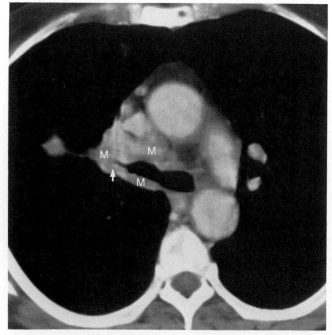

FIGURE 3–14 ■ Small-cell carcinoma invading the right hilum. CT scan demonstrates a mass (M) anterior, lateral, and posterior to the right main bronchus and crossing the midline. The right upper lobe bronchus is occluded (arrow). Thickening of the posterior wall of the right main bronchus is always abnormal.

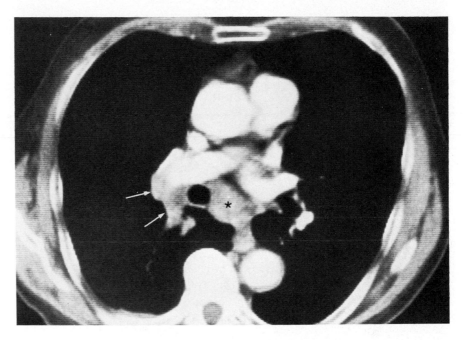

FIGURE 3–15 ■ Metastatic bronchogenic carcinoma to the right midhilum. CT scan during injection of contrast material shows a tumor mass *(arrows)* with an irregular contour lateral to the intermediate bronchus and proximal interlobar pulmonary artery. Subcarinal adenopathy *(asterisk)* is seen.

axial image. The CT appearance of the anterior right hilar contour is a composite of the superior pulmonary vein and the pulmonary artery; the contour normally is lobulated. A focal bulge laterally or anteriorly is a reliable indicator of abnormality. A uniform increase in size of the anterior hilum is difficult to detect, and dynamic scanning is useful in separating vessels from an adjacent mass (Fig. 3–15).

At the level of the origin of the right middle lobe bronchus, lung continues to contact the posterior bronchial wall. The interlobar artery lies lateral to the bronchial tree in the angle between the origin of the right middle lobe bronchus and the superior segmental bronchus. When viewed at lung window settings, the pulmonary artery frequently appears slightly larger than the adjacent lower lobe bronchus. The origins of branching vessels cause the pulmonary artery to appear slightly irregular. As Webb and colleagues[19] demonstrated, lobulation at this level suggests lymphadenopathy or a mass (Fig. 3–16).

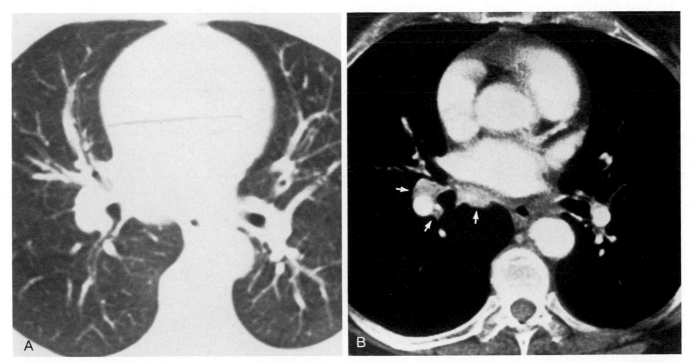

FIGURE 3–16 ■ Metastatic breast carcinoma to right hilar lymph nodes. *A,* CT scan at lung window settings demonstrates asymmetric enlargement of the right hilum at the level of the right middle lobe bronchus. Convex bulge medial to the right lower lobe bronchus is abnormal. *B,* CT scan following injection of contrast material confirms adenopathy *(arrows)* lateral and medial to the right lower lobe bronchus. Left hilum shows normal fat and vessels.

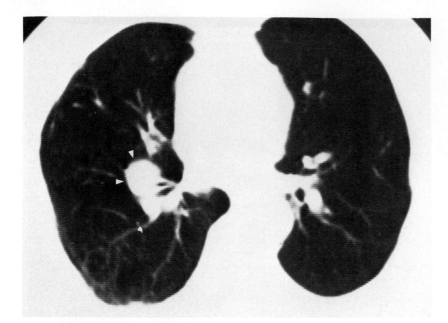

FIGURE 3–17 ■ Metastatic bronchogenic carcinoma to right inferior hilum. CT scan demonstrates nodal metastases to the right inferior hilar lymph nodes *(arrowheads)* that are considerably larger than the adjacent bronchi or normal segmental arteries.

The diagnosis of bronchial narrowing or an endo-bronchial mass at this level must be made with caution, because the superior segmental bronchus of the lower lobe and the right middle lobe bronchus both course obliquely across the plane of view. Only a short segment of each of these bronchi is present on a single scan.

The right pulmonary artery divides into its basal segmental branches about 1 cm below the level of the right middle lobe bronchus. The CT appearance of the pulmonary arterial branches varies as they course through the plane of the image. These branches often appear as small knobs or rounded densities, and they should not be much larger than the adjacent bronchial branches. Abnormal tissue at

this level appears as a focal enlargement of the inferior hilum (Fig. 3–17). At about the same level, the right inferior pulmonary vein courses from lateral to medial across the posterior hilum. The anterior hilum, however, is devoid of vascular structures, and lymphadenopathy or a mass will appear as an additional density.

ABNORMAL LEFT HILUM

The superior left hilum is analogous to that on the right, with a bronchus and one or two vessels of similar size to the bronchus. The apical posterior bronchus is seen in cross section. A hilar mass or lymphadenopathy must be larger than the normal vessels in the area to be recognized. Narrowing or

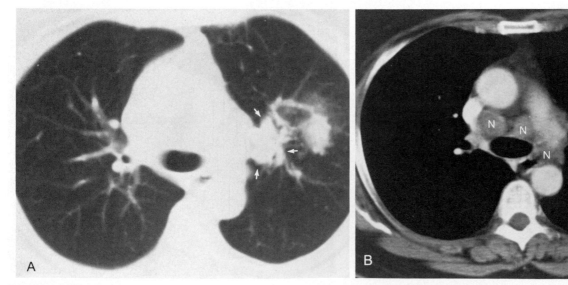

FIGURE 3–18 ■ Left upper lobe bronchogenic carcinoma metastatic to left superior hilum. *A*, CT scan at lung window settings demonstrates a left upper lobe mass and left hilar adenopathy *(arrows)*. *B*, CT scan at the same level, after contrast administration, confirms the hilar adenopathy *(arrows)*. Extensive aortic-pulmonic window adenopathy (N) and pretracheal adenopathy (N) are seen.

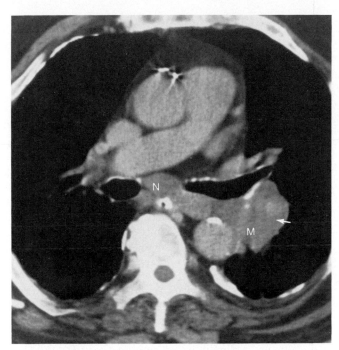

FIGURE 3–19 ■ Bronchogenic carcinoma with left hilar and mediastinal adenopathy in a patient with asbestos exposure. CT scan at the level of the left main bronchi demonstrates a large mass (M) encasing the descending left pulmonary artery *(arrow)*. The mass fills the left retrobronchial space between the left pulmonary artery and the aorta, thus gaining access to the mediastinum. Enlarged lymph nodes (N) are present in the subcarinal space. Extensive bilateral pleural calcifications are asbestos related. Contrast material is seen in the esophagus.

ance. However, the common trunk that gives rise to the anterior and apical posterior segmental bronchi and the apical posterior bronchus forms the lateral boundary of the hilum. A density lateral to the bronchus and larger than a normal vessel is abnormal (Fig. 3–18). The anterior left hilum has a distinctive convexity produced by the left superior pulmonary vein before it enters the mediastinum. Absence of this contour indicates an anterior left hilar mass effacing the normal venous convexity (see Fig. 3–18).

At the level of the bifurcation of the left main bronchus into its upper and lower lobe bronchi, the left hilar contour is similar to the right hilar contour at the level of the right middle lobe bronchus. The left lower lobe bronchus is visible, as is the descending left pulmonary artery lateral to it. The normal left pulmonary artery at this level should not be more than about one-and-one-half times the size of the adjacent bronchus. Extending forward at about 45° is the lingular bronchus with the superior pulmonary vein medial to it, joined by its middle pulmonary vein tributary.

Abnormalities of contour at this level appear as larger-than-expected masses or as abnormal lobulation (Fig. 3–19). Lymphadenopathy posterior to the left main and left lower lobe bronchi is readily detected between the descending pulmonary artery and the aorta. Only a small amount of soft tissue may be normally present in this location.

Below the origin of the lingular bronchus, the left hilum is similar to the inferior right hilum. The left inferior pulmonary vein courses across the posterior hilum and may contact the descending aorta. As on the right, only short segments of the basal pulmonary arteries are present on a single image. They appear as small, lobulated densities near the basal bronchi. Abnormal contours in the inferior hilum appear as focal enlargements greater in size than the anticipated vascular structures (Fig. 3–20).[19a]

obliteration of the bronchus is strong supportive evidence that the hilum is abnormal.

At a slightly lower level, the left pulmonary artery arches over the left main bronchus, producing a laterally convex contour. Arterial branches to the upper left lobe give the hilum an irregular appear-

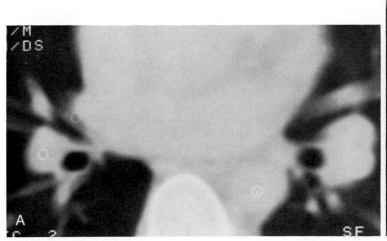

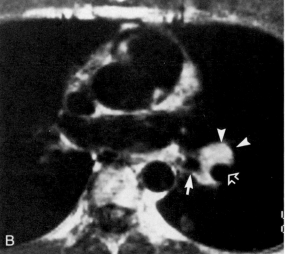

FIGURE 3–20 ■ Left inferior hilar bronchial adenoma. *A*, CT scan at the level of lower lobe basal trunk demonstrates asymmetric enlargement on the left, which appeared to opacify with contrast material. *B*, MR scan at the same level demonstrates the basal bronchus *(arrow)*, pulmonary artery *(open arrow)*, and tumor mass *(arrowheads)*.

ASSOCIATED HILAR ABNORMALITIES

Hilar masses, or adenopathy, are frequently accompanied by CT findings that help establish the hilum as abnormal. These findings may also suggest the cause of the abnormality and the most appropriate method of further diagnosis. In the study by Webb and colleagues,[20] more than 50 per cent of patients with an abnormal hilar contour had additional CT findings confirming the abnormality. These included obscuration of normal bronchial walls and hilar vessels, bronchial narrowing, and local abnormalities in the adjacent lung (see Figs. 3–13, 3–14, and 3–18).

The right lung contacts the posterior wall of the distal right main bronchus, the right upper lobe bronchus, and the intermediate bronchus in all patients. The left lung contacts the posterior wall of the distal left main bronchus and the posteromedial wall of the left lower lobe bronchus in about 90 per cent of patients. Thickening of the bronchial wall or masses at these sites are readily detected with CT.

Schnur and colleagues[21] investigated 36 patients with thickening of the posterior wall of the intermediate bronchus on lateral chest radiographs. The maximal normal thickness of the intermediate bronchus was 3 mm. Two patterns of abnormal thickening were found: uniform and lobulated. Both patterns were found in patients with metastatic carcinoma or lymphoma. Congestive heart failure, however, was the most common cause of uniform thickening. CT scans clearly define the bronchial wall, which is uniformly less than 2 mm thick. Hilar fat and the pleural surfaces do not add to the normal thickness of the bronchial wall.

Both Webb and colleagues[19] and Naidich and associates[22] reported that obscuration of the contour of the posterior hilum is a frequent and sensitive indicator of hilar abnormality. Nonvascular enlargement of a hilum is often accompanied by a decrease in the definition of the hilar contours. Seven of 25 patients with bronchogenic carcinoma or lymphoma had this finding.[19] Bronchial narrowing by a mass was also present in many of these patients, and the poor hilar definition may have been caused by tumor infiltration of the perihilar lung or lymphatic obstruction.

CT scans in the transverse axial plane readily demonstrate subtle degrees of bronchial narrowing. Bronchial narrowing may arise from intrinsic tumor, extrinsic compression from lymphadenopathy, or compression by vessel enlargement.[22a] The apparent diameter of the normal hilar bronchi is critically dependent on the window width and level at which they are viewed. Bronchial narrowing must be evaluated at various settings. The optimal window settings for measuring bronchial dimensions is a level of about -175 H and a fairly narrow width. With CT, it is often impossible to determine whether the mass narrowing the hilar bronchus has an endobronchial component that has disrupted the bronchial mucosa and is visible bronchoscopically.

MR Signs of Hilar Abnormalities

In general, MR is better able to distinguish between hilar mass and vessels than comparable CT scans.[5, 23] Small lymph nodes about 1 cm in diameter are also more easily detected with MR than with CT. The demonstration of hilar masses with MR employs the same morphologic findings as does CT. The mass or lymphadenopathy, however, is directly imaged against the background of signal void from vessels and bronchi (see Fig. 3–20B). T2-weighted spin-echo images have better signal-to-noise ratios, and masses are more intense than on T1-weighted images. Thus the contrast between the mass and vessels or bronchi is better. With these pulse sequences, however, masses cannot be differentiated from hilar fat, and for practical purposes, T1-weighted images suffice. T1-weighted images also allow demonstration of extension of hilar mass into the mediastinum. The T1 relaxation times of tumors or enlarged lymph nodes are longer than those of hilar or mediastinal fat, and thus the mass can be differentiated from fat on T1-weighted images.

The walls and caliber of the bronchi in the hila are better demonstrated with CT than MR. Bronchial narrowing and obstruction frequently cannot be precisely defined with MR. Artifacts from respiration during image acquisition can also produce false bronchial narrowing adjacent to a hilar mass. For these reasons, MR has not become generally accepted for imaging of hilar masses.[16]

Vascular Lesions of the Hila

DEVELOPMENT OF THE HILAR PULMONARY ARTERIES

The central pulmonary arteries are derived from the paired sixth (pulmonary) primitive aortic arches, which are formed by a ventral bud from the aortic sac and a dorsal bud from the dorsal aorta.[24–26] The pulmonary arch then joins the splanchnic plexus of vessels, which arises with the lung bud off the ventral esophagus. The portion of the splanchnic plexus giving rise to the lung vessels is referred to by Huntington as the "pulmonary postbrachial plexus."[27] The ventral buds, with contributions from the postbrachial plexus, form the pulmonary arteries. The dorsal buds form the left and right ductus arteriosus; normally only the left ductus persists until birth, after which it becomes the ligamentum arteriosus. Numerous vascular channels form communications between the distal aorta and the postbrachial plexus. Some of these persist as the bronchial arteries, whereas others form potential systemic pulmonary anastomoses in later life.

After absorption of the segment of the aortic arches that does not persist, the primitive truncus arteriosus rotates counterclockwise. The left pulmonary artery is pulled anteriorly, and the right pulmonary artery migrates posteriorly and to the left. Thus the main pulmonary artery is derived largely from the primitive left pulmonary artery, and the right pulmonary artery appears as a branch vessel of the main and left pulmonary arteries.

CONGENITAL ANOMALIES OF THE HILAR PULMONARY ARTERIES

Congenital Unilateral Absence of a Pulmonary Artery ■ This is a rare anomaly that has been called by many names; *proximal interruption, agenesis, aplasia, hypoplasia,* and *absence of the left or right pulmonary artery* are terms frequently used interchangeably. The embryologic malformation giving rise to absence of a pulmonary artery is probably a failure of the development of the ventral buds of the primitive aortic arch.[28] The intraparenchymal pulmonary vessels derived from the postbrachial plexus are present and patent. Blood is supplied to the lung by the bronchial arteries or by anomalous vessels from the aorta or from one of the great vessels.

The interrupted pulmonary artery is most frequently located opposite the aortic arch. When the absent pulmonary artery is on the same side as the aorta, there is a high incidence of cardiac anomalies, particularly tetralogy of Fallot and septal defects. Absence of the right pulmonary artery is frequently associated with a patent ductus arteriosus.

The radiographic features of absence of the pulmonary artery, first described by Danelius,[29] strongly suggest the diagnosis. The affected lung is frequently small, with decreased vascularity and a small hilum. The "lacy" pattern of pulmonary vessels has been attributed to enlarged bronchial arteries. Expiratory radiographs do not reveal delayed expiration on the affected side. Ventilation-perfusion radionuclide scans demonstrating absent pulmonary perfusion with nearly normal ventilation should confirm the diagnosis and distinguish this anomaly from the acquired Swyer-James syndrome. Madoff and colleagues[30] first reported the angiographic findings, which are typical.

Naidich and colleagues[22] described the CT appearance in a patient with an absent right pulmonary artery (Fig. 3–21). The right lung was small, and as anticipated, the mediastinum was displaced. The ipsilateral bronchi appeared intact, but the main and interlobar pulmonary arteries were absent. The contralateral pulmonary arteries and veins were both enlarged, reflecting a long-standing increase in pulmonary flow.

MR scans should be as accurate as CT in detecting absence of a pulmonary artery, and the same morphologic findings are well displayed by MR. Fletcher and Jacobstein[31] studied six patients with suspected narrowing of the central pulmonary arteries. MR provided complete imaging of the main and branch pulmonary arteries. Hypoplasia was clearly documented using a combination of transverse and coronal ECG-gated MR images.

Pulmonary Artery Dilation ■ The central pulmonary arteries dilate in response to a long-standing increase in intraluminal pressure or blood flow. Segmental dilatation of a pulmonary artery, often called a *pulmonary artery aneurysm*, usually results from turbulence within the pulmonary artery.[32–34] Both pulmonary valvular stenosis and subvalvular stenosis can produce a jet of turbulent blood directed toward the left pulmonary artery. Typically, the main and left pulmonary arteries are markedly enlarged, but the right hilar vessels are normal. Congenital pulmonary valvular insufficiency, however, is often associated with dilatation of both central pulmonary arteries and a ventricular septal defect. Segmental dilatation of the central pulmonary arteries may also be seen with mycotic aneurysms, syphilis, trauma, and diseases of defective connective tissue, such as Marfan's syndrome.

True congenital aneurysms of the pulmonary arteries are rare and are almost invariably associated with more common malformations of the lung, especially arteriovenous fistula and pulmonary sequestration.[32, 34] Guthaner and co-workers[35] used CT to measure the normal diameter of the central pulmonary arteries, which fell within a narrow range. The main pulmonary artery measured 2.8 ± 0.3 cm, the left pulmonary artery 2.0 ± 0.2 cm, and the right pulmonary artery 2.0 ± 0.4 cm. O'Callaghan and colleagues,[36] also using CT, measured the diameter of the right pulmonary artery between the anterior wall of the right main bronchus and the posterior wall of the superior vena cava. They found a mean diameter of 1.33 ± 0.15 cm in 25 adult patients without evidence of pulmonary vascular disease. Kuriyama and co-workers,[37] in a study of normal subjects and patients with pulmonary hypertension, found that the upper limit of normal (i.e., mean plus two standard deviations) for the main pulmonary artery was 28.6 mm (Fig. 3–22). The main pulmonary artery was the most accurate of the central arteries for detecting pulmonary hypertension, and a pulmonary artery diameter above 28.6 mm readily predicted pulmonary hypertension. The CT findings in segmental central pulmonary artery dilatation can be detected easily with CT scanning after contrast opacification of the vessels.

Pulmonary Artery Stenosis ■ Pulmonary artery stenosis without concomitant cardiac disease is a rare anomaly of the pulmonary vascular system. The stenotic segments, or coarctations, can be single or multiple, central or peripheral, short or long, unilateral or bilateral. Poststenotic dilatation is common, and when it is strategically placed, it may be seen as a hilar mass on CT scans.

Coarctations of the pulmonary artery are most frequently associated with congenital cardiac disease. Two major forms of congenital coarctation involve the main pulmonary artery. One is a short web immediately above the pulmonary valve; the other is a longer segment of stenosis extending to the bifurcation of the main pulmonary artery or even farther (Fig. 3–23). Pulmonary valvular stenosis, or tetralogy of Fallot, is commonly present with either form.[32, 38, 39] Stenosis of the pulmonary arteries distal to the bifurcation of the main pulmonary artery is part of

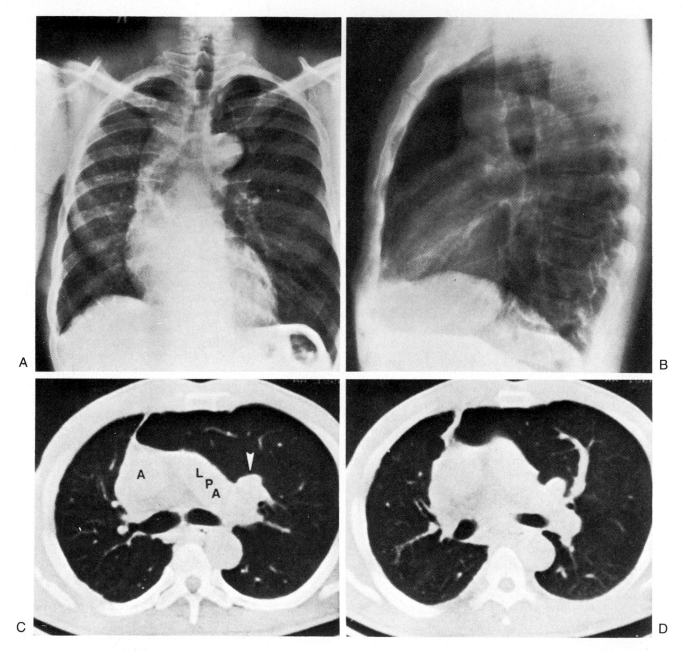

FIGURE 3–21 ■ Congenital absence of the right pulmonary artery. Frontal *(A)* and lateral *(B)* chest radiographs show a small right lung with a small right hilum. C, CT scan at the level of the tracheal carina confirms the small right lung. The mediastinum is shifted to the right. The bronchi are of normal caliber. The right hilum shows no right pulmonary artery, although the right posterior pulmonary vein is in normal position. The left pulmonary artery (LPA) and vein *(arrowhead)* are prominent. A represents the ascending aorta. *D*, CT scan at the level of the intermediate bronchus fails to show an interlobar pulmonary artery. (From Naidich DP, Khouri NF, Stitik FP, McCauley DI, Siegelman SS: J Comput Assist Tomogr 5:468, 1981. Reprinted by permission.)

several syndromes. In familial pulmonary artery stenosis, supravalvular aortic stenosis is commonly present. When stenosis arises from maternal rubella, other stigmata of the syndrome can be found. In the Williams-Beuren syndrome, pulmonary artery stenosis is associated with supravalvular aortic stenosis, mental retardation, and goblin facies.[38] When pulmonary artery stenosis is associated with Takayasu's arteritis or the Ehlers-Danlos syndrome, additional features of these entities are present.[40]

Chest radiographs may show hilar masses as a result of poststenotic dilatation of segments of the central pulmonary arteries. In the presence of peripheral stenoses, focal or diffuse regions of lung oligemia may be evident. When pulmonary stenosis is severe, chest radiographs will demonstrate the findings of pulmonary arterial hypertension and cor pulmonale. The CT appearance of pulmonary artery stenosis has not been described, but CT scans should be able to suggest the malformation. CT may be performed in these patients to clarify hilar abnormalities detected on conventional radiographs. In

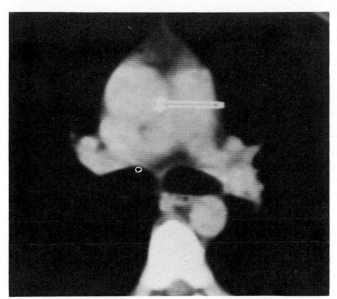

FIGURE 3–22 ■ CT scan at the midthorax showing the site of measurement of main pulmonary artery for predicting pulmonary hypertension. Cursor on the main pulmonary artery indicates the site where measurements should be obtained for determining the size of the main pulmonary artery.

patients in whom surgery is contemplated, detailed pulmonary and cardiac angiography is required to detect multiple lesions.

ANOMALOUS ORIGIN OF THE PULMONARY ARTERIES

Anomalous origin of the pulmonary arteries is a complex malformation of the embryonic ventral and

TABLE 3–1 ■ Anomalous Origin of Pulmonary Arteries
Descending aorta via patent ductus arteriosus
Ipsilateral to aortic arch
Contralateral to aortic arch
Innominate or subclavian artery via patent ductus arteriosus
Contralateral to aortic arch
Ascending aorta
Right pulmonary artery with left arch
Left pulmonary artery with right arch (rare)
Left pulmonary artery from right pulmonary artery
Persistent bronchial arteries

dorsal aortic arches and their communication with the postbrachial vascular plexus.[32] Most cases are associated with congenital heart disease, which usually dominates the clinical picture. The more common varieties are described in Table 3–1.

Stone and associates[41] described the CT findings in two patients with anomalous origin of the left pulmonary artery. The malformed artery arose from the posterior surface of the midportion of the right pulmonary artery and passed from right to left between the lower trachea and esophagus to enter the left hilum. Most patients with this anomaly have airway obstruction before the age of 2 years.[42] Airway obstruction may occur from compression by the maldeveloped pulmonary artery sling. In about 50 per cent of patients, however, an independent anomaly of complete tracheal cartilaginous rings is present, causing severe intrinsic tracheal stenosis.

Anomalous origin of the pulmonary arteries in

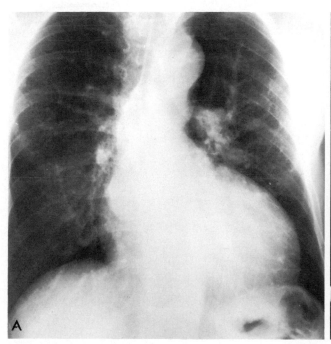
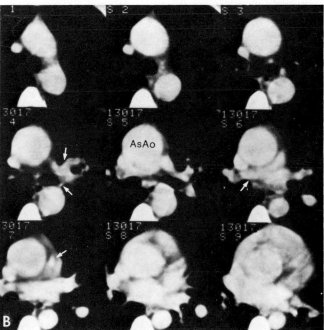

FIGURE 3–23 ■ Pulmonary artery atresia in a 23-year-old man. A, Frontal radiograph shows an enlarged heart with absence of the main pulmonary artery trunk and a narrow cardiac root. The intrapulmonary vessels are increased in size. B, Serial scans through the mediastinum from superior to inferior reveal a dilated ascending aorta (AsAo). The main pulmonary artery is atretic (S7, arrow). The ductus arteriosus is visible (S4, posterior arrow). Both the left (S4, anterior arrow) and the right (S6, arrow) pulmonary arteries are seen. At cardiac catheterization, a large ductus arteriosus connected the descending aorta to the left pulmonary artery. Both left and right pulmonary arteries were present and dilated. The main pulmonary artery was atretic.

adults is rare, but in the few cases that have been described, an asymptomatic mediastinal or hilar mass was present. Chest radiographs show a right hilar mass that displaces or indents the right main bronchus or lower trachea. CT studies may be obtained to characterize the abnormal hilum. In the patients reported by Stone and colleagues,[41] the abnormal origin and course of the maldeveloped left pulmonary artery was clearly documented by CT scans.

PULMONARY ARTERIAL HYPERTENSION

Radiologists have been intrigued for some time as to whether the caliber of vessels visible on chest radiographs reflects pulmonary hemodynamics. The pulmonary vascular bed is a low-pressure system; the upper limit of normal pressure is close to 30 mm Hg, and the mean pressure is 15 to 18 mm Hg.[43] Pressure within the pulmonary circuit is a function of flow and resistance. Flow is determined by cardiac output and resistance by the cross-sectional area of the pulmonary vascular bed. The pulmonary vascular bed contains a large volume of viscous liquid at low pressure that moves in a pulsatile manner.[44] The pulmonary vessels are variably distensible, with active and elastic tension in their walls. They are surrounded by the lungs, which continually change volume and thereby affect the transmural pressure across the pulmonary vessels. The pulmonary circuit can compensate for a two- to threefold increase in flow by decreasing resistance and allowing pressure to remain stable.[45]

A long-standing increase in flow causes adaptive changes in the pulmonary arteriolar walls that result in a radiographically visible increase in pulmonary artery caliber. Pulmonary hypertension, a sustained increase in systolic pulmonary arterial pressure above the normal 30 mm Hg,[46] with few exceptions occurs only when the cross-sectional area of the pulmonary vascular bed is reduced and pulmonary vascular resistance is increased. Pulmonary hypertension arises from a primary change in the structure or hemodynamics of the pulmonary vascular system (Table 3–2).

Altered Structure of the Pulmonary Vasculature ■ Diseases of the pulmonary artery wall, lungs, pleura, and chest wall may all result in increased pulmonary arterial pressure. Focal hypoxia may be a significant stimulus for vasoconstriction. Initially, transient pulmonary hypertension may occur that can be reversed by supplying 100 per cent oxygen. Later, pulmonary hypertension becomes irreversible. Other factors contributing to pulmonary hypertension include polycythemia, hypervolemia, and systemic pulmonary arterial anastomoses.

Primary pulmonary hypertension is an uncommon condition seen predominantly in young females.[47] The prognosis varies, but most patients do not survive longer than one decade from the time of diagnosis. Primary pulmonary hypertension designates a distinctive syndrome resulting from intrinsic idiopathic obstructive disease of the small pulmonary

TABLE 3–2 ■ Classification of Pulmonary Hypertension

Altered structure
  Vascular
    Primary pulmonary hypertension
    Thromboembolic disease
      Thrombotic emboli
      Neoplastic emboli
      Parasitic emboli
      Foreign body emboli
    Pulmonary arteritis
  Pulmonary
    Obstructive lung disease
      Emphysema
      Chronic bronchitis
    Restrictive and cicatricial lung disease
  Chest wall deformity
  Alveolar hypoventilation
Altered hemodynamics
  Increased flow
    Left-to-right shunt
  Increased venous pressure
    Cardiac
      Left ventricular failure
      Mitral stenosis
      Atrial obstruction
    Pulmonary venous obstruction

arteries. The cause of the initial elevation in pulmonary arterial pressure is unknown, but vasoconstriction does play some part. Once hypertension has been present for some time, morphologic changes in the vascular wall lead to sustained, nonreactive pulmonary hypertension. The radiographic features are distinctive. The caliber of the central hilar pulmonary arteries is uniformly increased, and the caliber of the peripheral vessels is decreased; right ventricular enlargement may also be evident (Fig. 3–24).

Pulmonary hypertension is a common sequela of both advanced emphysema and chronic bronchitis.[48]

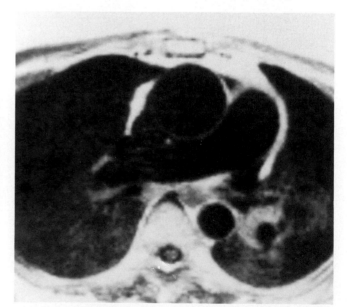

FIGURE 3–24 ■ Primary pulmonary arterial hypertension. Cardiac-gated MR scan shows marked enlargement of the main and right pulmonary arteries. The aorta is normal. The study is gated to vascular systole, and the vessels are void of signal.

The pathophysiology of the elevated pulmonary pressure in these conditions has not been completely clarified. The potential causative factors include hypoxia, destruction of the pulmonary vascular bed, and small pulmonary emboli.[49] Emphysema does not involve the lung uniformly, and the more affected regions show a marked decrease in caliber of the vessels subtending them. The more normal areas of the lungs contain normal-appearing vessels, as in the upper lobes in lower lobe emphysema caused by alpha₁-antitrypsin deficiency. Patients with chronic bronchitis may have significant airway obstruction and pulmonary hypertension without the radiographic features of the airway disease.

Advanced restrictive and cicatricial lung diseases frequently result in significant pulmonary hypertension. The radiographic features of pulmonary hypertension are often obscured by the concomitant pulmonary disease. Dilated central pulmonary arteries are the only radiographic clue to the developing pulmonary hypertension. Clinically, the diagnosis may not be apparent until right-sided heart failure supervenes. CT may be able to detect the pulmonary vessel abnormalities at an earlier stage than can chest radiographs, although this has not been determined.

Alveolar hypoventilation exists when alveolar ventilation is insufficient for the metabolic needs of the body. There are several causes of hypoventilation (Table 3–3). The term *alveolar hypoventilation syndrome* is used to designate lesions in which the lungs are normal and ventilatory insufficiency is from neurologic, muscular, or skeletal causes. All of these conditions can result in pulmonary hypertension.

Severe pulmonary hypertension may occur in children with upper airway obstruction,[50, 51] in obese patients with the pickwickian syndrome,[52] and in patients with autonomic dysfunction.[53] The radiographic features are those of pulmonary hypertension with otherwise normal-appearing lungs.

Pulmonary hypertension and cor pulmonale are major but infrequent complications of congenital, paralytic, or idiopathic spinal curvature. Pulmonary hypertension does not usually become clinically manifest until late middle age and should not be given primary consideration in children with kyphoscoliosis. The radiographic manifestations of severe kyphoscoliotic cardiopulmonary disease are extremely difficult to evaluate. The heart and mediastinum are distorted and rotated. The orientation of the main pulmonary arteries is abnormal, and even the intrapulmonary vasculature is difficult to assess.

Approximately 2 per cent of patients with pulmonary emboli have recurrent emboli, which may cause pulmonary hypertension and cor pulmonale.[54-56] A clinical history of repeated acute attacks is usually available. Recurrent showers of small blood clots that produce pulmonary hypertension without acute clinical attacks are extremely rare. Radiographic manifestations of pulmonary hypertension from recurrent pulmonary emboli are usually different from those seen in other conditions; the central pulmonary arteries are enlarged, whereas the peripheral pulmonary artery alteration is focal and asymmetric (Fig. 3–25). In affected areas, the lung parenchyma is often markedly oligemic and the vessels are attenuated; these changes are well demonstrated with CT (see Fig. 3–25D). The vessels in other areas of the lung maintain a nearly normal appearance or are increased in diameter.

Neoplastic emboli can affect the lungs in two ways. Large tumor emboli may be swept into the pulmonary arterial bed and produce acute attacks, simulating thrombotic emboli. These tumor emboli usually originate in abdominal viscera, especially the liver and kidneys, with large vessels that communicate directly with the inferior vena cava. Emboli consisting of small clumps of tumor cells, mainly from malignant trophoblastic disease and breast carcinoma, can cause insidious pulmonary hypertension without acute attacks.[57] The radiographic features are those of pulmonary hypertension without underlying disease.

Rare causes of pulmonary hypertension include parasites, such as those found in schistosomiasis; talc; cotton particles; or even mercury droplets in drug addicts. The radiograph shows symmetric vascular changes without evidence of lung abnormality, unless other diseases coexist.

Conditions that involve the pulmonary arterial walls and cause arterial hypertension may be from morphologic changes in the arterial wall or from vasoconstriction. Pulmonary arteritis from the collagen vascular diseases, including scleroderma, rheumatoid lung disease, systemic lupus erythematosus, and polyarteritis nodosa, can result in pulmonary hypertension without lung parenchymal fibrosis.[58] Drugs such as aminorex and poisons such as fumarate and cobalt have been implicated in the development of pulmonary hypertension, although their mechanisms of action have not been defined.[59]

Altered Pulmonary Vascular Hemodynamics ■ Congenital cardiac defects with left-to-right shunts can occur at the level of the pulmonary veins, atria,

TABLE 3–3 ■ Causes of Alveolar Hypoventilation

Respiratory center depression
  Anesthesia
  Morphine
  Barbiturates
  Trauma
  Anoxia
Neural conduction defect
  Spinal trauma
  Poliomyelitis
  Curare
  Myasthenia gravis
Respiratory muscle disease
Chest wall restriction
  Arthritis
  Deformity
Pleural restriction
  Fibrothorax
Pulmonary disease
  Restrictive lung disease
  Obstructive lung disease

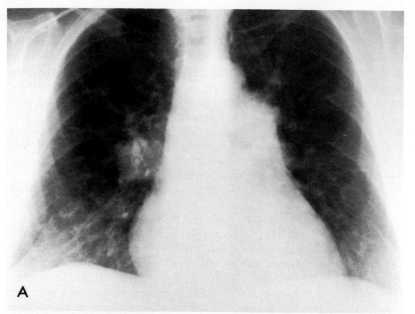

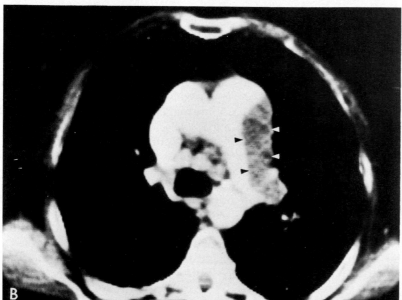

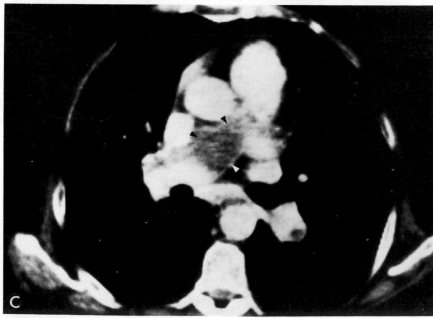

FIGURE 3–25 ■ Recurrent pulmonary emboli causing pulmonary hypertension in a 57-year-old woman. *A,* Frontal radiograph shows cardiomegaly and marked enlargement of the central pulmonary arteries. *B,* CT scan reveals massive enlargement of the left pulmonary artery and a large embolus *(arrowheads)* occluding more than 50 per cent of the left pulmonary artery. *C,* CT scan 2 cm inferior to the level shown in *B* demonstrates a large embolus *(arrowheads)* occluding the majority of the right pulmonary artery. Embolectomy was performed, confirming the diagnosis.

142

ventricles, or aorta. Pulmonary blood flow can be substantially increased for a considerable time before pulmonary hypertension develops. The radiographic features are those associated with increased pulmonary blood flow.[60] In about 10 per cent of patients with atrial septal defects, but rarely in other patients with left-to-right shunts, pulmonary vascular resistance increases and pulmonary hypertension supervenes (the Eisenmenger reaction).

The pathophysiology of the increase in pulmonary vascular resistance is not well understood, but the evidence suggests that reversible vasoconstriction occurs initially and that morphologic changes in the pulmonary vessels develop later.[61] The radiographic manifestations are difficult to see until the condition becomes well established. The central pulmonary vessels dilate, whereas the peripheral pulmonary arteries become narrower. Not until late in the disease do the pulmonary arteries show the severe peripheral attenuation seen in conditions characterized by pulmonary hypertension without increased flow.

Increased pulmonary venous pressure develops from obstruction to flow at the level of the pulmonary veins, left atrium, or mitral valve. Left ventricular failure can also increase pulmonary venous pressure. An increase in venous pressure of long duration leads to interstitial pulmonary edema and fibrosis in the small pulmonary vessels and reduces the cross-sectional area of the pulmonary vascular bed. Reflex pulmonary arterial constriction may also occur. Both factors cause pulmonary arterial hypertension.[62] The usual radiographic features of pulmonary arterial hypertension coexist with the venous changes. In some cases of mitral stenosis, arterial hypertension is the predominant radiographic feature and is accompanied by central artery enlargement, peripheral artery attenuation, and right ventricular prominence. Left atrial enlargement and some radiographic evidence of venous hypertension should be recognizable.

The radiographic features of pulmonary arterial hypertension vary with the cause of the hypertension.[63] Enlargement of the central pulmonary arteries, however, is common to all situations in almost all patients with chronic pulmonary hypertension. Pulmonary hypertension is one of the few conditions in which the caliber of vascular structures can be measured from the chest radiograph. An increase in the diameter of the right descending pulmonary artery is an indicator of elevated pulmonary arterial pressure in mitral stenosis, obstructive lung disease, and primary pulmonary hypertension.[48, 53, 64] The diameter of the right interlobar pulmonary artery is usually less than 16 mm. In patients with chronic pulmonary hypertension, this vessel is usually more than 20 mm in diameter.

The central pulmonary arteries in the mediastinum and hila can be measured precisely from CT scans. O'Callaghan and co-workers[36] found that the diameter of the right pulmonary artery was 16.6 to 26.6 mm in a small group of patients with pulmonary hypertension. Kuriyama and colleagues[37] found that the caliber of the main pulmonary artery, measured from CT, is a more accurate predictor of pulmonary artery pressure than the caliber of the right or interlobar arteries. In 32 patients with pulmonary hypertension but no left-to-right shunting, the calculated cross-sectional area of the main and interlobar pulmonary arteries (normalized for body surface area) predicted mean pulmonary artery pressure with a correlation coefficient (r) of 0.89. A main pulmonary artery diameter greater than 28.6 mm readily predicted the presence of pulmonary hypertension.

Gated MR imaging is as accurate as CT in determining the caliber of the mediastinal and hilar pulmonary arteries. It should be of similar precision in detecting pulmonary hypertension when vessel size is used for diagnosis (see Fig. 3–24). MR can also demonstrate abnormal decreased blood velocity within the dilated pulmonary arteries in pulmonary hypertension. With severe hypertension, it can show right ventricular enlargement and displacement of the interventricular septum. Using multiphasic spin-echo MR, von Schulthess and colleagues[65] demonstrated intraluminal signal in the right pulmonary artery during a major portion of the cardiac cycle, reflecting the decreased velocity of blood flow (Fig. 3–26). In normotensive patients, signal is evident only during late diastole, when blood flow is normally slow. Patients with hypertension showed a linear correlation between the duration of MR signal and pulmonary vascular resistance. In almost all patients with a pulmonary systolic pressure greater than 90 mm Hg, intraluminal signal is visible on multiphasic gated MR images obtained during both systole and diastole. Only about 30 per cent of those with a pressure below 90 mm Hg have this finding. White and co-workers,[66] in differentiating between severe hypertension and central pulmonary emboli, showed that the abnormal systolic MR signal increased in intensity from first to second echo images (Fig. 3–27). The signal intensity from thrombus was fixed throughout the cardiac cycle and did not significantly increase from first to second echo images.

Occasionally a patient with pulmonary arterial hypertension demonstrates hilar enlargement that is indistinguishable from hilar lymphadenopathy or other soft tissue mass. In these circumstances, CT or MR scans can show that the hilar enlargement results from enlarged pulmonary arteries and thus direct further evaluation of the patient.

Hilar Lymphadenopathy

The patterns of pulmonary lymph drainage are complex and variable. The hilar lymph nodes form the major pathway for lymph drainage from the lungs. From the hila, lymph flows through a maze of interconnecting paratracheal, mediastinal, and subdiaphragmatic lymphatic vessels and lymph nodes.[67] Direct pathways also course from the lungs

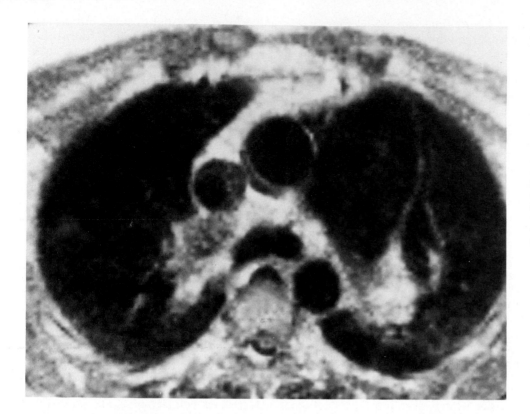

FIGURE 3–26 ■ Slow flow in pulmonary arterial hypertension. MR scan gated to the systolic portion of the cardiac cycle shows massive enlargement of the central pulmonary arteries with abnormal intravascular signal caused by the slow flow of blood.

directly to the aortic pulmonic window and the subcarinal and paraesophageal nodes, bypassing the hila.

CT and MR can provide a precise topographic display of the hilar nodes. Recognition of hilar lymph node enlargement requires an understanding of the position of the lymph nodes within the hila. Most descriptions of hilar lymph nodes are based on dissection of specimens in which the anatomy is distorted. In his original anatomic description, Sukiennikow[68] portrayed the hilar lymph nodes as grouped exclusively around the bronchial tree. Although Engel[69] disproved Sukiennikow's observations, this misconception still persists. Descriptions of hilar adenopathy based on radiographic studies frequently emphasize the bronchial relationships of hilar nodes, dismissing the importance of the perivascular nodes that are also present.

In his detailed description, Engel[69] divided the hilar (bronchopulmonary) lymph nodes into anteromedial and posterolateral groups. The anteromedial nodes are in the bifurcations between the upper and lower

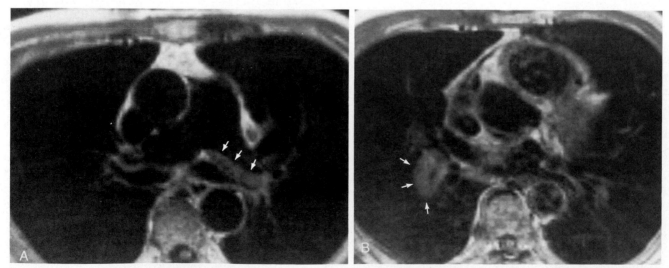

FIGURE 3–27 ■ Emboli in a patient with chronic pulmonary emboli. A, Cardiac-gated MR scan at the level of the left pulmonary artery demonstrates chronic emboli (arrows) lining the wall of the artery. The main pulmonary artery is enlarged. B, MR scan several centimeters caudal to the level seen in A shows almost complete occlusion of the right interlobar pulmonary artery by emboli (arrows).

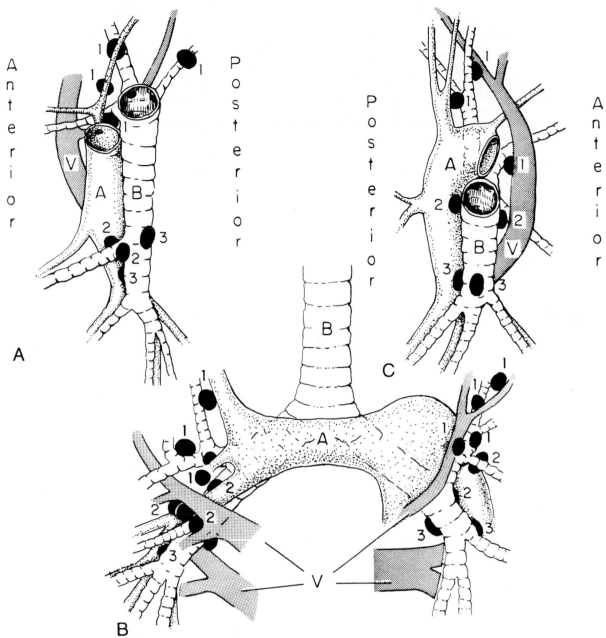

FIGURE 3–28 ■ Schema of hilar lymph nodes in relationship to bronchi, arteries, and veins. *A*, Right side viewed from medial perspective. *B*, Frontal view. *C*, Left side viewed from medial perspective. 1, Upper lobe nodal groups; 2, interlobar nodal groups; 3, lower lobe nodal groups; A, artery; B, bronchi; V, veins. (Modified from Sone S, Higashihara T, Morimoto S, Ikezoe J, Arisawa J, et al: AJR 140:887, 1983.)

lobe bronchi on both sides. On the right side, they are also medial to the intermediate bronchus and lower lobe bronchus; on the left, they are medial to the lower lobe bronchus. The posterolateral nodes are portrayed in his diagrams as situated in the bifurcations between the upper and middle lobe pulmonary artery and posterolateral to the interlobar and lower lobe pulmonary arteries on the right. On the left, the posterolateral nodes are similarly positioned posterior and lateral to the pulmonary arteries. Chang and Zinn[70] described the hilar lymph nodes only in relationship to the bronchial tree. They divided both the left and right hilar lymph nodes into

superior, inferior, anterior, and posterior groups. The lymph nodes around the main bronchi, lobar bronchi, and segmental bronchi were assigned either an anterior or a posterior position.

Sone and colleagues,[71] in their studies on cadavers and patients, provided the most complete description to date of the hilar lymph nodes (Fig. 3–28). As they indicate, lymph nodes are positioned in relationship to the hilar bronchi and vessels. On the right side, four sets of nodes are grouped (1) around the upper lobe and segmental bronchi and arteries, (2) medial and lateral to the intermediate bronchus and interlobar pulmonary artery, (3) around the origin of the middle lobe bronchus and artery, and (4) around the basal trunk of the lower lobe and inferior pulmonary vein. On the left, there are three groupings: (1) around the upper lobe and lingula bronchi and lateral to the left pulmonary artery, (2) posterior to the left main bronchus and medial to the descending left pulmonary artery, and (3) around the basal trunk and inferior pulmonary vein. When enlarged, all of these nodal groups can be observed on CT or MR scans. Good quality scans at suitable window settings in normal individuals can show aggregates of soft tissue up to 1.5 cm in diameter containing normal nodes at three sites: on the right at the bifurcation of the right pulmonary artery into the anterior trunk and interlobar artery; at the origin of the middle lobe; and on the left between the left upper lobe artery and the descending pulmonary artery. Webb and colleagues[5] demonstrated that these collections of soft tissue consist of fat and small lymph nodes.

Of the internal organs, the lungs are in most direct contact with the environment. The hilar lymph nodes form an important part of the lymphatic system, and numerous infectious, inflammatory, and neoplastic diseases involve these lymph nodes.

Hilar lymphadenopathy, which may be marked, is present in almost all patients with primary pulmonary tuberculosis but is rare in postprimary disease.[72] The lung on the side of the adenopathy is virtually always abnormal. The distribution of lymph node involvement varies in patients with tuberculosis. Hilar lymph node enlargement is unilateral in approximately 80 per cent of patients and is associated with mediastinal adenopathy in about half of these. In the remaining 20 per cent, bilateral (but usually asymmetric) hilar lymph node enlargement is present.

Most of the common bacterial pneumonias are not associated with hilar or mediastinal lymphadenopathy. Patients with unusual bacterial pneumonias may have lymph node enlargement, which can be unilateral or bilateral (Table 3–4). Hilar lymphadenopathy in mycoplasma and viral pneumonia is frequent and usually bilateral.

Histoplasmosis and coccidioidomycosis, both fungal infections, may cause either unilateral or bilateral hilar lymphadenopathy.[73–75] In histoplasmosis, hilar node involvement occurs in the benign form of the disease as well as in the more severe pneumonic form. Occasionally bilateral hilar lymph node enlargement is found without parenchymal disease. In the late healing phase, enlarged lymph nodes may compress the hilar bronchi. Hilar node calcification is a common sequela of histoplasmosis. Enlargement of the hilar nodes is common in the acute phase of coccidioidomycosis. It may be unilateral or bilateral and occurs in conjunction with mediastinal adenopathy in about 50 per cent of instances. Colwell and Tillman[76] suggested that involvement of mediastinal lymph nodes indicates imminent dissemination of the disease; this suggestion has been questioned.

The neoplasm most commonly involving the hilar

TABLE 3–4 ■ Causes of Hilar Adenopathy

	Unilateral	Bilateral
Infectious	Coccidioidomycosis	Anthrax
	Cystic fibrosis	Chicken pox
	Histoplasmosis	Coccidioidomycosis
	Mycoplasma	Cystic fibrosis
	Tuberculosis	Histoplasmosis
	Tularemia	Mononucleosis
	Whooping cough	Mycoplasma
		Plague
		Tropical eosinophilia
		Tuberculosis
Neoplastic	Bronchogenic carcinoma	Extrathoracic metastases
	Extrathoracic metastases	Histiocytic lymphoma
	Histiocytic lymphoma	Hodgkin's disease
	Hodgkin's disease (uncommon)	Immunoblastic lymphadenopathy
		Leukemia
Environmental		Berylliosis
		Extrinsic allergic alveolitis
		Silicosis
Idiopathic	Sarcoidosis (uncommon)	Eosinophilic granulomatosis
		Pulmonary hemosiderosis
		Sarcoidosis

Source: Modified from Fraser ERG, Pare JAP: Diagnosis of Diseases of the Chest, 2nd ed. Philadelphia, WB Saunders, 1979, pp 2300–2305.

nodes is bronchogenic carcinoma, discussed later in this chapter. Metastases to hilar and mediastinal lymph nodes do occur in patients with extrathoracic malignancy and are not rare. McLoud and co-workers[77] studied the frequency and types of extrathoracic malignancy that produce intrathoracic lymph node metastases (Fig. 3–29). Of 1021 patients with extrathoracic malignant neoplasms, 163 had an abnormal chest radiograph, and 25 (15.3 per cent of these) had hilar or mediastinal metastases or both. The hila were the most frequent site for metastatic adenopathy; seven patients had bilateral and ten patients unilateral lymph node enlargement. The most common sites of primary malignancy were the head and neck (including the thyroid), the genitourinary tract, the breast, and melanoma arising from the skin.[77, 78]

Tumors of the stomach and pancreas also can metastasize to the hilar lymph nodes. In his study of intrathoracic lymph node metastases from melanoma, Webb emphasized the frequency of symmetric bilateral hilar node involvement.[79] However, extrathoracic malignancy is an uncommon cause of bilateral adenopathy in unselected patients. Winterbauer and colleagues[80] found that only 2 of 100 patients had bilateral hilar adenopathy resulting from extrathoracic malignancy.

Filly and associates[81] described the incidence of hilar lymphadenopathy in patients with untreated lymphoma. Hilar nodal enlargement was demonstrated by conventional chest radiographs or tomograms in approximately 22 per cent of patients with Hodgkin's disease and approximately 10 per cent of additional sites of disease will affect treatment.[83, 84] In 20 to 60 per cent of patients additional diseases can be found with CT.[85, 86]

Sarcoidosis is a multisystem granulomatous disorder in which mediastinal and hilar adenopathy and pulmonary involvement are frequent. Sarcoidosis is characterized pathologically by the presence of non-caseating epithelioid cell tubercles (though some fibrinoid necrosis may be present at the centers of a few tubercles) in all affected organs or tissues. Either the condition resolves or the epithelioid cell tubercles are converted into avascular, acellular hyaline fibrous tissue.[87] This complex definition reflects the obscure origin and protean manifestations of the disease.

Kirks and associates[88] found abnormalities on the chest radiograph in 93 per cent of 162 patients in whom sarcoidosis was proved by biopsy. Lymphadenopathy was present in 84 per cent of those who had abnormal chest radiographs, and in 90 per cent of these, involvement included the hilar nodes bilaterally. The classic description of the thoracic lymph node distribution in sarcoidosis is one of bilateral and right paratracheal lymphadenopathy. Paratracheal lymphadenopathy with unilateral hilar node involvement, as in tuberculosis, is unusual with sarcoidosis, but it has been recorded in up to 5 per cent of patients (Fig. 3–31).[89] A more diffuse distribution of the lymphadenopathy has been shown in sarcoidosis. Subcarinal or anterior and posterior mediastinal lymph node enlargement may be present in up to 20 per cent of patients.[90, 91]

Winterbauer and associates[80] emphasized that the hilar lymphadenopathy was symmetric in almost all patients. Clinical correlations demonstrated that bilateral hilar adenopathy in the asymptomatic patient with a normal physical examination could be considered presumptive evidence of sarcoidosis without the need for further confirmation. Most pulmonologists, however, confirm the diagnosis by bronchoscopy and transbronchial biopsy.

CT studies of sarcoidosis have dealt mainly with the pulmonary parenchymal abnormalities but have confirmed the presence of widespread mediastinal lymphadenopathy.[92–94] The hilar lymph node involvement in patients with sarcoidosis is usually obvious from radiographs, and CT is not required for its detection. In a small percentage of patients, confluent lung disease or fibrosis obscures or distorts the hila; in these patients, CT or MR can detect hilar nodal enlargement.[93] In patients with advanced lung disease, CT can differentiate nodal hilar enlargement from enlarged central pulmonary arteries.

Bronchogenic Carcinoma

The spread of bronchogenic carcinoma has interested surgeons, internists, pathologists, and radiologists for many years. Lung cancer may spread by direct extension and also by lymphatic and hematogenous routes. Direct extension occurs into the adjacent pulmonary parenchyma and visceral pleura,

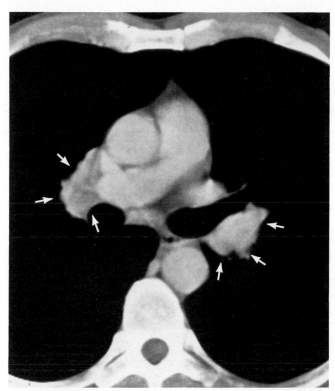

FIGURE 3–29 ■ Melanoma metastatic to hilar nodes. Contrast-enhanced CT scan shows bilateral hilar adenopathy anterolateral to the pulmonary artery on the right and posteromedial on the left (arrows).

patients with non-Hodgkin's lymphoma. In all but three of their patients, hilar adenopathy was visible on plain chest radiographs.

Winterbauer and colleagues[80] studied 212 patients with lymphoma and an abnormal chest radiograph and found unilateral hilar disease in 7.1 per cent and bilateral adenopathy in 3.8 per cent. An additional 12 patients developed adenopathy during the course of their disease. This incidence is less than that in Filly's study, probably reflecting differences in patient selection.[81] All patients with intrathoracic lymphoma had symptoms when first seen, and physical examination showed extrathoracic disease, which tended to differentiate them from patients with sarcoidosis.

In patients with lymphoma, the low yield of conventional frontal tomography in detecting hilar adenopathy not visible on chest radiographs suggests that CT will provide little additional information. However, evaluation of the pulmonary hila in the presence of bulky mediastinal adenopathy is difficult, and the finding of hilar lymph node enlargement in lymphoma may be of critical importance (Fig. 3–30). In many institutions, the radiotherapy ports in these patients are altered to include the ipsilateral lung, and those patients with Hodgkin's disease may require the addition of chemotherapy.[82] CT examination of the thorax should be obtained in all patients, both those with Hodgkin's disease and those with non-Hodgkin's lymphoma, in whom detection of

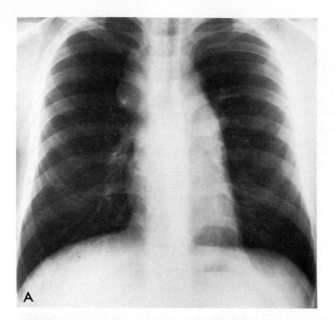

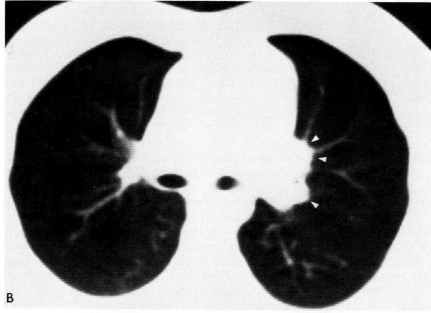

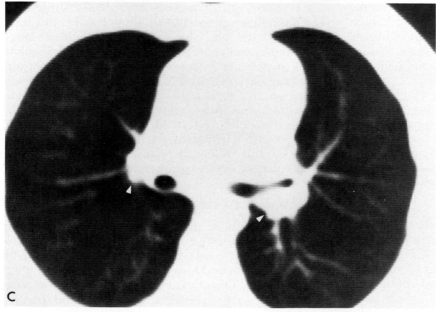

FIGURE 3–30 ■ Hodgkin's disease with hilar adenopathy in a 23-year-old woman. *A,* Frontal radiograph shows a bulky mass projecting to both sides of the upper mediastinum. Hilar adenopathy is not seen. *B,* CT scan at the level of the superior hila shows adenopathy *(arrowheads)* anterior, lateral, and posterior to the apical posterior bronchus on the left. The bronchus is compressed. *C,* CT scan 1 cm caudal to the level seen in *B* shows the left hilum still abnormal, with lobulation laterally and posterior enlargement *(arrowhead).* Adenopathy is also present on the right side *(arrowhead).*

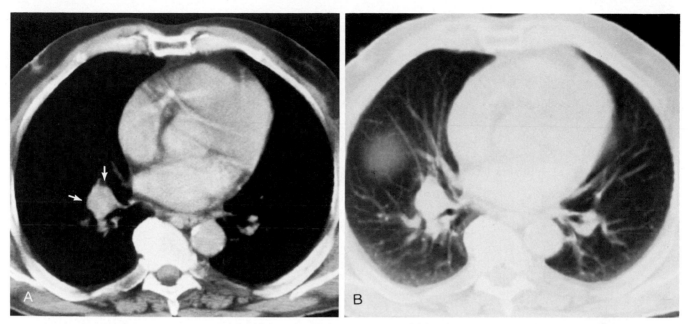

FIGURE 3–31 ■ Sarcoidosis presenting as unilateral hilar adenopathy in a 26-year-old female. CT scans at soft tissue setting *(A)* and at lung window setting *(B)* demonstrate unilateral right inferior hilar adenopathy *(arrows)*. Because of the atypical distribution of the adenopathy, further evaluation is warranted.

across interlobar fissures, along the bronchus from which the tumor originates, and also into the thoracic cage. Lymphatic dissemination of bronchogenic carcinoma is most commonly to hilar lymph nodes, but the carcinoma also spreads directly to mediastinal lymph nodes.[95–97] The presence of hilar disease not only influences treatment, but also may determine prognosis in bronchogenic carcinoma.

Lymphatic metastases occur frequently in patients with lung cancer, and the incidence of hilar lymph node involvement is 15 to 40 per cent in patients undergoing pulmonary resection.[98–101] The cell type of the primary tumor affects the incidence of lymphatic spread. In order of increasing frequency, squamous cell carcinoma, adenocarcinoma, large-cell carcinoma, and small-cell carcinoma all exhibit lymphatic metastases.[101]

The intrapulmonary lymph nodes occur at the bifurcations of the segmental bronchi and their accompanying pulmonary artery branches. Bronchopulmonary lymph nodes are referred to as *hilar* when they are situated along the lower portions of the lobar bronchi and *interlobar* when situated around the angles formed by the divisions of the right and left main bronchi into their lobar branches.[98] This distinction is usually not necessary, and all central lymph nodes that interface with the lungs can be considered hilar.

Nohl[98] has mapped in detail the hilar and mediastinal lymph nodes involved with bronchogenic carcinoma arising in various locations. On the right side, tumor drainage from all three lobes is into the lymph nodes around the intermediate bronchus, which Borrie[102] called the *lymphatic sump* (Fig. 3–32). These nodes are lateral and medial to the intermediate bronchus, anterior (between the intermediate

bronchus and the right interlobar pulmonary artery), and posterior (in the angle between the intermediate bronchus and the apical segmental bronchus of the lower lobe). Right upper lobe carcinomas also metastasize to the right superior hilar, azygos, right paratracheal, pretracheal, and posttracheal lymph nodes (Fig. 3–33). Carcinomas in the right upper lobe rarely involve lymph nodes below the level of the origin of the right middle lobe bronchus or the subcarinal lymph nodes.

Right lower and middle lobe carcinomas metastasize to the lymph nodes of the lymphatic sump, medially to the intermediate bronchus, to the subcarinal area, and to the paraesophageal nodes at the upper extent of the inferior pulmonary ligament. In general, bronchogenic carcinomas arising in the right lower lobe tend to involve the hilar lymph nodes more widely than do upper lobe tumors, and metastases to the right superior hilum are not uncommon.

On the left side, tumors in both the upper and lower lobes drain into the lymphatic sump formed by the lymph nodes between the upper and lower lobe bronchi, those anterior and posterior to the proximal lower lobe bronchus, and also those lateral to the proximal descending left pulmonary artery (Fig. 3–34). The lymph nodes above the superior segmental bronchus of the left lower lobe, below the lingular bronchus, and between the lingular and anterior segmental bronchi are also frequently involved by tumors arising in both the left upper and left lower lobes. Contralateral mediastinal spread of carcinoma, as noted in Chapter 2, is different for the two lungs. From the right lung, contralateral mediastinal nodal metastases is only about 5 per cent. On the left side, the incidence is 10 to 30 per cent,[103, 104] with a higher incidence from the left lower lobe.

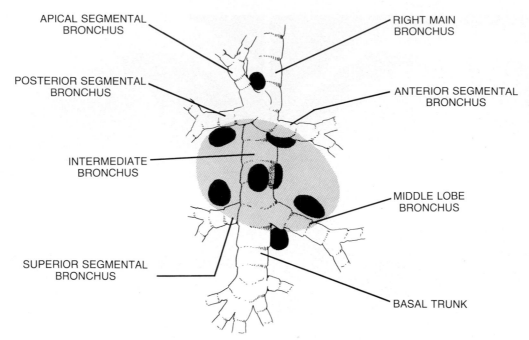

FIGURE 3–32 ■ Right lymphatic sump *(shaded area)*. Schema shows the relationship of the sump lymph nodes to the bronchial tree. (Modified from Shield TW: General Thoracic Surgery. Philadelphia, Lea & Febiger, 1972; p 76, with permission.)

Carcinomas arising in the left upper lobe frequently involve the lymph nodes listed earlier, as well as lymph nodes in the left superior hilum and left mediastinum. Unlike tumors in the right upper lobe, left upper lobe carcinomas do involve the subcarinal lymph nodes. However, involvement of nodes in the inferior left hilum below the lingular and superior segmental bronchi is rare. Tumors arising in the left lower lobe, in addition to draining upward to involve the sump nodes and other nodes listed previously, have a strong tendency to metastasize to the subcarinal, paraesophageal, and inferior pulmonary liga-

ment lymph nodes. Left lower lobe carcinomas tend not to involve the left superior mediastinum, but when advanced, they may cross over to involve the right paratracheal nodes.

On both the right and left sides, lymph nodes around the main bronchi are frequently involved by tumor. The posterior surfaces of both main bronchi are in contact with lung, and lymphadenopathy is readily detected with CT (Fig. 3–35).[4, 71] The anterior surfaces of both main bronchi are contiguous with vascular structures. On the right, the pulmonary artery and its anterior trunk are directly in front of

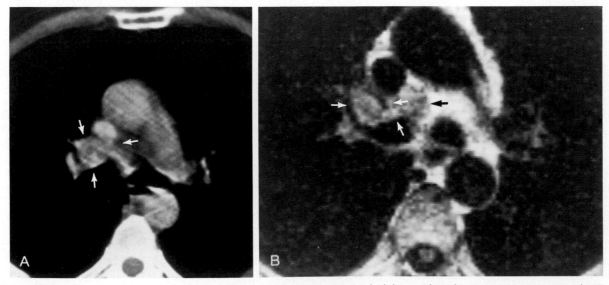

FIGURE 3–33 ■ Right upper lobe bronchogenic carcinoma with metastasis to right hilum and mediastinum. CT scan *(A)* and MR scan *(B)* demonstrate hilar nodes *(white arrows)* anterior to the right main bronchus compressing the anterior trunk of the right pulmonary artery *(black arrow)* and extending to the midline.

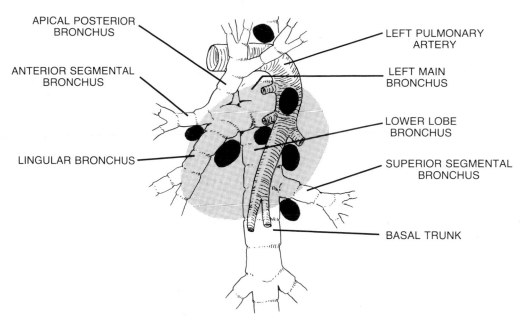

APICAL POSTERIOR
BRONCHUS

ANTERIOR SEGMENTAL
BRONCHUS

LINGULAR BRONCHUS

LEFT PULMONARY
ARTERY

LEFT MAIN
BRONCHUS

LOWER LOBE
BRONCHUS

SUPERIOR SEGMENTAL
BRONCHUS

BASAL TRUNK

FIGURE 3–34 ■ Left lymphatic sump *(shaded area).* Schema shows the relationship of the sump lymph nodes to the bronchial tree and left pulmonary artery. (Modified from Shield TW: General Thoracic Surgery. Philadelphia, Lea & Febiger, 1972, p 76, with permission.)

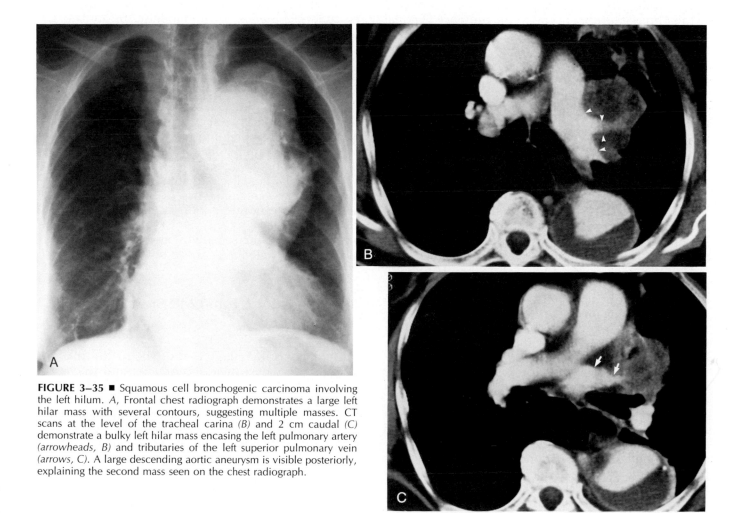

FIGURE 3–35 ■ Squamous cell bronchogenic carcinoma involving the left hilum. *A,* Frontal chest radiograph demonstrates a large left hilar mass with several contours, suggesting multiple masses. CT scans at the level of the tracheal carina *(B)* and 2 cm caudal *(C)* demonstrate a bulky left hilar mass encasing the left pulmonary artery *(arrowheads, B)* and tributaries of the left superior pulmonary vein *(arrows, C).* A large descending aortic aneurysm is visible posteriorly, explaining the second mass seen on the chest radiograph.

the right main bronchus. On the left, the superior pulmonary vein is directly anterior to the left main bronchus. Without intravenous contrast, the vascular structures cannot be easily distinguished from the surrounding mediastinal tissue, and subtle enlargement of lymph nodes is difficult to detect. Opacification of these vessels with a bolus of contrast medium during rapid sequential scanning is frequently necessary to obtain satisfactory CT images and detect lymph nodes in these regions.

The significance of metastases to hilar lymph nodes in patients with non–small-cell bronchogenic carcinoma remains controversial. As a general rule, tumor in the ipsilateral hilar nodes does not preclude resection if the procedure is technically feasible. Hilar lymphadenopathy frequently necessitates a more extensive resection (i.e., either resection of two lobes on the right or a pneumonectomy).

The prognosis for the patient with non–small-cell carcinoma metastatic to hilar lymph nodes is unclear. The reported prognosis ranges from poor[105–107] to relatively favorable.[99, 101, 108–111] The prognosis for the patient with hilar adenopathy also varies for different histologic cell types, although again there is no consensus. Classification of lung cancer according to the definitions of stage grouping rules developed by the American Joint Committee for Cancer Staging and End-Results Reporting contains factors related to the primary tumor (T) and to the presence of nodal metastases (N). For each more advanced stage of primary tumor (T), the presence of hilar node metastases worsens the prognosis.[99] In studies showing that ipsilateral hilar node metastases (N1) affect prognosis, the 5-year survival rate is intermediate between that associated with absence of nodal metastasis (N0) and that associated with metastasis to mediastinal nodes (N2 and N3). Among patients who undergo resection, those without lymph node metastases (N0) have a 35 to 60 per cent 5-year survival rate, whereas those with ipsilateral hilar node metastases (N1) have a 15 to 40 per cent 5-year survival rate. The prognosis of patients with adenocarcinoma and hilar metastases is particularly poor, which may be one of the factors explaining the wide discrepancies in the results of different studies.[110]

The use of CT or MR to detect mediastinal lymph node involvement by tumor has been extensively investigated in patients with non–small-cell bronchogenic carcinoma (see Chapter 2). These and other studies clearly show that metastases can exist in normal-sized lymph nodes and that moderately enlarged lymph nodes may not contain metastatic tumor.[98, 111a] The same difficulties and reservations are applicable to hilar lymph nodes. The interpretation of lymphadenopathy must always be tempered with the understanding that visibility of a node is not diagnostic of tumor involvement. Glazer and colleagues[112] found that both CT and MR were sensitive for detecting hilar adenopathy in patients with bronchogenic carcinoma. Both methods readily detected lymph nodes greater than 10 mm in diameter.

Nodes 10 to 16 mm in diameter were common but usually did not contain tumor. In this study, resected nodes that contained tumor were a mean of 27.6 mm (range, 5 to 50 mm) in diameter, whereas tumor-free nodes had a mean diameter of 9.5 mm (range, 2 to 16 mm). These data illustrate the difficulty in interpreting hilar CT and MR scans as indicative of metastases and severely limit the specificity of the results of the examination. The measured T1 and T2 relaxation times of enlarged nodes did not assist in discriminating between benign and malignant adenopathy. Other studies also have found comparable results for CT and MR in detecting hilar nodal enlargement.[5, 113, 114] These studies found that MR could more readily show small nodes in the range of 10 mm in diameter. However, these authors did not have the histologic correlations of the study by Glazer and colleagues,[108] and the true incidence of carcinoma in lymph nodes 10 to 15 mm in diameter remains problematic.

The CT appearance of changes in hilar contours as a result of lymph node enlargement has been described, as have the other CT appearances of lymphadenopathy.[119–122] The sensitivity, specificity, and accuracy of CT for detecting hilar lymphadenopathy metastasizing from bronchogenic carcinoma have been systematically investigated (Table 3–5).[108, 110–118] Most studies used a diameter of 1 cm as indicative of abnormal nodes. With modern, up-to-date CT scanners the sensitivity is about 90 per cent and the specificity about 70 per cent. These results probably reflect the biologic nature of lung tumors. Normal-sized or only slightly enlarged tumor-containing lymph nodes are present about 10 per cent of the time and limit the sensitivity of CT, and reactive hyperplasia or incidental enlargement of hilar lymph nodes not caused by tumor may occur in as many as 30 per cent of lymph nodes 10 to 15 mm in diameter, thus decreasing the specificity of the examination.

MR of hilar nodal enlargement in non–small-cell bronchogenic carcinoma has been less well evaluated. The detection of abnormal nodes employs the same size criteria as CT. The same limitations are applicable, and the sensitivity and specificity are, in all probability, similar to those of CT.

Indications for CT and MR Scans of the Hila

Generally speaking, CT and MR of the hila are indicated to detect hilar abnormality and to characterize or confirm an abnormality detected by other imaging modalities. Both of these indications must be modified by the clinical circumstances, and careful thought must be given to the potential impact that the information will have on patient management. The sensitivity, specificity, and accuracy of CT or MR relative to other imaging modalities must also be taken into consideration.

TABLE 3–5 ■ CT Detection of Hilar Lymphadenopathy in Patients With Lung Cancer

Author	Mintzer et al[116]*	Hirleman et al[117]	Faling et al[118]	Osborne et al[119]	Lewis[120]*	Glazer et al[122]	Frederick et al[121]	Heelan et al[114]	Glazer et al[112]
Year	1979	1980	1981	1982	1982	1983	1984	1985	1985
Scanner	EMI 5005	EMI 5005	Delta 2020	GMI	GMI	GECT/T8800	GECT/T2800	Technicare 2020	GECT/T9800
Scan time (sec)	19.0	19.0	2.0	5.0	2.0	4.8	5.8	—	2.0
Image thickness (mm)	13.0	13.0	15.0	10.0	—	10.0	10.0	10.0	10.0
No. patients	58	50	35	42	73	84	74	20	19
TP	13	25	10	11	—	56	35	14	8
FN	7	5	5	6	—	2	3	0	1
FP	—	5	2	3	—	3	4	2	5
TN	—	15	18	22	—	23	32	4	5
Sensitivity	0.65	0.83	0.67	0.65	0.73	0.96	0.92	1.0	0.89
Specificity	—	0.75	0.90	0.88	0.87	0.88	0.89	0.66	0.50
Accuracy	—	0.80	0.80	0.78	—	0.94	0.91	0.90	0.68
PV of + test	—	0.83	0.83	0.79	0.65	0.95	0.90	0.88	0.62
PV of − test	—	0.75	0.78	0.79	0.91	0.92	0.90	1.0	0.83

*Incomplete data.

Abbreviations: FN = false-negative results; FP = false-positive results; PV = predictive value; TN = true-negative results; TP = true positive results.

Definitions: $\text{Sensitivity} = \dfrac{TP}{TP + FN}$; $\text{Specificity} = \dfrac{TN}{FP + TN}$; $\text{Accuracy} = \dfrac{TP + FN}{TP + FN + FP + TN}$; $\text{PV of} + \text{Test} = \dfrac{TP}{TP + FP}$; $\text{PV of} - \text{Test} = \dfrac{TN}{TN + FN}$.

CT and MR Detection of Hilar Disease

The detection of hilar disease involves finding subtle hilar lymphadenopathy and masses. The accuracy of CT and MR in detecting hilar nodes and masses not suspected from chest radiographs has been well documented. With a thorough understanding of hilar anatomy, CT and MR have equal, high sensitivity in detecting disease in the medial, posterior, and anterior hilum. Lymph nodes lateral to the pulmonary arteries are probably also detected with equal sensitivity by the two techniques. However, collections of normal soft tissue and fat at these sites may cause difficulty in interpretation of the images.

The circumstances in which the detection of hilar nodes or masses affects patient management remain controversial. With most non-neoplastic diseases, subtle hilar adenopathy, found with CT but not with conventional radiography, may not assist in determining the cause of the adenopathy and will not influence patient management. In patients with non–small-cell bronchogenic carcinoma, CT and, less commonly, MR are used to determine the stage and resectability of the carcinoma (also see Chapters 1, 2, and 4). The status of the hila is valuable additional information, even though it may not directly influence the decision to perform surgery. Malignant hilar nodes, however, are extremely important in patients medically unable to undergo a resection greater than lobectomy. The demonstration of bronchial abnormalities in or adjacent to a hilum may also assist in the bronchoscopic localization of the tumor. CT-guided biopsy of hilar masses not diagnosed by bronchoscopy is also feasible.[123] In patients with lymphoma, especially Hodgkin's disease, with bulk mediastinal nodes, CT or MR may demonstrate hilar lymphadenopathy and affect the treatment regimen.

CT and MR Characterization of Hilar Disease

The CT attenuation values or MR relaxation times of hilar tissues rarely assist in diagnosis. Abnormalities of the hila are caused by enlarged nodes, soft tissue masses, or vessels. Fatty or cystic masses of the hila are rare. When unilateral or bilateral hilar enlargement results from a dilated or anomalous vessel, CT or MR clearly shows the vascular nature of the mass. Additionally, CT or MR may establish the cause of an abnormally small hilum when absence or atresia of a pulmonary artery is suspected. Very rarely, a neoplasm shows marked CT enhancement with contrast medium and may be mistaken for a vascular structure in the hilum.[124]

References

1. Webb WR, Glazer G, Gamsu G: Computed tomography of the normal pulmonary hilum. J Comput Assist Tomogr 5:476, 1981.
2. Naidich DP, Khouri NF, Scott WW Jr, Wang KP, Siegelman SS: Computed tomography of the pulmonary hila: 1. Normal anatomy. J Comput Assist Tomogr 5:459, 1981.
3. Glazer GM, Francis IR, Gebarski K, Samuels BI, Sorensen KW: Dynamic incremental computed tomography in evaluation of the pulmonary hila. J Comput Assist Tomogr 7:59, 1983.
4. Webb WR, Gamsu G: Computed tomography of the left retrobronchial stripe. J Comput Assist Tomogr 7:65, 1983.
5. Webb WR, Gamsu G, Stark DD, Moore EH: Magnetic resonance imaging of the normal and abnormal pulmonary hila. Radiology 152:89, 1984.
6. Dorland's Illustrated Medical Dictionary, 26th ed. Philadelphia, WB Saunders, 1981, p 609.
7. Naidich DP, Zinn WL, Ettenger NA, McCauley DI, Garay SM: Basilar segmental bronchi: thin-section CT evaluation. Radiology 169:11, 1988.
8. Gamsu G, Webb WR, Sheldon P, Kaufman L, Crooks LE, et al: Nuclear magnetic resonance imaging of the thorax. Radiology 147:473, 1983.
9. Boyden EA, Scannell JG: An analysis of variations in the bronchovascular pattern of the right upper lobe of fifty lungs. Am J Anat 82:27, 1948.
10. Boyden EA, Hamre CJ: An analysis of variations in the bronchovascular patterns of the middle lobe in fifty dissected and twenty injected lungs. J Thorac Surg 21:172, 1951.
11. Smith FR, Boyden EA: An analysis of the segmental bronchi of the right lower lobe of fifty injected lungs. J Thorac Surg 18:195, 1949.

12. Boyden EA, Hartmann JF: An analysis of variations in the bronchopulmonary segments of the left upper lobes of fifty lungs. Am J Anat 79:321, 1946.
13. Mencini RA, Proto AV: The high left and main pulmonary arteries: a CT pitfall. J Comput Assist Tomogr 6:452, 1982.
14. Yamashita H: Roentgenologic Anatomy of the Lung. Tokyo, Igaku-Shoin, 1978, pp 84–87.
14a. Lang EV, Friedman PJ: The anterior wall stripe of the left lower lobe bronchus on the lateral chest radiograph: CT correlative study. AJR 154:33, 1990.
15. Heitzman ER: Computed tomography of the thorax: current perspectives. AJR 136:2, 1981.
16. Gamsu G, Sostman S: Magnetic resonance imaging of the thorax. Am Rev Respir Dis 139:254, 1989.
17. Spritzer C, Gamsu G, Sostman HD: Magnetic resonance imaging of the thorax: techniques, current applications, and future directions. J Thorac Imag 4:1, 1989.
18. Posteraro RH, Sostman HD, Spritzer CE, Herfkens RJ: Cine-gradient-refocused MR imaging of central pulmonary emboli. AJR 152:465, 1989.
19. Webb WR, Gamsu G, Glazer G: Computed tomography of the abnormal pulmonary hilum. J Comput Assist Tomogr 5:485, 1981.
19a. Park C-K, Webb RW, Klein JS: Inferior hilar window. Radiology 178:163, 1991.
20. Webb WR, Gamsu G, Speckman JM: Computed tomography of the pulmonary hilum in patients with bronchogenic carcinoma. J Comput Assist Tomogr 7:218, 1983.
21. Schnur MJ, Winkler B, Austin JHM: Thickening of the posterior wall of the bronchus intermedius. Radiology 139:551, 1981.
22. Naidich DP, Khouri NF, Stitik FP, McCauley DI, Siegelman SS: Computed tomography of the pulmonary hila: 2. Abnormal anatomy. J Comput Assist Tomogr 5:468, 1981.
22a. Foster WL Jr, Roberts L Jr, McLendon RE, Hill RC: Localized peribronchial thickening: a CT sign of occult bronchogenic carcinoma. AJR 144:906, 1985.
23. Glazer GM, Gross BH, Aisen AM, Quint LE, Francis IR, Orringer MB: Imaging of the pulmonary hilum: a prospective comparative study in patients with lung cancer. AJR 145:245, 1985.
24. Bremer JL: On the origin of the pulmonary arteries in mammals. Am J Anat 1:137, 1902.
25. Bremer JL: On the origin of the pulmonary arteries in mammals. II. Anat Rec 3:334, 1909.
26. Bremer JL: An acknowledgment of Federow's work on the pulmonary arteries. Anat Rec 6:491, 1912.
27. Huntington GS: The morphology of the pulmonary artery in the mammalia. Anat Rec 17:165, 1919.
28. Pool PE, Vogel JHK, Blount SG: Congenital unilateral absence of a pulmonary artery: the importance of flow in pulmonary hypertension. Am J Cardiol 10:706, 1962.
29. Danelius G: Absence of the hilar shadow. AJR 47:870, 1942.
30. Madoff IM, Gaensler EA, Strieder JW: Congenital absence of the right pulmonary artery: diagnosis by angiocardiography with cardiorespiratory studies. N Engl J Med 247:149, 1952.
31. Fletcher BD, Jacobstein MD: MRI of congenital abnormalities of the great arteries. AJR 146:941, 1986.
32. Ellis K, Seaman WB, Griffiths SP, Berdon WE, Baker DH: Some congenital anomalies of the pulmonary arteries. Semin Roentgenol 2:325, 1967.
33. Good CA: Certain vascular abnormalities of the lungs. AJR 65:1009, 1961.
34. Trell E: Pulmonary arterial aneurysm. Thorax 28:644, 1973.
35. Guthaner DF, Wexler L, Harrell G: CT demonstrations of cardiac structures. AJR 133:75, 1979.
36. O'Callaghan JP, Heitzman ER, Somogyi JW, Spirt BA: CT evaluation of pulmonary artery size. J Comput Assist Tomogr 6:101, 1982.
37. Kuriyama K, Gamsu G, Stern RG, Cann CE, Herfkens RJ, Brundage BH: CT-determined pulmonary artery diameters in predicting pulmonary hypertension. Invest Radiol 19:16, 1984.
38. Hoeffel JC, Henry M, Jiminez J, Pernot C: Congenital stenosis of the pulmonary artery and its branches. Clin Radiol 25:481, 1974.
39. Baum D, Khoury GH, Ongley PA, Swan HJC, Kincaid OW: Congenital stenosis of the pulmonary artery branches. Circulation 29:680, 1964.
40. Lees MH, Menashe VD, Sunderland CO, Morgan CL, Dawson PJ: Ehlers-Danlos syndrome associated with multiple pulmonary artery stenoses and tortuous systemic arteries. J Pediatr 75:1031, 1969.
41. Stone DN, Bein ME, Garris JB: Anomalous left pulmonary artery: two new adult cases. AJR 135:1259, 1980.
42. Turner AF, Pacuilli JR, Lau FYK, Mikity VG, Johnson JL: Partial tracheal obstruction due to anomalous origin of the left pulmonary artery. Calif Med 114:59, 1971.
43. Keele CA, Neil E, Wright S: Applied Physiology, 11th ed. New York, Oxford University Press, 1965.
44. Harris P, Heath D, Apostopoulous A: Extensibility of the pulmonary trunk in heart disease. Br Heart J 27:660, 1965.
45. Caro CG: Physics of blood flow in the lungs. Br Med Bull 19:66, 1963.
46. Fowler NO, Westcott RN, Scott RC: Normal pressure in the right heart and pulmonary artery. Am Heart J 46:264, 1953.
47. Walcott G, Burchell HB, Brown AL: Primary pulmonary hypertension. Am J Med 49:70, 1970.
48. Matthay RA, Schwartz MI, Ellis JH Jr, Steele PP, Siebert PE, et al: Pulmonary artery hypertension in chronic obstructive pulmonary disease: determination by chest radiography. Invest Radiol 16:95, 1981.
49. Baum GL, Fisher FD: The relationship of fatal pulmonary insufficiency with cor pulmonale, right-sided mural thrombi, and pulmonary embolism. Am J Med Sci 240:609, 1960.
50. Gerald B, Dungan WT: Cor pulmonale edema in children secondary to chronic upper airway obstruction. Radiology 90:679, 1963.
51. Bland JW Jr, Edwards FK: Pulmonary hypertension and congestive heart failure in children with chronic upper airway obstruction. New concepts of etiologic factors. Am J Cardiol 23:830, 1969.
52. Burwell CS, Robin ED, Whaley RD, Bichelmann AS: Extreme obesity associated with alveolar hypoventilation: a pickwickian syndrome. Am J Med 21:811, 1956.
53. Ravin CE, Greenspan RH, McLoud TC, Lange RC, Langou RA, Putman CE: Redistribution of pulmonary blood flow secondary to pulmonary arterial hypertension. Invest Radiol 15:29, 1980.
54. Paraskos JA, Adelstein SJ, Smith RE, Rickman FD, Grossmam N, et al: Late prognosis of acute pulmonary embolism. N Engl J Med 289:55, 1973.
55. Dalen JE, Alpert JS: Natural history of pulmonary embolism. Progr Cardiovasc Dis 17:257, 1975.
56. Dantzker DR, Bower JS: Partial reversibility of chronic pulmonary hypertension caused by pulmonary thromboembolic disease. Am Rev Respir Dis 124:129, 1981.
57. Evans KT, Cockshott WP, Hendrickse PdeV: Pulmonary changes in malignant trophoblastic disease. Br J Radiol 38:161, 1965.
58. Steckel RJ, Bein ME, Kelly PM: Pulmonary arterial hypertension in progressive systemic sclerosis. AJR 124:461, 1975.
59. Follath F, Burkart F, Schweizer W: Drug induced pulmonary hypertension? Br Med J 1:265, 1971.
60. Abrams H: Radiologic aspects of increased pulmonary artery pressure and flow. Stanford Med Bull 14:97, 1956.
61. Kimball KG, McIlroy MB: Pulmonary hypertension in patients with congenital heart disease. Am J Med 41:883, 1966.
62. Selzer A, Cohn KE: Natural history of mitral stenosis: review. Circulation 45:878, 1972.
63. Sidd JJ, Dervan RA, Leland OS, Sasahara AA: Correlation of hemodynamic data and pulmonary angiography in mitral stenosis. Circulation 35:373, 1967.
64. Turner AF, Lau FYK, Jacobson G: A method for the estimation of pulmonary venous and arterial pressures from the routine chest roentgenogram. AJR 116:97, 1972.

65. Von Schulthess GK, Fisher MR, Higgins CB: Pathologic blood flow in pulmonary vascular disease as shown by gated magnetic resonance imaging. Ann Intern Med 103:317, 1985.
66. White RD, Winkler ML, Higgins CB: MR imaging of pulmonary arterial hypertension and pulmonary emboli. AJR 149:15, 1987.
67. Dyon JF: Contribution a l'etude du drainage des lymphatiques du poumon. Thesis. Grenoble, Université Scientifique et Médical de Grenoble, 1973.
68. Sukiennikow W: Dissertation. Berl Klin Wochenschr, 1903. Cited by Engel S: Lung Structure. Springfield, IL, Charles C Thomas, 1962, pp 74–80.
69. Engel S: Lung Structure. Springfield, IL, Charles C Thomas, 1962, pp 74–80.
70. Chang CHJ, Zinn TW: Roentgen recognition of enlarged hilar lymph nodes: an anatomical review. Radiology 120:291, 1976.
71. Sone S, Higashihara T, Morimoto S, Ikezoe J, Arisawa J, et al: CT anatomy of hilar lymphadenopathy. AJR 140:887, 1983.
72. Weber AL, Bird KT, Janower ML: Primary tuberculosis in childhood with particular emphasis on changes affecting the tracheobronchial tree. AJR 103:123, 1968.
73. Curry FJ, Wier JA: Histoplasmosis: a review of one hundred consecutively hospitalized patients. Am Rev Tuberc 77:749, 1958.
74. Murray JF, Howard D: Laboratory acquired histoplasmosis. Am Rev Respir Dis 93:47, 1966.
75. Greendyke WH, Resnick DL, Harvey WC: The varied roentgen manifestations of primary coccidioidomycosis. AJR 109:491, 1970.
76. Colwell JA, Tillman SP: Early recognition and therapy of disseminated coccidioidomycosis. Am J Med 31:676, 1961.
77. McLoud TC, Kalisher L, Stark P, Greene R: Intrathoracic lymph node metastases from extrathoracic neoplasms. AJR 131:403, 1978.
78. Reinke RT, Higgins CB, Niwayama G, Harris RH, Friedman PJ: Bilateral pulmonary hilar lymphadenopathy. Radiology 121:49, 1976.
79. Webb WR: Hilar and mediastinal lymph node metastases in malignant melanoma. AJR 133:805, 1979.
80. Winterbauer RH, Belic N, Moores KD: Clinical interpretation of bilateral hilar adenopathy. Ann Intern Med 78:65, 1973.
81. Filly R, Blank N, Castellino RA: Radiographic distribution of intrathoracic disease in previously untreated patients with Hodgkin's disease and non-Hodgkin's lymphoma. Radiology 120:277, 1976.
82. Hagemeister FB, Fuller LM, Sullivan JA, North L, Velasquez W, et al: Treatment of stage I and II mediastinal Hodgkin disease. Radiology 141:783, 1981.
83. Castellino RA, Blank N, Hoppe RT, Cho C: Hodgkin disease: contribution of chest CT in the initial staging evaluation. Radiology 160:603, 1986.
84. Khoury MB, Godwin JD, Halvorsen R, Hanun Y, Putman CE: Role of chest CT in non-Hodgkin lymphoma. Radiology 158:659, 1986.
85. Hopper KD, Diehl LF, Lesar M, Barnes M, Granger E, Baumann J: Hodgkin disease: clinical utility of CT in initial staging and treatment. Radiology 169:17, 1988.
86. Castellino RA: Hodgkin disease: imaging studies and patient management. Radiology 169:269, 1988.
87. Scadding JG: Sarcoidosis. London, Eyre & Spottiswoode, 1967, p 41.
88. Kirks DR, McCormick VD, Greenspan RH: Pulmonary sarcoidosis. Roentgenologic analysis of 150 patients. AJR 117:777, 1973.
89. Rabinowitz JG, Ulreich S, Soriano C: The usual unusual manifestations of sarcoidosis and the "hilar haze"—a new diagnostic aid. AJR 120:821, 1974.
90. Bein ME, Putman CE, McLoud TC, Mink JH: A reevaluation of intrathoracic lymphadenopathy in sarcoidosis. AJR 131:409, 1978.
91. Schabel SI, Foote GA, McKee KA: Posterior lymphadenopathy in sarcoidosis. Radiology 129:591, 1978.
92. Bergin CJ, Bell DY, Coblentz CL, Chiles C, Gamsu G, et al: Sarcoidosis: correlation of pulmonary parenchymal pattern at CT with results of pulmonary function tests. Radiology 171:619, 1989.
93. Muller NL, Kullnig P, Miller RR: The CT findings of pulmonary sarcoidosis: analysis of 25 patients. AJR 152:1179, 1989.
94. Kuhlman JE, Fishman EK, Hamper UM, Knowles M, Siegelman SS: The computed tomographic spectrum of thoracic sarcoidosis. Radiographics 9:449, 1989.
95. Martini N, Flehinger BJ: The role of surgery in N2 lung cancer. Surg Clin North Am 67:1037, 1987.
96. Libshitz HI: Patterns of mediastinal metastases in bronchogenic carcinoma. Chest 90:229, 1986.
97. Hata E, Troidl H, Hasegawa T (eds): In vivo Unterschungen der Lymphdrainage des Bronchialsystem beim menschen mit der Lymphoszintigraphie-eine neue diagnostische Technik. In Hata E, Troidl H, Hasegawa T (eds): Behandlung des Bronchialkarzinoms: Resignation oder neue Ansatze: symposium Kiel. New York, G Thieme Verlag, 1981.
98. Nohl HC: An investigation into the lymphatic and vascular spread of carcinoma of the bronchus. Thorax 11:172, 1956.
99. Naruke T, Suemasu K, Ishikawa S: Lymph node mapping and curability at various levels of metastasis in resected lung cancer. J Thorac Cardiovasc Surg 76:832, 1978.
100. Martini N: Prospective study of 445 lung carcinomas with mediastinal lymph node metastases. J Thorac Cardiovasc Surg 89:390, 1980.
101. Rubinstein I, Baum GL, Kalter Y, Pauzner Y, Lieberman Y, Bubis JJ: The influence of cell type and lymph node metastases on survival of patients with carcinoma of the lung undergoing thoracotomy. Am Rev Resp Dis 119:253, 1979.
102. Borrie J: Primary carcinoma of the bronchus: prognosis following surgical resection. Ann R Coll Surg Engl 10:165, 1952.
103. Nohl-Oser HC: Lymphatics of the lung. In Shields TW (ed): General Thoracic Surgery, 3rd ed. Philadelphia, Lea & Febiger, 1988.
104. Greschuchna D, Maassen W: Die lymphogenen Absiedlungswege des Bronchialkarzinoms. Stuttgart, G Thieme Verlag, 1973.
105. Higgins GA, Beebe GW: Bronchogenic carcinoma. Factors in survival. Arch Surg 94:539, 1967.
106. Vincent RG, Takita H, Lane WW, Gutierrez AC, Pickren JW: Surgical therapy of lung cancer. J Thorac Cardiovasc Surg 71:581, 1976.
107. Weiss W, Boucot KR, Cooper DA: The histopathology of bronchogenic carcinoma and its relation to growth rate, metastasis, and prognosis. Cancer 26:965, 1970.
108. Bergh NP, Schersten T: Bronchogenic carcinoma. A followup study of a surgically treated series with special reference to the prognostic significance of lymph node metastasis. Acta Chir Scand (Suppl) 347:1, 1965.
109. Shields TW, Yee J, Conn JH, Robinette CD: Relationship of cell type and lymph node metastasis to survival after resection of bronchial carcinoma. Ann Thorac Surg 20:501, 1975.
110. Kirsh MM, Rotman H, Argenta L, Bove E, Cimmino V, et al: Carcinoma of the lung: results of treatment over ten years. Ann Thorac Surg 21:371, 1976.
111. Martini N: Prognostic significance of N1 disease in carcinoma of the lung. J Thorac Cardiovasc Surg 86:646, 1983.
111a. Webb WR, Gatsonis C, Zerhouni EA, Heelan RT, Glazer GM, et al: CT and MR imaging in staging non–small cell bronchogenic carcinoma: report of the Radiologic Diagnostic Oncology Group. Radiology 178:705, 1991.
112. Glazer GM, Gross BH, Aisen AM, Quint LE, Francis IR, Orringer MB: Imaging of the pulmonary hilum: a prospective comparative study in patients with lung cancer. AJR 145:245, 1985.
113. Webb WR, Jensen BG, Sollitto R, de Geer G, McCowin M, et al: Bronchogenic carcinoma: staging with MR compared with staging with CT and surgery. Radiology 156:117, 1985.
114. Heelan RT, Martini N, Westcott JW, Bains MS, Watson RC, et al: Carcinomatous involvement of the hilum and mediastinum: computed tomographic and magnetic resonance evaluation. Radiology 156:111, 1985.

115. Levitt RG, Glazer HS, Roper CL, Lee JKT, Murphy WA: Magnetic resonance imaging of mediastinal and hilar masses: comparison with CT. AJR 145:9, 1985.
116. Mintzer RA, Malave SR, Neiman HL, Michaelis LL, Vanecko RM, Sanders JH: Computed vs. conventional tomography in evaluation of primary and secondary pulmonary neoplasms. Radiology 132:653, 1979.
117. Hirleman MT, YiuChiu VS, Chiu LC, Schapiro RL: The resectability of primary lung carcinoma: a diagnostic staging review. Comput Tomogr 4:146, 1980.
118. Faling LJ, Pugatch RD, JungLegg Y, Daly BDT Jr, Hong WK, et al: Computed tomographic scanning of the mediastinum in the staging of bronchogenic carcinoma. Am Rev Resp Dis 124:690, 1981.
119. Osborne DR, Korobkin M, Ravin CE, Putman CE, Wolfe WG, et al: Comparison of plain radiography, conventional tomography, and computed tomography in detecting intrathoracic lymph node metastases from lung carcinoma. Radiology 142:157, 1982.
120. Lewis JW, Madrazo BL, Gross SC, Eyler WR, Magilligan DJ, et al: The value of radiographic and computed tomography in the staging of lung carcinoma. Ann Thoracic Surg 34:553, 1982.
121. Frederick HM, Bernardino ME, Baron M, Colvin R, Mansour K, Miller J: Accuracy of chest computerized tomography in detecting malignant hilar and mediastinal involvement by squamous cell carcinoma of the lung. Cancer 54:2390, 1984.
122. Glazer GM, Francis IR, Shirazi KK, Bookstein FL, Gross BH, Orringer MB: Evaluation of the pulmonary hilum: comparison of conventional radiography, 55° posterior oblique tomography, and dynamic computed tomography. Comput Assist Tomogr 7:983, 1983.
123. Sider L, Davis TM: Hilar masses: evaluation with CT-guided biopsy after negative bronchoscopic examination. Radiology 164:107, 1987.
124. Komaiko MS, Lee ME, Birnberg FA: The contrast enhanced paravascular neoplasm: a potential CT pitfall. J Comput Assist Tomogr 4:516, 1980.

CHAPTER 4

THE LUNGS

GORDON GAMSU

The conventional chest radiograph is a sensitive, readily available, and inexpensive imaging modality. Air within the lungs provides natural contrast not available in other parts of the body, and the radiographic sensitivity for detection of pulmonary abnormalities is thus considerably greater for the lungs than for other organ systems. The radiographic patterns of pulmonary parenchymal disease are moderately specific indicators of disease processes involving the lungs. Many lung abnormalities can therefore be diagnosed from the plain chest radiograph. Improvement in spatial resolution of computed tomography (CT), however, has greatly extended imaging of the lung parenchyma. High-resolution CT (HRCT) permits detailed display of lobular and sublobular anatomy and is more sensitive and specific for the diagnosis of lung disease than are chest radiographs. CT and HRCT have largely replaced radiologic procedures such as bronchography and pulmonary angiography for evaluation of parenchymal lung disease. CT-based pulmonary nodule densitometry can provide specific quantitative information. In addition, improvements in nonradiologic diagnostic methods and in the treatment of pulmonary disease have decreased the indications for radiologic studies such as bronchography or tomography. For instance, advances in fiberoptic bronchoscopy and percutaneous transthoracic needle biopsy have led to a direct approach to the diagnosis of many pulmonary abnormalities. Thus the imaging of lung disease has been simplified and has become more focused on CT. In most medical centers, 30 to 40 per cent of body CT studies are of the thorax.

Magnetic resonance (MR) imaging of the lungs has suffered from poor spatial and temporal resolution. The modality also has intrinsic difficulties in the lung. The structure of the lung with its vast air-liquid interphase has unpredictable local magnetic susceptibilities that distort the characteristics of the tissues being imaged. Nevertheless, rapid technical advances in MR are occurring and may overcome these problems.

Anatomy

With CT, the individual lobes of the lung can be localized by their position within each hemithorax. Although the interlobar fissures are usually not seen on 10-mm-thick scans, their position can be determined in at least 90 per cent of patients. These fissures traverse a 2- to 3-cm-wide band of lung characterized by the absence of large vessels (Fig. 4-1).[1-3] They course from posterosuperior to inferoanterior for the major fissures and from posterior to anterior in the right midlung for the minor fissure. The latter has been referred to as the *right midlung window* and should not be mistaken for an abnormal paucity of vessels in this region (see Fig. 4-1B).[4] With HRCT, interlobar and accessory fissures are demonstrated as pencil-thin white lines (see Fig. 4-1C).[5-7]

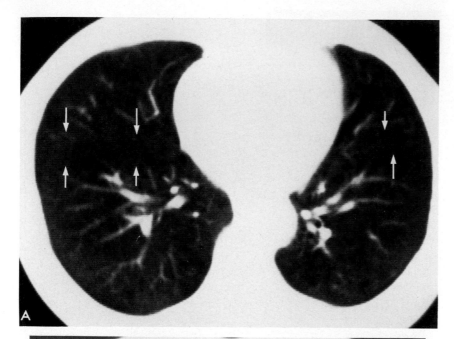

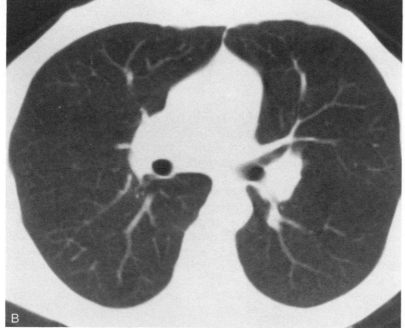

FIGURE 4–1 ■ Interlobular fissures. *A*, CT scan through the lower thorax demonstrates the "avascular" planes *(arrows)* of both major fissures. *B*, The plane of the minor fissure, shown in a 10-mm collimated CT scan, is an "avascular" area in the right midlung field.

Cardiac and vascular pulsations usually do not obscure the fissures except in the left lower lobe. On occasion, the major fissure, most often the left, will be imaged as a double line reflecting movement in its position between diastole and systole during acquisition of the image (Fig. 4–2).[8]

The individual bronchopulmonary segments are not separated by boundaries that can be seen on CT scans. Their approximate site within each lobe can be determined from the position and orientation of the segmental bronchus subtending each segment and from their general position within each lobe.

The intraparenchymal bronchi divide dichotomously into two daughter branches and are accompanied by branches of the pulmonary artery. Most bronchi beyond the segmental or subsegmental di-

visions are not demonstrated on conventional CT scans. They become visible only when surrounded by consolidation of the lung parenchyma, or when dilated or thickened by disease. A bronchus lying in the plane of the CT scan then appears as a tubular lucency against the increased CT density of the consolidated lung. More often, the bronchus lies in an oblique or vertical plane to the CT scan and appears as a small circular lucency within the consolidated lung.

With HRCT, normal bronchi are routinely visible in the inner two thirds of the lung. Their normal wall thickness can be recognized, and with experience, thickening of the peripheral bronchi and bronchioles and their surrounding interstitium can be appreciated. Bronchioles within the normal secon-

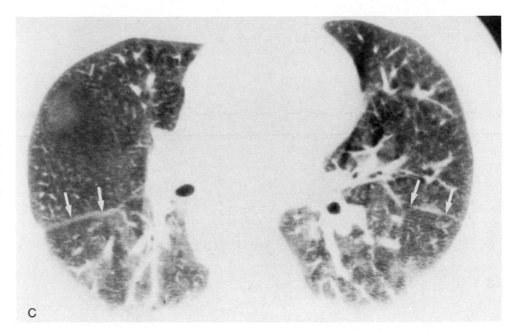

FIGURE 4–1 *Continued* ■ *C,* Expiratory CT scan demonstrates multiple small peripheral vessels in the plane of the minor fissure that should not be mistaken for small nodules. Both major fissures *(arrows)* are also seen.

dary pulmonary lobules can be occasionally demonstrated on HRCT. In general, demonstration of numerous subpleural peripheral intralobular bronchioles is indicative of abnormality.

The blood vessels seen on conventional CT scans of the lung are pulmonary arteries and veins. The general pattern of these vessels is a decrease in caliber from the hila to the periphery of the lungs. In the outer 1 to 2 cm of the lungs and adjacent to the fissures, there is a paucity of vessels. The caliber of the vessels seen on CT scans obtained at end-expiration is different from that seen at end-inspiration. At low lung volumes, the normal hydrostatic gradient of the blood volume in the lungs is reflected on CT scans as a prominence of the vessels in the dependent portions of the lung. At high lung volumes, this gradient is less apparent. At low lung

volumes, the most dependent 1 to 4 cm of the lungs may appear airless and consolidated (Fig. 4–3).[9] This misleading appearance of abnormality can be eliminated by scanning the patient in the prone or decubitus position. A hydrostatic gradient is also seen on CT scans of the lungs in the CT density (attenuation values) of the lung tissue itself. This will be reviewed more extensively in the subsequent section on CT densitometry of the lungs.

On HRCT scans, the peripheral pulmonary anatomy is shown with exquisite detail approaching that demonstrated on lung sections (Fig. 4–4). The basic structure imaged in the periphery of the lung is the secondary pulmonary lobule.[5, 10] The peripheral secondary lobule has the shape of a truncated pyramid with its base on the pleura. It is from 1 cm to about 4 cm on a side and contains a variable number of

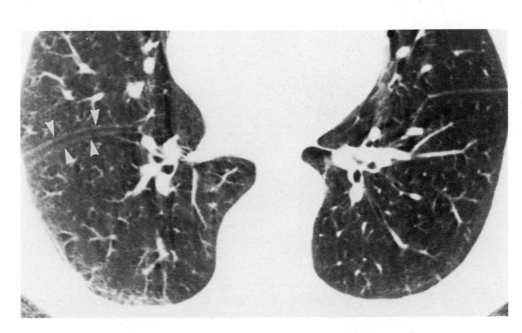

FIGURE 4–2 ■ Double fissure sign. The right major fissure *(arrowheads)* is shown in two positions, reflecting a change in its position during scanning between diastole and systole. Honeycombing is present on the right posteriorly.

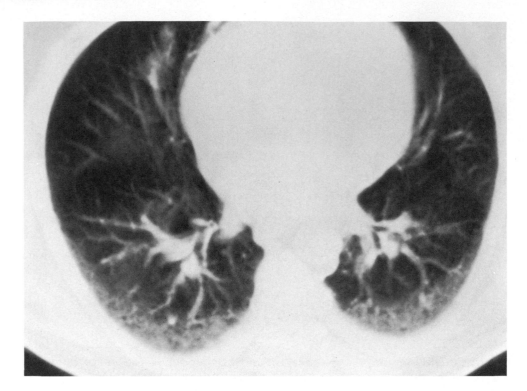

FIGURE 4–3 ■ Dependent density. The dependent portions of the lower lobes demonstrate a band of ill-defined hazy density that can be found in normal individuals when they are lying on their back.

FIGURE 4–4 ■ Schema of lung anatomy for HRCT. *A*, Central pulmonary interstitium. The interstitial space surrounds the central bronchi and pulmonary arteries. The space extends peripherally as far as the terminal bronchiole. *B*, Peripheral interstitial morphology. An interstitial space surrounds the secondary pulmonary lobule and the centrilobular bronchiole and arteriole. Lymphatics and veins course through the interlobular septa. The dependent interlobular septa are more prominent than nondependent septa because of venous distention. *C*, A single secondary pulmonary lobule with all the structures indicated.

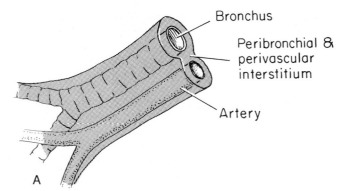

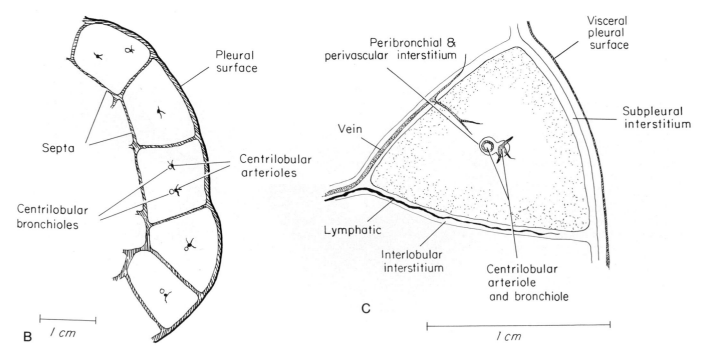

acini, usually three to five but as many as 20. The pulmonary acinus is a smaller unit of lung, subtended by a terminal bronchiole. Secondary pulmonary lobules are invested by connective tissue interlobular septa containing the peripheral tributaries of the pulmonary veins and lymphatics. These veins are distensible, and thus the septa are more prominent in dependent lung than in nondependent lung. Within the central complex of the secondary lobule, terminal or preterminal bronchioles are accompanied by pulmonary arterioles and lymphatics, all contained in a connective tissue interstitium. On HRCT, these centrilobular core structures appear as a small branching structure or dot 5 to 10 mm from the pleural surface (see Fig. 4–2).[9, 10] They do not extend to the pleural surface when normal. The core bronchus is only occasionally visible. The lobules and interlobular septa are not uniformly distributed. They are most prominent in the lung periphery, especially in the lower lobes and anterior, lateral, and mediastinal surfaces of the upper lobes, middle lobe, and lingula.[11, 12] On HRCT normal septa are thin, nontapering, and about 1 to 2 cm in length. They normally do not branch. Near the diaphragm, septa can be seen in cross section as polyhedral structures.

Techniques of Examination

CT Imaging

When the lungs are the region of primary concern, patients are usually scanned in the supine position with their arms above their head to reduce streak artifacts from the shoulder girdle. CT scans with the patient in the prone position can aid in distinguishing a suspected parenchymal nodule from a vessel in the dependent portion of the lung and can eliminate dependent lung density.[13]

The optimum lung volume for CT scanning of the lungs has been debated at length.[14] In our experience, full inspiration (total lung capacity) is reproducible and easily achieved by most patients. In older or dyspneic patients, a few deep breaths before each scan can help with breath holding for the required time. With slow scanners, some patients may not be able to suspend respiration for the time required to complete a single scan; in such instances, good quality CT scans can still be obtained during quiet breathing. In patients having difficulty holding their breath or cooperating, a nose clip can help suspend respiration.

Intravenously infused iodinated contrast material does not assist in the diagnosis of most focal or diffuse abnormalities of the lungs. Nevertheless, because CT scanning of the lungs is part of an examination of the entire thorax, intravenous contrast medium is injected or infused to delineate the blood vessels of the mediastinum and hila. When CT scanning is used to evaluate a suspected vascular lesion of the lungs, such as an arteriovenous malformation, high levels of intravascular contrast can be attained by the rapid injection of a bolus of 20 to 40 mL of 76 per cent contrast material. For this type of examination, rapid sequential (dynamic) scanning through the area of abnormality is usually required.

A wide range in CT density is present on any CT scan of the thorax. The density differences among chest wall, mediastinum, and lung parenchyma require viewing of the images at least at two window settings. Both the window level and window width must be manipulated to achieve optimum density for evaluation of the thorax. In general, the lungs are photographed at a window level between −400 and −700 Hounsfield units (H) and a window width between 1000 and 1500 H. Window settings extended up to 4000 H can be used to demonstrate the mediastinum, lungs, and chest wall on the same scan (Fig. 4–5). These images, however, are excessively gray, and object contrast is reduced. Narrower window widths decrease the gray scale and increase object contrast. With scan times in the 2- to 5-sec range, CT images of the lung do not appear degraded by cardiac motion or pulsation of the pulmonary arteries. Scans obtained with longer scan times will show artifacts from the motion of vascular structures.

In most instances, CT scans of the lungs are obtained at 1-cm intervals using 1-cm collimation. These scans are usually sufficient to demonstrate most abnormalities. Scans 1 to 5 mm thick may be used in special circumstances. For instance, when a pulmonary nodule is suspected from the thicker scans, thinner scans through the area of suspected abnormality should be used. Highly collimated scans can improve resolution for such special procedures as nodule densitometry. A preliminary projection CT radiograph (scout view) is often used to locate a focal pulmonary abnormality. With many scanners, the levels for scanning can be selected automatically from the projection CT radiograph.

HRCT of the lungs can be performed as an adjunct to conventional CT or as a stand-alone examination. HRCT for diffuse lung disease is obtained with 1- to 2-mm collimation. Thicker scans will result in a decrease in spatial resolution of the image. A high-resolution reconstruction algorithm is used (as for all thoracic imaging), and the peak kilovolts (kV[p]) and milliamperes (mA) are increased to compensate for low photon flux caused by the thin collimation (Fig. 4–6).[15, 15a] Appropriate levels for obtaining HRCT scans vary depending on the clinical application. For characterization of nodules or other focal radiographic opacities, thin sections are performed through the area of abnormality. For diffuse parenchymal lung disease, we have developed a sampling program that obtains scans every 4 cm, starting 2 cm above the aortic arch and extending to the lung bases. Scans are obtained at full inspiration in both the supine and prone positions. The prone position eliminates dependent vascular distention and compressive changes frequently found at the lung bases.[9] When the indication for CT is for the detection of bronchiectasis, we obtain HRCT scans at 1-cm inter-

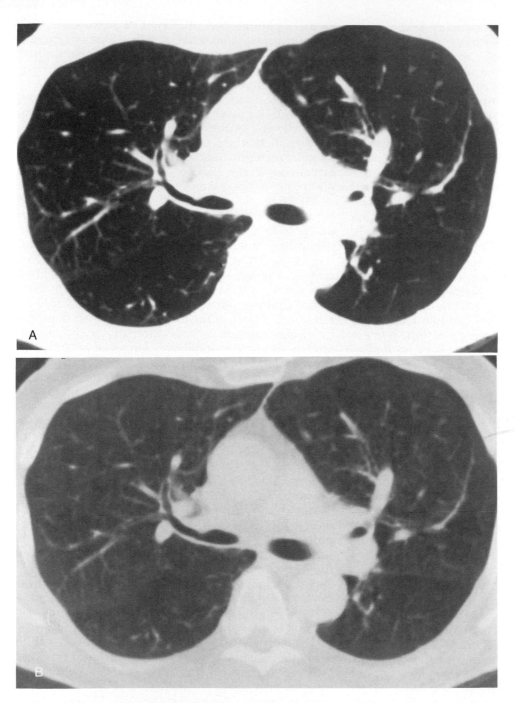

FIGURE 4–5 ■ Effect of varying window level and width on the caliber of pulmonary vessels. Scans are with 5-mm collimation. *A*, At a window level of −500 H and width of 750 H the larger pulmonary vessels are shown, but the smaller peripheral vessels are not seen. *B*, With the window level unchanged at −500 H but the window width increased to 2000 H, the gray scale changes but the caliber of the vessels remains constant.

vals throughout the lungs in the supine position only.[16]

The time necessary to complete data acquisition from one CT image varies with different scanners. Optimal reduction in pulmonary motion is achieved with scan times of 2 sec or less. In pediatric patients or others who are unable to cooperate, scan times may be reduced and data are acquired from less than the full rotation cycle of the gantry. This reduces respiratory motion but increases visible noise in the denser portions of the thorax. Furthermore, high-resolution reconstruction algorithms cannot be used with less than the full data set because of a marked increase in aliasing artifact with this technique.

MR Imaging

The techniques for MR of the lungs have not been standardized and are tailored for individual clinical situations. Most commonly, transaxial T1-weighted spin-echo images (short repetition time [TR] and short echo delay time [TE]) are used for the mediastinum and lungs. Spin-echo techniques are sensitive to nuclear density and flow. T1-weighted images will provide good contrast between mediastinal fat and mediastinal masses or enlarged lymph nodes (Fig. 4–7).[17, 18]

For thoracic imaging, ECG-synchronized acquisition of the images is essential. This technique mark-

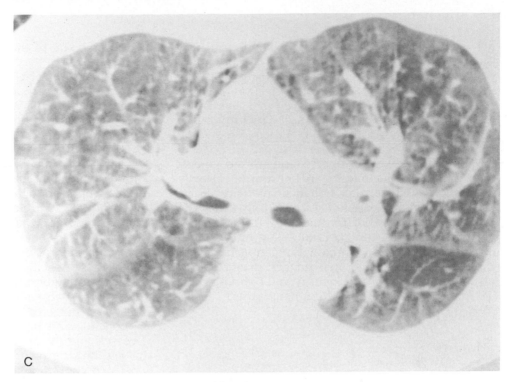

FIGURE 4–5 *Continued* ■ *C,* Changing the window level to −1000 H but keeping the window width at 750 H increases the caliber and visibility of all vessels.

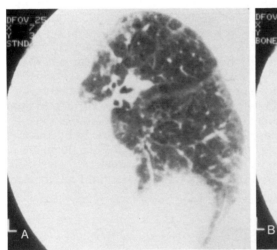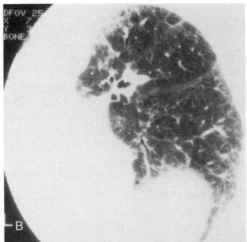

FIGURE 4–6 ■ Effect of reconstruction algorithm. *A,* HRCT scan with standard reconstruction algorithm shows reduced resolution of small structures because of smoothing in reconstruction of the image. *B,* HRCT scan with bone reconstruction algorithm demonstrates the peripheral structures of the lung more clearly.

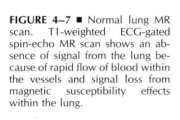

FIGURE 4–7 ■ Normal lung MR scan. T1-weighted ECG-gated spin-echo MR scan shows an absence of signal from the lung because of rapid flow of blood within the vessels and signal loss from magnetic susceptibility effects within the lung.

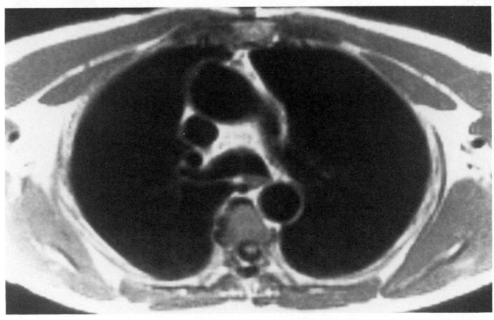

edly improves display of the mediastinal and hilar structures and also increases the signal-to-noise ratio. With ECG synchronization to every heart beat, the effective TR is about 600 ms. Detection of lung nodules and masses is improved by using T2-weighted images achieved by ECG synchronization to every other heart beat to lengthen TR and by using a TE of about 60 ms. Because MR directed to focal or diffuse lung lesions has not found clinical application, these techniques are not routine. Heavily T2-weighted images may enhance intensity differences between tumors and surrounding atelectatic lung, but these are not routine. Respiratory gating for thoracic disease can be undertaken but also has limited application and prolongs imaging time. For lung cancer staging, coronal images may assist in detecting mediastinal adenopathy and defining chest wall invasion of peripheral lung neoplasms.

Pathology

Patterns of Abnormality

ALVEOLAR (AIR SPACE) DISEASE

Air space disease is present when an increase in lung density stems from a replacement of the gas within the distal air spaces by tissue-equivalent material. The material may be liquid, blood, cellular elements, or a combination of these. Key to the concept is that the architecture of the lung parenchyma remains essentially intact. More specifically, the alveolar walls are not disrupted. In most circumstances, the bronchi within the involved area contain gas. When the subtending bronchus is occluded, the appearance is of a drowned or airless lobe or seg-

ment, and some of the features of air space disease are not evident.

The CT appearances of air space disease have been described by Naidich and colleagues[19] in their classic article and are similar to those shown in chest radiographs. Air space diseases manifest different CT appearances depending on the degree of replacement of air by liquid or tissue. The earliest finding is poorly marginated nodules. These may form rosettes or nodules about 1 cm in diameter. They are sublobular and may represent opacification of single acini; hence the term *acinar* nodules. With increasing consolidation, the nodules coalesce to form larger areas of opacity (Fig. 4–8). On CT and HRCT, the lack of superimposition of densities allows the detailed display of these opacities. Not infrequently, this extent of lung consolidation conforms to lobular boundaries, causing a "patchwork quilt" appearance. As more lobules are involved and if the bronchi are patent, air bronchograms become evident, with obscuration of vessels and the appearance of branching, tubular, air-filled bronchi or bronchioles. The increase in CT density of consolidation is clearly marginated at lobar, segmental, or lobular borders (Fig. 4–9). In less well-delineated sites, the denser consolidation is bordered by acinar or sublobular nodules. As with the chest radiograph, air bronchograms are a characteristic, although not invariable, feature of air space disease.

An appearance not uncommonly seen on HRCT is a hazy, subtle increase in CT density, corresponding to the radiographic ground-glass appearance (Fig. 4–10). This appearance probably is caused by incomplete filling of air spaces at the alveolar level by a mixture of air and soft tissue–equivalent material. It is seen most commonly with edema fluid or blood in

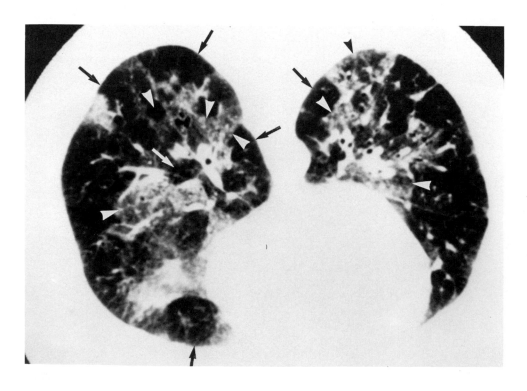

FIGURE 4–8 ■ Desquamative interstitial pneumonitis. HRCT shows a mosaic of consolidated secondary pulmonary lobules, lobules showing a ground-glass appearance *(arrowheads)*, and normal-appearing lobules *(arrows)*.

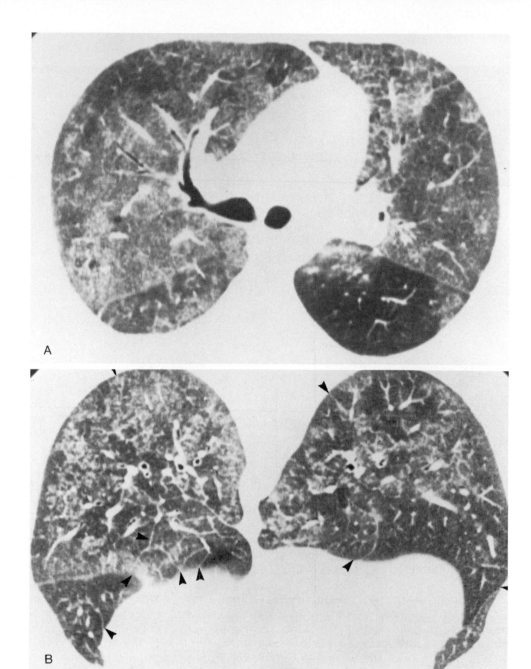

FIGURE 4–9 ■ Pulmonary alveolar proteinosis. *A*, HRCT scan through the midlung shows a typical diffuse ground-glass pattern. The pulmonary vessels are visible, and only minor air bronchograms are seen in the affected areas. *B*, Prone HRCT scan through the lower lobes shows a more granular pattern with mild peripheral interlobular septal thickening *(arrowheads)*.

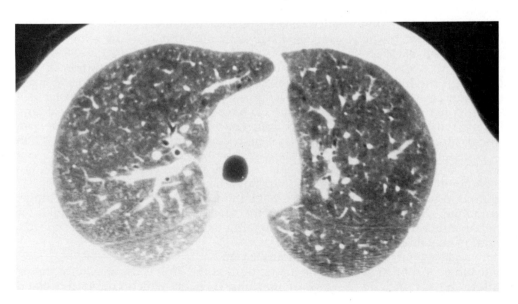

FIGURE 4–10 ■ Diffuse alveolar damage from a viral pneumonia. The HRCT scan shows a diffuse ground-glass pattern without specific features. An open lung biopsy showed diffuse alveolar wall thickening but no abnormality within the alveolar spaces.

165

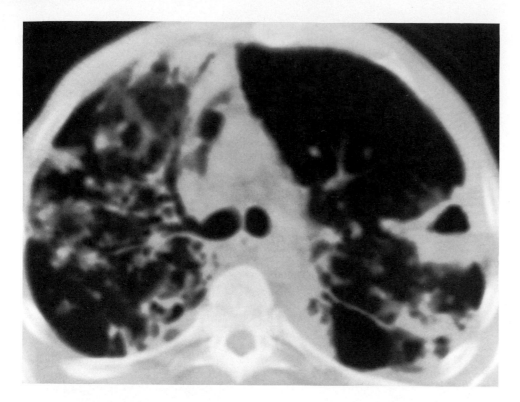

FIGURE 4–11 ■ Tuberculosis with transbronchial spread. CT scan through the midlung shows a fluid-containing left upper lobe cavity and multiple ill-defined acinar nodules up to 10 mm in diameter. (Courtesy of P. Schnyder, MD, Lausanne, Switzerland.)

the air spaces but is nonspecific and may also be found in conditions considered to be interstitial, such as interstitial viral pneumonia or other infections (e.g., *Pneumocystis carinii* pneumonia). In these circumstances, the hazy appearance is probably a combination of alveolar wall thickening and interstitial fluid, desquamated cells, and exudate lining the air spaces.

Itoh and colleagues[20] have emphasized that some air space nodules can be shown on CT around small bronchi, especially with tuberculous bronchopneumonia or transbronchial spread of tuberculosis (Fig. 4–11). We have not found this finding to have diagnostic value, perhaps because CT is uncommonly obtained in our patient population with acute pulmonary tuberculosis. However, we have seen this finding in several instances of sarcoidosis, extrinsic allergic alveolitis, and other causes of early air space disease.

Pneumonia tends to spread through the lung via collateral channels that are present in both alveolar walls and bronchioles. Lobar pneumonia frequently progresses to dense consolidation, which respects the boundaries of lobes unless the fissures are incomplete. If the proximal bronchus is patent, branching air bronchograms will be seen on CT and vessels will be invisible within the lung consolidation. Pulmonary infarction with hemorrhage and fluid in the infarcted lung can appear similar to pneumonia. The areas of opacity are usually pleural, based on either the costal pleural margin or a fissure. Cavitation may be evident if necrosis has occurred within the area of infarction.

Noninfectious causes of chronic lung consolidation that can show an alveolar pattern on CT include sarcoidosis, alveolar proteinosis, bronchoalveolar cell carcinoma, and the spectrum of lymphoma and pseudolymphoma (lymphocytic interstitial pneumonia). Newell and co-workers[21] and McCook and colleagues[22] described similar findings in pulmonary alveolar proteinosis consisting of air space nodules, air bronchograms, and diffuse, hazy densities (Figs. 4–9 and 4–12). In two cases we have studied with HRCT, a distinct interstitial component was also evident, a finding first described by Godwin and colleagues.[23] CT can show a peripheral predominance to the airspace consolidation in chronic eosinophilic pneumonia.[23a]

CT can be a key examination in patients with bronchoalveolar cell carcinoma.[24, 25] The CT appearance consists of hazy densities, acinar nodules, and consolidation with air bronchograms. Im and co-workers[25a] described visible opacified vessels after intravenous contrast material administration (a "CT angiogram sign"). Although these authors considered this finding specific for bronchoalveolar cell carcinoma, we have seen it in other instances of lung consolidation. The multifocal form of this neoplasm can be resected when limited to one lobe. When more extensive, the tumor is nonresectable. CT can define sites of tumor not evident on chest radiographs that show the lesion as nonresectable (Fig. 4–13). HRCT, at 1-cm intervals throughout the lungs, is probably the ideal examination to undertake for this purpose, although this has not been described.

INTERSTITIAL DISEASE

The interstitium of the lung is the structural framework of the lung through which course the blood vessels and airways. It constitutes an extravascular compartment in which fluid or cellular elements may collect and fibroblasts may proliferate. For the purposes of interpretation of CT and especially HRCT, a useful concept is of three interconnecting interstitial spaces: (1) central, (2) peripheral, and (3) alveolar wall (Fig. 4–14).

The central interstitial space has two components. One surrounds the bronchi and blood vessels and radiates from the hila to the pulmonary lobules. The second consists of long channels that directly connect the peripheral interlobular interstitium to the interstitium around the proximal bronchi and vessels. Thickening of the central interstitium produces apparent bronchial wall widening and long bands running through the lung.

The peripheral interstitial space consists of the interlobular interstitium surrounding the secondary pulmonary lobule and the centrilobular interstitium surrounding the bronchioles and arterioles within its

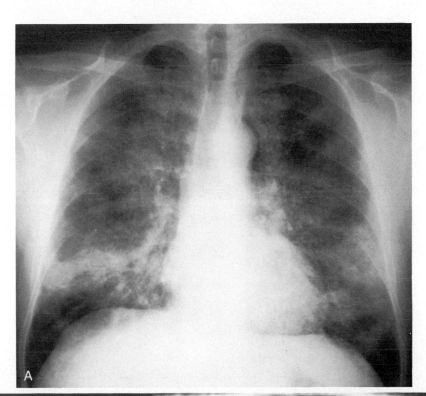

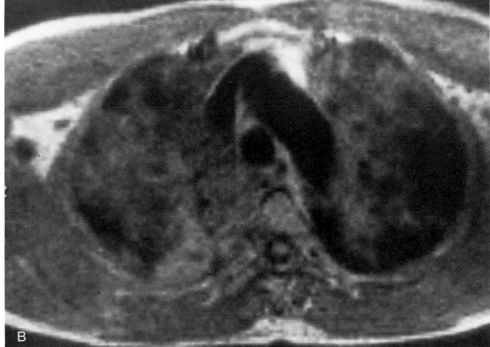

FIGURE 4–12 ■ Pulmonary alveolar proteinosis. *A*, Chest radiograph shows diffusely abnormal lungs with a nonspecific pattern of diffuse consolidation and linear opacities. *B*, MR scan using a T2-weighted spin-echo sequence shows diffuse low-intensity signal from both lungs.

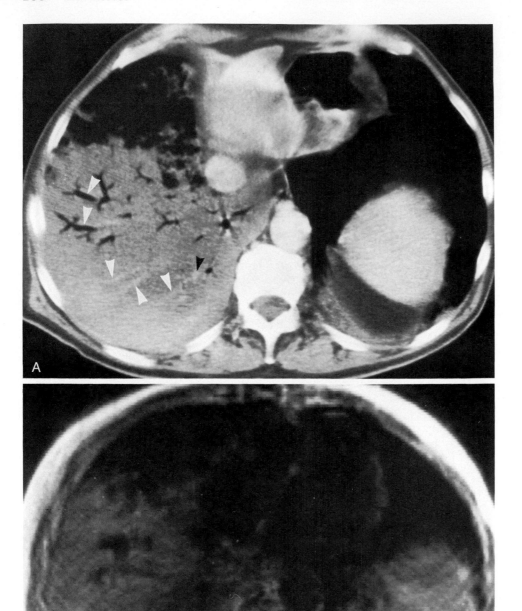

FIGURE 4–13 ■ Bronchiolar-alveolar cell carcinoma in a 38-year-old woman initially diagnosed as having alveolar proteinosis. *A,* CT scan shows dense consolidation involving the right lower lobe. Air bronchograms and opacified vessels *(arrowheads)* are present within the consolidated lobe. *B,* T1-weighted MR scan at the same level as *A* shows amorphous low-intensity signal within both lower lobes.

FIGURE 4–14 ■ Schema of HRCT features of different diseases. *A,* Ground-glass density is found with air space disease or thickening of alveolar walls. *B* through *H,* Features of interstitial disease. *B,* Thickening of interlobular septa and centrilobular interstitial spaces. *C,* Subpleural line. This parallels the pleural surface and, when present in nondependent lung, indicates interlobular thickening and distortion of secondary lobules. *D,* Several features seen with pulmonary fibrosis include interlobular fibrosis, honeycombing, architectural distortion, visceral subpleural thickening, and thin-walled cysts. *E,* Traction or cicatricial bronchiectasis is found in areas of marked fibrosis, especially honeycombing. *F,* Interstitial nodules may appear within septa, around the centrilobular structures, or within the parenchyma of the secondary lobule. *G,* Thin-walled cystic spaces containing gas can be seen with interstitial disease, usually when advanced, and also with emphysema. Geographic cysts are found with histiocytosis X and lymphangiomyomatosis. *H,* Parenchymal bands or long scars are found with various interstitial fibrotic diseases. They terminate at the pleural surface in interlobular septa. *I* and *J,* Features of airway disease. *I,* Bronchiectasis and bronchiolectasis are seen as dilated, thickened, walled bronchi or bronchioles. *J,* Emphysema. Early panlobular emphysema tends to involve the periphery of the secondary lobule, whereas centrilobular emphysema involves the center. More advanced emphysema of either type appears similar and involves the whole lobule. *K,* Lymphangitic spread of carcinoma. HRCT features are relatively specific, with peribronchial and peribronchiolar thickening and beaded interstitial thickening without architectural distortion.

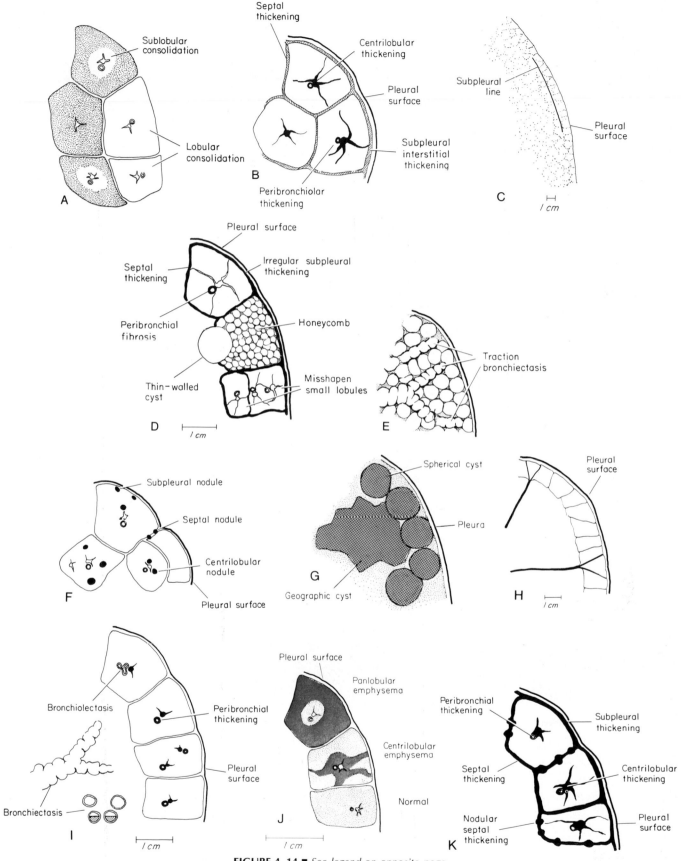

FIGURE 4–14 ■ *See legend on opposite page*

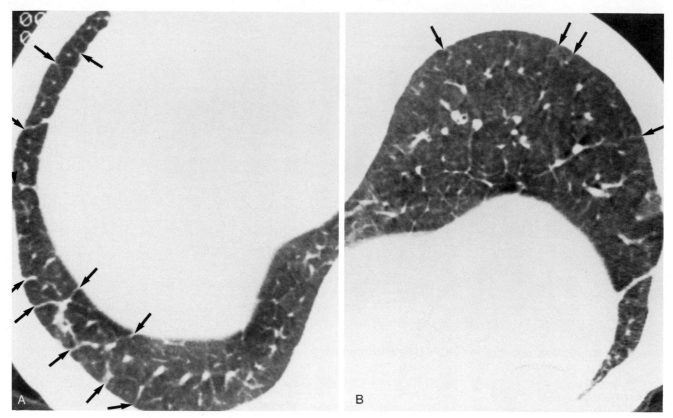

FIGURE 4–15 ■ Chronic left heart failure with interlobular, septal, and alveolar wall thickening. *A*, Supine HRCT scan shows extensive interlobular septal thickening *(arrows)* in the right lower lobe. *B*, Prone HRCT scan at the same level as *A* shows that the septal thickening has decreased *(arrows)* and thus represents dilated veins, lymphatics, and interstitial edema. The ground-glass hazy density is probably caused by chronic alveolar wall edema and capillary distention. Diagnosis was confirmed by lung biopsy.

center. Thickening of this space produces interlobular septal lines, subpleural or visceral pleural thickening, and centrilobular thickening.

The third interstitial space is within the alveolar walls and cannot be resolved with CT. Thickening of this space produces nonspecific, hazy increases in CT density, and when alveolar walls are markedly swollen, the CT features are similar to air space consolidation.[19]

The CT features of interstitial lung disease reflect

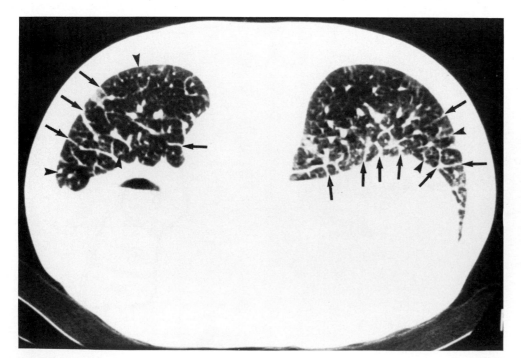

FIGURE 4–16 ■ Idiopathic pulmonary fibrosis with interstitial fibrosis. Prone HRCT scan shows extensive interlobular septal thickening *(arrows)*. Intralobular (centrilobular) structures *(arrowheads)* are prominent and extend toward the pleura, representing fibrosis around the peripheral pulmonary arteries and their accompanying small bronchi.

thickening, infiltration, or distortion of the interstitium of the lung. The involved structures are most easily appreciated on HRCT, now the standard CT examination for interstitial lung disease. The original descriptions by Zerhouni and his group[5] have been elaborated on by many authors.[26-30]

The most common HRCT finding in interstitial lung disease is thickening of interlobular (septal) and centrilobular (core) structures. Septal thickening is best appreciated in the subpleural and juxtadiaphragmatic regions, where septa are well developed (Fig. 4–16). Abnormal septa are thicker than 1 mm, and an increased number are visible in diseases involving the interlobular pulmonary interstitium. Adjacent to the diaphragm, abnormal lobules imaged in cross section have a characteristic polygonal shape. Within the more central regions of the lung, where lobules are not as well developed, linear opacities 1 to 2 cm in length, representing obliquely oriented septa, are evident. Sometimes a lattice of fine lines is seen within the central portion of the pulmonary lobule radiating from the core toward the lobular borders. These lines most likely represent thickening of the intralobular peribronchiolar interstitium. The perilobular interstitium includes a space that is contiguous with the pleura. Extension of fibrosis or infiltration to this subpleural interstitial space produces irregular thickening of the pleura that can be seen on HRCT.

Subpleural lines are 2- to 10-cm-long, thin, curvilinear lines and are another manifestation of interstitial lung disease. They are found within 1 cm of the pleural surface, paralleling the chest wall (Fig. 4–17). They were originally described in patients with asbestosis but also occur in other forms of pulmonary fibrosis.[31] They are most frequent in the posterior lower lobes, usually with other evidence of interstitial fibrosis. Subpleural lines that disappear when that portion of lung is nondependent are found in normal individuals, probably represent compressed lung, and are not of significance. Those that do not clear in the nondependent position probably represent fibrosed septa of disrupted lobules or occasionally the inner margin of fine subpleural honeycombing.

Long lines (scars) or parenchymal bands are linear, nontapering opacities 2 to 5 cm in length coursing through the lung, usually terminating in interlobular septa at the pleural surface (Fig. 4–18).[9] These bands are usually indicative of interstitial fibrosis but are also found with lymphangitic infiltration of the central interstitial space by neoplasm. They can be distinguished from vessel and interlobular septa by their length, thickness, direction, absence of branches, and association with parenchymal distortion. They probably represent large fibrotic scars coursing through the pulmonary interstitium.[32] They occur commonly in patients with asbestosis but are also seen with other causes of pulmonary fibrosis. When caused by lymphangitic carcinomatosis they frequently have a characteristic nodular appearance.[5]

Honeycombing appears on HRCT and CT as small (6- to 10-mm) cystic spaces with thick walls, most commonly in the lower lobes, and represents fibrosis from various causes (Fig. 4–19). In milder cases of pulmonary fibrosis, honeycombing may be localized to a subpleural location.

Irregularity of lung interfaces has been described as an HRCT manifestation of interstitial disease and is visible along the fissures and bronchovascular structures. The irregularity of the margins of these structures reflects abnormality of the subpleural or central interstitium.[5] This finding is subjective and requires experience to detect its presence.

Architectural distortion results from extensive fibrosis and is seen in end-stage fibrotic diseases such as idiopathic pulmonary fibrosis, sarcoidosis, silicosis, and asbestosis. The normal lung architecture

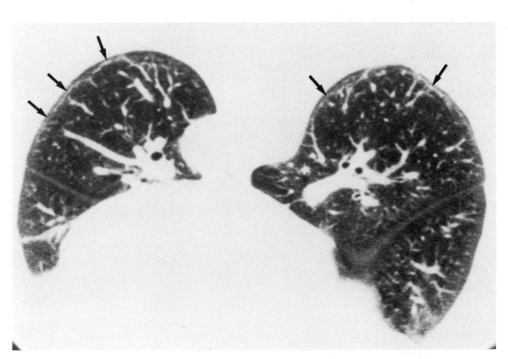

FIGURE 4–17 ■ Asbestosis with subpleural lines. Prone HRCT scan shows bilateral subpleural lines (arrows) at nondependent sites. These are abnormal when in a nondependent portion of the lung. Subpleural lines can be seen with other causes of interstitial fibrosis and are a manifestation of interstitial fibrosis.

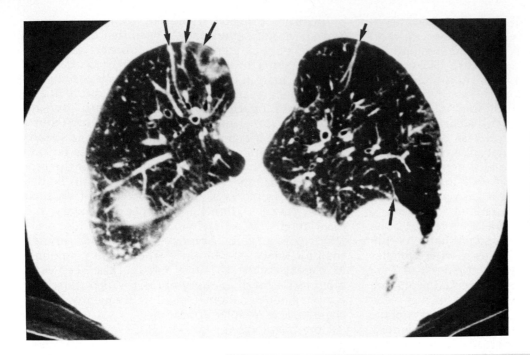

FIGURE 4–18 ■ Interstitial fibrosis with long scars (parenchymal bands). HRCT scan demonstrates long lines *(arrows)* extending to the pleura and not conforming to the morphology of blood vessels. Minor interstitial septal thickening is also seen.

FIGURE 4–19 ■ Rheumatoid lung disease with peripheral honeycombing in a 66-year-old man. *A,* Prone HRCT scan at the level of the inferior hila shows multifocal areas of honeycombing *(arrows).* Bilateral interlobular septal thickening and a cyst on the right side are seen. *B,* Prone HRCT scan taken 3 cm caudal to *A* shows that the lung bases are almost completely replaced by honeycomb lung. Beaded appearance *(arrowheads)* is probably cicatricial bronchiectasis.

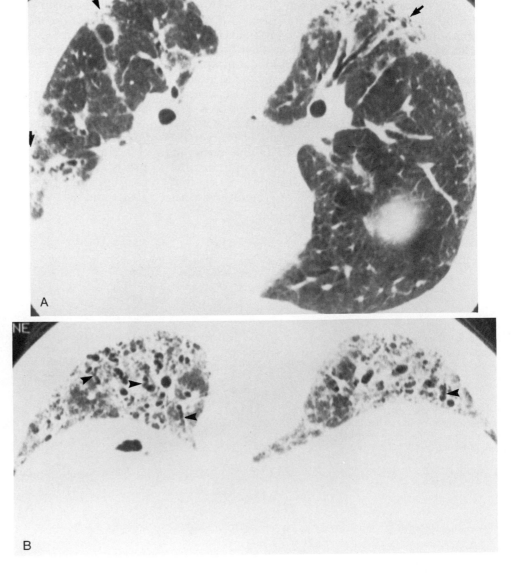

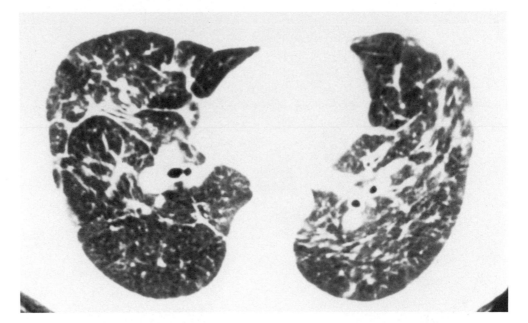

FIGURE 4–20 ■ Advanced sarcoidosis with architectural distortion. Supine HRCT scan shows extensive septal thickening. In addition, the normal lung morphology is distorted, with crowding and irregular branching of vessels in the middle third of both lungs.

is distorted, and the secondary lobules are shrunken and misshapen (Fig. 4–20). This distortion is more easily appreciated on transaxial HRCT images than on conventional radiographs.

Peribronchial interstitial thickening is from fibrosis or infiltration of the central peribronchial interstitium and manifests on HRCT as an apparent thickening of bronchial walls. This finding is more common in certain diseases such as sarcoidosis and lymphangitic spread of carcinoma than in idiopathic fibrosis or asbestosis.

Cicatricial bronchiectasis is seen on HRCT as bronchial dilatation, distortion, thickening, and beading in areas of severe pulmonary fibrosis (Fig. 4–21).[33] These findings are secondary to the increased traction

on small bronchi and do not imply primary bronchial disease.

Interstitial nodules 1 to 3 mm in diameter can be demonstrated on HRCT but when small may be difficult to distinguish from small vessels seen in cross section or points of confluence of linear structures. They are most easily identified when present within the lobular core. Remy-Jardin and co-investigators,[33a] have described small nodules less than 7 mm in diameter in a subpleural location as a feature of interstitial lung disease. They found these were nonspecific but increased in frequency in sarcoidosis, lymphangitic carcinomatosis, and coal worker's pneumoconiosis. They have also been found in asbestosis.

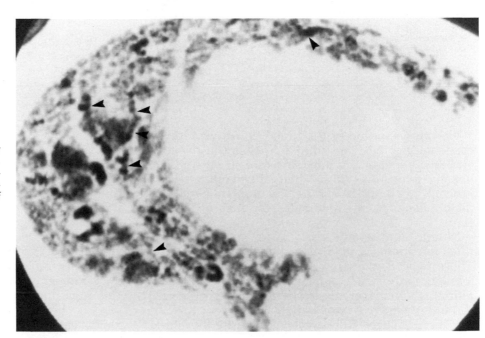

FIGURE 4–21 ■ Idiopathic pulmonary fibrosis with cicatricial bronchiectasis. HRCT scan shows extensive honeycombing with linear beaded lucencies (arrowheads) representing the dilated bronchi of cicatricial bronchiectasis.

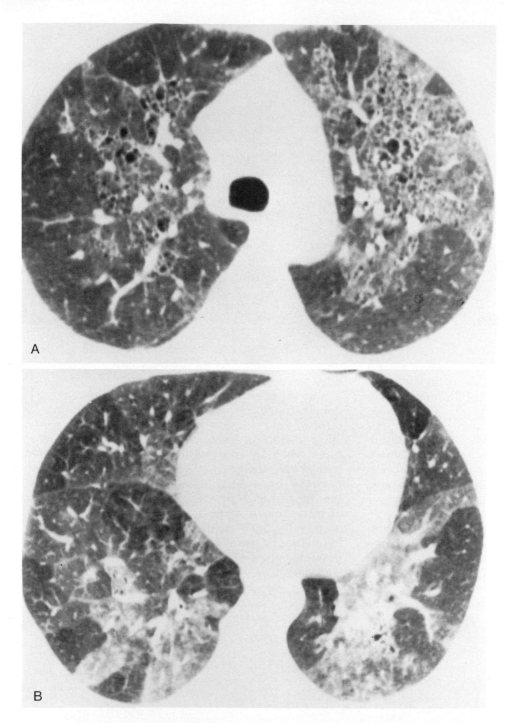

A

B

FIGURE 4–22 ■ Idiopathic pulmonary fibrosis with active alveolitis. *A*, HRCT scan through the upper lobes demonstrates honeycombing, interlobular septal thickening, and ground-glass opacities. *B*, HRCT scan through the lower lobes shows areas of ground-glass opacity mixed with normal lung lobules. Bronchoalveolar lavage showed activated lymphocytes and other features of active alveolitis.

Fibrotic distortion of the lung parenchyma causes cystic spaces that vary from 1 to 10 cm in diameter and are devoid of any lung structure. Their walls are usually pencil-line thin. Their appearance in conjunction with other features of interstitial fibrosis distinguishes them from bullae or sites of emphysema.

Multifocal areas of increased density can be identified in patients with diffuse interstitial lung disease. These regions, which in some instances conform to lobular borders, are similar to very fine air space filling. Pulmonary vessels tend to be preserved through the increased opacity, and air bronchograms are absent. These hazy areas represent either thickening of alveolar walls or incomplete filling of the alveolar air spaces and in the presence of interstitial disease may be indicative of an active inflammatory process (Fig. 4–22).[34] Bronchiolitis obliterans organizing pneumonia can show patchy combined airspace and interstitial abnormalities with a predominantly subpleural distribution.[34a]

HRCT has clearly demonstrated great sensitivity for detection of interstitial and air space parenchymal lung disease. It can detect abnormality when the chest radiograph is normal or minimally abnormal. The description of HRCT features in individual diseases is currently in process; the specificity of these combinations of findings is also being addressed.[35–38a]

It appears that for many interstitial diseases, the patterns of abnormality are better displayed or more easily perceived and classified on HRCT than on chest radiographs. The specificity for diagnosis, or at least compartmentalization, is undoubtedly better with HRCT than has been possible with chest radiographs.

Focal Lung Disease

PULMONARY NODULES

Pulmonary Metastasis ■ Detection of pulmonary nodules is a common clinical indication for CT of the lungs. CT scanning is valuable in detecting pulmonary nodules, because the transverse display of CT images is ideal for separating thoracic structures that overlap on radiographs and obscure these nodules. Nodules that are subpleural, high in the apices of the lungs, in the costophrenic angles, or obscured by mediastinal structures are especially difficult to appreciate from chest radiographs but are readily apparent on CT scans. Many nodules 0.5 to 1 cm in diameter are not apparent on chest radiographs, whereas CT allows visualization of most pulmonary nodules larger than 2 to 3 mm in diameter (Fig. 4–23). Pulmonary nodules can be detected on CT scans when they are larger than the pulmonary blood vessels in that portion of the lung. Nodules in the outer third of the lung are therefore more conspicuous than those closer to the hilum. Close observation of contiguous scans is often necessary to distinguish small nodules from vessels. Vessels can usually be seen on adjacent scans as they branch and course through the lungs. The eye can integrate information from serial scans and follow the course of pulmonary vessels. Small nodules appear as disjointed densities with no vascular connection. The anterior end of the

first rib and its costal cartilage can be mistaken for a lung nodule on CT scans, although this pitfall is now routinely recognized.

In their original studies, Muhm and colleagues[39] found that in 32 of 91 patients, CT scans demonstrated more nodules than were seen on conventional whole lung tomograms. In 5 of these 32 patients, conventional tomograms failed to show any nodules, whereas CT scans revealed one or more nodules. Shaner and co-workers[40] confirmed these findings in a study of 25 patients with sarcoma or melanoma. Conventional tomograms showed each patient to have one to four pulmonary nodules, whereas CT scans defined additional nodules, usually 3 to 6 mm in diameter, in 12 (48 per cent) of the patients. All 25 patients underwent thoracotomy, and CT scans had correctly demonstrated 78 per cent of all resected nodules greater than 3 mm in diameter. These results have been confirmed by others.[41, 42] For instance, Vanel and colleagues[41] studied 32 patients with osteosarcoma and found that CT was much more sensitive than other imaging modalities. They had only one false-positive CT scan.

The clinical significance of pulmonary nodules detected only by CT in a patient with a thoracic or extrathoracic primary neoplasm is controversial. Although the Shaner study[40] found that 60 per cent of these small nodules were benign granulomas or intrapulmonary lymph nodes, Muhm's group[39] found that only 10 to 15 per cent of the nodules in their study were benign. The latter result is most likely the more correct figure in industrialized countries with a low incidence of infectious granulomatous disease. In a comprehensive and detailed study, Peuchot and Libshitz[42a] showed that in patients with previously treated extrathoracic malignancies, only 73 per cent of resected nodules would be demonstrated with CT. Of the resected nodules, 87 per cent

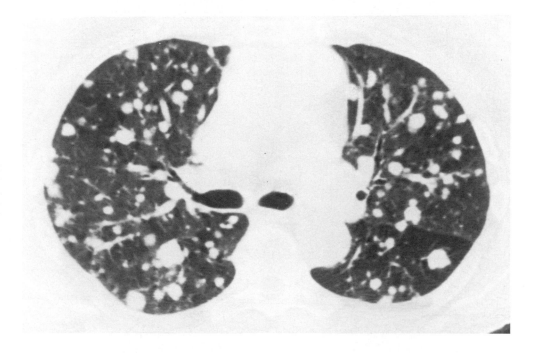

FIGURE 4–23 ■ Metastatic leiomyosarcoma. CT scan shows numerous nodules, many of which could not be resolved on chest radiographs. Some nodules show a small pulmonary vessel entering them, a finding that has been suggested as indicating a hematogenous route of spread to the lungs.

TABLE 4–1 ■ Neoplasms Likely to Have Nodular Pulmonary Metastases

Bone and soft tissue
Lung
Melanoma
Colon
Genitourinary tract
Head and neck

were metastases, 9 per cent benign lesions, and 4 per cent incidental bronchogenic carcinomas. For practical purposes, it must be appreciated that nodules detected only on CT scans, especially in a patient with a malignant neoplasm, are most likely but not always metastases. Depending on the clinical circumstances, additional evaluation may be necessary for diagnosis. In some situations, CT-guided percutaneous aspiration biopsy or thoracotomy may be required. Alternatively, repeat CT scanning after 6 to 10 weeks may show enlargement of the nodule or nodules. In our experience, the high sensitivity of CT scanning should be used in the search for metastatic pulmonary nodules, especially in patients with tumors that have a propensity for metastasizing to the lungs (Table 4–1). In almost all circumstances, CT has replaced conventional radiographs and whole lung tomography for this purpose.

Zerhouni[43] has emphasized the importance of the vascular relationship to focal lung nodules or masses, specifically hematogenous metastases and septic emboli. In his experience, a vessel can be imaged with thin sections entering the mass in up to 30 per cent of cases (Fig. 4–24). With multiple septic emboli, the vessel will generally enter a roughly wedge-shaped lesion situated on a pleural surface. Noninfected infarcts can have a similar CT appearance, although they will usually be larger and less well defined. Septic infarcts will frequently cavitate, a finding readily identified on CT.

Solitary Pulmonary Nodules ■ The role of CT in the evaluation of the patient who presents with a noncalcified solitary pulmonary nodule on a chest radiograph has been extensively investigated and is now reasonably clarified. There is considerable variation in clinical management of the patient with a solitary pulmonary nodule. The decision whether to follow the patient with periodic imaging studies or to obtain tissue from the nodule frequently depends on the radiologist's degree of confidence that the nodule is benign. A nodule can be assumed benign if it shows stability on serial chest radiographs over at least 2 years. When previous radiographs are unavailable, detection of calcium within the nodule is important in determining its probability of benignity, as most calcified pulmonary nodules are benign.[44, 45] The pattern of calcification is also important. Diffuse or central calcification within a pulmonary nodule usually indicates benignity. In a small proportion of patients, a bronchogenic carcinoma can engulf a calcified nidus, and thus an eccentric focus of calcification does not exclude malignancy (Fig. 4–25). Bronchogenic carcinomas themselves occasionally calcify, but the calcification is often very fine and invisible on radiographs or CT scans. Of 72 patients with a malignant solitary pulmonary nodule studied by O'Keefe and colleagues,[45] ten had calcification visible on radiographs of the resected specimens, but in only one instance was the calcification seen on conventional chest radiographs. In the same study 50 per cent of benign lesions, consisting mainly of granulomas and hamartomas, contained calcification. In only 35 per cent of these patients was calcification

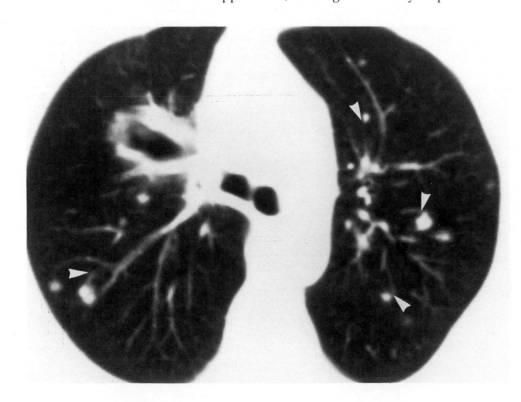

FIGURE 4–24 ■ Hematogenous spread of tuberculosis. CT scan shows multiple nodules, most of which show a vessel (arrowheads) entering them, suggesting hematogenous dissemination to the lungs.

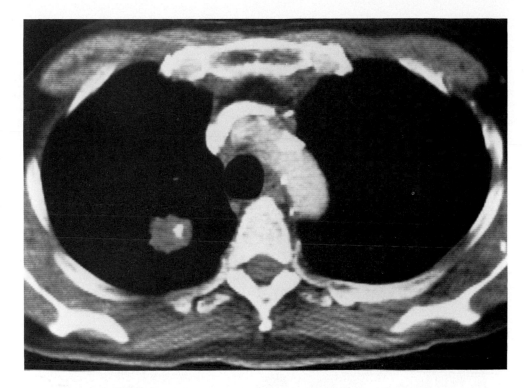

FIGURE 4–25 ■ Adenocarcinoma with an engulfed granuloma. Right upper lobe bronchogenic carcinoma shows an eccentric calcified nidus, representing an engulfed calcified granuloma. This type of calcification does not indicate that the mass is benign.

visible on chest radiographs. Metastatic malignant tumors, particularly osteogenic sarcoma, chondrosarcoma, and thyroid carcinoma, can also show stippled or homogenous calcification.

These circumstances, however, are uncommon and the majority of noncalcified solitary pulmonary nodules found from radiographs are indeterminate for malignancy. In these patients, the clinical choices include observation of the nodule for evidence of growth, percutaneous biopsy of the nodule, or surgical removal.

Since the 1950s, numerous studies in the radiology and surgery literature have established our basic understanding of the pulmonary nodule.[46–49] Most noncalcified nodules less than 2 cm in diameter are granulomas and should not be resected if the correct diagnosis can be established. However, the surgical mortality rate for resection of a solitary pulmonary nodule is low, particularly when the nodule is benign. Several factors can influence the decision on thoracotomy for nodule removal. Age can help in deciding management of the asymptomatic patient with a solitary pulmonary nodule, as pulmonary nodules are rarely malignant in asymptomatic patients younger than 35.[47] In most circumstances, a nodule in a patient younger than 35 years is followed with serial radiographs. After the age of 35, the incidence of malignancy in solitary pulmonary nodules increases significantly. Up to 50 per cent of resected solitary pulmonary nodules in older patients are primary or metastatic malignant tumors, and resection does result in an improved prognosis for the patient.[50, 51] This indicates that even without the information derived from CT a significant selection of patients for thoracotomy is possible, based on radiographic features alone. For those in whom the

nodule remains indeterminate, a convincing argument can be made for resection of the solitary pulmonary nodule in all patients older than 35 years. Few clinicians now follow patients with a nodule that is at all suspicious for malignancy. Percutaneous aspiration biopsy of the nodule is an intermediate course in deciding management, particularly in areas endemic for tuberculosis or fungal disease and when aspiration of organisms or inflammatory tissue would prevent an unnecessary thoracotomy.[52] A simple noninvasive method for distinguishing benign from malignant solitary pulmonary nodules would nevertheless be of benefit.

The appearance of a solitary pulmonary nodule on CT is similar to that on chest radiographs. Granulomas and carcinomas can be ill defined, lobulated, or well defined. Morphologic criteria are not very sensitive in distinguishing benign from malignant lesions, whether from chest radiographs or CT scans. Kuriyama and colleagues[53] described the HRCT morphology in 18 peripheral carcinomas less than 3 cm in diameter. They found a high incidence of spiculation (78 per cent), a notch in the mass (83 per cent), retraction of the pleura to the mass producing a pleural tag (78 per cent), and convergence of vessels toward the nodule (83 per cent). Heterogeneity of the tumor and a lower density halo were also common. One or a combination of these findings should be suspicious for a neoplasm, even though many of these features can be seen with benign nodules. Kuhlman and co-workers[54] found similar morphologic findings in a group of patients with solitary bronchioloalveolar cell carcinoma. In general, nodules that have a starburst appearance and are spiculated, inhomogeneous, notched, contain a cavity, or larger than 2 cm in diameter are likely to be malignant and should be resected. An additional finding on CT that may be indicative of malignancy is a bronchus extending to the margin of a nodule or mass or traversing the nodule.[55]

The high-contrast resolution of CT scans can provide important information about the density of solitary pulmonary nodules. Phantom studies by Cann and colleagues[56] showed that CT scanners are accurate densitometers. In simulated lung nodules, they found that differences of as little as 15 mg/mL of potassium phosphate could be detected using CT densitometry. Using a phantom, Godwin and co-workers[57] studied the relationship of nodule size to the degree of CT scanner collimation and the number

of CT voxels free of partial volume artifacts from surrounding aerated lung. With the resolving element of most scanners, nodules less than 1 cm in diameter require narrow collimation (1 to 2 mm) to obtain voxels from within the nodule for analysis, and thus narrow collimation scans are essential for CT nodule evaluation.

Early investigations using CT densitometry to distinguish benign from malignant nodules were controversial. Siegelman and associates[58] were the first to use CT nodule densitometry in a series of patients. With careful calibration of the scanner, narrow collimation (2 to 5 mm), and numeric printouts of the CT numbers, an average CT number was obtained from

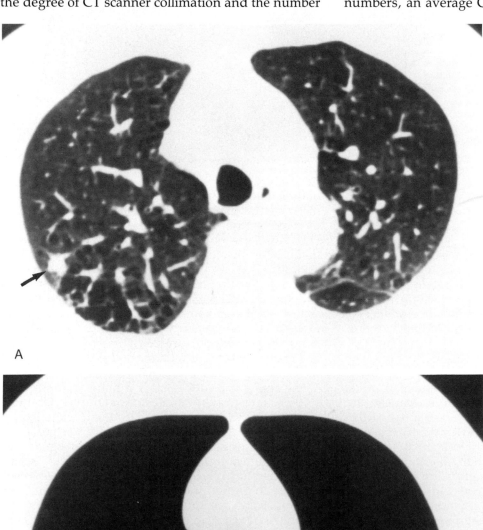

A

B

FIGURE 4–26 ■ Nodule densitometry with a phantom. *A*, HRCT scan shows a 1.2-cm nodule in the right upper lobe *(arrow)*. *B*, Scan of the phantom with a rod similar in size to the nodule and in the same position within the phantom as the nodule.

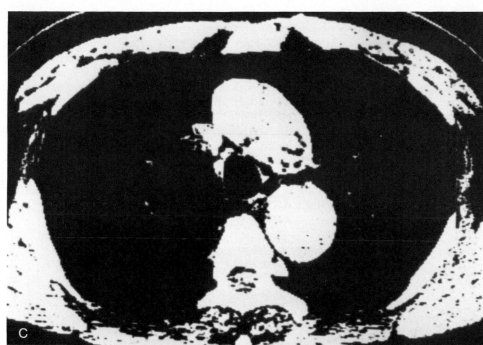

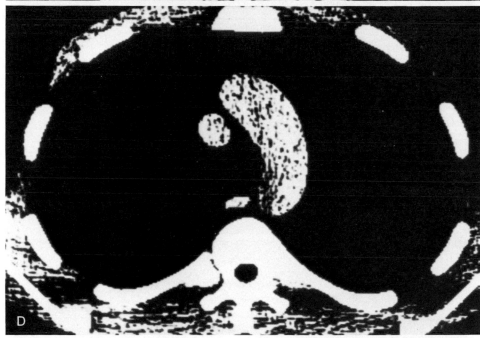

FIGURE 4–26 *Continued* ■ *C,* Using a narrow window width, the nodule in the patient disappeared at a window level of 34 H. *D,* The rod in the phantom disappeared at a window level of 37 H, indicating the nodule is indeterminate for malignancy. The resected right upper lobe contained a nodular adenocarcinoma.

a set of contiguous voxels having the highest CT density. The CT number suggested to distinguish benign from malignant nodules was 164 H. Of 91 nodules that were not calcified on radiographs, 45 were nodular bronchogenic carcinomas and had a representative CT number between 57 and 139 H (mean, 92 ± 18 H). Another 13 were nodular metastases having representative CT numbers ranging from 57 to 147 H (mean, 98 H). The remaining 33 nodules were classified as benign and fell into three groups on the basis of CT nodule densitometry. Twenty-seven per cent were indistinguishable from malignant lesions; 60 per cent had a representative CT number above 164 H and were readily distin-

guishable from the malignant lesions; and 13 per cent had a representative CT number between 147 and 162 H, an intermediate range between benign and malignant. A few overtly calcified nodules all had a representative CT number above 600 H. Thus about 20 per cent of solitary pulmonary nodules could be classified as benign based on CT densitometry data alone. The high CT numbers are assumed to reflect fine diffuse calcification not visible on radiographs, although high concentrations of collagen (with a CT value of about 400 H) could produce similar findings.

Early scanners other than the one used by Siegelman and colleagues[58] were poor densitometers, and their results were difficult to reproduce.[59-61] CT numbers varied with different scanners and at different times on the same scanner. They also varied with size and location of a nodule within the chest.[62] The difficulties in accurate in vivo CT densitometry in the thorax have been extensively discussed. Early commercial CT scanners also varied widely in their algorithms and corrections for producing CT numbers. The CT number for high atomic number materials depends on effective x-ray energy, corrections for filtration and dynamic range, scanner configuration, and other factors. All of these functions have become better standardized for virtually all scanners.[62, 63] In the thorax, differing quantities of air, soft tissue, and

bone, as well as cardiopulmonary motion, also influence the recorded CT number. By using thin-section scans and short scanning times to minimize motion effects, the reproducibility of CT numbers has improved significantly. A thorax phantom that enables standardization of nodule densities can further improve the reproducibility and reliability of nodule densitometry (Fig. 4–26).[64, 65]

Five years after Siegelman's initial observation, and with improvements in CT scanners, Proto and Thomas[66] reported results supporting the initial work of Siegelman and colleagues.[58] Meanwhile, in a large series, Siegelman and co-workers[67] examined 634 solitary pulmonary nodules and, using 200 H as the

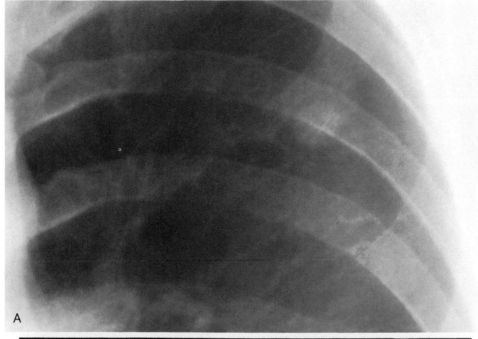

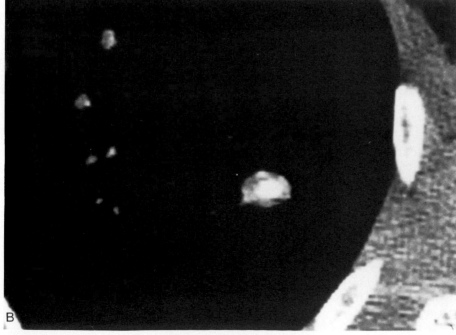

FIGURE 4–27 ■ Nodule densitometry without a phantom. *A*, Chest radiograph shows a well-circumscribed 2-cm left upper lobe nodule. *B*, HRCT scan demonstrates that the nodule contains a densely calcified center.

	X 380	381	382	383	384	385	386	387	388
Y									
260	-3	86	103	122	95	60	25	23	95
261	17	53	42	34	51	137	119	68	111
262	18	2	101	230	277	326	236	174	118
263	64	82	95	285	401	529	502	403	215
264	27	109	141	247	395	530	526	453	222
265	65	133	208	324	380	440	472	367	174
266	98	77	126	185	186	199	172	156	80
267	79	97	47	82	78	70	12	-50	-66
268	6	-17	8	71	22	54	45	45	14

FIGURE 4–27 *Continued* ■ *C*, A region-of-interest chart from within the nodule shows numerous contiguous CT numbers between 200 and 530 H. The nodule is a benign granuloma.

number dividing benign nodules from those that were indeterminate for malignancy, correctly identified 176 as benign, with no false-positive results.

From the results of a multicenter cooperative study, Zerhouni and co-workers[64] have defined an approach to CT characterization of the apparently noncalcified solitary pulmonary nodule. Using a standardized method of nodule densitometry, together with the morphologic features of the nodules, they identified 65 of 118 otherwise indeterminate nodules as benign. The nodule was visibly dense on CT images in 28 of the 65 patients, and it then was unnecessary to use a phantom or do quantitative nodule densitometry (Fig. 4–27). In the remaining 37 patients, densitometry with a phantom showed high CT numbers, even though the CT scans had not shown visible calcification. In this study, the density of nodules was compared with attenuation values of a comparably sized reference cylinder in a standardization phantom. To be characterized as benign, a group of contiguous voxels representing at least 10 per cent of the cross-sectional area of the nodule had to be higher than the pixels in the reference cylinder. Features causing a nodule to be characterized as indeterminate for benignity included low CT attenuation values, size greater than 3 cm, and irregular or spiculated borders. In this group, some calcium was seen in 12 (7 per cent) malignant nodules. The calcium in malignant nodules tended to be eccentric when compared with a central or diffuse distribution in benign nodules. Only one calcified malignant nodule was falsely diagnosed as benign. Nodules containing a cavity are unsuitable for densitometry. Although Zerhouni's group[64] favors using a reference phantom and stresses that no absolute CT number reliably distinguishes a benign pulmonary nodule, in our experience newer scanners do not require the standardization phantom, and densitometry can be done using the absolute CT numbers. A mean CT number of 150 to 200 H from the appropriate number of contiguous voxels in a morphologically benign-appearing nodule defines a lower limit for the CT density indicative of benignity (Table 4–2).[66, 68]

An additional reason for CT scanning in a patient with a solitary pulmonary nodule has been proposed.[39] A solitary pulmonary nodule may be a metastasis and the only radiographic manifestation of an occult extrathoracic malignancy. Detection of multiple nodules with CT could suggest the possibility of metastases and initiate a search for the primary neoplasm. This reasoning cannot be considered valid, as the frequency of metastasis presenting on chest radiographs as a solitary pulmonary nodule is only 3 to 6 per cent.

Several investigators, however, have studied whether CT is beneficial in staging patients with a solitary pulmonary nodule or mass suspected of being a primary bronchogenic carcinoma.[69-71] The incidence with which occult metastases or other significant abnormalities are found in this circumstance is up to 20 per cent. Although controversial,

TABLE 4–2 ■ **Method for CT Pulmonary Nodule Densitometry**

1. Smoothly bordered nodule less than 2 cm in diameter
2. Exclude cavitated nodules
3. Thin section (1.0 to 2.0 mm)
4. Standard mA, kVp, time, field-of-view
5. High resolution reconstruction algorithm
6. Nodule contains visible central or diffuse calcification: nodule is benign
7. Nodule contains fats: nodule is a hamartoma
8. Measure nodule size; determine number of pixels in nodule
9. Measure mean CT number from 15 per cent of highest contiguous pixels in nodule
10. Mean CT number above 200 H; nodule is benign
11. Mean CT number below 200 H; nodule is indeterminate

it does appear that CT can find occult mediastinal, abdominal, or contralateral lung abnormalities in sufficient instances that full thoracic and upper abdominal CT scans should be obtained in patients with suspected primary lung carcinoma, presenting as a solitary nodule.

A benign solitary pulmonary neoplasm that can be diagnosed with accuracy from CT is a pulmonary hamartoma (Fig. 4–28). Hamartomas arise from connective tissue in the bronchial wall and account for about 7 per cent of resected nodules.[72] CT has demonstrated fat and calcium within these tumors.[73] Siegelman and colleagues[74] studied 47 pulmonary

hamartomas, using HRCT. Their diagnostic criteria were (1) a diameter less than 2.5 cm, (2) a smooth edge, and (3) focal collections of fat or fat and foci of calcium. Those criteria were met in 28 of the 47 hamartomas and proved accurate for the correct diagnosis. Neither pulmonary bronchogenic carcinoma nor metastasis shows these features.

Pulmonary arteriovenous malformations are readily recognized with CT or MR. With CT, the lesion enhances after a bolus injection of contrast material, and its vascular connections are evident.

MR is limited for the examination of pulmonary nodules. The greater spatial resolution of CT enables

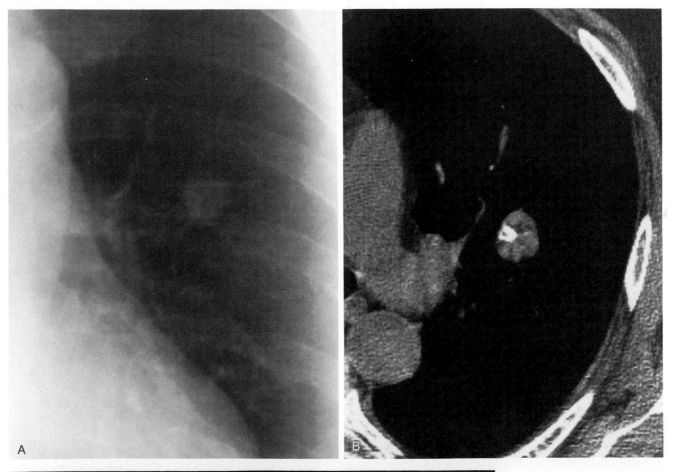

	X 358	359	360	361	362	363	364	365	366
Y									
297	71	252	183	10	-90	45	63	-4	-34
298	-26	113	82	-24	-86	13	35	30	40
299	80	114	210	89	-63	4	0	28	4
300	.267	225	353	162	12	45	60	61	66
301	849	799	548	140	6	10	47	11	7
302	1117	1166	440	-55	-40	-43	-15	14	60
303	367	266	149	-31	-58	-46	-16	22	75
304	24	-40	-50	-50	-7	24	40	20	36
C 305	-3	-67	-64	-31	23	30	-7	23	31

FIGURE 4–28 ■ Pulmonary hamartoma. *A,* Chest radiograph shows a 2.5-cm left lung nodule. *B,* HRCT scan shows the nodule containing dense calcification and adjacent low-density fat. *C,* A region-of-interest chart from within the nodule demonstrates CT numbers up to 1166 H, indicating calcification, and negative numbers as low as −58 H, indicating fat within the nodule.

more sensitivity than MR in nodule detection. Most nodules larger than 1 cm are detected by both techniques, whereas CT detects more nodules less than 1 cm in diameter. Muller and his colleagues[75] have shown that by identifying the solid nature of the nodules, MR is able to detect nodules close to the hila that could be mistaken for pulmonary vessels. This has application only when detection of nodules is key, for example, in planning resection of pulmonary metastases. We have studied the suitability of MR for quantifying calcium within pulmonary nodules[76] and have found that within the range of calcium found in pulmonary nodules, MR was limited by the type of calcium salt and its concentration. **Occult Nodules or Masses** ■ Confirming the presence and intrapulmonary location of a small nodule or mass suspected from chest radiographs can be difficult. The problem may be resolved with oblique chest radiographs or fluoroscopy with spot films of the area. Nodules or masses located in the apex of the lung, subpleurally, or in the retrocardiac region may not be demonstrated even with these techniques. When the presence of a mass remains unresolved, CT is sensitive for detecting and localizing a focal mass or nodule within the pulmonary parenchyma. We have seen numerous instances of CT scans demonstrating even large masses that were not visible using more conventional imaging modalities. The frequency of this situation is difficult to determine, and in practice, CT should be applied with due consideration of the clinical circumstances. CT can also demonstrate an occult cavity or a mycetoma within a lung mass and help elucidate the cause of hemoptysis (Fig. 4–29).[77, 78] In fact, Naidich and colleagues[78a] found that CT could find a specific cause for hemoptysis in 28 of 58 patients.

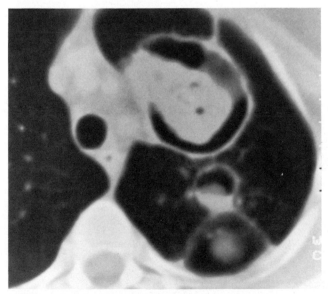

FIGURE 4–29 ■ Mycetomas within old tuberculous cavities. CT scan shows three masses within cavities, one attached to the wall of the largest cavity and one lying free in a dependent position within the smaller cavity. The largest mycetoma shows air within its center. (Courtesy of P. Schnyder, MD, Lausanne, Switzerland.)

TABLE 4–3 ■ **Extrathoracic Manifestations of Bronchogenic Carcinoma**

Endocrine and metabolic
  Cushing's syndrome
  Hypercalcemia
  Excessive antidiuretic hormone
  Carcinoid syndrome
  Estrogen excretion
Neuromuscular
  Peripheral neuropathy
  Cortical cerebellar degeneration
  Carcinomatous myopathy
  Subacute spinocerebellar degeneration
  Mental aberration
Skeletal and connective tissue
  Clubbing
  Pulmonary hypertrophic osteoarthropathy
  Acanthosis nigricans
  Dermatomyositis
Vascular and hematologic
  Migratory thrombophlebitis
  Nonbacterial verrucous endocarditis
  Anemia
  Fibrinolytic purpura

Sputum cytologic screening of patients with pulmonary symptoms or of those at risk for the development of bronchogenic carcinoma has been widely adopted. Some individuals have malignant cells in their sputum, although their chest radiograph shows no abnormality.[79, 80] Many such bronchogenic carcinomas are small and centrally located within a bronchus. Detailed fiberoptic bronchoscopy can show more than half of these lesions. In the remainder, CT scanning may demonstrate the occult neoplasm or may show a suspicious area for subsequent bronchial biopsy, brushing, or washing.

A related problem occurs in the patient who manifests a paraneoplastic syndrome thought to be caused by a bronchogenic carcinoma. Bronchogenic carcinoma can cause a variety of paraneoplastic syndromes that manifest as neuromuscular, endocrine, metabolic, skeletal, connective tissue, vascular, or hematologic disease (Table 4–3).[81, 82] In most patients, the responsible tumor will be seen on chest radiographs. The syndrome, however, can antecede the radiographic appearance of tumor by months or even years. In these instances, CT scanning may disclose the primary carcinoma or confirm a suspicious nodule or mass.

Focal Inflammatory Masses ■ Several focal or multifocal inflammatory entities produce CT findings that are highly suggestive of their causes. Lipoid pneumonia from the aspiration of instilled oily nose drops can produce chronic foci of air space consolidation. CT and HRCT scans show characteristic fat-density regions within an irregular mass or areas of consolidation, usually at the lung bases.[83] The MR findings of lipoid pneumonia have not been described but should also be characteristic for fat.

The invasive form of aspergillosis found in immunocompromised patients is characterized pathologically by angioinvasion with thrombosis and infarction of lung tissue. At an early stage, the inflammatory mass of dense consolidation and in-

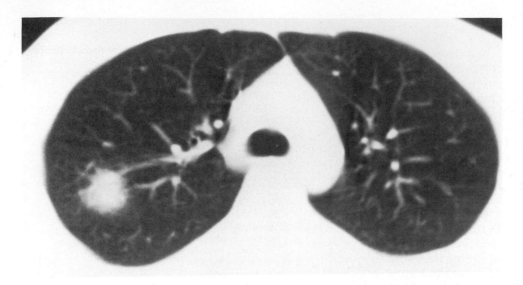

FIGURE 4–30 ■ Invasive aspergillosis in an immunocompromised renal transplant patient. Chest radiograph showed a vague right upper lobe opacity. CT scan shows an ill-defined mass in the right upper lobe. CT-guided biopsy demonstrated aspergillosis.

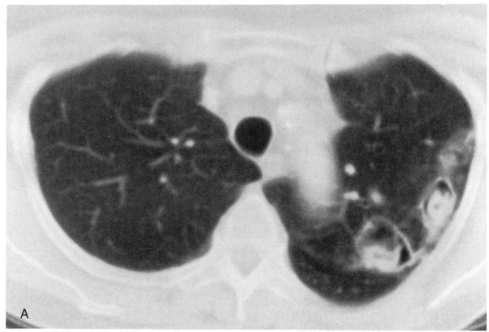

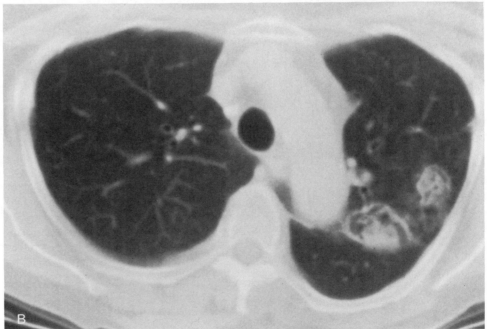

FIGURE 4–31 ■ Developing mycetomas. CT scans through the left upper lobe demonstrate fungus balls developing in preexisting cavities. The mycetomas are still ill defined, and several are attached to the wall of the cavities.

farction sometimes can show a lower density halo of fluid or blood on CT.[84] In our experience, this halo effect can be seen also in some hemorrhagic metastases and even mucus-producing adenocarcinomas. However, in the correct clinical setting, the halo sign on CT is highly suggestive of invasive aspergillosis (Fig. 4–30). At a later stage in the infection, the mass may develop a peripheral crescent of air surrounding a central sequestrum of dead lung tissue and infection.[85] Frequently as a neutropenic patient's white blood cell count returns toward normal, the crescent develops and frank cavitation ensues. With hematogenous fungal infections in immunocompromised patients, CT can show multiple nodules with cavitation, a halo, fluffy margins, or clusters of nodules.[84a] The usual fungi are *Aspergillus* or *Candida* species.

The term *aspergilloma* describes a discrete lesion consisting of a dense ball of fungal hyphae growing within a preexisting lung cavity.[86] The fungal ball, usually caused by *Aspergillus fumigatus,* can enlarge, invade the surrounding lung, and erode vessels, causing hemoptysis.[87, 88] Roberts and colleagues[89] described the CT findings in 26 patients with aspergilloma. They found that the fungus ball formed an ovoid or lobulated mass within the cavity (Fig. 4–31). When the cavity was large enough, the fungus ball could be shown to be mobile. Variations on the classic appearance included a fungus ball filling or nearly filling the cavity, fronds connecting the fungus ball to the cavity wall, air spaces and high density foci within the fungus ball, and multiple strands traversing the cavity prior to formation of a mature fungus ball. The cavity wall was frequently thick and irregular, and surrounded by compressed lung containing dilated bronchi (Fig. 4–32).

Laryngeal papillomatosis is a viral infection that spreads transbronchially to affect the trachea, bronchi, and lung parenchyma in about 5 per cent of cases. The radiographic and CT findings are characteristic of the entity. Large papillomas may cause segmental or lobar obstruction with distal lung collapse. Papillomas that are more distal produce masses or nodules that cavitate. The cavities are thick-walled, spherical, and may contain fluid. They may enlarge to several centimeters in diameter and may even be lobulated. They must be differentiated from cavitating metastases that can have similar appearances, but the clinical setting will be informative.

Huang and co-workers[89a] have suggested that CT of the lungs can assist in suggesting that multiple pulmonary nodules are septic pulmonary emboli. The CT findings in 15 patients included demonstration of a feeder vessel in 10 and subpleural wedge-shaped densities, with or without cavitation, in 11. Demonstration of a similar feeder vessel has been reported in nodular pulmonary metastases.[89b] We have not found this of diagnostic value in clinical studies of patients with either septic emboli or pulmonary metastatic disease.

Inflammatory masses that invade transpleurally into the chest wall are rare. Tuberculosis and actinomycosis are the two infections that are capable of this route of spread. In both circumstances, percutaneous aspiration of the lesion demonstrates the offending organism.

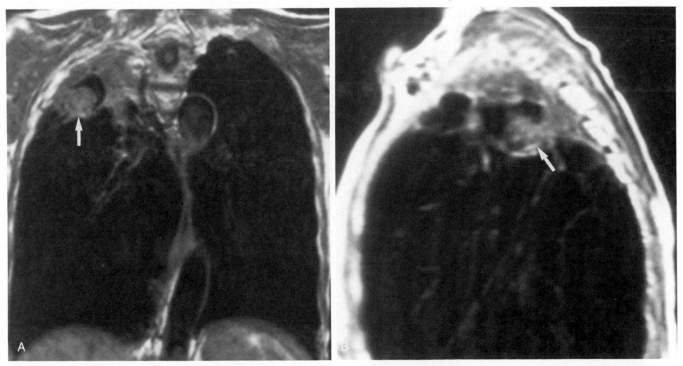

FIGURE 4–32 ■ Mycetoma with surrounding consolidation and pleural thickening. Coronal *(A)* and sagittal *(B)* MR scans show a fungus ball *(arrows)* within a cavity surrounded by inflammatory consolidation and pleural thickening. This combination is sometimes referred to as *semiinvasive aspergillosis.*

In the majority of inflammatory lung infiltrates, the CT scan will not show characteristic features. However, CT may be important in localizing the lesion for biopsy and, by demonstration of air bronchograms, may suggest the inflammatory nature of the lesions. It must be remembered, however, that bronchioloalveolar cell carcinoma, lymphoma, and some adenocarcinomas can have air bronchograms and be multifocal.

BRONCHOGENIC CARCINOMA

CT and MR of bronchogenic carcinoma have been discussed in Chapters 1 through 3. Topics that are not covered elsewhere are the determination of the extent of bronchogenic carcinoma, CT-guided aspiration biopsy of thoracic masses, radiotherapy planning, radiation lung damage, and the CT appearance of the thorax after pneumonectomy. The following discussion will be limited to non–small-cell carcinoma of the lung.

Extent and Staging ■ The literature on CT and MR imaging of bronchogenic carcinoma primarily discusses the detection of hilar and mediastinal adenopathy and the direct invasion of the mediastinum by bronchogenic carcinoma. These aspects of the staging of bronchogenic carcinoma have been covered in previous chapters. Multiple findings on CT and MR of the thorax and abdomen can assist in determining the extent of bronchogenic carcinoma and profoundly affect management of the patient. These findings may unequivocally demonstrate that the patient is not a candidate for resection, or alternatively, they can direct biopsy procedures to areas of metastatic spread of the neoplasm.

The most recent classification of the stages of bronchogenic carcinoma has taken into account newer surgical techniques that allow more aggressive local resection of the tumor (see also Chapter 2).[90] In clinical practice, the surgical approach to lung cancer and the criteria for resectability vary in different medical institutions. Therefore the significance of CT findings must always be interpreted in collaboration with the patient's surgeon.

Contralateral Tumor ■ In virtually all situations, the presence of metastasis to the contralateral lung is indicative of advanced disease not treatable by surgery. CT or MR may show contralateral tumor not seen on chest radiographs (Fig. 4–33). A mass or nodule in the contralateral lung invariably requires biopsy for histologic confirmation of metastasis. Occasionally synchronous primary bronchogenic carcinomas occur and can be resected. This is always a difficult clinical problem and requires careful discussion among all of the patient's physicians.

Spine or Sternum Destruction ■ Tumor destruction of the sternum or spine indicates advanced disease and nonresectability. The frequency with which CT scans first detect this finding is difficult to establish. We have seen cases of spine (Fig. 4–34) and sternum destruction that had not been appreciated before the CT or MR scan was obtained. MR may be more accurate than CT in demonstrating bony invasion or metastasis to the spine or sternum (Fig. 4–35).

Chest Wall Invasion ■ Focal tumor invasion of the chest wall is stage IIIA and is considered resectable.[90–92] Many surgeons undertake a block resection of the chest wall when the tumor has crossed the pleura without diffuse seeding of the pleural surface, as indicated by a malignant pleural effusion. We, however, have seen several instances in which carcinoma against the chest wall produced edema in the adjacent soft tissues that could have been misinterpreted as chest wall invasion. Thus CT scans of chest wall invasion must be interpreted with caution.

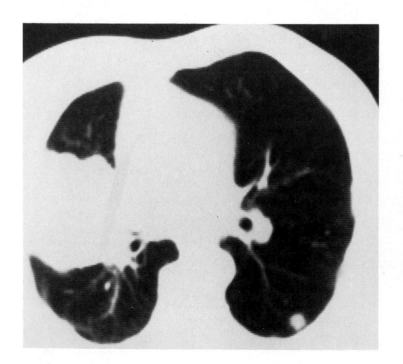

FIGURE 4–33 ■ Bronchogenic carcinoma with contralateral metastasis. CT scan demonstrates a large right lung mass and a small contralateral nodule not apparent on chest radiographs. CT-guided aspiration biopsy of this nodule revealed that it was a metastasis.

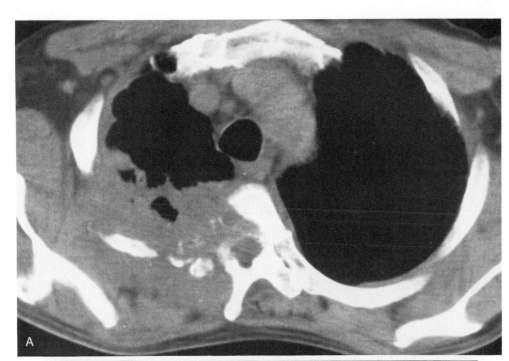

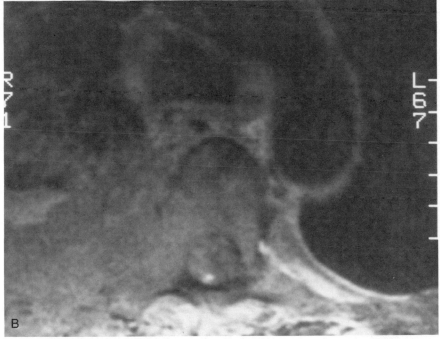

FIGURE 4–34 ■ Nonresectable bronchogenic carcinoma invading the spine and chest wall. *A,* CT scan shows a right upper lobe carcinoma with destruction of the adjacent rib, vertebral body, pedicle, and transverse process. Asymmetric thickening of the soft tissues of the chest wall is present. *B,* MR scan using a surface coil shows the tumor mass invading the spinal canal.

Glazer and colleagues,[93] Ekholm and co-workers,[94] and Rendina and co-investigators,[95] in small series, all showed a low predictive value for CT in detecting chest wall invasion by bronchogenic carcinoma. This was confirmed by Pennes and colleagues[96] in a study of 33 patients with peripheral tumors adjacent to the chest wall. They found an accuracy of only 39 per cent, using as their criteria pleural thickening, increased density of extrapleural fat, asymmetry of extrapleural soft tissues, rib destruction, and apparent mass invading the chest. MR for this purpose has not been studied in detail. High-resolution T2-weighted MR with surface coils can produce detailed images with excellent contrast between tumor and extrapleural fat. It is likely that MR can detect transpleural extension of tumor more accurately than CT. Haggar and co-workers[97] studied 19 patients with potential chest wall invasion. In all 10 cases with invasion, abnormalities were found on MR. Indicative of abnormality on T2-weighted images were extension of high signal intensity into the chest wall from the tumor; increased signal intensity within the chest wall, with thickening of the muscles; and diffusely increased signal intensity in the chest wall without morphologic distortion. It appears likely that MR with surface coils or images tangent to the contact

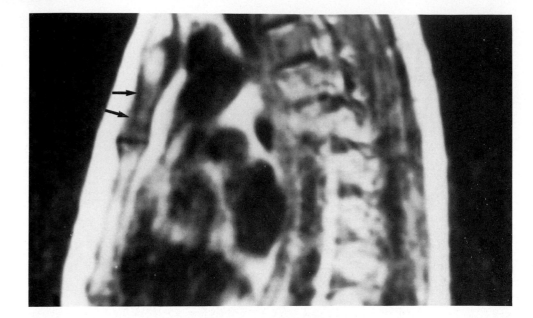

FIGURE 4–35 ■ Bronchogenic carcinoma with metastasis to the manubrium. Chest radiographs and CT scans had shown an apparently resectable left upper lobe bronchogenic carcinoma. Sagittal MR scan shows replacement of the normal high signal intensity by low signal intensity within the marrow cavity of the manubrium (arrows). A marrow aspirate from this site revealed malignant cells.

between tumor and chest wall should replace CT for pleural-based bronchogenic carcinoma. Although the prognosis, perioperative mortality, and surgical approaches are different, focal chest wall invasion does not alter resectability in many instances.

Superior sulcus tumors are a subset of bronchogenic carcinomas with a high propensity for invasion into the soft tissues over the cupola of the lung (see Chapter 5). They may invade the brachial plexus, producing shoulder, back, or arm pain with or without Horner's syndrome from involvement of the stellate ganglion. Improved survival can be achieved with a combination of preoperative radiation and block resection of the tumor, upper lobe, and involved chest wall. Precise determination of the local extent of tumor and exclusion of tumor invasion of mediastinal structures, vessels, and the spine, as

well as exclusion of distant metastases, must be undertaken before this aggressive approach can be advocated. Webb and colleagues[98] and O'Connell and co-workers[99] have evaluated CT for this purpose. CT was equal to or more accurate than conventional radiographs for detecting the mass, vertebral body invasion, rib destruction, and encasement of the subclavian artery.

Reports of the value of MR for superior sulcus tumors have been limited.[97, 100] Haggar and colleagues[97] found that in two cases multiplanar MR clearly demonstrated the extrapleural extent of tumor. In our experience sagittal MR images using a surface coil can precisely localize the relationship of the tumor to the subclavian vessels, brachial plexus, and vertebral bodies (Fig. 4–36).

Adrenal and Liver Metastases ■ The incidence of

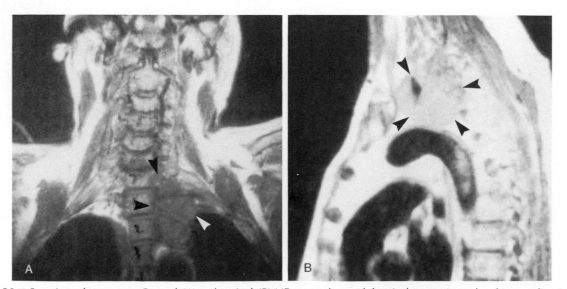

FIGURE 4–36 ■ Superior sulcus tumor. Coronal (A) and sagittal (B) MR scans show a left apical tumor (arrowheads) extending into the soft tissues and surrounding the lower brachial plexus. On the sagittal image, the tumor surrounds the subclavian artery.

silent liver and adrenal metastases from bronchogenic carcinoma has been studied by several investigators.[101–103] The published incidence varies with the cell type of the carcinoma. Silent liver metastasis occurs in 10 to 40 per cent of patients, and adrenal metastasis may be found in 15 to 40 per cent. In our experience and that of others 10 to 15 per cent is a more realistic figure for these lesions at the time of evaluation of patients for bronchogenic carcinoma.[104, 105] The CT examination of a patient with bronchogenic carcinoma should always include the upper abdomen. The examination must be interpreted with caution. For instance, Oliver and co-workers[105] reported that in two thirds of patients with non–small-cell carcinoma, an adrenal mass was a benign adenoma and not a metastasis. They therefore advocated that all such masses should be biopsied (Fig. 4–37). In their series, neither size nor the

CT characteristics of the adrenal mass were helpful in separating metastasis from adenoma. Berland and co-workers[106] and Hussain and colleagues[107] on the other hand have listed the CT findings that help differentiate between a benign and malignant adrenal mass with some success. Several studies have used T2-weighted MR of the adrenal, trying to differentiate between benign adenomas and malignant lesions.[108–110] Unfortunately MR lacks specificity, and the signal intensity ratios of mass to liver or fat are limited and even less apparent with high field strength (1.5 T) magnets.[111]

Pleural Effusion ■ CT and MR are both highly sensitive in demonstrating pleural effusions. The clinical significance of pleural fluid in the presence of a bronchogenic carcinoma depends on the contents of the fluid and not just its presence.[112, 113] Malignant cells in the fluid indicate nonresectability in more

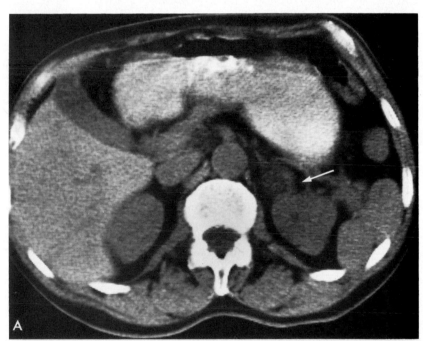
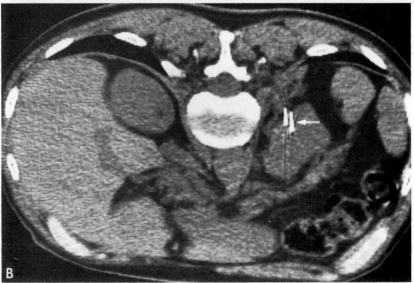

FIGURE 4–37 ■ Silent adrenal metastasis. *A,* CT scan through the upper abdomen in a patient with bronchogenic carcinoma shows a left adrenal mass *(arrow). B,* CT scan taken in the prone position demonstrates the tips of two needles *(arrow)* for biopsy of the metastasis.

than 90 per cent of patients. The finding of unsuspected pleural effusion is thus extremely important but does not by itself indicate that the tumor is not resectable. The MR characteristics of the fluid cannot differentiate between benign and malignant effusions,[114] and pleurocentesis is indicated in most circumstances. Occasionally CT and MR show tumor nodules studding the pleura. MR is probably more sensitive for this purpose, but the circumstances in which this is clinically useful are limited.

CT-Guided Aspiration Biopsy ■ Percutaneous, fine-needle aspiration has become widely accepted for the biopsy of focal intrathoracic lesions.[115–117] (See also Chapter 8.) The key to a successful biopsy is precise needle placement within the nodule or mass. In most situations, exact placement of the needle tip can be achieved by using fluoroscopic guidance, preferably in two planes. CT scanning can be used initially to locate a pulmonary mass that subsequently undergoes biopsy using fluoroscopically guided needle placement.[118, 119] The patient should be scanned in the position that will subsequently be used for the biopsy. The depth and distance from surface landmarks of the mass can be precisely measured with the CT monitor. This technique works well when the lung lesion is large enough to be demonstrated fluoroscopically in at least one plane. The same technique can also be used for hilar and mediastinal masses.

Certain thoracic masses should undergo biopsy using CT rather than fluoroscopic guidance.[120–123] These are lung lesions that cannot be precisely located fluoroscopically, necrotic or cavitary lesions in which the wall of the mass must be sampled (Fig. 4–38), or small hilar and central mediastinal masses. Lung nodules as small as 0.8 cm can be successfully aspirated with this technique. The results of CT-guided aspiration biopsy are equal in accuracy to those of fluoroscopically guided biopsy. If a coaxial system[124] is used, the procedure takes 20 to 40 minutes, and the incidence of pneumothoraces is small and equal to that in fluoroscopy. Pinstein and colleagues[121] have shown that for suspected necrotic masses, administration of intravascular contrast material can help define the solid enhancing portion of the mass that should be biopsied. We now perform most of our lung biopsies using CT guidance.

Radiotherapy Planning ■ The goal of radiotherapy is to minimize irradiation of normal tissues while adequately treating the tumor. Therapy planning normally uses all available information from the physical examination, radiography, bronchoscopy, and surgery. Radiotherapy planning for bronchogenic carcinoma relies heavily on radiographic techniques to determine tumor extent.

The superimposition of the thoracic skeleton, cardiovascular structures, and occasionally pleural effusion can make the radiographic assessment of tumor extent difficult. The transverse orientation of CT scans eliminates many of the problems of superimposition. In 40 to 75 per cent of patients, CT scans

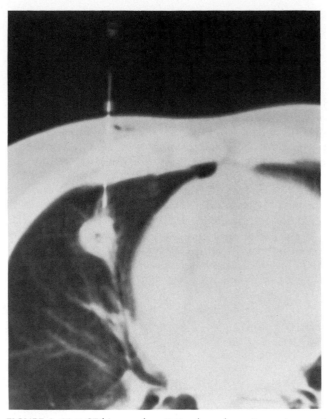

FIGURE 4–38 ■ CT biopsy of cavitating bronchogenic carcinoma. A thin-walled 19-gauge Greene outer needle of a coaxial biopsy system is positioned with its tip at the edge of the middle lobe mass. A small pneumothorax is seen anteriorly. Cavitation is present in the center of the mass.

more clearly delineate tumor extent than do chest radiographs.[125, 126] This information leads to either a decrease or an increase in treatment volume.

In the majority of patients in whom treatment volume is altered, CT scans show tumor that was unsuspected from conventional radiographic studies, resulting in a larger volume of irradiation to include all the tumor.[127, 128] In other patients, CT scans may reveal that a smaller volume of irradiation is sufficient to cover the tumor. When the decision is to decrease treatment volume, normal tissue is spared unnecessary irradiation. In some patients, CT scans show metastases in the mediastinum, adrenals, and liver that were unsuspected from chest radiographs. In these instances, the stage of the tumor is altered, and the entire therapy protocol may be changed. In many institutions, the data from CT are incorporated directly into the computers that determine the portals for radiotherapy. In these situations, the accuracy of defining the target volume can approach the precision with which modern radiotherapy machines can deliver irradiation.

Radiation Injury ■ The severity of radiation injury to the lung is determined primarily by the total radiation dose, fractionation, and the length of time the radiation is given. Chest radiographs are often used to follow the course of radiation lung injury. Radiographic changes are unusual with 30 gray or less. After a dose of 40 gray in 4 weeks, some patients demonstrate lung damage, and after 50 gray in 5 weeks, about 50 per cent of patients show lung damage.[129, 130] Almost all patients receiving 60 gray exhibit radiographic abnormalities. Symptoms of lung injury are often present when only a third to half of a lung is radiated.

Ionizing radiation damages cells capable of proliferation by inducing mitotic death. The morphologic changes in lung tissue following radiation occur on a continuum but can be divided into three phases that occur within the first 6 to 9 months after radiation.[131] An *exudative phase* is seen during the first 30 days; a *pneumonic phase* lasts through the second and third months; and a *reparative phase* occurs between the third and sixth to ninth months.[132, 133]

In the exudative phase, endothelial and epithelial damage appears with interstitial edema, alveolar proteinosis, and hyaline membranes. In the pneumonic phase, alveolar type II cells and macrophages fill the air spaces.[134] Capillary damage is extensive, and collagen deposition begins. In the reparative phase, many cells proliferate, with profound distortion of lung architecture. Mast cells, among others, predominate, and collagen production continues, leading to fibrosis. At 6 to 9 months and beyond, fibrosis of the alveolar walls develops, markedly reducing the number, size, and volume of the alveoli. The number of patent capillaries and small vessels is also greatly reduced.

The radiographic appearance of radiation lung injury conforms to the pathologic abnormalities.[135, 136] The first abnormalities usually appear 6 to 12 weeks after treatment is completed. The first manifestation is an ill-defined increase in density in the radiated field that obscures the pulmonary vessels (Fig. 4–39). This may progress to pulmonary consolidation or to a nodular or acinar pattern (Fig. 4–40). The pneumonic changes progress to dense linear streaks radiating from the area of involvement. Marked scarring causes volume loss in the radiated volume of the lung. The permanent changes of fibrosis take 6 to 24 months to evolve.

CT may be used to detect recurrent tumor follow-

ing radiation therapy, and it is therefore important to understand the CT features of radiation lung damage.[137–139] Libshitz and Shuman[137] have described the CT patterns of abnormality in the lung following completion of radiotherapy. The earliest changes are seen at 3 to 4 weeks, and these form a continuum of abnormalities similar to those identified radiographically. A homogeneous, slight increase in CT density, probably representing minimal radiation pneumonitis, is the least severe abnormality. The most common pattern is patchy air space consolidation that can be seen up to 15 months after radiation. Discrete, dense consolidation, often containing bronchiectasis, corresponds to the fibrotic phase of radiation lung damage. It invariably demonstrates a spiculated border, frequently conforming to the shape of the radiated field (Fig. 4–41). In no instance does the abnormality extend beyond the field of radiation. The early radiation abnormalities are found more frequently and earlier on CT than on chest radiographs and may be seen by 25 days following completion of treatment.[138]

In the fibrotic stage, involved lung characteristically shows shrinkage. We have found that a nearly straight edge to the region of increased density and dilated bronchi is typical of radiation fibrosis.

Following radiation to the lung or mediastinum, differentiation of radiation-induced fibrosis and recurrent tumor may be a difficult clinical problem. In patients with bronchogenic carcinoma, the available therapy may be limited, and clinical judgment is required as to whether to pursue the issue. In many cases, recurrent tumor is suspected from an enlarging mass on chest radiographs. Localization of the sites suspicious for tumor recurrence are important for biopsy prior to initiating additional treatment. CT is poor for detecting tumor in this circumstance. A discrete mass, abnormality beyond the confines of the radiation field, and cavitation are suggestive of recurrent tumor. MR has shown some promise in discriminating between recurrent tumor and radiation fibrosis. Glazer and colleagues[140] studied 12 patients with suspected recurrent tumor. Radiation fibrosis was low in signal intensity on both T1- and

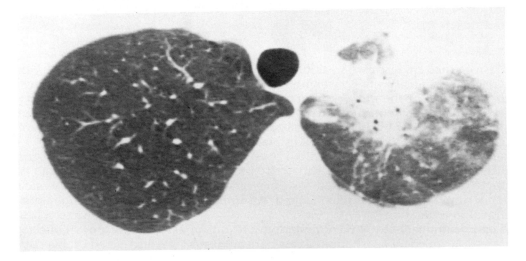

FIGURE 4–39 ■ Acute radiation pneumonitis in a 32-year-old female six weeks after 6000 rad superclavicular radiation for metastatic breast carcinoma. CT scan demonstrates patchy consolidation toward the periphery and dense consolidation with air bronchograms in the center of the left lung apex. The findings are not specific for radiation damage, but their site, limited to the field of radiation, and the clinical picture are highly suggestive of the diagnosis.

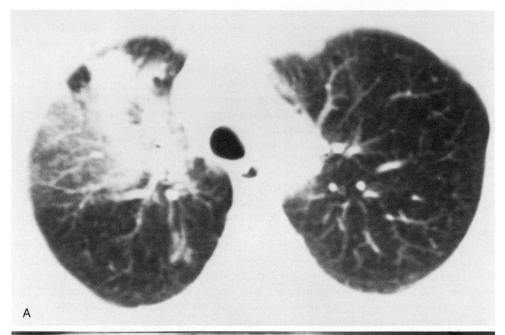

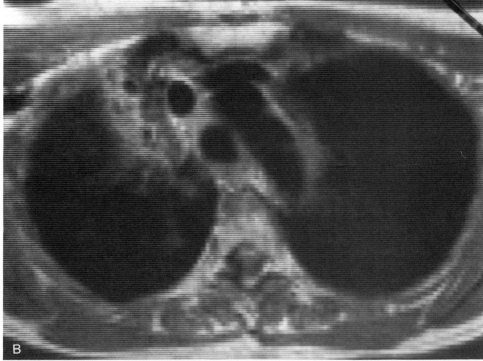

FIGURE 4–40 ■ Subacute radiation pneumonitis, following 5000 rad and chemotherapy for bronchogenic carcinoma. *A,* CT scan demonstrates right subapical dense consolidation. The consolidation conformed to the radiation port. *B,* T1-weighted spin-echo image demonstrates more inhomogeneity than the CT scan. The low-intensity areas represent residual tumor in the right upper mediastinum.

T2-weighted images, whereas tumor showed an increase in intensity on T2 weighting. This approach is not useful in the months prior to development of radiation fibrosis or in patients with infection or pneumonia. In our experience, detection of recurrent tumor in the hemithorax following pneumonectomy may be similarly facilitated with T2-weighted spin-echo images. MR spectroscopy may also prove useful for following patients treated for lung cancer.[141, 142] This approach is experimental and requires additional investigation.

Postpneumonectomy ■ Pneumonectomy results in a large, air-filled space bounded by parietal pleura.

The evacuated hemithorax contains gas and a variable amount of fluid, producing a single, large air-fluid level on chest radiographs. Unless complications occur, the pleural space progressively fills with fluid.[143, 144] Radiographs show filling of the pleural space with fluid in 3 to 24 weeks after pneumonectomy, usually associated with a gradual decrease in the volume of the hemithorax. The mediastinum shifts toward the side of pneumonectomy, and the ipsilateral hemidiaphragm becomes elevated.

Biondette and colleagues,[145] using CT to investigate the postpneumonectomy hemithorax in 22 patients, discovered some interesting and previously un-

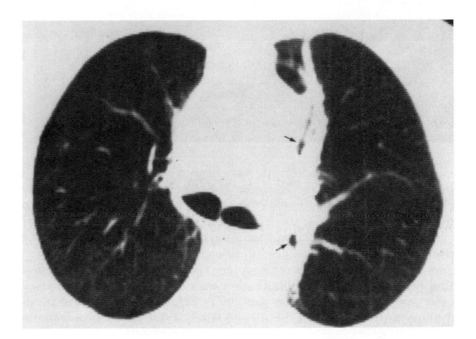

FIGURE 4–41 ■ Chronic radiation lung injury. CT scan five months after 6500 rad to the left medial hemithorax and mediastinum shows a nearly straight edge to the area of irradiation. Dilated bronchi *(arrows)* are visible within the radiation fibrosis.

documented findings. It had been assumed that the fluid in the postpneumonectomy space is resorbed and replaced by connective tissue. In 13 of the 22 patients, fluid was evident on CT scans even years after surgery (Fig. 4–42). They found that generally the postpneumonectomy space was obliterated and the fluid was absent when marked mediastinal shift had occurred. Also, after a right pneumonectomy, the mediastinum rotated to the right; after a left pneumonectomy, the mediastinum tended to shift to the left without rotating.

Bronchopleural fistula and empyema can occur as complications of resectional surgery in patients with bronchogenic neoplasms. Empyema is a dreaded complication with a mortality rate of 16 to 28 per cent.[146, 147] Vigorous therapy with drainage of the pleural space is usually necessary. An increase in the volume of the fluid-filled hemithorax can be detected from chest radiographs. CT can help delineate localized empyema following pulmonary resection. The encapsulated fluid can be readily distinguished from free-flowing pleural fluid and from the higher density pleural peel. CT, after infusion of intravenous contrast material and obtained with the patient in prone and decubitus positions, may help demonstrate an encapsulated fluid collection. Encapsulated fluid will be low in density and not move with change in position. An additional finding on CT is that as the

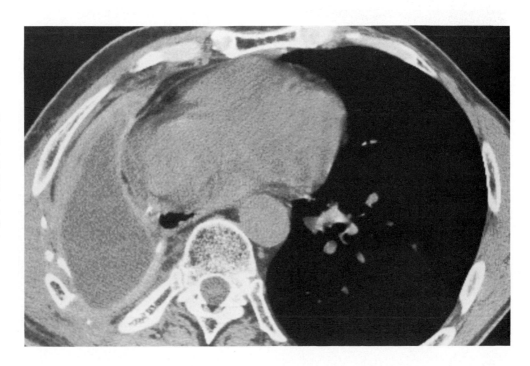

FIGURE 4–42 ■ Appearance eight years after right pneumonectomy. CT scan demonstrates reduction in size of the right hemithorax. Pleural calcification is visible within the parietal pleura. The contents of the right hemithorax are homogeneous and of low uniform density, probably representing fluid and fibrofatty tissue. The heart and mediastinum are displaced and rotated to the left.

empyema enlarges the concave interface of the postpneumonectomy space with the mediastinum can become convex.[148] An increase in the amount of air within the evacuated hemithorax also may indicate the development of a bronchopleural fistula.

Recurrence of bronchogenic carcinoma after pulmonary resection is common. Between 35 and 70 per cent of patients who die within 1 month after pulmonary resection are found to have had either metastatic spread or persistence of tumor within the thorax.[149, 150] At 1 year after resection, the incidence of tumor rises to 85 per cent. Recurrence of tumor in the ipsilateral hemithorax after pneumonectomy is difficult to detect from radiographs. A shift of the mediastinum toward the contralateral side may indicate a large tumor mass on the side of the pneumonectomy. CT scans can demonstrate recurrent tumor at an earlier stage than can chest radiographs.[151] Glazer and colleagues[151] found that enlarged mediastinal lymph nodes and a tumor mass were the two features indicating tumor recurrence. The tumor mass is denser than the fluid or fibroadipose tissue normally present after pneumonectomy.

In our limited experience, MR is superior to CT for detecting recurrent tumor following pneumonectomy. On T1-weighted spin-echo images, the tumor may be lower in intensity than the fluid-filled space. With invasion of the chest wall, the tumor is usually more intense than the chest wall muscles on T2-weighted images. Heelan and colleagues[152] have presented their experience with MR following pneumonectomy, and MR was equal to or better than CT for detecting tumor recurrence in five patients. In most circumstances, recurrent tumor following pneumonectomy is treated with radiation therapy. Early detection and precise localization are of major clinical importance in these patients (Fig. 4–43).

LUNG ABSCESS

An abscess is a focus of inflammation associated with tissue necrosis. In the lung, an abscess is usually caused by pyogenic bacteria and has a rounded configuration with organization and compression of lung tissues surrounding the inflammatory collection. An air-fluid level may develop within the necrotic center of the abscess and usually implies connection with an airway. An air-fluid level may also occasionally occur after percutaneous aspiration or bronchoscopy, with the creation of a communication between the abscess and a bronchus.

A lung abscess can be difficult to detect within an area of pneumonia on chest radiographs and non–contrast-enhanced CT scans when there is no air-fluid level. The presence of foci of decreased CT density within a rounded or oval masslike area is typical.[153] Intravascular contrast material may help to identify an abscess by showing enhancement of the abscess wall and may better demonstrate the low-attenuation necrotic sites.[154] Identification of an air-fluid level or central lucency is strongly suggestive of abscess formation in the appropriate clinical setting. A necrotic carcinoma also can show these features.

In general, an abscess has a thick cavity wall and an irregular inner margin. Air-containing abscesses can show residual strands of lung tissue traversing the abscess cavity. Infected aspiration, necrotizing pneumonia, bronchial obstruction with infection, and infected cavitated pulmonary infarction are all causes of a thick-walled abscess cavity with an irregular inner lining. An abscess can rupture into the pleural space, resulting in empyema. Chronic infection, such as tuberculosis or other granulomatous infections, causes areas of fibrosis and parenchymal distortion, as well as cavities with thick walls (Fig. 4–44).[154a] Air-

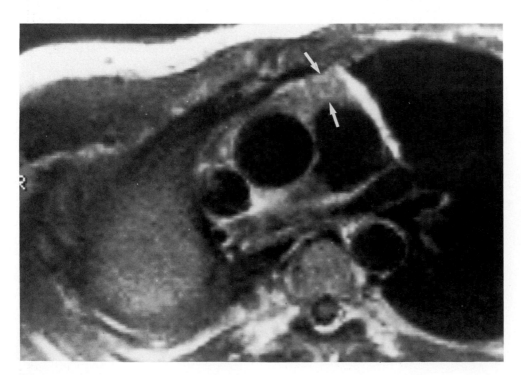

FIGURE 4–43 ■ Recurrent bronchogenic carcinoma following pneumonectomy. MR image reveals a homogeneous appearance to the right hemithorax after pneumonectomy. Replacement of normal high-intensity mediastinal fat by low-intensity tissue within the mediastinum *(arrows)* is strongly suspicious for tumor recurrence.

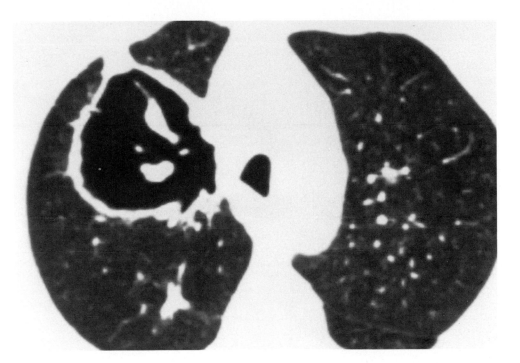

FIGURE 4–44 ■ Lung cavity following radiation for bronchogenic carcinoma. CT scan demonstrates an irregular thick-walled cavity containing the residue of pulmonary vessels and bronchi. The patient received 6500 rad to the right upper lobe for a large bronchogenic carcinoma. The tumor has undergone necrosis and liquefaction with cavitation.

fluid levels in preexisting bullae with or without infection usually have a smooth inner margin, although they may be surrounded by consolidated lung.

Many pulmonary abscesses resolve on medical therapy without surgical intervention. Invasive management may be indicated for large abscesses unresponsive to medical treatment or for an associated empyema. Percutaneous catheter drainage provides a less invasive alternative to thoracotomy for treatment of lung abscesses.[155, 156] CT is frequently used to localize the abscess and guide insertion of the drainage catheter. This form of treatment is limited to those abscesses contiguous with the pleural surface.

BULLAE AND CYSTS

The definitions of the different forms of abnormal air-containing spaces within the lung are imprecise, and their etiologies, locations, and appearances have given rise to different nomenclatures. When it is unclear precisely what the CT or radiographic appearance represents, it is usually appropriate to call the lesion a *thin-walled cystic space*. These are characterized by pencil-line-thin walls and an absence of internal structure.

A bulla is an abnormal respiratory space larger than 1 to 2 cm in diameter within the lung parenchyma and resulting from tissue destruction.[157] Bullae may be isolated or a component of emphysema or advanced fibrotic lung disease. The walls of a bulla are usually less than 1 mm in thickness and are frequently invisible on chest radiographs, appearing as areas of hyperlucency. On CT or HRCT, the walls of bullae are invariably seen, allowing them to be distinguished from focal emphysema.

Large bullae can occur as an isolated abnormality in normal lung parenchyma, usually in the upper lobes. Young men, usually smokers, are most commonly affected. In severe emphysema, confluent areas of parenchymal destruction form bullae in which the thin walls are composed of surrounding compressed lung; hence the term *bullous emphysema*. Severe symptoms of airway obstruction are common when large bullae are present.[158] Airway obstruction can be from loss of lung elastic recoil associated with the bullae themselves or can result from the concomitant emphysema.[159] Resection of large bullae may be considered to improve pulmonary function.[160, 161] The best results of bullectomy occur when the remainder of the lungs is near normal. When diffuse emphysema is also present, improvement may be marginal and temporary. Specialized function studies can aid in determining the component of functional impairment caused by the bullae. Chest radiographs, radionuclide ventilation and perfusion studies, and pulmonary angiograms have also been used to detect the extent of the bullae and concomitant emphysema.[162] CT and HRCT are more sensitive than these techniques for evaluating the extent of bullae and detecting associated emphysema. CT scans can also demonstrate the size and exact location of localized bullae and can assist in the planning of resection (Fig. 4–45).[163, 164] The presence of diffuse bullae or emphysema should discourage attempts at surgical resection.

Blebs are focal air-containing spaces within the layers of the visceral pleura. They are not associated with lung destruction and are frequently isolated findings on CT. Blebs are commonly found at autopsy on the surface of the lungs, usually over the apices and anterior upper surfaces. The rupture of blebs is thought to be the cause of spontaneous pneumothorax in young adults.[157]

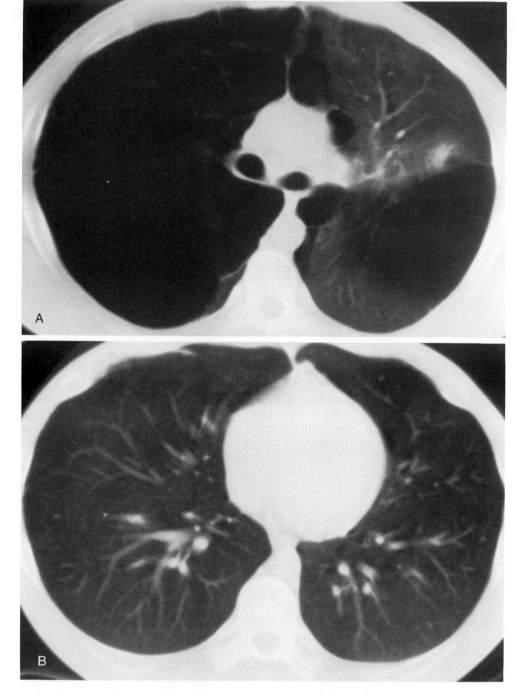

FIGURE 4–45 ■ Bullous lung disease in a patient with Ehlers-Danlos syndrome. *A,* CT scan through the midlung fields demonstrates massive bilateral upper lobe bullae. A few residual strands of tissue are visible on the right. The compressed left upper and lower lobes are seen. *B,* CT scan 6 cm caudal to *A* shows essentially normal lower lobe morphology.

Blebs appear thin-walled on CT and are always contiguous with the pleural surface. They do not become infected, nor do they contain fluid. The appearance of blebs may be similar to that of paraseptal emphysema, which is also peripheral but is usually multiple and occurs as a subpleural row of thin-walled spaces.

Lung cysts may be congenital or acquired and either single or multiple. Distinguishing lung cysts from thin-walled cavities is not always possible by radiographic or CT appearance. Cavitated pulmonary emboli and some infections, particularly coccidioidomycosis, are classic causes of thin-walled cavities.

Thick-walled cavities may form in granulomatous and nongranulomatous lung infections and in pulmonary neoplasms, most notably squamous cell carcinoma.

Cystic spaces associated with fibrotic lung disease are common in tuberculosis, sarcoidosis, and interstitial fibrosis. In idiopathic pulmonary fibrosis, the cystic spaces are peripheral, approximately 1 cm in size, and have a honeycomb appearance. In sarcoidosis, the cystic spaces are frequently in the mid- and upper lung zones and vary in size from 1 to 4 cm. The cystic spaces associated with tuberculosis and sarcoidosis may subsequently be colonized by aspergillus or other fungi, forming fungus balls within the cavities with a characteristic radiographic and CT appearance.

Bronchial (bronchogenic) cysts are derived from an abnormal bud from the developing bronchial tree. Most are situated within 5 cm of the tracheal carina, although a minority are entirely within the lung parenchyma.[165] Rarely they may be within the pleura or may even be infradiaphragmatic.[166] Those within the pulmonary parenchyma have a predilection for the inner third of the lungs and the lower lobes. They are rounded or oval, and smooth; on CT they have a uniform density (Fig. 4–46). Infected cysts, however, can be ill defined and may communicate with an adjacent airway, demonstrating an air-fluid level. After infection and excavation, the cyst may remain as a thin-walled cystic space.

Congenital cystic adenomatoid malformation consists of anomalous fetal development of the terminal airway structures. The resultant malformation is composed of a mass of cysts and bronchiolar elements.[167] Most cases involve a large portion of the lung and present at, or shortly after, birth. When localized, the malformation may present in childhood or adult life.[168] The CT appearances are single or multicystic masses with thick walls.[169, 169a] Differentiation from a pulmonary sequestration may not be possible from the CT appearances.

VASCULAR LESIONS

Rapid, sequential CT scanning after an intravenous bolus injection of contrast material or MR imaging frequently can precisely diagnose various vascular lesions of the lung. Normal mediastinal and hilar blood vessels show a predictable increase in CT density following the bolus of contrast material. Similarly, large abnormal vessels in the lung demonstrate enhancement by intravenous contrast material.[170]

Spin-echo MR imaging offers superb inherent contrast between vessels and adjacent soft tissue structures.[17, 18] Several variables determine the degree to which moving spins increase or decrease MR signal intensity. These variables include flow velocity, plane of section, TR, TE, flip angle, interslice gap, and location of the slice within a multislice series (Table 4–4).[171] In a spin-echo sequence, spins must be exposed to both a 90° (nutation) and a 180° (refocusing) radio frequency (RF) pulse. Spins that leave an image

TABLE 4–4 ■ Factors Influencing Intravascular MR Signal

Technical
    Pulse sequence
    Sectional position in multisection sequence
    Spin-echo type
    Imaging gradient
    Cardiac synchronization
Biologic
    Direction of flow
    Velocity of flow
    Acceleration/deceleration
    Velocity profile

volume before being refocused or that enter the image volume after the nutation pulse do not generate a signal. For example, when an 8-mm-thick section is obtained with a TR of 80 ms, all spins initially within the imaged volume perpendicular to the plane of section moving at a velocity greater than 10 cm/sec leave the slice during one imaging sequence. Thus no signal is detected from blood flowing at velocities greater than 10 to 15 cm/sec. Blood flow in large vessels is usually greater than 10 cm/sec, and therefore no signal is obtained. Turbulence also causes loss of signal in flowing blood. However, signal may be obtained from slow-flowing blood. As flow decreases, intensity of blood on T2-weighted sequences increases, reflecting the relatively short longitudinal relaxation time (T1) and long transverse relaxation time (T2) of unclotted blood. At velocities less than 3 cm/sec, blood may demonstrate "paradoxical enhancement," having an MR signal greater than stationary blood. This enhancement occurs when previously nonmagnetized protons enter the imaging field. These unsaturated protons can be more fully magnetized than protons remaining in the sites after a previous sequence. Therefore strong signal can be elicited when slow-flowing blood first enters a slice. This is also known as the *entry enhancement phenomenon* (Fig. 4–47).

The phenomenon of *even-echo rephasing* or *odd-echo dephasing* also affects the signal intensity within vessels when laminar flow of constant velocity is imaged in a linear gradient. Even-echo rephasing results in higher signal intensity for even echoes compared with interspersed odd echoes. It is caused by a loss of phase coherence in moving spins at the time of the first echo, which are then rephased by the second 180° RF pulse. This phenomenon can be used to distinguish vessels containing slowly flowing blood from vessels containing thrombus. A third phenomenon that increases signal intensity from flowing blood is diastolic pseudogating. Under certain circumstances, high signal intensity may be obtained from arteries. When MR acquisition is gated to the ECG, higher signal is obtained within arteries during diastole than during systole. Occasionally, with certain heart rates and TRs, the cardiac rate and MR repetition cycles can become synchronized without intentional cardiac gating. In this situation, images obtained during diastole demonstrate higher signal intensity, an effect called *diastolic pseudogating*. Thus in spin-echo sequences, high velocity, turbulence, and odd-echo dephasing lead to signal loss or "flow void" phenomena. Flow-related enhancement, even-echo rephasing, and diastolic pseudogating cause increased signal intensity within vessels.

These features can be useful in the chest to distinguish vessels from other structures, to identify vascular malformations, and to distinguish slow-flowing blood within vessels from intravascular thrombus.

Limited flip angle (LFA), gradient-recalled echo techniques such as fast, low-angle shot (FLASH); gradient-recalled acquisition in the steady state

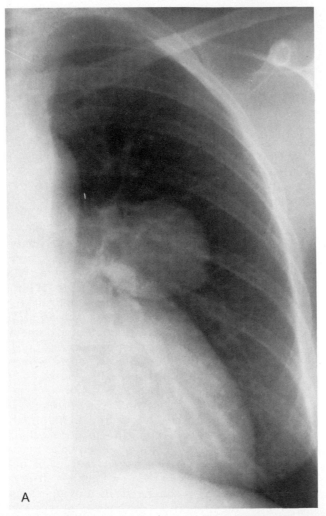

A

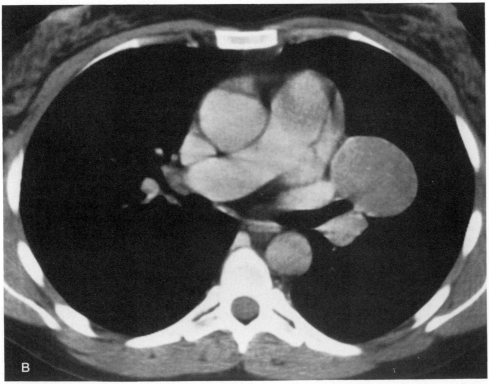

B

FIGURE 4–46 ■ Pulmonary sarcoma simulating a bronchogenic cyst in a 26-year-old female six years after renal transplantation. *A,* Chest radiograph demonstrates a well-defined, round, 5-cm mass in the left hilum. *B,* CT scan shows the mass is homogeneous and contacts the left upper lobe bronchus.

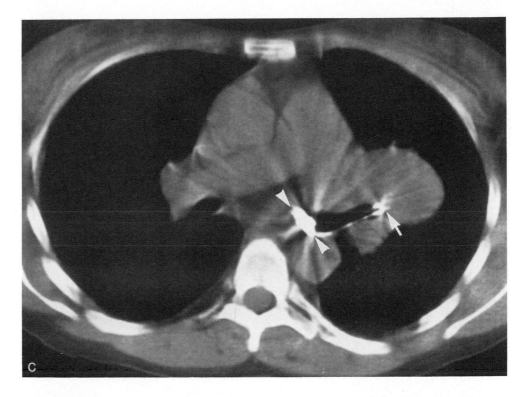

FIGURE 4–46 *Continued* ■ *C*, CT-guided transbronchial biopsy. The end of the bronchoscope *(arrowheads)* is visible. The tip of the Wang transbronchial biopsy needle *(arrow)* is shown entering the mass. Cytologic examination demonstrated malignant cells. The diagnosis of pulmonary sarcoma was made from the pneumonectomy specimen.

(GRASS); and fast imaging with steady-state precession (FISP) substitute an adjustable flip angle for the 90° RF pulse of spin-echo imaging. For TRs less than the tissue T1, the signal is maximized by a smaller flip angle as TR is decreased. Most LFA techniques do not employ a 180° RF pulse to refocus the protons but reverse the gradients to produce a signal.[172] This permits very short TEs (on the order of 10 ms), which also improves the signal-to-noise ratio.

For a given TR, adjusting either the flip angle or the TE changes the contrast. When the selected TR is shorter than the T2 of the tissue, the tissue T2 relaxation time also affects the signal (known as *steady-state free precession*).

Essentially, two contrast situations exist. In the first, the TRs are sufficiently long that T2 relaxation times may be ignored. Thus only T1 and spin density are important. The second situation occurs when the TRs approach the tissue T2 relaxation times. Then tissue contrast is dependent on T2, as well as on T1 and spin density. FLASH, GRASS, and FISP have different contrasts for a given TR, TE, and flip angle.

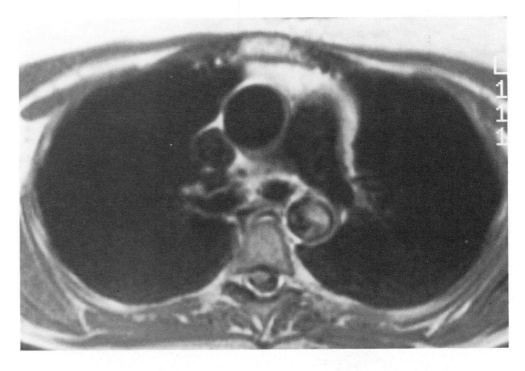

FIGURE 4–47 ■ Flow phenomena in the descending aorta. Cardiac-gated spin-echo image demonstrates intravascular signal within the descending aorta, a common occurrence because of the entry enhancement phenomenon.

FLASH images tend to be T1 weighted, whereas GRASS, and especially FISP, images tend to be T2 weighted.

Gradient refocused images are more likely than spin-echo images to be degraded from magnetic susceptibility effects and therefore are significantly limited in their application to imaging flow in lung blood vessels.

Cine-MR is an LFA, gradient-echo, fast imaging technique that is synchronized to the cardiac cycle.[173] Data from 20- to 40-ms segments of the cardiac cycle are used to create a cine-formatted image with a framing rate of 16 to 40 frames/min. Cine-MR has been used to evaluate cardiac and great vessel morphology, dynamic behavior, and blood flow. Cine-MR may also be used to image the more central pulmonary arteries.[173a] For a complete series of 8 to 12 10-mm-thick slices, the imaging time is about 15 minutes. The resultant images, when displayed in an endless loop on a television monitor, have nearly the temporal resolution of cine-angiocardiograms but slightly less spatial resolution than conventional MR. As with other fast gradient-echo methods, rapidly flowing blood produces a high signal intensity. A

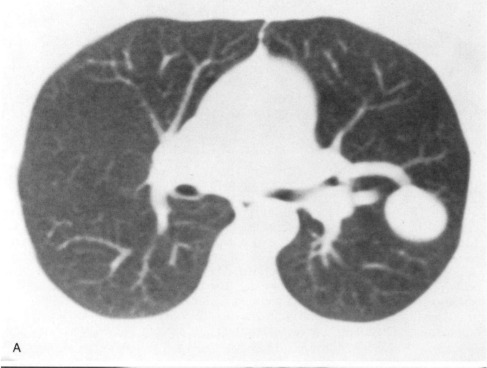

A

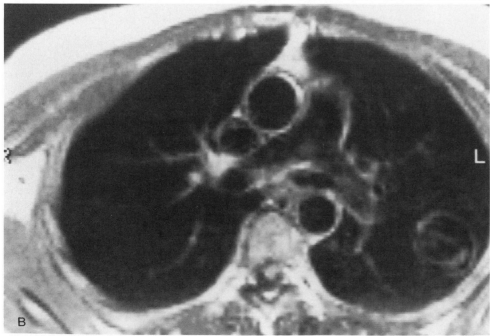

B

FIGURE 4–48 ■ Arteriovenous malformation. *A*, CT scan demonstrates a well-circumscribed mass in the left midlung, with a draining vessel arising from the mass. *B*, Cardiac-gated spin-echo image demonstrates the mass with minor signal within it.

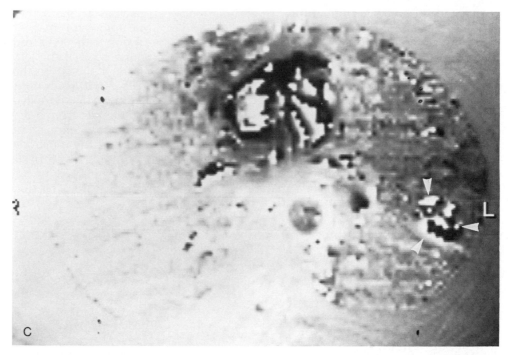

FIGURE 4–48 *Continued* ■ C, Gradient-echo image, sensitive to flow, demonstrates signal *(arrowheads)* within the mass, indicating flowing blood. Signal is also visible within the descending aorta and cardiac chambers.

dynamic signal void from the intravascular compartment at the appropriate site reflects vascular turbulence and is seen with valvular stenosis or regurgitation. Other causes of signal voids, with different dynamic behavior, include clots, calcification, and magnetic susceptibility artifacts.

Techniques for accurate quantification of blood flow utilize either time-of-flight or phase-shift phenomena.[173, 174] In conventional spin-echo sequences, the effect of blood moving through the acquisition volume and the dephasing effect of motion on protons within flowing blood degrade image quality. However, these effects are exploited in MR angiography to selectively detect flow and suppress signal from stationary tissues. These techniques have been used to demonstrate the carotid vessels, the cerebral circulation, flow within the heart and great vessels, and flow in the peripheral circulation. In the chest, blood flow has also been quantitated within the aorta and proximal pulmonary vessels, but techniques that utilize gradient-recalled echoes are limited for imaging of lung parenchyma.

Congenital and acquired abnormalities of the pulmonary vessels are uncommon. Among those that have been diagnosed from CT scans are arteriovenous fistulae, pulmonary vein varices, and pulmonary sequestration. The diagnosis of central pulmonary emboli by CT scanning has also been discussed in Chapter 3.

Pulmonary Arteriovenous Fistulae ■ A pulmonary artery–to–pulmonary vein fistula is only one type of abnormal vascular shunt within the lungs. Abnormal communication can also exist between pulmonary arteries and bronchial arteries and between pulmonary veins and bronchial veins.[175] Pulmonary arteriovenous fistulae can be congenital or posttraumatic. The congenital type is much more common. Usually the abnormal dilated vascular channel is supplied by a single artery and drained by a single vein.[176] Occasionally many feeding arteries and draining veins are present.[177] In about a third of cases, arteriovenous fistulae are multiple, but often only the dominant lesion is seen on chest radiographs. From 40 to 60 per cent of these patients have additional lesions outside the thorax, and the condition is then known as *hereditary hemorrhagic telangiectasia* (Rendu-Osler-Weber syndrome).

Pulmonary arteriovenous fistulae can usually be suspected or diagnosed from chest radiographs and appear as round or slightly lobular masses of less than one to several centimeters in diameter. They are most common in the inner third of the lung toward the hila. In many patients, the feeding artery emanating from the hilum and the draining vein coursing toward the left atrium are visible. Confirmation of the diagnosis can be obtained by pulmonary angiography or sometimes by radioisotope angiography, but dynamic CT is a more convenient, noninvasive method of confirming the diagnosis and provides a precise anatomic display of the abnormality.[178, 179] MR is a reasonable alternative to CT for imaging suspected pulmonary arteriovenous fistulae (Fig. 4–48). On spin-echo images, the wall of the fistula can usually be observed. Depending on the blood flow pattern and blood velocity within the fistula, signal within the fistula may be evident. With cine-MR, high-intensity flowing blood is seen within the fistula. In our experience, MR and CT obviate the need for angiography unless surgery or embolization of the fistula is being contemplated. Under these circumstances, angiography must be performed to detect any additional lesions, because MR and CT have not been shown capable of demonstrating small, radiographically inapparent fistulae. Carefully performed pulmonary angiography of all lung lobes is then required.

Pulmonary Vein Varicosities ■ Pulmonary vein varicosities are uncommon and can be congenital or acquired. They are usually asymptomatic, do not require treatment, and are most often detected from chest radiographs. The tortuous, dilated segment of the pulmonary vein appears as a smooth, round or oval density close to the left atrium.[180, 181] Its nature can be inferred from its characteristic shape and position. Dynamic CT and MR are both ideal methods for diagnosing pulmonary vein varicosities. After an intravenous bolus of contrast material, the varix

opacifies at about the same time as the left atrium. MR spin-echo images display the varix and its connection to the left atrium. A pulmonary arteriovenous fistula close to the left atrium may have CT and MR findings similar to those of a pulmonary vein varicosity.[182] It is doubtful whether CT and MR can routinely distinguish a medially situated arteriovenous fistula from a pulmonary vein varicosity.

Pulmonary Sequestration ■ Pulmonary sequestration is one of the most common congenital anomalies of the lung. The sequestered portion of lung is characterized by a lack of communication with the tracheobronchial tree and an abnormal systemic blood sup-

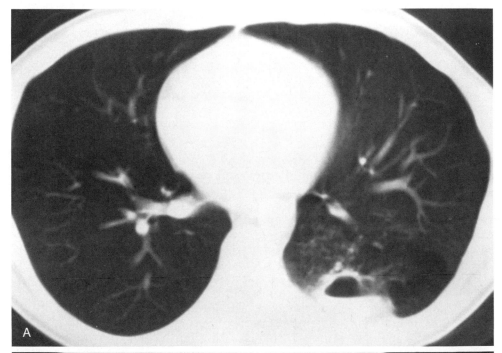

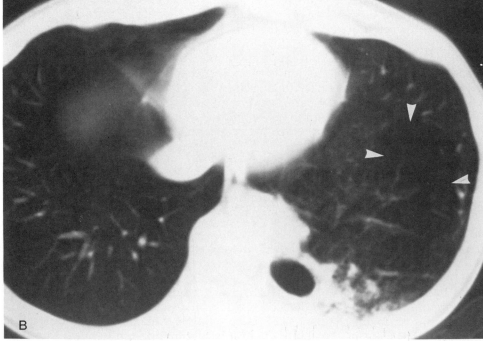

FIGURE 4–49 ■ Pulmonary sequestration in a 37-year-old man involving the left lower lobe with recurrent left lower lobe pneumonia and abscesses. *A,* CT scan at the level of the inferior hilum demonstrates a left lower lobe abscess with an air-fluid level. Patchy consolidation is present in the surrounding lung, which appears abnormally lucent. *B,* CT scan 4 cm caudal to the level seen in *A* shows a second abscess cavity with surrounding consolidation. The left lower lobe is hyperlucent *(arrowheads)* with diminished vessels. CT scan at a different level demonstrated an abnormal vessel extending from the aorta toward the abnormal lung, probably representing an aberrant arterial supply.

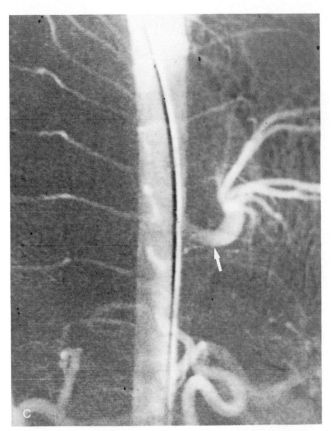

FIGURE 4–49 *Continued* ■ *C*, Digital subtraction angiogram shows an abnormal artery *(arrow)* arising from the aorta and supplying the entire abnormal left lower lobe, confirming the diagnosis.

ply. The abnormal systemic blood supply is from an anomalous vessel arising from the descending aorta in about 70 per cent of cases and from the abdominal aorta, bronchial arteries, intercostal arteries, or aortic arch in the other 30 per cent. When the sequestered lung is clearly within the normal visceral pleura and has its venous drainage to the pulmonary veins, it is referred to as *intralobar*. Much less commonly, the sequestered lung has its own envelope of pleura, has its venous drainage to systemic veins, and is called *extralobar*. However, intermediate forms of venous drainage are not uncommon.[183, 184] Pulmonary sequestration is only one of several causes of abnormal systemic blood supply to the lung.[185] Abnormal systemic blood supply to a portion of the lung can also be from anomalous vessels that arise from the aorta or its branches, transpleural vessels from the intercostal arteries, or hypertrophied bronchial arteries. The lung itself may be otherwise normal, or it may be dysplastic or damaged, usually from chronic infection.[186]

The radiographic appearance of an intralobar pulmonary sequestration depends on whether the sequestered lung is aerated. When the sequestration does not communicate with the rest of the lung, it appears as a sharply circumscribed, homogeneous density, usually in the posterior portion of the lower lobe and almost invariably contiguous with the dia-

phragm. A sequestration that communicates with the remainder of the lung, usually after being infected, appears cystic. It may exhibit one or more cystic spaces, with or without air-fluid levels (Fig. 4–49). The lung parenchyma surrounding a sequestered area may be abnormal.[187] We, and others,[187a] have seen several cases of extensive hyperlucency on CT in the lower lobe of a sequestration.

A definitive diagnosis of pulmonary sequestration usually depends on the presence of a masslike density in the posteroinferior lower lobe and the demonstration of the anomalous vessels. In some cases, CT can show a large vessel from the aorta feeding into the sequestration.[188] In one case we have studied, the septations between the cystic spaces of the sequestration enhanced after a bolus injection of contrast material immediately after the enhancement of the descending thoracic aorta, indicating systemic blood supply to the sequestration. Godwin and Webb[170] described an angioma and an inflammatory mass, both with systemic blood supply and showing contrast enhancement immediately after that of the descending thoracic aorta. Dynamic CT scanning can thus show systemic blood supply to the lung even when the feeding vessels are not demonstrated. Contrast enhancement of the abnormal portion of lung during the arterial phase after injection of an intravenous bolus of contrast material should indicate that aortography will show abnormal systemic blood supply to the lesion. Calcification within a pulmonary sequestration is unusual but can be central, peripheral, or both and can be demonstrated with CT.[189, 190]

Pulmonary Embolism ■ Pulmonary embolism is the most common acute pulmonary emergency for the hospitalized patient and accounts for an estimated 120,000 deaths per year in the United States. Autopsy studies show that pulmonary embolism is not diagnosed in 60 to 70 per cent of fatal cases. Pulmonary angiography is the definitive diagnostic modality but is not universally available and can have severe complications. An accurate, noninvasive method of diagnosis could improve the diagnostic accuracy for pulmonary embolism. Godwin and co-workers[191] have shown that central pulmonary emboli can be demonstrated on CT scans. After a bolus injection of contrast material, emboli as peripheral as lobar pulmonary arteries can be imaged (Fig. 4–50). Ovenfors and colleagues[192] were able to show autologous blood clots in segmental pulmonary arteries in dogs. Indirect evidence of pulmonary emboli might be found in some patients from the CT scan appearance of the lung distal to an occluded artery. Detection of pulmonary infarction distal to sites of pulmonary vascular occlusion has been studied both in humans and in animals. Grossman and colleagues[193] found an increase in CT density in one of six experimentally occluded vessels before infusion of contrast material and in three of six after infusion. In subsequent studies, this group demonstrated decrease in CT density ("oligemia") in areas of lung distal to a

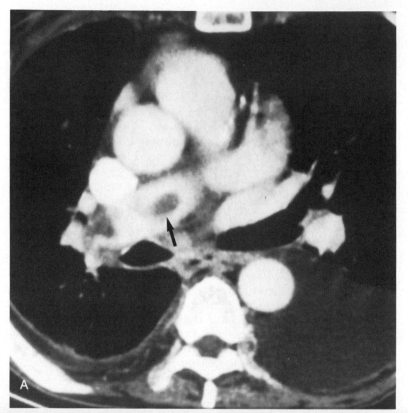

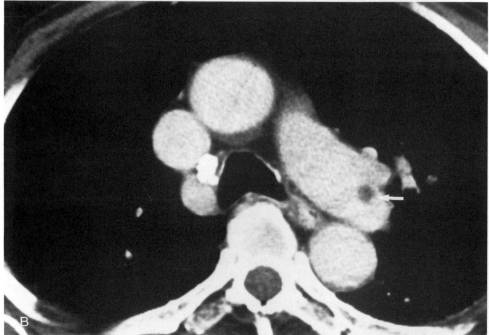

FIGURE 4–50 ■ Pulmonary emboli demonstrated on CT scan in two patients. *A*, Contrast-enhanced CT scan through the midthorax demonstrates a filling defect *(arrow)* in the right pulmonary artery, representing an unsuspected pulmonary embolus. A large left pleural effusion is seen. *B* and *C*, CT scans through the main and descending pulmonary artery in a second patient showed two pulmonary emboli *(arrows)*. The central pulmonary arteries are enlarged, and the patient has severe pulmonary arterial hypertension.

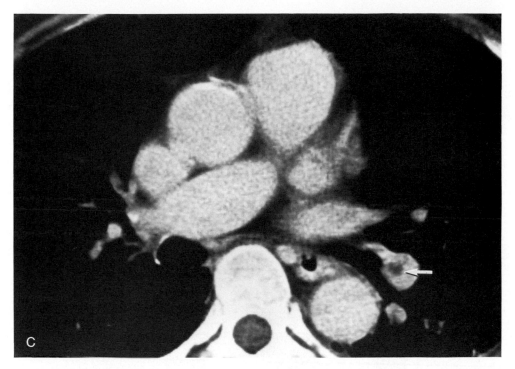

FIGURE 4–50 *Continued*

balloon occlusion of segmental pulmonary arteries.[194] This finding was consistently demonstrated only in the nondependent portion of the lung. Lourie and co-workers,[195] on the other hand, demonstrated areas of increased density on CT scans of 81 per cent of dogs that had verified infarctions after experimental pulmonary artery occlusion.

Sinner[196] described various patterns of peripheral wedge-shaped areas of increased CT density in patients with suspected pulmonary emboli. The exact nature of these findings and their specificity, however, were not documented. The clinical significance of this finding in patients with suspected pulmonary embolism awaits further clarification. In our opinion, CT scanning should be used for evaluating suspected chronic pulmonary emboli, as described in Chapter 3. Its routine use cannot be advocated for suspected acute pulmonary embolism.

Blood flowing at normal velocity shows an MR signal void in the pulmonary arteries on ECG-gated images obtained during systole; emboli within the pulmonary arteries can be detected with these imaging techniques. The MR signal intensity of pulmonary emboli, however, is variable, depending on the age of the clot.[197–200] Intraluminal MR signal may also be caused by slow flow in the pulmonary arteries, as in pulmonary arterial hypertension, or proximal to an anatomic or functional vessel occlusion. Emboli can be suspected on spin-echo images from a local intraluminal area of medium signal intensity, with little or no change in intensity from first to second echo images, and a constant appearance on images obtained at different phases of the cardiac cycle (Fig. 4–51).[201]

Problems with MR imaging of pulmonary embolism include spurious results caused by flow artifacts,

limited spatial resolution, motion artifacts, and inability to distinguish thrombus from airless lung.[197, 199, 200] The sensitivity and specificity for MR detection of pulmonary embolism have not been determined in patients, but in a study of 30 dogs, the sensitivity and specificity of MR for detecting proven pulmonary embolism were 82 and 88 per cent, respectively.[200] These figures are not sufficient to advocate MR either as a screening test or for definitive diagnosis. White and colleagues[201] made the diagnosis of central pulmonary emboli in several patients using MR. This technique, however, was not considered adequate for exclusion of emboli in more distal vessels. Recent experience suggests that cine-MR at 1.5 T can delineate large pulmonary emboli in main or lobar pulmonary vessels.[202] Spatial resolution is limited, and more peripheral pulmonary emboli are not accurately imaged. Reductions in TE and the use of thinner slices may improve these results.

Our recommendation is that MR imaging for suspected acute pulmonary embolism is still experimental and should not be undertaken clinically. The role of MR for chronic emboli is promising but unconfirmed.[203]

Pulmonary Hypertension ■ The severity of the anatomic and functional abnormalities demonstrated with MR in patients with pulmonary hypertension (see also Chapter 3) is dependent on the severity of the hypertension. The central pulmonary arteries in the mediastinum and hila can be measured precisely from CT and MR scans, and these diameters do reflect the pressure within the vessel in patients with pulmonary hypertension.[171] We have found that the caliber of the main pulmonary artery, measured from CT scans, is a useful predictor of pulmonary artery pressure. The upper limit of normal for the main

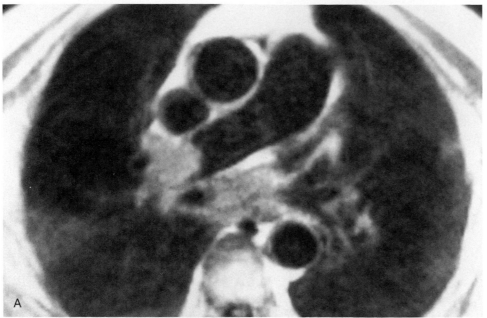

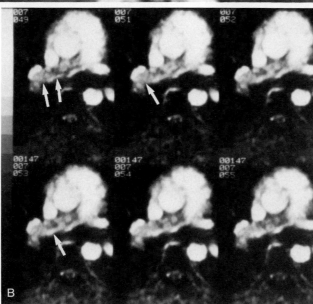

FIGURE 4–51 ■ MR demonstration of pulmonary emboli in two patients. *A,* Cardiac-gated spin-echo image during systole demonstrates a pulmonary embolus partially occluding the right pulmonary artery. *B,* Cine-MR scan shows extensive embolus *(arrows)* within the right pulmonary artery. Flowing blood is high, and the embolus is intermediate in signal intensity.

pulmonary artery is 28.6 mm. Pulmonary artery diameter correlates with pulmonary artery pressure with a coefficient of 0.89.[204] A diameter greater than 28.6 mm readily predicts pulmonary hypertension. Gated MR is as precise as CT in determining the caliber of the central pulmonary vessels.

Right ventricular hypertrophy, frequently with flattening or convexity of the interventricular septum toward the left ventricular chamber, is invariably present with severe pulmonary hypertension. Gated MR can readily demonstrate right ventricular enlargement and displacement of the interventricular septum. MR can also show evidence of decreased velocity of pulmonary blood flow in pulmonary hypertension. In normotensive subjects, MR signal is evident only during late diastole when blood flow is slow. During systole and early diastole, blood flow is normally too rapid to give a signal on spin-echo MR. Intraluminal signal during a major portion of the cardiac cycle is an MR finding of decreased blood velocity. Von Schulthess and colleagues[171] have shown that in patients with a pulmonary systolic pressure above 90 mm Hg, intraluminal signal is visible on gated MR scans obtained during systole, whereas in those patients with a pressure below 90 mm Hg, this finding is evident in only 30 per cent. Patients with pulmonary arterial hypertension show a linear correlation between the intensity of the MR signal from the central pulmonary arteries and the pulmonary vascular resistance.

MRI OF FOCAL LUNG DISEASE

MR has not gained application for evaluation of parenchymal lung disease largely because of its poor temporal and spatial resolution and magnetic susceptibility artifacts. This is mostly because the image is degraded by respiratory motion during the long imaging times.[205] Although some software advances have reduced-motion artifacts, the resolution is still less than that of CT. Artifacts from respiration and flowing blood in large vessels may be imaged in the lungs and mistaken for an infiltrate or mass. With fast imaging sequences that can be accomplished within one breath-holding period, contrast and resolution remain poor. The MR detection and characterization of focal lung lesions await MR scanners with better spatial resolution.

With spin-echo images of normal lung, little signal is obtained for the lung parenchyma. A few vessels or flowing blood can appear extending from the hila on cardiac-gated spin-echo sequences during systole. During diastole, blood-filled vessels, also radiating from the hila, can be imaged for several generations.

Fluid-filled structures in the lung such as an abscess or bronchogenic cyst may be recognized by their imaging characteristics. Fluid with low protein content and no blood has low signal intensity on T1-weighted images and increased signal intensity (medium or high) on T2 weighting. Cystic lesions containing blood or high protein content will show high intensity on T1- and T2-weighted images. Theoretically MR promises significantly greater ability than CT for tissue specificity in focal lung abnormalities. For instance, Huber and colleagues[206] show in experimental studies with excised lungs that T1 and T2 relaxation times of pneumonitis differ from those of collapsed lung in which there is no inflammation. An increase in T1 and T2 relaxation rates has been demonstrated in inflammatory diseases from multiple causes, including bacterial, viral, and *P. carinii* pneumonia and radiation pneumonitis.[207] Cohen and colleagues[208] demonstrated that lung abscesses and acute pneumonia showed a marked increase in signal intensity on T2-weighted images when compared with T1-weighted images. A single case report of pulmonary hemosiderosis showed higher signal intensity on T1- than on T2-weighted images.[209] The decreased signal intensity with T2 weighting is presumably from the paramagnetic effect of ferric iron in the lungs.

MR with T2-weighted images can at times distinguish between a central bronchogenic carcinoma and a peripheral obstructive pneumonitis.[210] The high water content of the distal obstructed lung sometimes displays a higher signal intensity than the proximal tumor. Unfortunately, pulmonary inflammation, obstructive pneumonitis, and lung tumors all show a marked overlap in their relaxation times. It is unlikely that relaxation values alone will discriminate among these disorders within the clinical setting.

Extension of infection or tumor from the lung parenchyma into the mediastinum or chest wall is well delineated by MR and is discussed in Chapter 5. Tumor and infection usually prolong T1 and T2 relaxation times and are therefore identified as low signal intensity areas on T1-weighted images, contrasting with mediastinal or chest wall fat. On T2-weighted images, infection and tumor are usually brighter in signal intensity than muscle, a property that can be utilized to depict the extent of disease in the chest wall.[97] The signal intensity ratio of tumor to fat on T2-weighted images can vary, but with a repetition time longer than 2 sec, signal intensity of tumors is usually brighter than that of fat.

Diffuse Lung Disease

INTERSTITIAL DISEASE

In the beginning of this chapter we discussed the CT anatomy and findings of alveolar air space filling processes and those that thicken or infiltrate the interstitium of the lung. The high sensitivity of CT and HRCT for the detection of diffuse lung disease has been established. The specificity with which a combination of findings can suggest a specific diagnosis is becoming evident.[9, 28, 34, 35, 37, 112a, 112b, 211, 212] In this section we will deal with entities in which the HRCT findings appear suggestive or highly suggestive of that specific disease.

Lymphangitic Carcinoma ■ Malignant neoplasms from thoracic or extrathoracic sites can access the interstitium of the lung by two routes. Hematogenous tumor can break through the wall of small vessels into the interstitium, or alternatively, tumor can disseminate through the lymphatics in a retrograde fashion from hilar lymph nodes. The involved lymphatic channels are those in the interlobular septa, centrilobular units, subpleural lymphatic plexus, peribronchial channels, and large lymphatic channels coursing from the periphery of the lung toward the hila.[213] The HRCT appearances are produced by tumor deposition, edema secondary to lymphatic obstruction, and a fibrotic response within the interstitial compartment. The HRCT appearances are frequently multifocal, with some segments and lobes involved and some spared. The characteristic features described by Munk and colleagues[214] and Stein and co-workers[215] are of irregular thickening of interlobular septa with a beaded or nodular appearance (Fig. 4–52). Thickening of centrilobular structures produces a spiderlike appearance in the center of secondary lobules. Toward the diaphragm, where lobules are imaged in cross section, thickened polygonal structures 1 to 2 cm in diameter are characteristic. Apparent thickening and irregularity of bronchial walls are caused by thickening of the peribronchial interstitium. Involvement of the subpleural plexus of lymphatics produces the appearance of irregular fissural thickening (Fig. 4–53).

Pulmonary lymphangitic spread of tumor is most commonly found with carcinoma of the breast, stomach, prostate, lung, and pancreas and adenocarcinoma from an unknown source. In our experience, within the appropriate clinical context and a known carcinoma at one of these sites, HRCT can be used to establish the diagnosis with a sufficiently high probability to obviate lung biopsy.

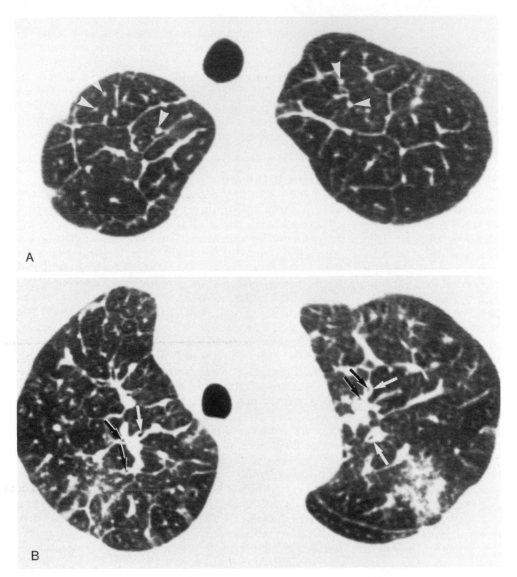

A

B

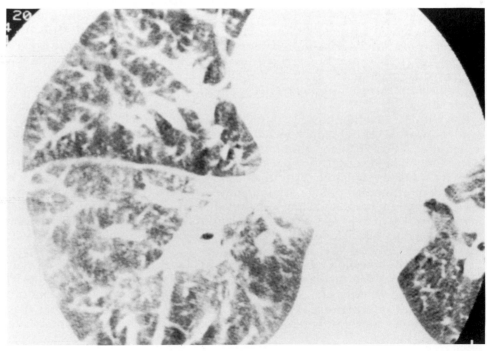

FIGURE 4–52 ■ Lymphangitic carcinomatosis from a primary breast carcinoma. HRCT scans through the upper and lower lobes demonstrate bilateral extensive irregular interlobular septal thickening. Architectural distortion is not present. Prominence of the centrilobular structures *(arrowheads)* is seen. Apparent bronchial wall thickening *(arrows)* is a result of tumor infiltration of the peribronchial interstitium.

FIGURE 4–53 ■ Extensive lymphangitic carcinomatosis. HRCT scan through the lower lung demonstrates massive interstitial thickening extending throughout the lung. Apparent thickening of the major fissure represents subpleural interstitial infiltration with tumor.

Idiopathic Pulmonary Fibrosis ■ Idiopathic pulmonary fibrosis (cryptogenic fibrosing alveolitis) is a chronic inflammatory disorder of the lower respiratory tract of unknown cause. It is characterized by a chronic inflammation involving the alveolar walls and interstitium of the lung.[216–218] The alveolar macrophage and neutrophil are the dominant cell types involved in the inflammatory reaction, producing fibroblastic proliferation and collagen deposition. Pathologically the lesions are multifocal and demonstrate inflammation at various stages of maturity.

Muller and co-workers,[28, 34] in two seminal articles, described some of the HRCT findings in idiopathic pulmonary fibrosis. The most characteristic finding was honeycombing, which had a strong tendency to be in a subpleural location (Fig. 4–54). The honeycomb cysts, measuring 5 to 20 mm in diameter, tended to be patchy, with interspersed normal-appearing lung parenchyma. At a later stage, the lung may be diffusely involved, often with traction bronchiectasis in the involved areas.[33] They also described "reticular changes" in many cases, although a precise definition of this term was not given. In our experience and that of others,[5, 26, 30, 37] idiopathic pulmonary fibrosis at a stage prior to the development of honeycombing predominantly involves the interlobular and centrilobular structures on HRCT (Fig. 4–55). Interlobular septal thickening is a prominent feature with distortion of the architecture of the secondary lobule (see Figs. 4–16 to 4–20). Fibrosis of the subpleural interstitium is seen as irregular thickening of the costal visceral pleura and as thickening of the interlobar fissures. Peribronchial interstitial thickening and apparent irregularity of the vessel walls are less prominent features (Fig. 4–56).[5] Toward the lung bases, thickened secondary lobules can have a polygonal appearance. This appearance is similar to that seen in lymphatic infiltration with tumor, but in that condition the interstitium appears more irregular and there is less architectural distortion. In advanced cases of interstitial fibrosis, long scars can be seen to course through the lungs, frequently extending to the pleural surface (see Fig. 4–18). A similar pattern of lung fibrosis can be seen in rheumatoid lung disease, systemic lupus erythematosus of the lung, scleroderma, and mixed connective tissue disease. In fact, there is considerable clinical and biochemical overlap between idiopathic pulmonary fibrosis and the collagen vascular diseases.

In some cases of idiopathic pulmonary fibrosis, a ground-glass air space density is seen peripherally, tending to conform to the lobular anatomy of the lungs (Fig. 4–57). In cases of known idiopathic pulmonary fibrosis and HRCT evidence of interstitial fibrosis, this finding may be indicative of the active alveolitis of interstitial fibrosis.[34] Although this hazy density has been related in some cases to pathologic activity of the inflammatory process, we have not found good correlation with the results of bronchoalveolar lavage. The inflammation and fibrosis in idiopathic pulmonary fibrosis are frequently at different stages of maturity in different parts of the lung. Additional studies are required to determine whether this hazy density is of clinical significance and whether it can predict a response to antiinflammatory agents.

The findings in pulmonary fibrosis are more apparent on HRCT scans than on chest radiographs, and the patterns of abnormality are more closely associated with functional abnormalities and patient symptoms.[35, 219] The specificity of the combinations of HRCT abnormalities for this specific entity is not known. Mathieson and colleagues[212] found an accuracy of 89 per cent, but in their study the choices of possible diagnoses were limited.

Granulomatous Disease

Sarcoidosis ■ Sarcoidosis is a chronic systemic granulomatous disease of unknown etiology. Histologically it has the hallmarks of a type IV immune reaction, with characteristic noncaseating granuloma formation. The thorax is most commonly involved, with a high propensity for involvement of hila and mediastinal lymph nodes. About a third of patients with lung involvement develop diffuse pulmonary fibrosis. Patients with intrathoracic sarcoidosis may be strikingly free of symptoms, and the disease may be first identified at various stages of development.

The chest radiographic and CT findings depend on the stage of the disease. In early parenchymal sarcoidosis, the findings are of multiple small nodules and patchy areas of air space disease (Fig. 4–58). An alveolar form of the disease can produce large, spherical, masslike alveolar opacities. At this stage, hilar and mediastinal adenopathy are frequently present. We have seen several instances in which transbronchial biopsy demonstrated sarcoid granulomas when HRCT of the lung parenchyma was entirely normal. As with other interstitial lung disease, patchy, hazy densities on the CT scan may be indicative of an active alveolitis.[220] As the disease progresses and fibrosis supervenes, interlobular septal thickening (Fig. 4–59) and long linear bands of fibrosis extending to the pleural surface (parenchymal bands) become prominent features. Architectural distortion manifests as misshapen and contracted lobules, and honeycombing develops (Fig. 4–60). Advanced disease may demonstrate severe honeycombing or cicatricial conglomeration of vessels and bronchi that tends to be more severe in the upper lobes than the lower lobes (Fig. 4–61). Cystic spaces between 1 and 10 cm in diameter are seen in advanced disease and are usually associated with marked lung destruction. Traction or cicatricial bronchiectasis can occur in areas of severe fibrosis and honeycombing.

Bergin and colleagues[221] and Muller and co-investigators[222] have shown that the extent of disease and type of abnormality are reasonably predictive of functional impairment. Patients whose HRCT scans show multiple discrete nodules or fibrotic changes

Text continued on page 215

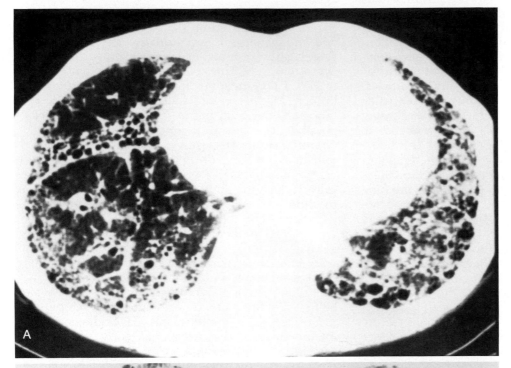

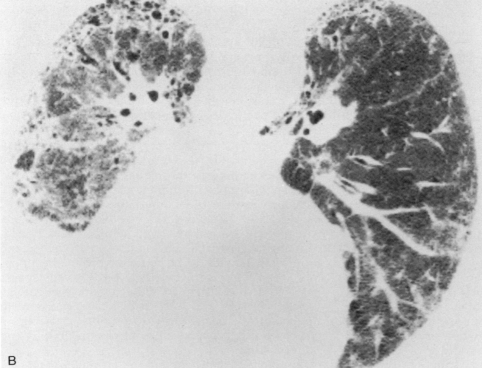

FIGURE 4–54 ■ Idiopathic pulmonary fibrosis with honeycombed lung in three patients. *A,* HRCT scan through the lower lungs demonstrates the typical subpleural distribution of honeycomb lung in a patient with idiopathic pulmonary fibrosis. Honeycombing in the right middle lobe is subpleural, adjacent to the major fissure. More extensive abnormalities are present on the left. *B,* Prone HRCT scan in another patient demonstrates subpleural honeycombing at both lung bases. The ground-glass appearance in the left lower lobe suggests an active alveolitis.

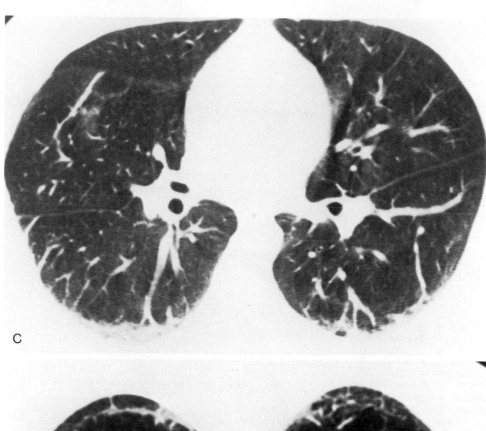

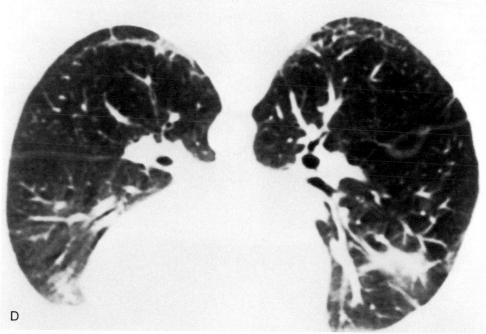

FIGURE 4–54 *Continued* ■ *C* and *D*, Supine and prone HRCT scan in a third patient shows 5 mm of dependent density posteriorly obscuring the lung bases in the supine position. In the prone position, the dependent density clears, revealing interstitial fibrosis at the left base and honeycombing at the right base.

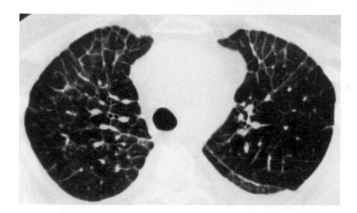

FIGURE 4–55 ■ Idiopathic pulmonary fibrosis with interstitial thickening. HRCT scan through the upper lobes demonstrates marked interlobular septal thickening visible in both dependent and nondependent portions of the lung. Mild prominence of centrilobular structures is also present. Peribronchial thickening around the larger bronchi is not seen and is not a frequent feature of idiopathic pulmonary fibrosis.

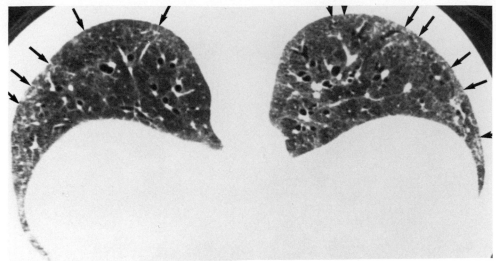

FIGURE 4–56 ■ Idiopathic pulmonary fibrosis with dominant peribronchiolar fibrosis. CT scan demonstrates a peripheral pattern of small ring shadows *(arrows)* representing peribronchiolar thickening, in this instance caused by fibrosis. Interlobular septal thickening is minimal, and the lung architecture does not demonstrate major distortion. The central larger bronchi appear dilated. Lung biopsy revealed predominantly peribronchiolar fibrosis.

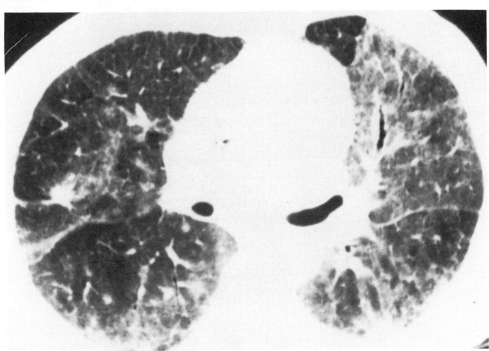

FIGURE 4–57 ■ Idiopathic pulmonary fibrosis with active alveolitis. CT scan shows multifocal interstitial thickening, especially visible anteriorly on the right side. In addition, multifocal areas of ground-glass opacity are visible posteriorly on both the left and right sides and anteriorly on the left side. Open lung biopsy revealed interstitial fibrosis with an active alveolitis.

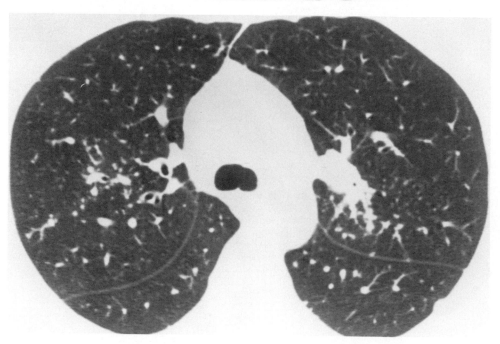

FIGURE 4–58 ■ Early sarcoidosis with multiple small lung granulomas. Chest radiograph showed hilar adenopathy with normal lungs. HRCT scan demonstrates numerous small nodules throughout both lungs. The prominent left superior hilum is caused by adenopathy.

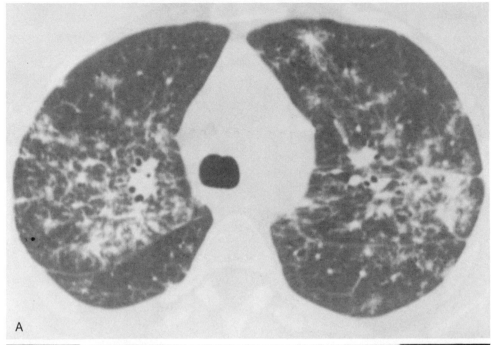

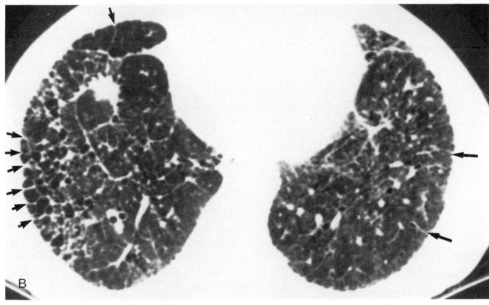

FIGURE 4–59 ■ Moderately advanced sarcoidosis in two patients. *A*, CT scan through the midlung demonstrates ill-defined nodular opacities, representing granulomas with surrounding inflammation, and mild interstitial prominence. Transbronchial biopsy demonstrated sarcoid granulomas. *B*, HRCT scan in a second patient shows predominantly interstitial thickening *(arrows)* involving the interlobular septa and centrilobular structures. Honeycombing is present at the right base laterally. Irregularity of the pleura is from subvisceral pleural interstitial fibrosis.

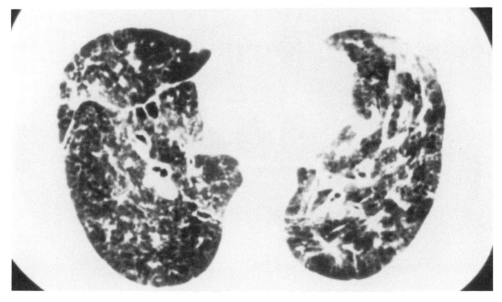

FIGURE 4–60 ■ Advanced sarcoidosis with architectural distortion. HRCT scan shows distortion of lung architecture with cicatricial changes in both lower lobes. Multiple nodules probably represent granulomas. Peribronchial thickening represents fibrosis or granulomas around the larger bronchi. Irregularity of the vessel walls indicates perivascular fibrosis.

213

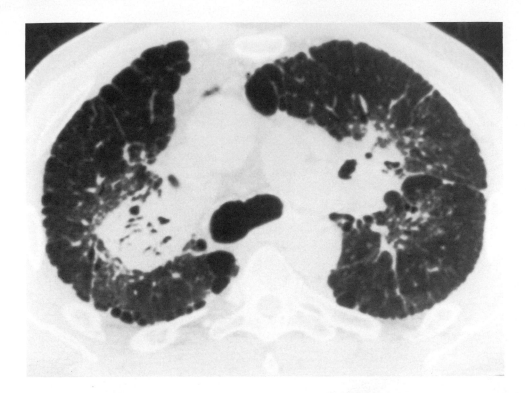

FIGURE 4–61 ■ Advanced sarcoidosis with marked fibrosis and architectural distortion. HRCT scan through the upper lobes demonstrates marked fibrosis adjacent to both hila with lung distortion and air bronchograms. The thin-walled subpleural cystic spaces anteriorly and posteriorly in the lung parenchyma probably represent paraseptal emphysema.

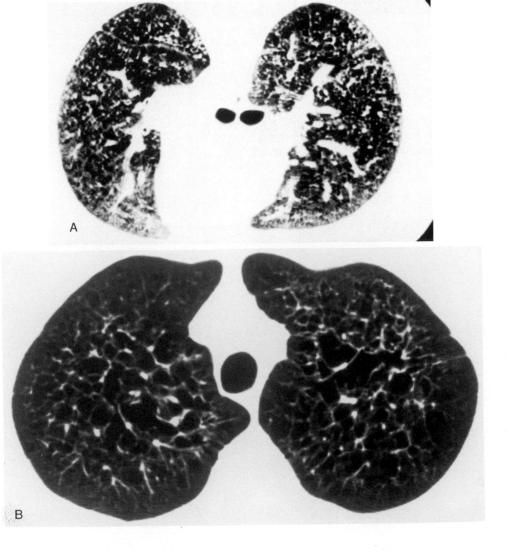

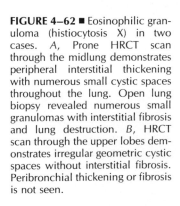

FIGURE 4–62 ■ Eosinophilic granuloma (histiocytosis X) in two cases. *A,* Prone HRCT scan through the midlung demonstrates peripheral interstitial thickening with numerous small cystic spaces throughout the lung. Open lung biopsy revealed numerous small granulomas with interstitial fibrosis and lung destruction. *B,* HRCT scan through the upper lobes demonstrates irregular geometric cystic spaces without interstitial fibrosis. Peribronchial thickening or fibrosis is not seen.

usually have restrictive dysfunction on pulmonary function studies.

Mathieson and colleagues[212] demonstrated that CT and HRCT features had a 77 per cent accuracy in diagnosis of sarcoidosis. In our experience, the main features distinguishing the lung parenchymal changes of advanced sarcoidosis from those of idiopathic pulmonary fibrosis are the former's upper lobe distribution; the presence of adenopathy, nodules, large cystic spaces, and cicatricial distortion of the lung parenchyma; involvement of the central interstitial space; and focal conglomeration of bronchi and vessels.[223, 224]

Eosinophilic Granulomatosis ■ Also known as pulmonary histiocytosis X, eosinophilic granulomatosis of the lung is an uncommon idiopathic disease afflicting mainly middle-aged adults, most of whom are smokers.[225, 226] It is responsible for only about 4 per cent of diffuse infiltrative lung disease and can be a diagnostic dilemma. In most circumstances, tissue is required for diagnosis and shows characteristic granulomas containing mononuclear histiocytes. In about 30 per cent of cases, granulomas are also present in organs other than the lung, especially bone and liver. The prognosis of eosinophilic granuloma of the lung is varied; it may resolve, remain static for many years, or progress to advanced pulmonary fibrosis and respiratory insufficiency.

CT and especially HRCT can depict the pulmonary abnormalities more clearly than can chest radiographs.[227, 228] The components of the disease that may be seen on CT include nodules, cysts, adenopathy, pneumothorax, large cystic spaces, peribronchial thickening, and hazy ground-glass opacities (Fig. 4–62).[217, 228] The nodules in histiocytosis X may show an upper lobe predominance but are usually generalized throughout the lung. They vary in size from 1 to 2 mm to several centimeters in diameter. In almost all cases, at least some of the nodules have cavitated. Small nodules may be centrilobular, next to a bronchiole within the secondary pulmonary lobule.

Air-containing cystic spaces are the most common finding of established eosinophilic granuloma of the lung. They vary in size and wall thickness. With advancing disease, cysts may enlarge up to several centimeters in diameter and may become confluent. In some cases, the cysts appear to arise next to a pulmonary artery branch, which invaginates the cyst or thickens one segment of its wall, a finding not frequently found in other diseases. In advanced disease, cystic spaces become the dominant finding, and nodules are less evident. Irregular shapes of the lung cysts are another typical finding in eosinophilic granulomatosis.

Interstitial fibrosis in eosinophilic granuloma is evident as interlobular septal thickening and irregularity of the interlobar fissures, indicating subpleural interstitial fibrosis or cellular infiltration.

There has been insufficient experience with eosinophilic granuloma of the lung to determine whether the findings on HRCT can give an indication of the prognosis. It is likewise unknown whether any HRCT features, such as the hazy ground-glass appearance, may indicate treatable active inflammation.

Pulmonary Lymphangiomyomatosis ■ Pulmonary lymphangiomyomatosis is a rare interstitial disease seen principally in adult females. Pathologically the disease is characterized by smooth muscle proliferation within the interstitium around lymphatics, airways, and smaller blood vessels.[229, 230] Chylous pleural effusion and recurrent pneumothorax are frequent associated findings. On chest radiographs, the lungs appear hyperinflated with a reticular interstitial pattern of abnormality.[230] CT and HRCT scans can demonstrate the interstitial components of the disease more clearly than can chest radiographs.[231–233] In early stages, the CT findings are of diffuse small cysts that appear to have a lobular distribution. Thickening of the interlobular septa is also demonstrated but is not a major feature. As the disease advances, the cystic spaces enlarge and have a well-defined thin wall (Fig. 4–63).[233a] Large cysts that are not round but have an undulating wall, similar to those found with eosinophilic granulomatosis, are sufficiently characteristic to be diagnostic in the appropriate clinical setting. The same lung CT findings can be seen in patients with pulmonary tuberous sclerosis.[233b]

PNEUMOCONIOSIS

Silicosis ■ Silicosis is a chronic nodular fibrotic response of part of the lungs to inhaled quartz (silica or silicon dioxide). Virtually all cases of silicosis in North America stem from occupational exposure in hard rock mining, sand blasting, or foundry work. Because of protective measures, the incidence of new cases is rapidly declining; nevertheless, because of the chronicity of the disease, large numbers of individuals are still being evaluated for compensation and disability.

The traditional imaging modality used for morphologic assessment of these patients is the chest radiograph. In simple silicosis, nodules are the predominant finding. They tend to be well defined, dense, and of uniform size within an individual. The size of the nodules varies between individuals, and their different sizes have been designated by specific letters in the ILO Classification of Pneumoconioses.[234] CT is equal to or better than chest radiographs for detecting the profusion and extent of nodules (Fig. 4–64).[235–237a] Akira and colleagues[237] have shown with HRCT that the smallest type of opacities tends to center in the middle of the secondary pulmonary lobule. They frequently have low attenuation, with centrilobular emphysema around them.

Bergin and colleagues[235] demonstrated that in patients with silicosis and obstructive pulmonary function, CT could detect diffuse emphysema not evident from chest radiographs and thus explain the abnormal physiology. Begin and co-workers[236] found that CT could detect areas of coalescence and large opacities that could represent conglomerate silicosis, su-

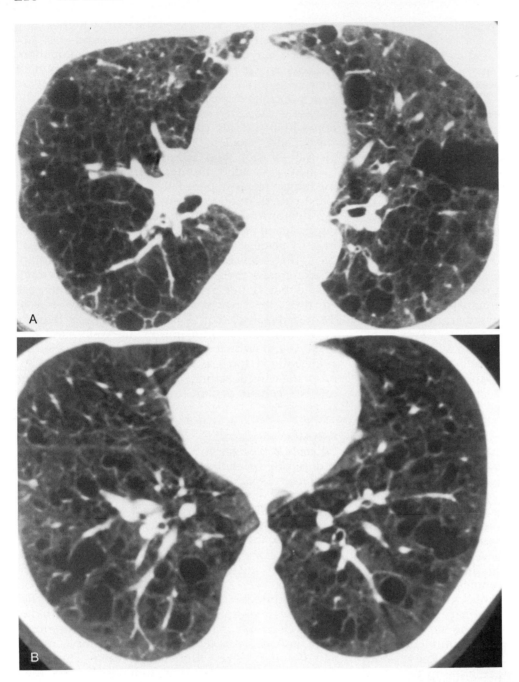

A

B

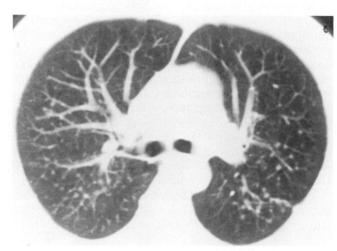

FIGURE 4–63 ■ Lymphangiomyomatosis in a middle-aged female. CT scans through the lower lobes demonstrate numerous thin-walled cystic spaces, most of which are round and some of which are irregular and geometric in shape. Interstitial fibrosis is minimal. The apparent CT density between the cystic spaces is probably normal or nearly normal lung parenchyma that contains increased quantities of diverted blood within dilated small vessels. (Courtesy of Denise Aberle, MD, Los Angeles.)

FIGURE 4–64 ■ Silicosis in a 70-year-old former Nevada gold miner. CT scan demonstrates numerous small nodular densities scattered throughout the lungs.

perimposed tuberculosis, or neoplasm, and were not seen on chest radiographs. Unless these opacities have the typical features of progressive massive fibrosis, further evaluation is necessary. These investigators[236] suggest that all patients in whom simple silicosis is discovered from chest radiographs should be screened with CT to detect nonevident masses. However, they did not suggest the time intervals at which this screening should be undertaken.

Complicated silicosis is present when conglomerate masses greater than 1 cm in diameter are present. These masses start as a coalescence of smaller nodules and can progress to large masses 10 cm or more in diameter. When serial chest radiographs do not show stability of the mass, CT is indicated for further investigation. CT is not capable of differentiating these conglomerate masses from other causes of masses. With progressive massive fibrosis, the fibrotic mass may be surrounded by a margin of emphysema, attesting to a chronic process and making neoplasm unlikely.

The precise role of CT in patients with suspected silicosis has yet to be defined. At present it appears that HRCT can detect early or minimal disease and also be useful in individuals with chest radiographic abnormalities and/or impaired pulmonary function.[238] In those with radiographic abnormality, HRCT may detect underlying obscured masses, and in the impaired, CT can help determine the cause of the functional abnormality. We suggest that HRCT be used instead of conventional CT and that the scans be obtained through the thorax at 1-cm intervals.

Asbestos-Related Disease ■ The term *asbestos* describes a group of hydrated fibrous silicates. Inhalation of these fibers causes disease in both the pleura and lung parenchyma. The pleural diseases include focal pleural fibrosis or plaques, pleural effusion, diffuse pleural thickening, and mesothelioma. Pleural effusion may antecede diffuse pleural fibrosis, although a history of effusion is not always obtained from patients with diffuse pleural thickening. The lung parenchymal abnormalities include pulmonary fibrosis or asbestosis, lung neoplasms, and cicatricial lung masses. Rounded atelectasis is a parenchymal abnormality usually seen in conjunction with diffuse pleural thickening; HRCT frequently shows concomitant lung fibrosis.

Pleural Disease ■ Pleural abnormalities are common in patients with occupational asbestos exposure. The most frequent lesions are pleural plaques that are discrete, elevated, opaque, shiny, fibrous areas. They are found mostly on the parietal pleura and characteristically on the posterior and lateral aspects of the costal pleura, over the lower lobes and hemidiaphragms.

CT and HRCT are more sensitive than chest radiographs for detection of pleural plaques.[36, 239, 240] On CT, pleural plaques form linear white densities of various thicknesses. They may be flat or irregularly marginated (Fig. 4–65). On HRCT, they must be differentiated from the normal endothoracic fascia and from the subjacent intercostal vein (see Chapter 5). On HRCT, calcification is seen within some plaques in about 10 per cent of individuals with pleural plaques. CT can also differentiate between extrapleural fat and pleural plaques, sometimes a difficult distinction with chest radiographs.[241]

Diffuse pleural thickening is more easily appreciated from CT than from chest radiographs.[36, 242] It is of lower density than pleural plaques, usually thicker and more irregular, and forms a continuous sheet at least 8 to 10 cm in a craniocaudal direction and 5 cm in a lateral direction (Fig. 4–66). The posterior and paraspinous regions are the most commonly affected sites. Extensive diffuse pleural thickening, unlike pleural plaques, can be associated with restrictive pulmonary dysfunction.

Parenchymal Disease ■ Asbestosis is the term reserved for pulmonary fibrosis caused by the inhalation of asbestos fibers.[243, 244] The fibrotic process usually starts at the centrilobular bronchiolar level and is multifocal, with normal parenchyma intervening. Subpleural areas are usually involved first, predominantly in the lower lobes. Subpleural honeycombing may be present but is seen in only about 10 per cent of patients with asbestosis.

During the 1980s, several groups of investigators studied the potential of CT for detecting parenchymal abnormalities in asbestos-exposed workers.[9, 31, 239, 240, 245, 246] In early studies, Katz and Kreel[240] found that CT demonstrated abnormalities about twice as frequently as radiographs. The abnormalities included honeycombing, reticulonodular densities, and fine linear densities. This increased sensitivity for detection of parenchymal abnormalities has been confirmed by several groups. Begin and colleagues,[246] however, found that CT and chest radiographs demonstrated findings of asbestosis with comparable frequency.

More recently, investigators have applied HRCT to detect and characterize asbestosis. Patients with asbestosis display many of the features of interstitial lung disease described in the early part of this chapter (Table 4–5). These include septal and centrilobular thickening (Figs. 4–67 through 4–69), long scars or parenchymal bands traversing the lung (see Figs. 4–67 and 4–69), honeycombing, subpleural lines (see Fig. 4–67B), and architectural distortion (Fig. 4–70). The interstitial changes frequently occur next to sites of pleural plaques and are usually most severe in the lower lobes posteriorly. In our experience, selected HRCT scans obtained in the supine and prone positions are most appropriate for demonstrating asbestosis (Table 4–6).

In most asbestos-exposed individuals with abnormal chest radiographs compatible with asbestosis, HRCT will demonstrate a multiplicity of abnormalities at several levels that conform to known pathologic abnormalities of asbestosis.[36, 239] Although the incidence of asbestosis without radiographically visible pleural plaques is about 15 per cent, we have found that virtually all patients with parenchymal

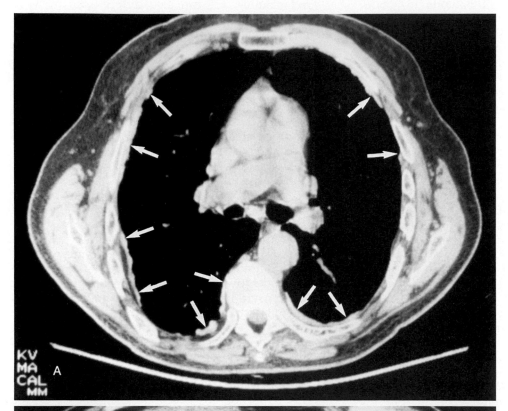

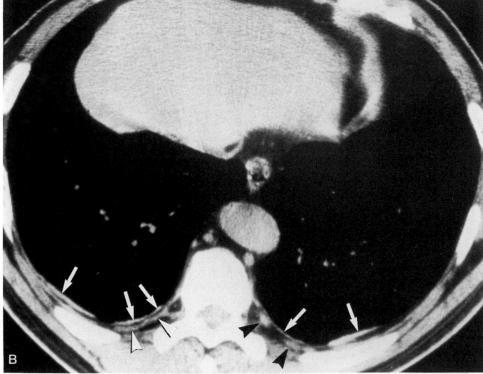

FIGURE 4–65 ■ Asbestos-related pleural plaques. *A,* HRCT scan demonstrates numerous large pleural plaques *(arrows)* posteriorly, laterally, and anteriorly. *B,* HRCT scan demonstrates smooth, flat plaques posteriorly *(arrows).* The plaques must be differentiated from extrapleural intercostal veins *(arrowheads).*

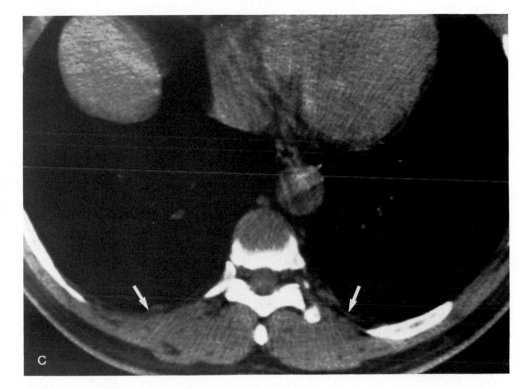

FIGURE 4–65 *Continued* ■ *C,* Minimal flat pleural plaques *(arrows)* are demonstrated posteriorly. The more prominent structures are the intercostal veins and subcostal muscles.

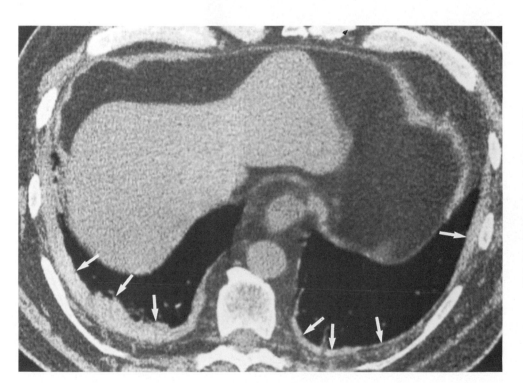

FIGURE 4–66 ■ Diffuse pleural thickening as a result of asbestos-related benign pleural effusion. HRCT scan demonstrates bilateral diffuse pleural thickening *(arrows)* more marked on the right than on the left. Hypertrophy with increased thickness of the extra-pleural fat is common with fibro-thorax. The patient had a history of asbestos exposure and bilateral pleuritis. The density of the fibrosis of diffuse pleural thickening usually is lower than that of pleural plaques.

TABLE 4–5 ■ HRCT Features of Asbestosis

Sign	Description	Significance	Probable Pathologic Correlate
Centrilobular thickening	Radiating fine lines within 1 to 2 cm of pleural surface	Common finding in mild/ moderate pulmonary fibrosis	Probably peribronchiolar fibrosis
Interlobular septal thickening	Parallel short lines perpendicular to pleura, extending 1 to 2 cm into lung	Mild/moderate fibrosis	Fibrous thickening of interlobular or intralobular septa
Curvilinear subpleural line	1- to 10-cm line within 1 cm of pleura and parallel to it	Common in dependent lung; suggests fibrosis when persistent in nondependent lung	Interlobular septal fibrosis on inner margin of subpleural honeycombing
Haze	Persistent ground-glass, increased density of nondependent lung	Uncommon; may indicate active lung inflammation	Alveolitis
Parenchymal bands	2- to 5-cm lines contacting pleural surface, extending into lung parenchyma	Interstitial lung fibrosis	Long fibrotic scars
Honeycombing	Cystlike spaces < 1 cm diameter with walls 1 to 3 mm thick	End-stage lung destruction	Destroyed lung, with air cysts and dilated bronchioles
Visceral pleural thickening	Thickened irregular pleural surfaces/fissures	Advanced fibrosis (usually with other signs)	Subpleural fibrosis

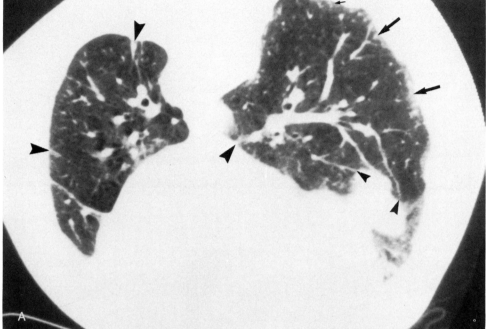

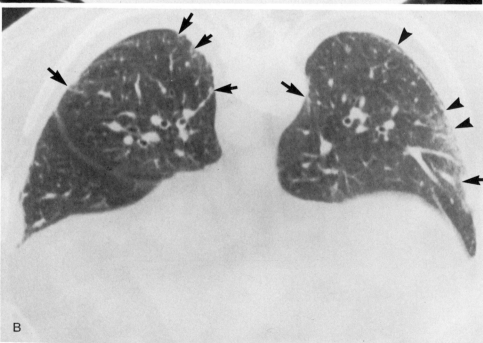

FIGURE 4–67 ■ Asbestosis in two patients. *A*, Prone HRCT scan shows multifocal areas of subpleural interstitial abnormality *(arrows)*. Abnormality consists of interstitial septal thickening, centrilobular thickening, and long scars *(arrowheads)*. *B*, Prone HRCT scan demonstrates a subpleural line *(arrowheads)* on the right side. Multifocal areas of interstitial, predominantly centrilobular, thickening *(arrows)* are seen.

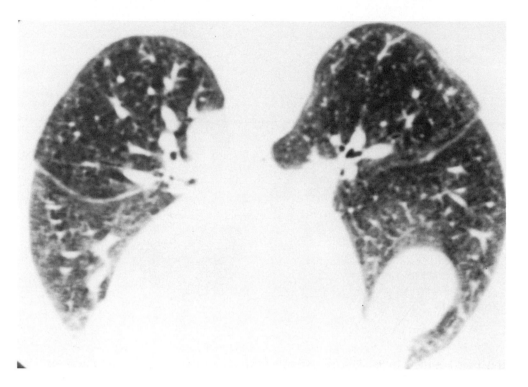

FIGURE 4–68 ■ Asbestosis in an occupationally exposed shipyard worker. HRCT scan demonstrates multifocal areas of peripheral interstitial thickening at nondependent sites. A subpleural line is visible on the right side.

disease demonstrate at least some plaques on HRCT. In occupationally exposed individuals, the incidence of HRCT abnormality suggestive of asbestosis when the chest radiograph shows normal lung parenchyma varies with the age of the population and the extent of exposure. In our experience in a population with heavy shipyard exposure and long latency, the percentage is between 15 and 25 per cent. This range would concur with the known incidence of pathologic fibrosis not seen on chest radiographs in this type of population. Aberle and colleagues[36] investigated 100 asbestos-exposed workers. They found that of 45 patients who fulfilled the usual clinical criteria

for asbestosis, HRCT demonstrated abnormal lung parenchyma in 43. In 55 patients with normal chest radiographs, parenchymal abnormalities were present in 30 and highly suggestive of asbestosis in 20. They also found a positive correlation between the results of HRCT and pulmonary function studies, indicating a restrictive pattern of respiratory dysfunction.

Staples and colleagues[247] studied asbestos-exposed individuals with normal chest radiographs to determine the functional importance of parenchymal disease found only with HRCT. HRCT of the lung parenchyma was normal in 76 patients and sugges-

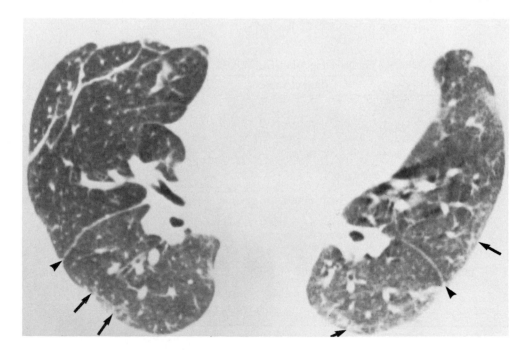

FIGURE 4–69 ■ Asbestosis with long scars. HRCT scan through the lower lobes shows bilateral posterior displacement of the major fissures (arrowheads). Focal areas of irregular interstitial thickening (arrows) are seen. Several long scars are present in the middle lobe, terminating in anterior pleural plaques.

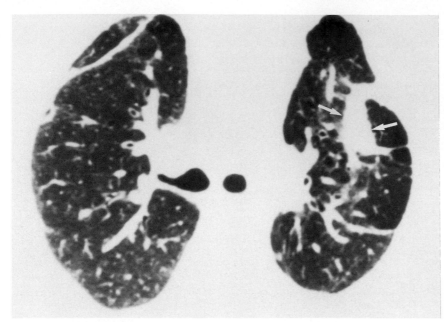

FIGURE 4–70 ■ Asbestos exposure with diffuse pleural thickening and an irregular cicatricial mass. HRCT scan demonstrates a diffusely abnormal lung. An irregular 2 × 4–cm mass (arrows) extends into the left upper lobe from an area of diffuse pleural thickening (seen on soft tissue window settings). The mass was unchanged over two years.

tive of asbestosis in 57. The 57 patients with abnormal findings on HRCT had significantly reduced lung function, indicative of a restrictive defect. This suggests that HRCT can show mild asbestosis not visible radiographically.

Individuals with occupational exposure to asbestos are at risk for developing lung masses. These masses include fissural pleural plaques, rounded atelectasis, fibrous masses, mesothelioma, and bronchogenic carcinoma (Figs. 4–70 and 4–71).[248–251] CT is useful for evaluating these patients and can frequently differentiate between benign and malignant masses. One such benign mass is rounded atelectasis; the CT features suggestive of this entity are contiguity of the mass with an area of diffuse pleural thickening, a lentiform or wedge shape to the mass, volume loss in the lobe containing the mass, and a "comet tail" of vessels and bronchi entering the mass.[249–251] On

CT, the mass of rounded atelectasis may have a lower density center, contain air bronchograms, and have calcific foci.

CT and especially HRCT have shown that visceral pleural plaques are more common than previously thought. Lynch and colleagues[250] found ten fissural plaques in 260 exposed individuals. HRCT can readily identify the plaques as intrafissural, and additional evaluation of the lung mass is not considered warranted.

CT has identified a spectrum of fibrotic or cicatricial masses in patients with asbestos exposure and diffuse pleural thickening.[250] Such masses do not have the typical features of rounded atelectasis and must be viewed with suspicion for neoplasms. On CT, benign masses tend to be contiguous with abnormally thickened pleura and have multiple long fibrotic scars radiating from them.

Patients with asbestos exposure are at risk for developing lung carcinoma and mesothelioma.[252, 253] Adenocarcinoma arising in the lower lobe is the most common and may be difficult to detect when pleural and parenchymal fibrosis is present. A high index of suspicion for malignancy must be maintained in these circumstances. Masses that do not demonstrate stability over time or do not have the features of benignity previously described should undergo aspiration needle-biopsy.

The role of CT and HRCT for detecting asbestos-related diseases is both medical and legal, as many of these patients are being evaluated for compensation. In patients with unequivocally abnormal radiographs, CT and HRCT probably do not add additional information. In patients with equivocally abnormal or normal chest radiographs, information can be obtained in a variable proportion of exposed individuals. CT and HRCT can clearly demonstrate pleural and parenchymal disease when chest radiographs are normal. They may also be helpful in

TABLE 4–6 ■ Technique for Detecting Asbestosis with HRCT*

Variable	Desired Value
kV(p)	120–140
mA	110–170
Scan time	2 to 3 sec
Collimation	1.0 to 1.5 mm
Matrix/field of view	512/full
Contrast	None
Positioning	Supine and prone
Scan area	Supine
	Scan 1: Through aortic arch
	Scan 2: Through carina
	Scan 3: Midway between carina and right dome of diaphragm
	Scan 4: Midway between scan 2 and dome of diaphragm
	Scan 5: At right dome of diaphragm
	Scan 6: Midway between right dome of diaphragm and base of right lung
	Prone
	Same as for supine series

*All scans are reconstructed using a high–spatial resolution algorithm.

explaining symptoms or abnormal pulmonary function studies in these subjects. For instance, HRCT can detect unsuspected areas of emphysema unrelated to the asbestos exposure. In exposed patients with a suspected lung mass, CT can help characterize the mass and provide a means for performing a biopsy on lesions suspicious for malignancy. Smoking in association with asbestos inhalation causes radiographic abnormality that can be mistaken for asbestosis.[254] In these cases, HRCT can differentiate between the effects of smoking and those of asbestos exposure.

EMPHYSEMA

Pulmonary emphysema is defined pathologically as an increase in the size of the air spaces distal to the terminal bronchiole, accompanied by destruction of alveolar walls.[255] The diagnosis of emphysema during life, without the availability of lung tissue, is always indirect. Pulmonary function studies rely on demonstrating an increase in airway resistance and a decrease in the surface area of the alveolocapillary membrane.[256, 257] These tests of function are only moderately sensitive and are nonspecific for the precise cause of airflow obstruction. The conventional chest radiograph is also insensitive for the detection of emphysema when hyperinflation and vascular attenuation are the criteria for diagnosis.[258, 259] CT is more sensitive than the chest radiograph in identifying emphysema and is more accurate in determining the extent of parenchymal destruction.[260-262] Emphysema on CT images is characterized by areas of low attenuation without definable walls, associated with diminished, attenuated, and frequently distorted pulmonary vessels (Fig. 4–72). We have observed that when emphysema involves an entire secondary lobule, the appearances may mimic that of a 1- to 2-cm cyst with its walls formed by the interstitial septa of the lobule.

The types of emphysema are classified pathologically by their sites within the lung and their position within the secondary pulmonary lobule. Four principal types are recognized: centrilobular, panacinar or panlobular, paraseptal, and irregular (Table 4–7).[255, 261]

Centrilobular emphysema involves destruction of the central portion of the lobule surrounding the respiratory bronchiole. In mild and moderate cases, it forms well-circumscribed holes within the lobules, surrounded by relatively normal parenchyma. The abnormalities seen on CT at lung window settings range from punctate dark grey or black holes against a normal homogeneous light grey background to more extensive areas of confluent destruction. In mild emphysema, the pulmonary vessels are normal, but with more severe destruction, the vessels are pruned and attenuated. An upper lobe distribution is characteristic. Hruban and colleagues[263] studied postmortem lung specimens with HRCT, and Foster and co-workers[264] studied 25 cases of pathologically proved centrilobular emphysema in individuals who had premortem CT scans. Both groups found a good correlation between the severity of emphysema on postmortem lung slices and certain CT features of emphysema. Of these features, nonperipheral areas of low attenuation had the best correlation with pathologic disease. In our experience, HRCT is better than conventional CT for detecting subtle low-density areas without definable walls and should be used for this purpose.

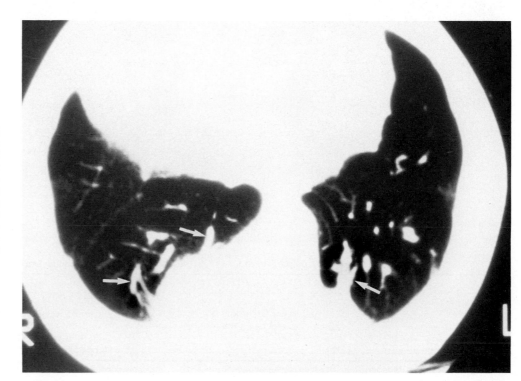

FIGURE 4–71 ■ Asbestos-related diffuse pleural thickening with bilateral rounded atelectasis. CT scan demonstrates bilateral lower lobe masses with vessels and bronchi *(arrows)* extending into the mass. Soft tissue window settings demonstrated bilateral diffuse pleural thickening. Both major fissures are displaced posteriorly, indicating volume loss in both lower lobes.

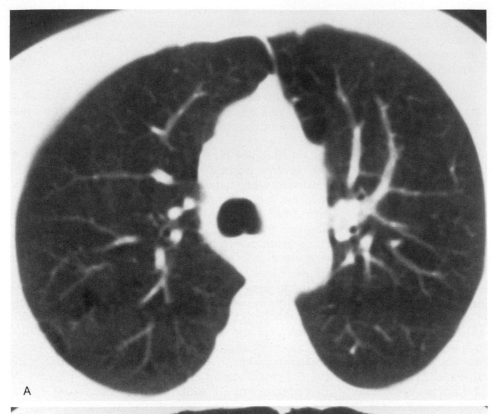

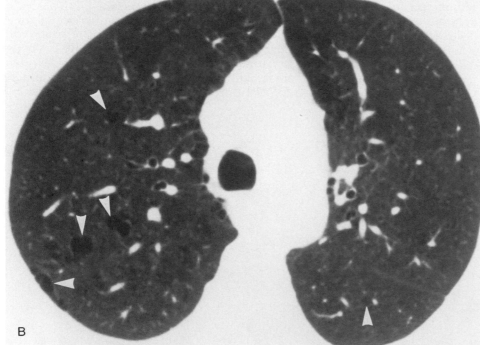

FIGURE 4–72 ■ Mild emphysema in an asymptomatic patient. *A*, Conventional CT scan demonstrates areas of hyperlucency representing emphysema. The lesions are not well seen. *B*, HRCT scan more clearly shows the areas of emphysema *(arrowheads)*. Several of the lucency spaces do not have visible walls. Lucent areas adjacent to the mediastinum represent paraseptal emphysema and not honeycomb lung.

TABLE 4–7 ■ Comparison of CT in Centrilobular (CLE) and Panlobular Emphysema (PLE)

	CLE	PLE
Distribution	Upper lobes	Lower lobes
Appearance	Scattered to confluent low-density areas with normal parenchyma intervening	Diffuse low-density areas with little normal parenchyma
Vascular pruning	In severe CLE	In moderate or severe PLE
Vascular branching angles	Usually < 80°	Frequently > 80°

Source: Adapted from The Journal of Thoracic Imaging, Vol. 1, No. 2, p. 94, with permission of Aspen Publishers, Inc., © 1986.

Panlobular emphysema is located predominantly in the lower lobes. This distribution may be seen on the chest radiograph but is better appreciated on CT. It is the result of uniform destruction of the pulmonary lobule and is seen as widespread areas of low CT density. The pulmonary vessels are usually narrower than normal, with fewer branches and increased branching angles.[261] Advanced panlobular emphysema is likely to be more diffuse in distribution but cannot be distinguished from advanced centrilobular emphysema. The classic form of panlobular emphysema is that associated with alpha₁-antitrypsin deficiency.

Paraseptal emphysema involves the peripheral portion of the acinus and is therefore most striking adjacent to the pleura, interlobular septa, vessels, and airways. HRCT is required to detect paraseptal emphysema when the emphysematous spaces are less than 0.5 cm in diameter (Fig. 4–73). Often, subpleural emphysema is not seen on the chest radiograph, but is visible as areas of low attenuation on CT. Subpleural bullae are considered to be a manifestation of paraseptal emphysema, although they may be seen in all types of emphysema and as an isolated phenomenon. CT commonly shows subpleural bullae at three sites: in the azygoesophageal

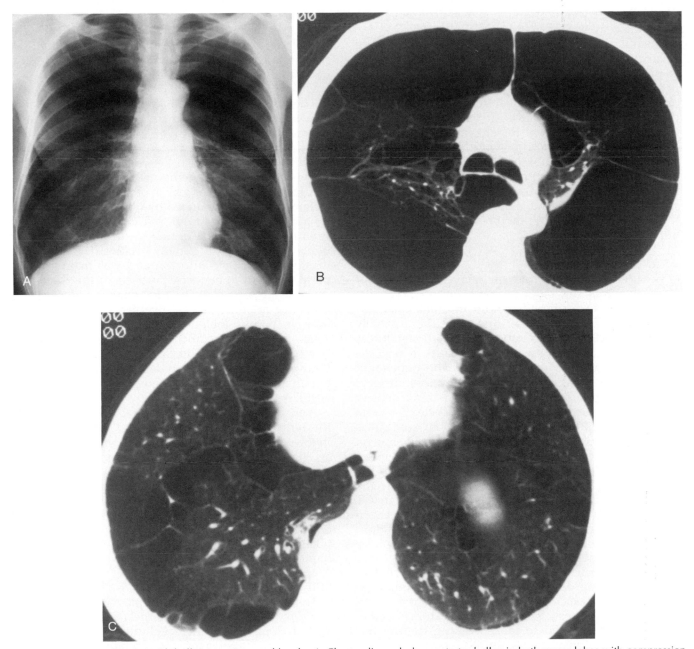

FIGURE 4–73 ■ Emphysema with bullae in a 43-year-old male. *A,* Chest radiograph demonstrates bullae in both upper lobes with compression of the lower lobes. *B* and *C,* HRCT scan through the middle and lower lungs demonstrates large avascular bullae in both upper and lower lobes. The lung compressed by the bullae also is markedly abnormal and contains numerous thin-walled cystic spaces and areas of confluent emphysema. The patient will not benefit from resection of the bullae because of extensive emphysema in both lungs.

recess behind the right main stem bronchus, adjacent to the left ventricle, and near the anterior junctional line.

Irregular or cicatricial emphysema is found around scars within the lung and involves the lobule irregularly. This type of emphysema may accompany many conditions causing lung scarring, such as sarcoidosis. It is seen prominently in patients with complicated silicosis who have developed progressive massive fibrosis.[236] Frequently the extent of irregular emphysema seen on chest radiographs is obscured by the scarring process, and emphysema associated with fibrosis is most easily recognized on CT. However, this type of emphysema may also be seen with microscopic fibrosis, in which case the distinction between irregular and centrilobular emphysema may be impossible.

Several authors have correlated the extent and severity of emphysema as seen on CT with the results of pulmonary function studies.[260, 265, 266] In general, a positive correlation is found with measures of airflow obstruction and alveolar wall destruction. The early detection of emphysema is of growing importance because of the potential for enzymatic replacement treatment of the disease[267–269] and as an inducement for patients to stop smoking. We have found a group of patients with normal chest radiographs and without airflow obstruction who demonstrate emphysema on HRCT. CT and especially HRCT may prove to be the most scientific method for the early detection of emphysema.

LUNG DENSITOMETRY

The density of the normal lung consists of four main elements: air; blood; walls of bronchi, vessels, and alveoli; and interstitial fluid in small quantity. The density of the normal lung is neither spatially nor temporally homogeneous. Gravitational forces on the lung cause a gradient that results in regional variation in air and blood volume. The dependent portion of the lung contains relatively less air (gas) and more fluid. Temporal changes in lung density occur during the normal respiratory cycle.[270, 271] The density of the lung and the gravitational gradient is greatest on expiration. Robinson and Kreel[271] showed that with patients in the supine position, the mean CT density (attenuation value) was −766.2 H in the posterior third of the lung and −844.4 H in the anterior third. This anteroposterior gradient in CT density varied from 36 to 188 H at suspended neutral respiration and from 20 to 68 H on deep inspiration. These CT findings are similar to those shown by other investigators.[272–274]

Many abnormalities of the lung are reflected in changes in lung density. The noninvasive quantitation of lung disease by the measurement of lung density has interested many investigators. Several methods can be used to measure lung density, including fluorodensitometry and videodensitometry, microwave transmission, electrical impedance, Compton scatter, and CT.[274–279] Of these methods,

only CT scanning precisely delineates the anatomic localization of the density measurement.[280] The lung is technically the most difficult region of the body for quantitative CT densitometry, because density varies greatly within the thorax and motion degrades the measurements.

Pulmonary emphysema is characterized pathologically by enlargement of the terminal air spaces of the lung with destruction of alveolar walls. As anticipated, CT densitometry in patients with advanced emphysema shows that the lungs are distinctly less dense than normal.[260, 281, 282] In the study by Rosenblum and colleagues,[282] the mean CT density of the lungs in patients with emphysema was −860 to −912 H, compared with a density of −742 H for normal patients. Similar reductions in mean CT numbers have been found by Goddard and associates[260] and Gould and co-workers.[281] Another feature is that the normal anteroposterior gravitational CT density gradient of the lungs was small and inconsistent.

Quantitation of pulmonary edema by quantitative CT densitometry has been studied only under experimental conditions in animals. Utell and colleagues[283] detected an increase in lung CT density in pulmonary edema induced by intravenous infusion of air. They found a close correlation between lung density and postmortem measurements of pulmonary edema. Hedlund and co-workers[284] studied normotensive pulmonary edema induced by oleic acid injury to the lung in dogs. They found that CT density increased from a mean of −802 H to a mean of −757 H. The initial increase in CT density occurred 15 to 30 minutes after oleic acid infusion and was mainly in the periphery and dependent portions of the lung. The increase in lung density presumably reflects accumulation of fluid in the alveolar spaces. The dog lung is poorly lobulated with a small interstitial space, and edema fluid will accumulate predominantly in the alveoli. The clinical application of quantitative CT densitometry in detection and assessment of pulmonary edema is not known, and the technique is still experimental.

A modification of quantitative CT densitometry of the lung was studied by Gur and associates[285] and involved the inhalation of inert xenon gas. They used an 80 per cent concentration of xenon and found CT density typically increased by 50 to 90 H at 2 minutes. Serial CT scans were used to measure the washout of xenon from the lungs over time. Damaged areas of lung demonstrated decreased CT enhancement and delayed washout. The exciting possibility of obtaining regional ventilation with high spatial resolution requires further study.[286]

MRI OF DIFFUSE LUNG DISEASE

The lung represents a unique challenge to MR imaging. The lungs are the largest organ in the body with a combined average volume of 8.6 L, most of which is air.[287] However, the combined weight of the two lungs is only approximately 1000 grams, giving an average density of 0.23, less than any other organ in the body. Furthermore, the 300 million alveoli that make up the lung have a surface area of approximately 143 m², creating a huge tissue-air interface. At any one instant, the lungs contain a total blood volume of 200 mL and therefore less than 1.4 mL of blood per m² of lung surface area. Apart from the blood vessels and contained blood, the lung parenchyma is predominantly collagen and elastin, which constitute the supporting structures of the lung. The interstitium also contains a small amount of extracellular fluid.

MR signal intensity depends on the proton density and relaxation properties of imaged tissue. In the larger pulmonary vessels, most of the signal comes from flowing blood. Techniques for imaging larger pulmonary vessels and quantitating flow within them are discussed earlier in this chapter. GRASS and other gradient-recalled sequences can provide acceptable signal-to-noise ratios for imaging proximal pulmonary vessels. Hatabu and colleagues[288] have demonstrated sixth- and seventh-order pulmonary vessels using GRASS images obtained during breath holding with dual surface coils and ECG gating. Phase contrast imaging techniques have also been developed to use the phenomenon of phase shift in moving spins to estimate arterial blood flow.[289]

The precise structures that contribute to the low but measurable MR signal from normal lung parenchyma are not well understood. One suggestion is that static lung tissue including collagen, elastin, and extracellular fluid accounts for 85 to 88 per cent of the observed signal and that slowly moving blood in the capillary network accounts for approximately 12 to 15 per cent on ECG-gated images.[290] The MR signal from normal lung parenchyma, using conventional MR sequences, is limited, in part because of the low proton density of the lung and the short T2 relaxation times of static lung tissue. The major limitation in obtaining signal from normal lung parenchyma, however, is the effect of magnetic susceptibility.[17, 18] The magnetic susceptibility effect in MR imaging refers to inhomogeneity of the magnetic field created by differences in diamagnetic susceptibilities between two substances, as in air-tissue interfaces in the lung. This local inhomogeneity of the magnetic field causes a marked decrease and degradation of the signal from lung structures. This effect can be quantitated by measuring the tissue-induced free induction decay (FID) rate $(T'_2)^{-1} \times (T'_2)^{-1} = K.B._0 + 1/T2$, when K = a constant and B_0 = the magnetic field strength.

The FID rate increases with increasing field strength (B_0) and with lung inflation.[291] Signal loss from magnetic susceptibility affects gradient-recalled images more than spin-echo images because of the lack of a refocusing pulse with the former technique. Therefore gradient-recalled sequences can demonstrate blood flow in larger vessels but have greater loss of signal from the lung parenchyma. MR techniques to image lung parenchyma must minimize the effects of magnetic susceptibility. One of several possible approaches to this problem is to use very short echo times to decrease the effects of magnetic susceptibility and increase signal from tissues with very short T2 relaxation times. The quantitation of lung tissue signal by MR offers potential application for certain abnormalities such as pulmonary edema. Lung water content has been shown to correlate with signal intensity and T1 and T2 relaxation times.[292-294] Carroll and colleagues[295] have shown a gravity-dependent gradient of signal intensity in lungs of normal volunteers and in sheep with increased hydrostatic pulmonary pressures. A linear relationship has been found between relaxation times and extravascular lung water in permeability edema induced in rats.[296] Schmidt and colleagues[292] induced permeability edema by intravenous injection of oleic acid in rats and compared signal intensity and relaxation rates in different types of pulmonary edema. They found differences in distribution of edema, greater increase in signal intensity, and longer T2 relaxation rates in rats with increased permeability pulmonary edema when compared with rats with hydrostatic edema. These studies suggest an experimental role for MR for determining severity of pulmonary edema and possibly for demonstrating differences between the two types of edema. The complexity of MR, however, precludes its clinical use for monitoring pulmonary edema.

Variations in signal intensity and relaxation parameters have been reported in various lung disorders. An increase in T2 values has been observed in rat lungs after bleomycin-induced lung injury in the absence of increased water content.[297, 298] An increase in cellularity in bleomycin-damaged lungs was found by Taylor and colleagues,[297] who postulated that the prolonged T2 was the result of a change in intracellular water and in the macromolecular composition of the lung. No change was observed in T1 relaxation rates. In the later stages of bleomycin-induced inflammation, Vinitski and colleagues[298] found a decrease in T1 and T2 values as the alveolitis developed into fibrosis.

Limited attempts have been made to correlate signal intensity with diffuse inflammatory lung diseases in patients. T1 shortening was reported in alveolar proteinosis by Moore and colleagues (see Fig. 4–12).[299] Preferential T2 shortening has been described in pulmonary hemosiderosis associated with increased signal on T1-weighted images.[209] The marked T2 shortening is caused by deposition of paramagnetic ferric irons in the lungs of these patients. Specificity of the signal characteristics described in these diseases remains to be determined.

As yet there has been little documentation of the MR appearance of diffuse fibrotic lung diseases, but MR offers the potential for distinguishing active inflammation from fibrosis.[300] The MR appearance of focal pulmonary fibrosis has been described and frequently is different from the signal characteristics of tumor.[140] There remains considerable overlap in relaxation rates, and therefore the reliability of distinguishing fibrosis from tumor has yet to be established. MR features of diffuse pulmonary hemorrhage also have yet to be determined.

Accurate documentation of MR patterns of signal abnormalities in diffuse lung disease awaits the development of techniques with shorter echo times and other methods for improving MR image resolution in the lungs.

Pulmonary Parenchymal Versus Pleural Disease

It can be difficult to distinguish between abnormalities of the pleural space and those of the peripheral lung parenchyma. This distinction is important, because the diagnosis and treatment of disease in the pleural space often differs from that involving the lung. For example, an empyema requires immediate drainage, whereas a lung abscess may respond to conservative therapy with antibiotics.[301] CT scanning is indicated whenever chest radiographs and fluoroscopy do not clearly establish the site of abnormality.

Pugatch and co-workers[302] studied 75 patients with diagnostically problematic disease of the pleura, pulmonary parenchyma, or both. In 28 per cent of the patients, information from the CT scans aided in diagnosis or altered management of the patient. In another 40 per cent, CT scans helped clarify the site and extent of the disease but did not alter therapy.

CT guidelines have been established for distinguishing pleural from parenchymal disease. Obtuse angles with the chest wall and sharp interphases with the lung parenchyma characterize pleural or extraparenchymal lesions. Parenchymal lesions usually form acute angles with the chest wall, and their margins are well or poorly defined. Several investigators[153, 154, 303] have tested additional criteria for improving the distinction between a lung abscess and an empyema (Fig. 4–74). A lung abscess tends to be spherical and without significant change in shape with patient position. In contrast, an empyema conforms to the pleural space, is generally more lentiform in shape, and is more mobile with change in position. A pleural mass or fluid collection displaces lung structures, compressing and distorting adjacent bronchi vessels, in contrast to an abscess, in which adjacent structures are involved and less likely to be displaced. The walls of a lung abscess are most frequently thick and irregular, whereas the walls of an empyema tend to be thin and smoother. Stark and co-workers[153] found, in addition, that with empyemas, when intravenous contrast material is administered, the separated visceral and parietal pleura are enhanced and visible on CT. Features that are not helpful in distinguishing lung abscess from empyema include air within the lesion, multiple lesions, additional free-flowing pleural fluid, septations within the lesion, and subjacent pulmonary consolidation.

In our experience, CT scans are better than sonograms in localizing empyema for drainage. The CT finding of multiple septations within an empyema can indicate that a simple thoracostomy tube will not be successful for drainage. The site of the empyema should be marked on the patient's skin while the patient is still in position on the scanner table. Diagnostic aspiration of an empyema can also be undertaken using CT guidance (see also Chapter 8).

Marked pleural thickening or a large pleural effu-

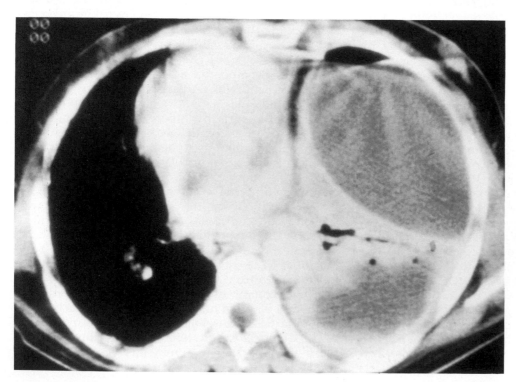

FIGURE 4–74 ■ Empyema and lung abscess. CT scan demonstrates both an empyema and a lung abscess on the left side. The anteriorly situated empyema shows a smooth inner margin and an enhancing pleural wall. Posteriorly, the lung abscess has an irregular inner margin and no enhancing pleural wall. The compressed left lower lobe containing the abscess does enhance with contrast material. The empyema was drained and the lung abscess treated with antibiotics. Both lesions contain air, which does not help differentiate one from another.

sion can make conventional radiographs uninterpretable. In these situations, CT scans can often demonstrate any parenchymal, hilar, or mediastinal abnormalities that may be present. Extension of the pleural process to the chest wall may also be detected first from CT scans.

Indications for CT and MRI of the Lungs

Since 1980, major advances have been made in the application of CT and HRCT to the evaluation of thoracic disease. The promise of MR imaging, however, remains elusive, awaiting further improvements in scanner technology.

In patients with proved or suspected malignancy, CT is a primary imaging modality. In patients with extrathoracic neoplasms, CT is the most sensitive technique for the detection of pulmonary metastases. Most pulmonary nodules 2 to 4 mm in diameter are visible on CT, whereas noncalcified nodules of less than 6 to 10 mm in diameter can remain undetected on conventional chest radiographs. MR can occasionally demonstrate a central nodule that has been mistaken for a blood vessel on CT. However, MR has not replaced CT for the detection of pulmonary nodules. In an occasional patient being evaluated for resection of metastatic pulmonary nodules, both imaging modalities may be considered. HRCT for detection of lymphangitic dissemination of tumor within the lungs has application and in the appropriate setting can be diagnostic for that condition.

CT scanning to detect an occult primary lung tumor can benefit those patients who present with malignant cells in their sputum and a normal chest radiograph or patients with a paraneoplastic syndrome and no convincing neoplasm on chest radiographs. HRCT, with or without nodule densitometry, has a role in characterizing solid nodules less than 2 cm in diameter as benign. Visual demonstration of certain patterns of calcification or of fat can indicate benignity. For the remainder, nodule densitometry, using a standard phantom or the numeric printout of the CT pixel values, may show the nodule as diffusely, finely calcified. This technique is standard practice for evaluation of solitary pulmonary nodules indeterminate for malignancy on conventional radiographs.

In most patients with proved or suspected bronchogenic carcinoma, CT scans are obtained to determine the extent of disease; the extent of invasion of the chest wall, mediastinum, and diaphragm; and the presence of occult extrathoracic metastasis to liver and adrenal glands. MR may be marginally better than CT for demonstrating the degree of chest wall or mediastinal invasion but has no clear advantages over CT.

A frequent clinical problem is an abnormality on a chest radiograph suspicious for a mass. In our experience, CT usually clarifies the situation and resolves the enigma, frequently demonstrating that the suspected lesion is part of a rib or a benign confluence of vessels.

CT-guided biopsy of pulmonary masses or nodules is well established. In our practice, we use CT more frequently than fluoroscopy. The rapid reconstruction times of new scanners have resulted in a procedure that is as quick, convenient, low in complications, and more precise than biplane fluoroscopy.

The use of CT scanning of the thorax for radiation therapy planning is routine. Many radiation oncology departments have their own CT scanners with direct coupling to therapy units. This application has largely moved out of the realm of diagnostic radiology.

Detection of recurrent intrathoracic tumor after resection is a complex clinical problem. Both CT and MR can detect enlarged hilar or mediastinal nodes and chest wall masses. In our experience, confirmed by unpublished studies, MR is preferable for finding recurrent tumor in the chest wall or pleural space after pneumonectomy. The high tumor-to–chest wall contrast of MR facilitates detection of tumor.

Detection and characterization of focal inflammatory lesions, especially in the immunocompromised patient, has not been widely reported using CT. However, CT is able to detect focal masses that may be septic emboli. Certain characteristics of inflammatory masses, such as a lower density around the mass and the relationship of the mass to adjacent blood vessels, may suggest the likelihood of an infection. CT may also detect early cavitation or abscess formation in an area of pneumonia. In the appropriate clinical setting, CT is very useful for evaluating complex pleuroparenchymal infection. CT can readily detect an empyema obscured by an indolent pneumonia. It also can frequently distinguish between a lung abscess and an empyema. MR has not shown any advantages over CT for these purposes.

HRCT has rapidly gained acceptance in the evaluation of many interstitial lung processes. In certain diffuse lung diseases, the HRCT findings are sufficiently characteristic to be highly suggestive of that specific disease. In fibrotic diseases, HRCT can distinguish between those abnormalities that are indicative of an end-stage, often burned out, fibrotic process and a more active inflammation that may be responsive to treatment.

In patients being treated for known diffuse lung disease, HRCT can be used to follow the course of the disease. For instance, in the treatment of sarcoidosis or idiopathic pulmonary fibrosis, HRCT at 3- to 6-month intervals can demonstrate a change in the pattern, extent, and severity of morphologic abnormality. The abnormalities responsive to treatment include nodules, interstitial thickening, and ground-glass densities. Long scars, honeycombing, and destructive lung cysts are usually not responsive.

Amongst the pneumoconioses, both silicosis and asbestosis have been studied using CT and HRCT. In silicosis, CT may detect occult masses that do not have the characteristic features of benign fibrotic masses. CT may also detect occult emphysema and elucidate the cause of dyspnea in a patient with silicosis. In asbestosis, HRCT is more sensitive than chest radiographs for detecting lung and pleural disease. CT and HRCT may also distinguish between benign and malignant lung or pleural masses seen in association with asbestos inhalation.

In the detection of emphysema, HRCT has been shown to be more sensitive than chest radiographs and may be more sensitive than pulmonary function studies. HRCT can define the extent of abnormalities and grade the severity of emphysema. In patients with obstructive pulmonary physiology or a low carbon monoxide diffusing capacity, HRCT may explain the abnormal function by demonstrating sites of emphysema.

Vascular lesions of the lung that have been studied with CT and MR include pulmonary emboli and various vascular malformations. CT and MR can noninvasively establish the diagnosis of an arteriovenous malformation in most instances. Both CT and MR can demonstrate central pulmonary emboli. This is useful for patients in whom recurrent emboli is the suspected cause of chronic pulmonary hypertension. Neither CT nor MR has gained acceptance for evaluation of patients with suspected acute pulmonary emboli.

HRCT has become the definitive imaging modality for suspected bronchiectasis, replacing bronchography. In many patients with chronic cough, HRCT is able to detect and locate radiographically unapparent sites of bronchiectasis.

CT and HRCT are the established imaging modalities for many patients with focal, multifocal, or diffuse lung diseases. We have used these modalities to detect and localize diseases, as well as to explain chest symptoms or abnormal results of pulmonary function studies. The specificity of HRCT for individual diseases is now being established. Although MR has gained widespread use in neurologic and musculoskeletal imaging, its application in the lung is limited and experimental. The small amounts of normal tissue and magnetic susceptibility problems have restricted its use in pulmonary imaging.

References

1. Frija J, Schmit P, Katz M, Vadrot D, Laval-Jeantet M: Computed tomography of the pulmonary fissures: normal anatomy. J Comput Assist Tomogr 6:1069, 1982.
2. Proto AV, Ball JB Jr: Computed tomography of the major and minor fissures. AJR 140:439, 1983.
3. Marks BW, Kuhns LR: Identification of the pleural fissures with computed tomography. Radiology 143:139, 1982.
4. Goodman LR, Golkow RS, Steiner RM, Teplick SK, Haskin ME, et al: The right mid-lung window: a potential source of error in computed tomography of the lung. Radiology 143:135, 1982.
5. Zerhouni EA, Naidich DP, Stitik FP, Khouri NF, Siegelman SS: Computed tomography of the pulmonary parenchyma. Part 2: interstitial disease. J Thorac Imaging 1:54, 1985.
6. Godwin JD, Tarver RD: Accessory fissures of the lung. AJR 144:39, 1985.
7. Berkmen YM, Auh YH, Davis SD, Kazam E: Anatomy of the minor fissure: evaluation with thin-section CT. Radiology 170:647, 1989.
8. Mayo JR, Muller NL, Henkelman RM: The double-fissure sign: a motion artifact on thin-section CT scans. Radiology 165:580, 1987.
9. Aberle DR, Gamsu G, Ray CS, Feuerstein IM: Asbestos-related pleural and parenchymal fibrosis: detection with high-resolution CT. Radiology 166:729, 1988.
10. Bergin C, Roggli V, Coblentz C, Chiles C: The secondary pulmonary lobule: normal and abnormal CT appearances. AJR 151:21, 1988.
11. Reid L: The connective tissue septae in the adult human lung. Thorax 14:138, 1959.
12. Heitzman ER. Subsegmental anatomy of the lung. In Heitzman ER (ed): The Lung: Radiologic-Pathologic Correlations, 2nd ed. St Louis, CV Mosby, 1984, p 42.
13. Spirt BA. Value of the prone position in detecting pulmonary nodules by computed tomography. J Comput Assist Tomogr 4:871, 1980.
14. Heitzman ER. Computed tomography of the thorax: current perspectives. AJR 136:2, 1981.
15. Mayo JR, Webb WR, Gould R, Stein MG, Bass I, et al: High-resolution CT of the lungs: an optimal approach. Radiology 163:507, 1987.
15a. Zwirewich CV, Terriff B, Muller NL: High-spatial-frequency (bone) algorithm improves quality of standard CT of the thorax. AJR 153:1169, 1989.
16. Grenier P, Maurice F, Musset D, Menu Y, Nahum H: Bronchiectasis: assessment by thin-section CT. Radiology 161:95, 1986.
17. Gamsu G, Sostman D: Magnetic resonance imaging of the thorax. Am Rev Respir Dis 139:254, 1989.
18. Spritzer C, Gamsu G, Sostman HD: Magnetic resonance imaging of the thorax: techniques, current applications, and future directions. J Thorac Imag 4:1, 1989.
19. Naidich DP, Zerhouni EA, Hutchins GM, Genieser NB, McCauley DI, Siegelman SS: Computed tomography of the pulmonary parenchyma. Part I: distal air-space disease. J Thorac Imag 1:39, 1985.
20. Itoh H, Tokunaga S, Asamoto H, Furuta M, Funamoto Y, et al: Radiologic pathologic correlations of small lung nodules with special reference to peribronchiolar nodules. AJR 130:223, 1978.
21. Newell JD, Underwood GH Jr, Russo DJ, Bruno PP, Wilkerson GR, Black ML: Computed tomographic appearance of pulmonary alveolar proteinosis in adults. J Comput Assist Tomogr 8:21, 1984.
22. McCook TA, Kirks DR, Merten DF, Osborne DR, Spock A, Pratt PC: Pulmonary alveolar proteinosis in children. AJR 137:1023, 1981.
23. Godwin JD, Muller NL, Takasugi JE: Pulmonary alveolar proteinosis: CT findings. Radiology 169:609, 1988.
23a. Mayo JR, Muller NL, Road J, Sisler J, Lillington G: Chronic eosinophilic pneumonia: CT findings in six cases. AJR 153:727, 1989.
24. Metzger RA, Mulhern CB, Arger PH, Coleman BG, Epstein DM, Gefter WB: CT differentiation of solitary from diffuse bronchioloalveolar carcinoma. J Comput Assist Tomogr 5:830, 1981.
25. Epstein DM, Gefter WB, Miller WT: Lobar bronchioloalveolar cell carcinoma. AJR 139:463, 1982.
25a. Im J, Han MC, Yu EJ, Han JK, Park JM, Kim C, Seo JW, Yoon Y, Lee JD, Lee KS: Lobar bronchioloalveolar carcinoma: "angiogram sign" on CT scans. Radiology 176:749, 1990.
26. Nakata H, Kimoto T, Nakayama T, Kido M, Miyazaki N, Harrada S: Diffuse peripheral lung disease: evaluation by high-resolution computed tomography. Radiology 157:181, 1985.
27. Bergin CJ, Muller NL: CT in the diagnosis of interstitial lung disease. AJR 145:505, 1985.
28. Muller NL, Miller RR, Wenn WR, Evans KG, Ostrow DN:

Fibrosing alveolitis: CT-pathologic correlation. Radiology 160:585, 1986.

29. Meziane MA, Hruban RH, Zerhouni EA, Wheeler PS, Khouri NF, et al: High resolution CT of the lung parenchyma with pathologic correlation. Radiographics 8:27, 1988.

30. Webb WR, Stein MG, Finkbeiner WE, Im J-G, Lynch D, Gamsu G: Normal and diseased isolated lungs: high-resolution CT. Radiology 166:81, 1988.

31. Yoshimura H, Hatakeyama M, Otsuji H, Maeda M, Ohishi H, et al: Pulmonary asbestosis: CT study of subpleural curvilinear shadow. Radiology 158:653, 1986.

32. Sison RF, Hruban RH, Moore GW, Kuhlman JE, Wheeler PS, Hutchins GM: Pulmonary disease associated with pleural "asbestos" plaques. Chest 95:831, 1989.

33. Westcott JL, Cole SR: Traction bronchiectasis in end-stage pulmonary fibrosis. Radiology 161:665, 1986.

33a. Remy-Jardin M, Beuscart R, Sault MC, Marquette CH, Remy J: Subpleural micronodules in diffuse infiltrative lung diseases: evaluation with thin-section CT scans. Radiology 177:133, 1990.

34. Muller NL, Staples CA, Miller RR, Vedal S, Thurlbeck WM, Ostrow DN: Disease activity in idiopathic pulmonary fibrosis: CT and pathologic correlation. Radiology 165:731, 1987.

34a. Muller N, Staples CA, Miller R: Bronchiolitis obliterans organizing pneumonia: CT features in 14 patients. AJR 154:983, 1990.

35. Staples CA, Muller NL, Vedal S, Abboud R, Ostrow D, Miller RR: Usual interstitial pneumonia: correlation of CT with clinical, functional, and radiologic findings. Radiology 162:377, 1987.

36. Aberle DR, Gamsu G, Ray CS: High-resolution CT of benign asbestos-related diseases: clinical and radiographic correlation. AJR 151:883, 1988.

37. Bergin CL, Coblentz CL, Chiles C, Bell DY, Castellino RA: Chronic lung diseases: specific diagnosis using CT. AJR 152:1183, 1989.

38. Naidich DP: Pulmonary parenchymal high-resolution CT: to be or not to be. Radiology 171:22, 1989.

38a. Schurawitzki H, Stiglbauer R, Graninger W, Herold C, Polzleitner D, Burghuber OC, Tscholakoff D: Interstitial lung disease in progressive systemic sclerosis: high-resolution CT versus radiography. Radiology 176:755, 1990.

39. Muhn JR, Brown LR, Crowe JK, Sheedy PF II, Hattery RR, Stephens DH: Comparison of whole lung tomography and computed tomography for detecting pulmonary nodules. AJR 131:981, 1978.

40. Shaner EG, Chang AE, Doppman JL, Concle DM, Flye MW, Rosenberg SA: Comparison of computed and conventional whole lung tomography in detecting pulmonary nodules: a prospective radiologic-pathologic study. AJR 131:51, 1978.

41. Vanel D, Henry-Amar M, Lumbroso J, Lemalet E, Couanet D, et al: Pulmonary evaluation of patients with osteosarcoma: roles of standard radiology, tomography, CT, scintigraphy, and tomoscintigraphy. AJR 143:519, 1984.

42. Heaston DK, Putman CE, Rodan BA, Nicholson E, Ravin CE, et al: Solitary pulmonary metastases in high-risk melanoma patients: a prospective comparison of conventional and computed tomography. AJR 141:169, 1983.

42a. Peuchot M, Libshitz HI: Pulmonary metastatic disease: radiologic-surgical correlation. Radiology 164:719, 1987.

43. Zerhouni EA: Computed tomographic characterization of focal pulmonary lesions. In Margulis AR, Gooding CA (eds): Diagnostic Radiology. San Francisco, University of California, 1987, p 349.

44. Bateson EM: An analysis of 155 solitary lung lesions illustrating the differential diagnosis of mixed tumors of the lung. Clin Radiol 16:51, 1965.

45. O'Keefe ME, Good CA, McDonald JR: Calcification in solitary nodules of the lung. Am J Roentgenol Radium Ther Nucl Med 77:1023, 1957.

46. Davis EW, Peabody JW Jr, Katz S: The solitary pulmonary nodules. J Thorac Surg 32:728, 1956.

47. Steele JD: The solitary pulmonary nodule. J Thorac Cardiovasc Surg 46:21, 1963.

48. Vance JW, Good CA, Hodgson CH, Kirklin JW, Gage RP: The solitary circumscribed pulmonary lesion due to bronchogenic carcinoma. Dis Chest 36:231, 1959.

49. Walske DR: The solitary pulmonary nodule. Dis Chest 49:302, 1966.

50. Jackman RJ, Good CA, Clagett OT, Woolner LB: Survival rates in peripheral bronchogenic carcinomas up to 4 centimeters in diameter presenting as solitary nodules. J Thorac Cardiovasc Surg 57:1, 1969.

51. Mountain CF: Surgical management of pulmonary metastases. Postgrad Med 48:128, 1970.

52. Lillington GA: The solitary pulmonary nodule—1974. Am Rev Respir Dis 110:699, 1974.

53. Kuriyama K, Tateishi R, Doi O, Kodama K, Tatsuta M, et al: CT-pathologic correlation in small peripheral lung cancers. AJR 149:1139, 1987.

54. Kuhlman JE, Fishman EK, Kuhajda FP, Meziane MM, Khouri NF, et al: Solitary bronchioalveolar carcinoma: CT criteria. Radiology 167:379, 1988.

55. Naidich DP, Sussman R, Kutcher WL, Aranda CP, Garay SM, Ettenger NA: Solitary pulmonary nodules: CT-bronchoscopic correlation. Chest 93:595, 1988.

56. Cann CE, Gamsu G, Birnberg FA, Webb WR: Quantification of calcium in solitary pulmonary nodules using single- and dual-energy CT. Radiology 145:493, 1982.

57. Godwin JS, Fram EK, Cann CE, Gamsu G: CT densitometry of pulmonary nodules: a phantom study. J Comput Assist Tomogr 6:254, 1982.

58. Siegelman SS, Zerhouni EA, Leo FP, Khouri NF, Stitik FP: CT of the solitary pulmonary nodule. AJR 135:1, 1980.

59. Godwin JD, Speckman JM, Fram EK, Johnson GA, Putman CE, et al: Distinguishing benign from malignant pulmonary nodules by computed tomography. Radiology 144:349, 1982.

60. Freundlich IM, Horsely WW, Udall C: Evaluation of pulmonary masses by CT number: a modification of the Siegelman method. Presented at the 67th Annual Meeting of the Radiological Society of North America. Chicago, November 15–19, 1981.

61. Levi C, Gray JE, McCullough EC, Hattery RR: The unreliability of CT numbers as absolute values. AJR 139:443, 1982.

62. Zerhouni EA, Spivey JF, Morgan RH, Leo FP, Stitik FP, Siegelman SS: Factors influencing quantitative CT measurements of solitary pulmonary nodules. J Comput Assist Tomogr 6:1075, 1982.

63. Cann CE: Quantitative CT applications: comparisons of current scanners. Radiology 162:257, 1987.

64. Zerhouni EA, Stitik FP, Siegelman SS, Naidich DP, Dagel SS, et al: CT of the pulmonary nodule: a cooperative study. Radiology 160:319, 1986.

65. Huston J III, Muhm JR: Solitary pulmonary nodules: evaluation with a CT reference phantom. Radiology 170:653, 1989.

66. Proto AV, Thomas SR: Pulmonary nodules studied by computed tomography. Radiology 156:149, 1985.

67. Siegelman SS, Khouri NF, Leo FP, Fishman EK, Braverman RM, Zerhouni EA: Solitary pulmonary nodules: CT assessment. Radiology 160:307, 1986.

68. Im J-G, Gamsu G, Gordon D, Stein MG, Webb WR, et al: CT densitometry of pulmonary nodules in a frozen human thorax. AJR 150:61, 1988.

69. Pearlberg JL, Sandler MA, Beute GH, Madrazo BL: $T_1N_0M_0$ Bronchogenic carcinoma: assessment by CT. Radiology 157:187, 1985.

70. Heavey LR, Glazer GM, Gross BH, Francis IR, Orringer MB: The role of CT in staging radiographic $T_1N_0M_0$ lung cancer. AJR 146:285, 1986.

71. Conces DJ, Klink JF, Tarver RD, Moak GD: T1N0M0 lung cancer: evaluation with CT. Radiology 170:643, 1989.

72. Bateson EM: So-called hamartoma of the lung: a true neoplasm of fibrous connective tissue of the bronchi. Cancer 31:1458, 1973.

73. Ledor K, Fish B, Chaise L, Ledor S: CT diagnosis of pulmonary hamartomas. Comput Tomogr 5:343, 1981.

74. Siegelman SS, Khouri NF, Scott WW, Leo FP, Hamper UM, et al: Pulmonary hamartoma: CT findings. Radiology 160:313, 1986.

75. Muller NL, Gamsu G, Webb WR: Pulmonary nodules: detection using magnetic resonance imaging and computed tomography. Radiology 155:687, 1985.

76. Gamsu G, de Geer G, Cann C, Muller N, Brito A: A preliminary study of MRI quantification of simulated calcified pulmonary nodules. Invest Radiol 22:853, 1987.

77. Kruglik GD, Wayne KS: Occult lung cavity causing hemoptysis: recognition by computed tomography. J Comput Assist Tomogr 4:407, 1980.

78. Breuer R, Baigelman W, Pugatch RD: Occult mycetoma. J Comput Assist Tomogr 6:166, 1982.

78a. Naidich DP, Funt S, Ettenger NA, Arranda C: Hemoptysis: CT-bronchoscopic correlations in 58 cases. Radiology 177:357, 1990.

79. Grzybowski S, Coy P: Early diagnosis of carcinoma of the lung. Cancer 25:113, 1970.

80. Pearson FG, Thompson DW, Delarue NC: Experience with the cytologic detection, localization, and treatment of radiographically undemonstrable bronchial carcinoma. J Thorac Cardiovasc Surg 54:371, 1967.

81. Bower BF, Gordon GS: Hormonal effects of nonendocrine tumors. Ann Rev Med 16:83, 1965.

82. Nathanson I, Hall TC: A spectrum of tumors that produce paraneoplastic syndromes. Lung tumors: how they produce their syndromes. Ann NY Acad Sci 230:367, 1974.

83. Wheeler PS, Stitik FP, Hutchins GM, Klinefelter HF, Siegelman SS: Diagnosis of lipoid pneumonia by computed tomography. JAMA 245:65, 1981.

84. Kuhlman JE, Fishman EK, Burch PA, Karp JE, Zerhouni EA, Siegelman SS: CT of invasive pulmonary aspergillosis. AJR 150:1015, 1988.

84a. Mori M, Galvin JR, Barloon TJ, Gingrich RD, Stanford W: Fungal pulmonary infections after bone marrow transplantation: Evaluation with radiography and CT. Radiology 178:721, 1991.

85. Kuhlman JE, Fishman EK, Siegelman SS: Invasive pulmonary aspergillosis in acute leukemia: characteristic findings on CT, the CT halo sign, and the role of CT in early diagnosis. Radiology 157:611, 1985.

86. Deve F: Une nouvelle forme anatomo-radiologique de mycome pulmonaire primitive. Arch Med Chir App Respir 13:337, 1938.

87. Rafferty P, Biggs AB, Crompton GK, Grant IWB: What happens to patients with pulmonary aspergillosis? Analysis of 23 cases. Thorax 38:579, 1983.

88. Jewkes J, Kay P, Paneth M, Citron KM: Pulmonary aspergilloma: analysis of prognosis in relation to hemoptysis and survey of treatment. Thorax 38:572, 1983.

89. Roberts CM, Citron KM, Strickland B: Intrathoracic aspergilloma: role of CT in diagnosis and treatment. Radiology 165:123, 1987.

89a. Huang R-M, Naidich DP, Lubat E, Schinella R, Garay SM, McCauley DI: Septic pulmonary emboli: CT-radiographic correlation. AJR 153:41, 1989.

89b. Milne ENC, Zerhouni EA: Blood supply of pulmonary metastases. J Thorac Imag 2:15, 1987.

90. American Joint Committee on Cancer: In Oliver OH, Henson DE, Hutter RVP, Myers MH (eds): Manual for Staging of Cancer, 3rd ed. Philadelphia, JB Lippincott, 1988.

91. Scott IR, Muller NL, Miller RR, Evans KG, Nelems B: Resectable stage III lung cancer: CT, surgical, and pathologic correlation. Radiology 166:75, 1988.

92. Friedman PJ: Lung cancer: update on staging classifications. AJR 150:261, 1988.

93. Glazer HS, Duncan-Meyer J, Aromberg DJ, Moran JF, Levitt RG, Sagel SS: Pleural and chest wall invasion in bronchogenic carcinoma: CT evaluation. Radiology 157:191, 1985.

94. Ekholm S, Albrechtsson U, Kugelberg J, Tylen U: Computed tomography in preoperative staging of bronchogenic carcinoma. J Comput Assist Tomogr 4:763, 1980.

95. Rendina EA, Bognolo DA, Mineo TC, Gualdi GF, Caterino M, et al: Computed tomography for the evaluation of intrathoracic invasion by lung cancer. J Thorac Cardiovasc Surg 94:57, 1987.

96. Pennes DR, Glazer GM, Wimbish KJ, Gross BH, Long RW,

97. Orringer MB: Chest wall invasion by lung cancer: limitations of CT evaluation. AJR 144:507, 1985.

97. Haggar AM, Pearlberg JL, Froelich JW, Hearshen DO, Beute GH, et al: Chest-wall invasion by carcinoma of the lung: detection by MR imaging. AJR 148:1075, 1987.

98. Webb WR, Jeffrey RB, Godwin JD: Thoracic computed tomography in superior sulcus tumors. J Comput Assist Tomogr 5:361, 1981.

99. O'Connell RS, McLoud TC, Wilkins EW: Superior sulcus tumor: radiographic diagnosis and workup. AJR 140:25, 1983.

100. Heelan RT, Demas BE, Caravelli JF, Martini N, Bains MS, et al: Superior sulcus tumors: CT and MR imaging. Radiology 170:637, 1989.

101. Vas W, Zylak CJ, Mather D, Figueredo A: The value of abdominal computed tomography in the pre-treatment assessment of small cell carcinoma of the lung. Radiology 138:417, 1981.

102. Nielsen ME Jr, Heaston DK, Dunnick NR, Korobkin M: Preoperative CT evaluation of adrenal glands in non-small cell bronchogenic carcinoma. AJR 139:317, 1982.

103. Sandler MA, Pearlberg JL, Madrazo BL, Gitschlag KF, Gross SC: Computed tomographic evaluation of the adrenal gland in the preoperative assessment of bronchogenic carcinoma. Radiology 145:733, 1982.

104. Poon PY, Feld R, Evans WK, Ege G, Yeoh JL, McLoughlin ML: Computed tomography of the brain, liver, and upper abdomen in the staging of small cell carcinoma of the lung. J Comput Assist Tomogr 6:963, 1982.

105. Oliver TW, Bernardino ME, Miller JI, Mansour K, Greene D, Davis WA: Isolated adrenal masses in nonsmall-cell bronchogenic carcinoma. Radiology 153:217, 1984.

106. Berland LL, Koslin DB, Kenney PJ, Stanley RJ, Lee JY: Differentiation between small benign and malignant adrenal masses with dynamic incremented CT. AJR 151:95, 1988.

107. Hussain S, Belldegrun A, Seltzer SE, Richie JP, Gittes RF, Abrams HL: Differentiation of malignant from benign adrenal masses: predictive indices on computed tomography. AJR 144:61, 1985.

108. Reinig JW, Doppman JL, Dwyer AJ, Frank J: MRI of indeterminate adrenal masses. AJR 147:493, 1986.

109. Glazer GM, Woolsey EJ, Borrello J, Francis IR, Aisen AM, et al: Adrenal tissue characterization using MR imaging. Radiology 158:73, 1986.

110. Chang A, Glazer HS, Lee JKT, Ling D, Heiken JP: Adrenal gland: MR imaging. Radiology 163:123, 1987.

111. Kier R, McCarthy S: MR characterization of adrenal masses: field strength and pulse sequence considerations. Radiology 171:671, 1989.

112. Brinkman GL: The significance of pleural effusion complicating otherwise operable bronchogenic carcinoma. Dis Chest 36:152, 1959.

112a. Muller NL, Miller RR: Computed tomography of chronic diffuse infiltrative lung disease, part 1. Am Rev Respir Dis 142:1206, 1990.

112b. Muller NL, Miller RR: Computed tomography of chronic diffuse infiltrative lung disease, part 2. Am Rev Respir Dis 142:1440, 1990.

113. Byrd RB, Carr DT, Miller WE, Payne WS, Woolner LB: Radiographic abnormalities in carcinoma of the lung as related to histological cell type. Thorax 24:573, 1969.

114. Tscholakoff D, Sechtem U, de Geer G, Schmidt H, Higgins CB: Evaluation of pleural pericardial effusions by magnetic resonance imaging. Eur J Radiol 7:169, 1987.

115. Dahlgren S, Nordenstrom B: Transthoracic Needle Biopsy. Chicago, Year Book Medical, 1966, p 29.

116. Zelch JV, Lalli AP, McCormack LJ, Belovich DM: Aspiration biopsy in diagnosis of pulmonary nodules. Chest 63:149, 1973.

117. Levy JM, Gordon B, Nykamp PW: Computed tomography guides percutaneous transthoracic lung biopsy. Comput Tomogr 2:217, 1978.

118. Zavala DC, Schoell JE: Ultrathin needle aspiration of the lung in infectious and malignant disease. Am Rev Respir Dis 123:125, 1981.

119. Gobien RP, Skucas J, Paris BS: CT-assisted fluoroscopically

guided aspiration biopsy of central hilar and mediastinal masses. Radiology 141:443, 1981.

120. Fink I, Gamsu G, Harter LP: CT-guided aspiration biopsy of the thorax. J Comput Assist Tomogr 6:958, 1982.

121. Pinstein ML, Scott RL, Salazar J: Avoidance of negative percutaneous lung biopsy using contrast-enhanced CT. AJR 140:265, 1983.

122. vanSonnenberg E, Lin AS, Deutsch AL, Mattrey RF: Percutaneous biopsy of difficult mediastinal, hilar, and pulmonary lesions by computed-tomographic guidance and a modified coaxial technique. Radiology 148:300, 1983.

123. vanSonnenberg E, Casola G, Ho M, Neff CC, Varney RR, et al: Difficult thoracic lesions: CT-guided biopsy experience in 150 cases. Radiology 167:457, 461.

124. Greene R: Transthoracic needle aspiration biopsy. In Athanasoulis CA, Pfister RC, Greene RE, Roberson GH (eds): Interventional Radiology. Philadelphia, WB Saunders, 1982, p 587.

125. Emani B, Melo A, Carter BL, Munzenrider JE, Prio AJ: Value of computed tomography in radiotherapy of lung cancer. AJR 131:63, 1978.

126. Seydal HG, Kutcher GJ, Steiner RM, Mohiuddin M, Golberg B: Computed tomography in planning radiation therapy for bronchogenic carcinoma. Int J Radiat Oncol Biol Phys 6:601, 1980.

127. Munzenrider JE, Pilepich M, Rene-Ferrero JB, Tchakarova I, Carter BL: Use of body scanner in radiotherapy treatment planning. Cancer 40:170, 1977.

128. Ragan DP, Perez CA: Efficacy of CT-associated two-dimensional treatment planning: analysis of 45 patients. AJR 131:75, 1978.

129. Libshitz HI, Southard ME: Complications of radiation therapy: the thorax. Semin Roentgenol 9:41, 1974.

130. Salazar OM, Rubin P, Brown JC, Feldstein ML, Keller BE: The assessment of tumor response to irradiation of lung cancer: continuous versus split-course regimens. Int J Radiat Oncol Biol Phys 1:1107, 1976.

131. Gross NJ: Pulmonary effects of radiation therapy. Ann Intern Med 86:81, 1977.

132. Jennings FL, Arden A: Development of radiation pneumonitis—time and dose factors. Arch Pathol 74:351, 1962.

133. Moosavi H, McDonald S, Rubin P, Cooper R, Stuard ID, Penney D: Early radiation dose-response in lung: an ultrastructural study. Int J Radiat Oncol Biol Phys 2:291, 1977.

134. Phillips TL, Benak S, Ross G: Ultrastructural and cellular effects of ionizing radiation. In Vaeth JM (ed): Frontiers of Radiation Therapy and Oncology, Vol 6. Radiation Effects and Tolerance, Normal Tissue. Baltimore, University Park Press, 1972, p 21.

135. Fried JR, Goldberg H: Post-irradiation changes in lungs and thorax: a clinical, roentgenological and pathological study, with emphasis on late and terminal stages. AJR 43:877, 1940.

136. Prato FS, Kurdyak R, Saibil EA, Rider WD, Aspin N: Physiological and radiographic assessment during the development of pulmonary radiation fibrosis. Radiology 122:389, 1977.

137. Libshitz HI, Shuman LS: Radiation-induced pulmonary change: CT findings. J Comput Assist Tomogr 8:15, 1984.

138. Ikezoe J, Takashima S, Morimoto S, Kadowaki K, Takeuchi N, et al: CT appearance of acute radiation-induced injury in the lung. AJR 150:765, 1988.

139. Nabawi P, Mantravadi R, Breyer D, Capek V: Computed tomography of radiation-induced lung injuries. J Comput Assist Tomogr 5:568, 1981.

140. Glazer HS, Lee JKT, Levitt RG, Heiken JB, Ling D, et al: Radiation fibrosis: differentiation from recurrent tumor by MR imaging. Work in progress. Radiology 156:721, 1985.

141. Margulis AR, James TL: Localized tissue MR spectroscopy. AJR 147:1327, 1986.

142. Naruse S, Horikawa Y, Tanaka C, Phalen JT: Evaluation of the effects of photoradiation therapy on brain tumors with in vivo P-31 MR spectroscopy. Radiology 160:827, 1986.

143. Andersen JC, Egedorf J, Stougard J: The pleural space succeeding pneumonectomy: a roentgenological and clinical study of 167 cases of bronchogenic carcinoma. Scand J Thorac Cardiovasc Surg 2:70, 1968.

144. Christiansen KH, Morgan SW, Karich AF, Takaro T: Pleural space following pneumonectomy. Ann Thorac Surg 1:298, 1965.

145. Biondette PR, Fiore D, Sartori F, Colognato A, Ravasini R, Romani S: Evaluation of the post-pneumonectomy space by computed tomography. J Comput Assist Tomogr 6:238, 1982.

146. Hood RM, Kirksey TD, Calhoom JH, Arnold HS, Tate RS: The use of automatic stapling devices in pulmonary resection. Ann Thorac Surg 16:85, 1973.

147. Zumbro JI Jr, Treasure R, Geiger JP, Green DC: Empyema after pneumonectomy. Ann Thorac Surg 15:615, 1973.

148. Heater K, Revzani L, Rubin JM: CT evaluation of empyema in the postpneumonectomy space. AJR 145:39, 1985.

149. Spjut JH, Mateo LF: Recurrent and metastatic carcinoma in surgically treated carcinoma of the lung: an autopsy survey. Cancer 18:1462, 1955.

150. Weiss W, Gillick JS: The metastatic spread of bronchogenic carcinoma in relation to the interval between resection and death. Chest 71:725, 1977.

151. Glazer HS, Aronberg DJ, Sagel SS, Emami B: Utility of CT in detecting postpneumonectomy carcinoma recurrence. AJR 142:487, 1984.

152. Heelan RT, Burt M, Caravelli JF, Bains MS, Martini N, Panicek DM: MR imaging in the postpneumonectomy chest. Radiology 173P:210, 1989.

153. Stark DD, Federle MP, Goodman PC, Podrosky AE, Webb WR: Differentiating lung abscess from empyema: radiography and computed tomography. AJR 141:163, 1983.

154. Baber CE, Hedlund LW, Oddson TA, Putman CE: Differentiating empyemas and peripheral pulmonary abscesses. The value of computed tomography. Radiology 135:755, 1980.

154a. Kuhlman JE, Deutsch JH, Fishman EK, Siegelman SS: CT features of thoracic mycobacterial disease. RadioGraphics 10:413, 1990.

155. Parker LA, Melton JW, Delany DJ, Yankaskas BC: Percutaneous small bore catheter drainage in the management of lung abscesses. Chest 92:213, 1987.

156. Yellin A, Yellin EO, Liberman Y: Percutaneous tube drainage: the treatment of choice for refractory lung abscess. Ann Thorac Surg 39:266, 1985.

157. Thurlbeck WM: Chronic Airflow Obstruction in Lung Disease. Major Problems in Pathology, Vol 5. Philadelphia, WB Saunders, 1976.

158. Rogers RM, DuBois AB, Blakemore WS: Effect of removal of bullae on airway conductance and conductance volume ratios. J Clin Invest 47:2569, 1968.

159. Gelb AF, Gold WM, Nadel JA: Mechanisms limiting air-flow in bullous lung disease. Am Rev Respir Dis 107:571, 1973.

160. Harris J: Severe bullous emphysema: successful surgical management despite poor preoperative blood gas levels and marked pulmonary hypertension. Chest 70:658, 1976.

161. Gaensler EA, Angell DW, Knudson RJ, Fitzgerald MX: Surgical management of emphysema. Clin Chest Med 4:443, 1983.

162. Wesley JR, Macleod WM, Mullard KS: Evaluation and surgery of bullous emphysema. J Thorac Cardiovasc Surg 63:945, 1972.

163. Fiore D, Biondette PR, Sartori F, Calabro F: The role of computed tomography in the evaluation of bullous lung disease. J Comput Assist Tomogr 6:105, 1982.

164. Morgan MDL, Strickland B: Computed tomography in the assessment of bullous lung disease. Br J Dis Chest 78:10, 1984.

165. Reed JC, Sobonya RE: Morphologic analysis of foregut cysts in the thorax. AJR 120:851, 1974.

166. Sumiyoshi K, Shimizu S, Enjoji M, Iwashita A, Kawakami K: Bronchogenic cyst in the abdomen. Virchows Arch Pathol Anat 408:93, 1985.

167. Miller RR, Sieber WK, Yunis EJ: Congenital adenomatoid malformation of the lung. A report of 17 cases and review of the literature. In Sommers SC, Rosen PP (eds): Pathology Annual, Part I. New York, Appleton-Century-Crofts, 1980, p 387.

168. Avitabile AM, Greco MA, Hulnick DH, Feiner HD: Congenital cystic adenomatoid malformation of the lung in adults. Am J Surg Pathol 8:193, 1984.

169. Hulnick DH, Naidich DP, McCauley DI, Feiner HD, Avitabile AM, et al: Late presentation of congenital cystic adenomatoid malformation of the lung. Radiology 151:569, 1984.

169a. Mata JM, Caceres J, Lucaya J, Garcia-Conesa JA: CT of congenital malformations of the lung. RadioGraphics 10:651, 1990.

170. Godwin JD, Webb WR: Dynamic computed tomography in the evaluation of vascular lung lesions. Radiology 138:629, 1981.

171. von Schulthess GK, Fisher MR, Higgins CB: Pathologic blood flow in pulmonary vascular disease as shown by gated magnetic resonance imaging. Ann Intern Med 103:317, 1985.

172. Wehrli FW, Shimakawa A, Gullberg GT, MacFall JR: Time-of-flight MR flow imaging: selective saturation recovery with gradient refocusing. Radiology 160:781, 1986.

173. Sechtem U, Pflugfelder PW, White RD, Gould RG, Holt W, et al: Cine-MRI: potential for the evaluation of cardiovascular function. AJR 148:239, 1987.

173a. Gefter WB, Hatabu H, Dinsmore BJ, Axel L, Palevsky HI, Reichek N, Schiebler ML, Kressel HY: Pulmonary vascular cine MR imaging: a noninvasive approach to dynamic imaging of the pulmonary circulation. Radiology 176:761, 1990.

174. Walker MF, Souza SP, Dumoulin CL: Quantitative flow measurement in phase contrast MR angiography. J Comput Assist Tomogr 12:304, 1988.

175. Kirks DR, Kane PE, Free EA, Taybi H: Systemic arterial supply to normal basilar segments of the left lower lobe. AJR 126:817, 1976.

176. Stork WJ: Pulmonary arteriovenous fistulas. AJR 74:441, 1955.

177. Abbott OA, Haebich AT, Van Fleit WE: Changing patterns relative to the surgical treatment of pulmonary arteriovenous fistulas. Am Surg 25:674, 1959.

178. Rankin S, Faling LJ, Pugatch RD: CT diagnosis of pulmonary arteriovenous malformations. J Comput Assist Tomogr 6:746, 1982.

179. Webb WR, Gamsu G, Golden JA, Crooks LE: Nuclear magnetic resonance of pulmonary arteriovenous fistula: effects of flow. J Comput Assist Tomogr 8:155, 1984.

180. Bartram C, Strickland B: Pulmonary varices. Br J Radiol 44:927, 1971.

181. Kelvin FM, Boone JA, Peretz D: Pulmonary varix. J Can Assoc Radiol 23:227, 1972.

182. Nelson WP, Hall RJ, Garcia E: Varicosities of the pulmonary veins simulating arteriovenous fistulas. JAMA 195:13, 1986.

183. Iwai K, Shindo G, Hajikano H, Tajima H, Morimoto M, et al: Intralobar pulmonary sequestration, with special reference to developmental pathology. Am Rev Respir Dis 109:911, 1973.

184. Stocker JT, Kagan-Hallet K: Extralobar pulmonary sequestration: analysis of 15 cases. Am J Clin Pathol 72:917, 1979.

185. Chopin RH, Siegel MJ: Pulmonary sequestration: six unusual presentations. AJR 134:695, 1980.

186. Landing BH, Dixon LG: Congenital malformations and genetic disorders of the respiratory tract (larynx, trachea, bronchi, and lungs). Am Rev Respir Dis 120:151, 1979.

187. Felson B: Pulmonary sequestration revisited. Med Radiol Photogr 64:1, 1988.

187a. Ikezoe J, Murayama S, Godwin JD, Done SL, Vershakelen JA: Bronchopulmonary sequestration: CT assessment. Radiology 176:375, 1990.

188. Webb WR: CT of solitary pulmonary vascular lesions. Semin Roentgenol 19:189, 1984.

189. Wojtowycz M, Gould HR, Atwell DT, Pois A: Calcified bronchopulmonary sequestration. J Comput Tomogr 8:171, 1984.

190. Van Dyke JA, Sagel SS: Calcified pulmonary sequestration: CT demonstration. J Comput Assist Tomogr 9:372, 1985.

191. Godwin JD, Webb WR, Gamsu G, Ovenfors CO: Computed tomography of pulmonary embolism. AJR 135:691, 1980.

192. Ovenfors CO, Godwin JD, Brito AC: Diagnosis of peripheral pulmonary emboli by computed tomography in the living dog. Radiology 141:519, 1981.

193. Grossman ZD, Thomas FD, Gagne G, Mauceri R, Cohen WN, et al: Transmission computed tomographic diagnosis of experimentally produced acute pulmonary vascular occlusion in the dog. Radiology 131:767, 1979.

194. Grossman ZD, Ritter CA, Tarner RJ, Somogyi JW, Johnson AC, et al: Successful indentification of oligemic lung by transmission computed tomography after experimentally produced acute pulmonary arterial occlusion in the dog. Invest Radiol 16:275, 1981.

195. Lourie GL, Pizzo C, Putman C, Thompson WM: Experimental pulmonary infarction in dogs: a comparison of chest radiography and computed tomography. Invest Radiol 17:224, 1982.

196. Sinner WN: Computed tomographic patterns of pulmonary thromboembolism and infarction. J Comput Assist Tomogr 2:395, 1978.

197. Gamsu G, Hirji M, Moore EH, Webb WR, Brito A: Experimental pulmonary emboli detected using magnetic resonance. Radiology 153:467, 1984.

198. Thickman D, Kressel HY, Axel L: Demonstration of pulmonary embolism by magnetic resonance imaging. AJR 142:921, 1984.

199. Stein MG, Cruess JV, Bradley WG, Kortman KE, Andrues TA, et al: MR imaging of pulmonary emboli: an experimental study in dogs. AJR 147:1133, 1986.

200. Pope CF, Sostman D, Carbo P, Gore JC, Holcomb W: The detection of pulmonary emboli by magnetic resonance imaging. Evaluation of imaging parameters. Invest Radiol 22:937, 1987.

201. White RD, Winkler ML, Higgins CB: MR imaging of pulmonary arterial hypertension and pulmonary emboli. AJR 149:15, 1987.

202. Spritzer CE, Sussman SK, Blinder RA, Saeed M, Herfkens RJ: Deep venous thrombosis evaluation with limited-flip-angle, gradient-refocused MR imaging: preliminary experience. Radiology 166:371, 1988.

203. Fisher MR, Higgins CB: Central thrombi in pulmonary arterial hypertension detected by MR imaging. Radiology 158:223, 1986.

204. Kuriyama K, Gamsu G, Stern RG, Cann CE, Herfkens RJ, Brundage BH: CT-determined pulmonary artery diameters in predicting pulmonary hypertension. Invest Radiol 19:16, 1984.

205. Webb WR: Computed tomography and magnetic resonance imaging of the lung parenchyma. Presented at the American College of Radiology Categorical Course on Body Computed Tomography and Magnetic Resonance Imaging Correlation, Cincinnati, September 24, 1988.

206. Huber DJ, Kobzik L, Melanson G, Adam DF: Detection of inflammation in collapsed lung by alterations in proton nuclear magnetic relaxation times. Invest Radiol 20:460, 1985.

207. Moore EH, Webb WR, Muller N, Sollitto R: MRI of pulmonary airspace disease. AJR 146:1123, 1986.

208. Cohen MD, Eigen H, Scott PH, Tepper R, Cory DA, et al: Magnetic resonance imaging of inflammatory lung disorders: preliminary studies in children. Pediatr Pulmonol 2:211, 1986.

209. Rubin GD, Edwards DR, Reicher MA, Doemeny JM, Carson SH: Diagnosis of pulmonary hemosiderosis by MR imaging. AJR 52:573, 1989.

210. Tobler J, Levitt RG, Glazer HS, Moran J, Crouch E, Evens RG: Differentiation of proximal bronchogenic carcinoma from post-obstructive lobar collapse by magnetic resonance imaging: comparison with computed tomography. Invest Radiol 22:539, 1987.

211. Murata K, Khan A, Herman PG: Pulmonary parenchymal disease: evaluation with high-resolution CT. Radiology 170:629, 1989.

212. Mathieson JR, Mayo JR, Staples CA, Muller NL: Chronic diffuse infiltrative lung disease: comparison of diagnostic accuracy of CT and chest radiography. Radiology 171:111, 1989.

213. Bergin CJ, Muller NL: CT of interstitial lung disease: a diagnostic approach. AJR 148:8, 1987.

214. Munk PL, Muller NL, Miller RR, Ostrow DN: Pulmonary lymphangitic carcinomatosis: CT and pathologic findings. Radiology 166:705, 1988.

215. Stein MG, Mayo J, Muller N, Aberle DR, Webb WR, Gamsu G: Pulmonary lymphangitic spread of carcinoma: appearance on CT scans. Radiology 162:371, 1987.

216. Crystal RG, Fulmer JD, Roberts EC, Moss ML, Line BR, Reynolds HY: Idiopathic pulmonary fibrosis. Clinical histologic, radiographic, physiologic, scintigraphic, cytologic, and biochemical aspects. Ann Intern Med 85:769, 1976.

217. Turner-Warwick M, Burrows B, Johnson A: Cryptogenic fibrosing alveolitis: clinical features and their influence on survival. Thorax 35:171, 1980.

218. O'Donnell K, Keogh B, Cantin A, Crystal RG: Pharmacologic suppression of the neutrophil component of the alveolitis in idiopathic pulmonary fibrosis. Am Rev Respir Dis 136:288, 1987.

219. Sider L, Dennis L, Smith LJ, Dunn MM: CT of the lung parenchyma and the pulmonary function test. Chest 92:406, 1987.

220. Lynch DA, Webb WR, Gamsu G, Stulbarg M, Golden G: Computed tomography in pulmonary sarcoidosis. J Comput Assist Tomogr 13:405, 1989.

221. Bergin CJ, Bell DY, Coblentz CL, Chiles C, Gamsu G, et al: Sarcoidosis: correlation of pulmonary parenchymal pattern at CT with results of pulmonary function tests. Radiology 171:619, 1989.

222. Muller NL, Mawson JB, Mathieson JR, Abboud R, Ostrow DN, Champion P: Sarcoidosis: correlation of extent of disease at CT with clinical, functional, and radiographic findings. Radiology 171:613, 1989.

223. Muller NL, Kullnig P, Miller RR: The CT findings of pulmonary sarcoidosis: analysis of 25 patients. AJR 152:1179, 1989.

224. Brauner MW, Grenier P, Mompoint D, Lenoir S, de Cremoux H: Pulmonary sarcoidosis: evaluation with high-resolution CT. Radiology 172:467, 1989.

225. Marcy TW, Reynolds HY: Pulmonary histiocytosis X. Lung 163:129, 1985.

226. Friedman PJ, Liebow AA, Sokoloff J: Eosinophilic granuloma of lung: clinical aspects of primary pulmonary histiocytosis in the adult. Medicine 60:385, 1981.

227. Brauner MW, Grenier P, Mouelhi MM, Mompoint D, Lenoir S: Pulmonary histiocytosis X: evaluation with high-resolution CT. Radiology 172:255, 1989.

228. Moore ADA, Godwin JD, Muller NL, Naidich DP, Hammar SP, et al: Pulmonary histiocytosis X: comparison of radiographic and CT findings. Radiology 172:249, 1989.

229. Corrin B, Liebow AA, Friedman PJ: Pulmonary lymphangiomyomatosis. Am J Pathol 79:348, 1975.

230. Carrington CB, Cugell DW, Gaensler EA, Marks A, Redding RA, et al: Lymphangioleiomomatosis. Physiologic-pathologic-radiologic correlations. Am Rev Respir Dis 116:977, 1977.

231. Merchant RN, Pearson MG, Rankin RN, Morgan WKC: Computerized tomography in the diagnosis of lymphangioleiomyomatosis. Am Rev Respir Dis 131:295, 1985.

232. Rappaport DC, Weisbrod GL, Herman SJ, Chamberlain DW: Pulmonary lymphangioleiomyomatosis: high-resolution CT findings in four cases. AJR 152:961, 1989.

233. Sherrier RH, Chiles C, Roggli V: Pulmonary lymphangioleiomyomatosis: CT findings. AJR 153:937, 1989.

233a. Aberle DR, Hansell DM, Brown K, Tashkin DP: Lymphangiomyomatosis: CT, chest radiographic and functional correlations. Radiology 176:381, 1990.

233b. Lenoir S, Grenier P, Brauner MW, Frija J, Remy-Jardin M, Revel D, Cordier J: Pulmonary lymphangiomyomatosis and tuberous sclerosis: comparison of radiograph and thin-section CT findings. Radiology 175:329, 1990.

234. Russell AR (ed): Classification of radiographs of the pneumoconioses. Med Radiogr Photogr 57:2, 1981.

235. Bergin CJ, Muller NL, Vedal S, Chan-Yeung M: CT in silicosis: correlation with plain films and pulmonary function tests. AJR 146:477, 1986.

236. Begin R, Bergeron D, Samson L, Boctor M, Cantin A: CT assessment of silicosis in exposed workers. AJR 148:509, 1987.

237. Akira M, Higashihara T, Yokoyama K, Yamamoto S, Kita N, et al: Radiographic type p pneumoconiosis: high-resolution CT. Radiology 171:117, 123.

237a. Remy-Jardin M, Degreef JM, Beuscart R, Vioson C, Remy J: Coal worker's pneumoconiosis: CT assessment in exposed workers and correlation with radiographic findings. Radiology 177:363, 1990.

238. Begin R, Ostiguy G, Cantin A, Bergeron D: Lung function in silica-exposed workers: a relationship to disease severity assessed by CT scan. Chest 94:539, 1988.

239. Friedman AC, Fiel SB, Fisher MS, Radecki PD, Lev-Toaff AS, Caroline DF: Asbestos-related pleural disease and asbestosis: a comparison of CT and chest radiography. AJR 150:269, 1988.

240. Katz D, Kreel L: Computed tomography in pulmonary asbestosis. Clin Radiol 30:207, 1979.

241. Sargent EN, Boswell WD, Ralls PW, Markovitz A: Subpleural fat pads in patients exposed to asbestos: distinction from noncalcified pleural plaques. Radiology 152:273, 1984.

242. Gamsu G, Aberle DR, Lynch D: Computed tomography in the diagnosis of asbestos-related thoracic disease. J Thorac Imaging 4:61, 1989.

243. Murphy RL, Becklake RL, Brooks SM, Gaensler EA, Gee BL, et al: The diagnosis of nonmalignant diseases related to asbestosis. Am Rev Respir Dis 134:363, 1986.

244. Becklake MR: Asbestos-related diseases of the lung and other organs: their epidemiology and implications for clinical practice. Am Rev Respir Dis 114:187, 1976.

245. Sperber M, Mohan KK: Computed tomography—a reliable diagnostic modality in pulmonary asbestosis. Comput Radiol 8:125, 1984.

246. Begin R, Boctor M, Bergeron D, Cantin A, Berthiaume Y, et al: Radiographic assessment of pleuroparenchymal disease in asbestos workers: posteroanterior, four view films, and computed tomograms of the thorax. Br J Ind Med 41:373, 1984.

247. Staples CA, Gamsu G, Ray CS, Webb WR: High resolution computed tomography and lung function in asbestos-exposed workers with normal chest radiographs. Am Rev Respir Dis 139:1502, 1989.

248. Law MR, Gregor A, Husband JE, Kerr IH: Computed tomography in the assessment of malignant mesothelioma of the pleura. Clin Radiol 33:67, 1982.

249. Doyle TC, Lawler GA: CT features of rounded atelectasis of the lung. AJR 143:225, 1984.

250. Lynch DA, Gamsu G, Ray CS, Aberle DR: Asbestos-related focal lung masses: manifestations on conventional and high-resolution CT scans. Radiology 169:603, 1988.

251. McHugh K, Blaquiere RM: CT features of rounded atelectasis. AJR 153:257, 1989.

252. Kishimoto T, Okada K: The relationship between lung cancer and asbestos exposure. Chest 94:486, 1988.

253. Berry G, Newhouse ML, Antonis P: Combined effect of asbestos and smoking on mortality from lung cancer and mesothelioma in factory workers. Br J Ind Med 42:12, 1985.

254. Blanc PD, Gamsu G: The effect of cigarette smoking on the detection of small radiographic opacities in inorganic dust diseases. J Thorac Imaging 3:51, 1988.

255. ACCP-ATS Joint Committee on Pulmonary Nomenclature: Pulmonary terms and symbols. Chest 67:583, 1975.

256. Thurlbeck MW, Henderson JA, Fraser RG, Bates DV: Chronic obstructive lung disease—a comparison between clinical, roentgenologic, functional and morphological criteria in chronic bronchitis, emphysema, asthma and bronchiectasis. Medicine (Baltimore) 49:81, 1970.

257. American Thoracic Society: Chronic bronchitis, asthma, and pulmonary emphysema by the Committee on Diagnostic Standards for Nontuberculosis Respiratory Disease. Am Rev Respir Dis 85:762, 1962.

258. Gamsu G, Nadel JA: The roentgenologic manifestations of emphysema and chronic bronchitis. Med Clin North Am 57:719, 1973.

259. Pratt PC: Role of conventional chest radiography in diagnosis and exclusion of emphysema. Am J Med 82:998, 1987.

260. Goddard PR, Nicholson EM, Laszlo G, Watt I: Computed tomography in pulmonary emphysema. Clin Radiol 33:379, 1982.

261. Bergin CJ, Muller NL, Miller RR: CT in the qualitative assessment of emphysema. J Thorac Imaging 1:94, 1986.

262. Sanders C, Nath PH, Bailey WC: Detection of emphysema with computed tomography: correlation with pulmonary function tests and chest radiography. Invest Radiol 23:262, 1988.

263. Hruban RH, Meziane MA, Zerhouni EA, Khouri NF, Fishman EK, et al: High resolution computed tomography of inflation-fixed lungs. Am Rev Respir Dis 136:935, 1987.

264. Foster WL, Pratt PC, Roggli VL, Godwin JD, Halvorsen RA Jr, Putman CE: Centrilobular emphysema: CT-pathologic correlation. Radiology 159:27, 1986.

265. Sider L, Dennis L, Smith LJ, Dunn MM: CT of the lung parenchyma and the pulmonary function test. Chest 92:406, 1987.

266. Sakai F, Gamsu G, Im J-G, Ray CS: Pulmonary function abnormalities in patients with CT-determined emphysema. J Comput Assist Tomogr 11:963, 1987.

267. Powers JC: Synthetic elastase inhibitors: prospects for use in the treatment of emphysema. Am Rev Respir Dis 127(suppl):54, 1983.

268. Lucey EC, Stone PJ, Christensen TG, Breuer R, Calore JD, Snider GL: Effect of varying the time interval between intratracheal administration of eglin-c and human neutrophil elastase on prevention of emphysema and secretory cell metaplasia in hamsters: with observations on the fate of eglin-c and the effect of repeated instillations. Am Rev Respir Dis 134:471, 1986.

269. Wewers MD, Casolaro A, Sellers SE, Swayze SC, McPhaul KM, et al: Replacement therapy for alpha$_1$-antitrypsin deficiency associated with emphysema. N Engl J Med 316:1055, 1987.

270. Wegener OH, Koeppe P, Oeser H: Measurement of lung density by computed tomography. J Comput Assist Tomogr 2:263, 1978.

271. Robinson PJ, Kreel L: Pulmonary tissue attenuation with computed tomography: comparison of inspiration and expiration scans. J Comput Assist Tomogr 3:740, 1979.

272. Dohring W: Quantitative analyses of regional pulmonary ventilation using Compton densitometry and computed tomography. Prog Respir Res 11:48, 1979.

273. Rosenblum LJ, Mauceri RA, Wellenstein DE, Thomas FD, Bassano DA, et al: Density patterns in the normal lung as determined by computed tomography. Radiology 137:409, 1980.

274. Kourilsky R, Marchal M, Marchal MT: Recording respiratory function by x-rays: Basic principles. Thorax 20:428, 1965.

275. Silverman NR: Clinical videodensitometry: pulmonary ventilation analysis. Radiology 103:263, 1972.

276. Zelefsky MN, Schultz RJ, Freeman LM: Assessment of regional lung function and its clinical application: the combined use of lung scan and gamma densigraphy. Radiology 94:167, 1970.

277. Gamsu G, Kaufman L, Swann SJ, Brito AC: Absolute lung density in experimental canine pulmonary edema. Invest Radiol 14:261, 1979.

278. Bragg DG, Durney CH, Johnson CC, Pedersen PC: Monitoring and diagnosis of pulmonary edema by microwaves: a preliminary report. Invest Radiol 12:289, 1977.

279. Weng TR, Spence JA, Polgar G, Nyboer J: Measurement of regional lung function by tetrapolar electrical impedance plethysmography. Chest 76:64, 1979.

280. Hedlund LW, Putman CE: Analysis of lung density by computed tomography. In Putman CE (ed): Pulmonary Diagnosis: Imaging and Other Techniques. New York, Appleton-Century-Crofts, 1981, p 107.

281. Gould GA, MacNee W, McLean A, Warren PM, Redpath A, et al: CT measurements of lung density in life can quantitate distal airspace enlargement—an essential defining feature of human emphysema. Am Rev Respir Dis 137:380, 1988.

282. Rosenblum IJ, Mauceri RA, Wellenstein DE, Bassano DA, Cohen WN, Heitzman ER: Computed tomography of the lung. Radiology 129:521, 1978.

283. Utell MJ, Wandkte JC, Fahey PJ, Baker A, Fischner HW, Hyde RW: Lung weight in normal and edematous dogs by computerized tomography. Fed Proc 38:1326, 1979.

284. Hedlund LW, Effmann EL, Bates WM, Beck JW, Goulding PH, Putman CE: Pulmonary edema: a CT study of regional changes in lung density following oleic acid injury. J Comput Assist Tomogr 6:939, 1982.

285. Gur D, Drayer BP, Borovetz HS, Griffith BP, Hardesty RL, Wolfson SK: Dynamic computed tomography of the lung: regional ventilation measurements. J Comput Assist Tomogr 3:749, 1979.

286. Herbert DL, Gur D, Shabason L, Good WF, Rinaldo JE, et al: Mapping of human local pulmonary ventilation by xenon enhanced computed tomography. J Comput Assist Tomogr 6:1088, 1982.

287. Wang NS: Anatomy. In Dail DH, Hammer SP (eds): Pulmonary Pathology. New York, Springer-Verlag, 1988, p 27.

288. Hatabu H, Gefter WB, Kressel HY, Axel L, Lenkinski RE: Pulmonary vasculature: high resolution MR imaging. Work in progress. Radiology 171:391, 1989.

289. Donmalin CL, Souza MF, Walker MF, Yoshitome F: Time resolved magnetic resonance angiography. Magn Reson Med 6:285, 1988.

290. Lallemand DP, Brasch RC, Gooding CA, Wesbey GE, Higgins CB: NMR imaging of lung parenchyma. Presented at the Society of Magnetic Resonance in Medicine Second Annual Meeting, August 16–19, San Francisco, 1983. Abstract.

291. Kveder M, Zuparai I, Lahajnar G, Blinc R, Suput D, et al: Water proton NMR relaxation mechanisms in lung tissue. Magn Reson Med 7:432, 1988.

292. Schmidt HC, Tsay D-G, Higgins CB: Pulmonary edema: an MR study of permeability and hydrostatic types in animals. Radiology 158:297, 1986.

293. Cutillo AG, Morris AH, Alion DC, Case TA, Durney CH, et al: Assessment of lung water distribution by nuclear magnetic resonance: a new method for quantifying and monitoring experimental lung injury. Am Rev Respir Dis 137:1371, 1988.

294. Hayes CE, Case TA, Alion DC, Morris AH, Cutillo A, et al: Lung water quantitation by nuclear magnetic resonance imaging. Science 216:1313, 1982.

295. Carroll FE, Loyd JE, Nolop KB, Collins JC: MR imaging parameters in the study of lung water: preliminary study. Invest Radiol 20:381, 1985.

296. Skalina S, Kundel HL, Wolf G, Marshall B: The effect of pulmonary edema on proton nuclear magnetic resonance relaxation times. Invest Radiol 19:7, 1984.

297. Taylor CR, Sostman DH, Gore JC, Walker-Smith G: Proton relaxation times in bleomycin-induced lung injury. Invest Radiol 22:621, 1987.

298. Vinitski S, Pearson MG, Karlik SJ, Morgan WKC, Carey LS, et al: Differentiation of parenchymal lung disorders with *in vitro* proton nuclear magnetic resonance. Magn Reson Med 3:120, 1986.

299. Moore EH, Webb WR, Muller N, Sollitto R: MRI of pulmonary airspace disease: experimental model and preliminary clinical results. AJR 146:1123, 1986.

300. McFadden RG, Carr TJ, Wood TE: Proton magnetic resonance imaging to stage activity of interstitial lung disease. Chest 92:31, 1987.

301. Bartlett JG, Gorbach SL, Tally FP, Finegold SM: Bacteriology and treatment of primary lung abscess. Am Rev Respir Dis 109:510, 1974.

302. Pugatch RD, Faling LJ, Robbins AH, Snider GL: Differentiation of pleural and pulmonary lesions using computed tomography. J Comput Assist Tomogr 2:601, 1978.

303. Williford ME, Godwin JD: Computed tomography of lung abscess and empyema. Radiol Clin North Am 21:575, 1983.

CHAPTER 5

CHEST WALL, AXILLARY SPACE, PLEURAE, AND DIAPHRAGM

W. RICHARD WEBB ▪ *GORDON GAMSU*

Computed tomography (CT) plays an important role in the diagnosis of abnormalities involving the chest wall, axillary space, pleurae, and diaphragm. These structures can be involved by contiguous spread of disease from the neighboring lung or mediastinum, or diseases can originate from their intrinsic component tissues. The cross-sectional format and excellent density resolution provided by CT result in information about the chest wall that cannot be obtained with conventional radiographic techniques. Furthermore, the chest wall is visible on all CT scans of the thorax, and unsuspected pathologic conditions involving the chest wall may be detected in patients who are being evaluated for other reasons.

Magnetic resonance (MR) imaging of the thoracic cage and pleura has received scant attention, even though MR images show good contrast resolution of the structures of the chest wall. Pulmonary and pleural neoplasms are readily differentiated from the chest wall fat and muscles, and with improved spatial resolution MR could become an excellent method for demonstrating chest wall lesions.

Techniques of Examination

In general, the chest wall, axillary space, pleurae, and diaphragm are well evaluated using standard techniques for CT of the thorax. Scans are usually obtained at 1-cm intervals with 1-cm collimation during suspended respiration at full inspiration. In most instances, patients are positioned with their arms raised over the head, and the examination is performed form the apex to the base of the lungs. The diaphragm and posterior pleural spaces extend well below the lung bases, and scans inferior to the diaphragmatic cupula must be obtained to evaluate these structures completely. Scanning with the patient in the prone or decubitus position may be of assistance, particularly for evaluating pleural diseases. Free pleural effusions shift to the dependent portion of the pleural space when the patient is moved from the supine position to the prone or decubitus position, whereas loculated effusions or fibrosis show little or no change.[1] The movement of an effusion helps in the diagnosis of a pleural density seen on CT scans and can reveal underlying pulmonary parenchymal or pleural lesions that are otherwise obscured.[1] Baber and colleagues[2] have shown that in patients with a loculated collection of air and fluid in the pleural space from a bronchopleural fistula or empyema, movement of air with a change in patient position allows precise delineation of the size and shape of the cavity.

Mediastinal window settings (level, 20 to 50 Hounsfield units [H]; width, 500 to 1000 H) are most suitable for evaluating the soft tissues of the chest wall, pleurae, and diaphragm. However, lung window settings (level, −500 to −700 H; width, 1200 H) or extended window settings (level, 20 to 50 H; width, 2000 H) allow more accurate estimation of the size, contour, and appearance of pleural lesions at their interface with adjacent lung. Appropriate window settings must be used to evaluate bony lesions of the chest wall.

Occasionally, multiplanar reformation of images can clarify the relationship of chest wall or pleural processes to the lung or mediastinal structures (Fig. 5–1). These reformations are particularly helpful to nonradiologists who are more familiar with standard frontal or lateral radiographic projections.

Van Waes and Zonneveld[3] demonstrated that direct coronal CT images can help in the diagnosis of intrathoracic disease and provide better resolution than multiplanar reformations (Fig. 5–2). With the patient seated in the gantry and bending forward, both the upper and lower thorax can be evaluated, but the entire chest cannot be imaged on a single scan.

Reformatted CT images have been replaced by multiplanar MR imaging. The MR images are easier to obtain and also demonstrate anatomic relationships better than direct coronal CT scans. The patient is lying flat rather than bending forward, and MR can provide better tissue contrast than CT. In partic-

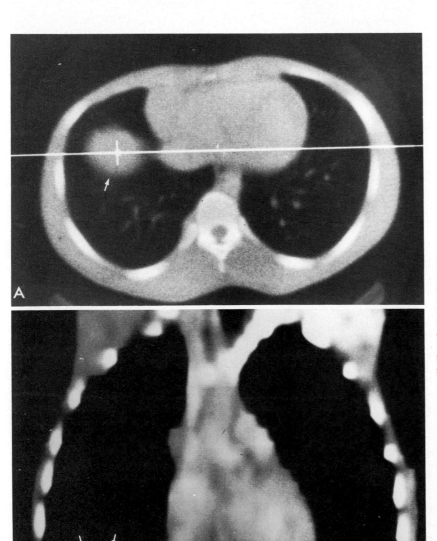

FIGURE 5–1 ■ Coronal reconstruction. Patient is a 20-year-old male with thymoma and myasthenia gravis. *A,* CT scan shows a density in inferior right hemithorax *(arrow).* On cross-sectional images it is unclear whether this represents liver or a pleural mass at the diaphragmatic surface. *B,* Coronal reconstruction along the plane indicated by the line in *A* shows that the mass *(arrows)* is less dense than the subjacent liver, and the pleural metastasis is separate from the normal liver.

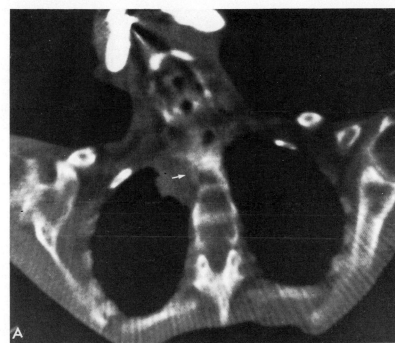

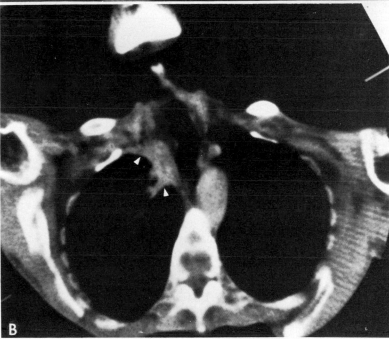

FIGURE 5–2 ■ Direct coronal CT scan in an elderly man with a right superior sulcus (Pancoast's) tumor using direct coronal CT at the levels of the vertebral column *(A)* and the trachea *(B)*. *A*, The tumor mass is visible medially at the right apex. The right cortical margin of a vertebral body *(arrow)* has been destroyed by the tumor. *B*, Tumor involves the right paratracheal mediastinum *(arrowheads)*.

ular, sagittal and coronal MR images define the relationship of masses at the lung apex or base to the chest wall, pleural surface, or diaphragm better than can transaxial CT images or CT reformations (Fig. 5–3).[4, 5]

High-resolution CT (HRCT) techniques can demonstrate the anatomy of the lung–pleura–chest wall interface better than conventional CT. This technique uses thin (1- to 1.5-mm) collimation, a high spatial frequency reconstruction algorithm, and usually an increase in peak kilovolts (kV[p]) and milliamperes (mA) settings to reduce image noise.[6] Image targeting to decrease pixel size in the final image probably does not improve diagnostic yield. Several HRCT scans are obtained selectively at the level of the focal abnormality or, in a patient with extensive disease, at spaced intervals from the lung apex to base. Scanning with the patient both prone and supine is valuable in distinguishing subtle pleural and parenchymal abnormalities from compression or transient atelectasis of the dependent lung. Thus with the patient prone, scans can be used to evaluate posterior pleural or parenchymal abnormalities. Free-flowing pleural effusions move with the patient prone, and the nondependent lung is expanded more fully.

MR imaging techniques for the thoracic cage are

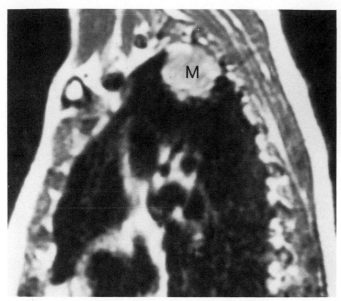

FIGURE 5–3 ■ Apical bronchogenic carcinoma. Coronal T1-weighted spin-echo MR scan, 6 cm from the midline, demonstrates the relationship of an apical tumor mass (M) to the chest wall. The tumor is not invading the chest wall.

similar to those used for the thorax as a whole and are described in Chapter 2. In general, spin-echo sequences are obtained at multiple levels during any single scanning procedure. Typically 5 to 20 levels are scanned, each 3- to 10-mm thick. The usual pixel matrix is 256 × 128 or 256 × 256, and each pixel is about 2 mm on a side. A distinct advantage of MR is the direct acquisition of images in coronal, sagittal, and oblique planes. Oblique MR images are particularly useful for defining the relationship of masses to the chest wall. Coronal images of the brachial plexus and lung apex also are useful.

Motion of the thorax during image acquisition is a problem. Methods for cardiac and respiratory synchronization and compensation are available and improve spatial resolution, signal intensity, and periodic "ghost artifacts." Fast imaging sequences with a low flip angle, gradient-echo technique have not been applied to the thoracic cage.

Surface coils placed directly on the chest wall improve the quality of MR images significantly. Coils for the lower neck can be used for imaging the brachial plexus. MR imaging of the breast likewise uses surface coils designed specifically for this purpose. Lesions as small as 2 mm can be detected with these coils. Usually T1-weighted and T2-weighted images with thin collimation and contiguous sections are obtained of each breast separately.

Chest Wall

Anatomy

The chest wall consists of the thoracic skeleton and its associated musculature. The axilla and its contents and the breast will be discussed separately.

THORACIC SKELETON

The thoracic vertebrae are intermediate in size between the small cervical vertebrae and the larger lumbar vertebrae. When viewed at the level of the neural canals, the vertebral bodies are rounded, with a posterior notch (Fig. 5–4). In adults, osteophytes often distort the contour of the thoracic vertebral bodies and most often occur anteriorly and on the right side.[7]

From their articulations with the transverse processes and vertebral bodies, the ribs extend laterally and then obliquely downward and anteriorly (Fig. 5–4A through H). Usually only a short segment of each rib is visible on a single CT scan; each progressively more anterior rib represents the one arising at a higher thoracic level. Thus the fifth rib lies anterior to the sixth and the fourth lies anterior to the fifth, and so forth. At the level of the lung apex, the first rib can be identified by its anterior position and by its articulation with the manubrium immediately below the sternoclavicular joint.

In some patients, a bony spur projects inferiorly from the undersurface of the first rib at its junction with the manubrium. In cross section, it appears to be surrounded by lung and can mimic a lung nodule.[8] This spur is usually lateral to the manubrium and bilaterally symmetric, providing a clue to its true nature. The "nodule" can also be seen to be of bone density when viewed at appropriate window settings, and its relationship to the first rib becomes apparent when successively higher images are examined (Fig. 5–5). Also, one or two small episternal ossicles posterior to the upper manubrium or suprasternal notch are visible on CT in about 1 per cent of patients. They should not be mistaken for fracture fragments or other pathologic processes.[9–12]

The manubrium is usually visible over a distance of 3 or 4 cm and is considerably wider than the body of the sternum, which is at lower levels (see Fig. 5–4E through H). Destouet and colleagues[13] have shown a clearly defined joint space between the clavicular head and the articular surface of the manubrium. The sternoclavicular joint contains a fibrocartilaginous disk that can be seen on CT scans when a normal vacuum phenomenon, with gas in the joint space, is present. At a level 1 cm caudal to the suprasternal notch, the first ribs articulate with the lateral surfaces of the manubrium at its widest point. At this level, the undersurfaces of the clavicular heads appear triangular in transaxial section. They are located medial to the end of the first rib and posterior to the manubrium (see Fig. 5–4F).

The junction between the manubrium and the sternal body lies in the axial plane and is not visible on CT scans. However, this level is defined by the articulations of the second ribs with the sternum. In cross section, the body of the sternum is narrower and more rectangular than the manubrium (see Fig. 5–4F through H). The articulations of the anterior ribs and sternal body are not visible unless their costal cartilages are calcified. Uncalcified costal cartilage can be difficult to distinguish from adjacent intercostal muscle.

Inferiorly, the xiphoid process is seen on CT scans as an extension of the sternal body and is usually ossified in adults. Except for the xiphoid process, the manubrium and sternum have well-defined cortices.

The variations in CT appearance of the normal sternum and its articulations have been reviewed in several articles.[9–12] CT features of postoperative, inflammatory, and neoplastic diseases affecting this portion of the thoracic skeleton have also been described.

In some patients, deformities of the thoracic skeleton such as pectus excavatum can mimic a mediastinal or hilar mass on plain radiographs. In such patients, CT can help establish the correct diagnosis.[14]

THORACIC MUSCULATURE

The muscles of the chest wall visible on CT are the shoulder girdle and intercostal muscles (see Fig. 5–4). Anatomically they also define the boundaries of the axillary space.

The pectoralis major muscle arises from the anterior surface of the sternal half of the clavicle, the anterior surface of the upper sternum, and the cartilages of the upper ribs (see Fig. 5–4). From these origins, the muscle fibers converge on a single tendinous insertion at the greater tuberosity of the humerus.[15] The pectoralis major varies in size depending on the patient's muscular development. Inferiorly the muscle is a thin sheet that is separated from the ribs by only a thin plane of fat. At higher levels, the muscle thickens and is farther from the thoracic cage. Both its sternal and its clavicular origins are usually visible.

The pectoralis minor muscle is thinner and lies behind the pectoralis major. It arises from the cranial margins and outer surfaces of the anterior third, fourth, and fifth ribs and inserts into the coracoid process of the scapula.[15] On CT scans, the pectoralis minor muscle is visible posterior to the upper portion of the pectoralis major (see Fig. 5–4). The two muscles are separated only by a layer of fat. The insertion of the pectoralis minor into the coracoid process is also usually visible (see Fig. 5–4A.)

Posteriorly several muscles are related to the scapula. These include the subscapularis, supra- and infraspinatus, teres major and minor, and latissimus dorsi muscles.[15]

On CT images, the subscapularis muscle lies anterior to the scapula and separates it from the thoracic cage (see Fig. 5–4). The subscapularis muscle arises from the axillary portion of the scapula and the subscapular fossa and inserts into the lesser tuberosity of the humerus and the capsule of the shoulder joint. Posterior to the scapula, the infraspinatus muscle is visible medial to the much smaller teres minor muscle (see Fig. 5–4). Both of these muscles arise from the medial border of the scapula and insert into the greater tubercle of the humerus. CT scans show

the teres minor and latissimus dorsi muscles lateral to the scapula, but they are difficult to separate at this level. The teres major muscle arises from the inferior angle of the scapula and inserts into the lesser tubercle of the humerus. The latissimus dorsi is a triangular muscle that covers the posterior chest and back (see Fig. 5–4B through H). It originates from a broad aponeurotic attachment to the spinous processes of the lower thoracic and lumbar vertebrae and inserts onto the humerus.

The serratus anterior is a thin sheet of muscle between the ribs and the scapula. It arises from the superior borders of the first eight or nine ribs and inserts into the ventral surface of the scapula.[15] The serratus anterior is difficult to distinguish from the subscapularis muscle on CT scans (see Fig. 5–4).

Within the posterior chest wall, a number of muscles are visible at successive levels. These include the trapezius, rhomboideus major and minor, and the complex group of extensor muscles of the vertebral column (see Fig. 5–4). The trapezius is a flat triangular muscle covering the upper posterior neck and shoulders. It arises from the spinous processes of the cervical and thoracic vertebrae and inserts into the posterior border of the lateral clavicle, the acromion, and the posterior border of the spine of the scapula. Its insertion into the spine of the scapula can easily be seen on CT scans. The rhomboideus major and minor muscles arise from the spinous processes of the lower cervical and upper thoracic vertebral bodies, pass beneath the trapezius muscle, and descend to attach to the medial margin of the scapula. CT scans below the level of the scapula still show the trapezius, but the rhomboideus muscles are no longer visible.

Deep within the chest wall, the intercostal muscles lie between the visible segments of adjacent ribs. The intercostal muscles are dealt with in greater detail later in this chapter.

Chest Wall Abnormalities

In both adults and children, metastatic tumors involve the thoracic skeleton more commonly than do primary tumors.[16, 17] In adults, adenocarcinomas are the most common; in children, neuroblastoma and leukemia predominate. In adults, the most common primary tumors arising from the thoracic skeleton are chondrosarcoma and myeloma; in children, Ewing's sarcoma is the most common primary tumor.[16, 17] In both groups, benign tumors occur less commonly than primary malignant neoplasms. Osteomyelitis can closely mimic tumor and must be considered in the differential diagnosis of thoracic skeletal lesions. Care must also be taken to avoid misdiagnosing a partially ossified anterior costal cartilage as a destroyed rib.

A majority of patients with malignant tumors of the thoracic skeleton experience chest pain. Other patients first notice a local mass. In most patients, routine radiographs are insufficient to establish the

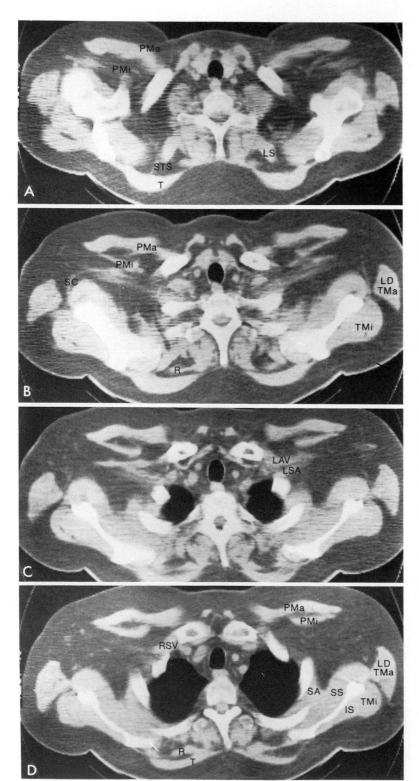

FIGURE 5–4 ■ Normal anatomy of the chest wall and axilla with arms positioned above the head. *A,* CT scan 20 mm above the lung apices shows the clavicular origins of the pectoralis major muscles (PMa) anteriorly. On the right, the insertion of the pectoralis minor muscle (PMi) into the coracoid process of the scapula marginates the cephalic extent of the axilla. Posteriorly, the fat-filled subtrapezial space (STS) is ventral to the trapezius muscle (T). The levator scapulae muscle (LS) can be seen clearly in the medial aspect of this space. *B,* CT scan 10 mm above the lung apices shows both the pectoralis major (PMa) and pectoralis minor (PMi) muscles, which together form the anterior margin of the axillary space. The axillary vessels and branches of the brachial plexus extend laterally within the cephalic portion of the axilla. On the right side, a circumflex scapular artery or vein (SC) is visible. The first two ribs arise posteriorly; the first is anterior to the second. The subtrapezial space remains visible at this level, with the rhomboideus major (R) muscle along its posterior aspect. *C,* CT scan at the level of the lung apices; the first two ribs are again visible. Both the left axillary artery (LSA) and the left axillary vein (LAV) are seen within the axilla. The vein lies anterior to the artery. Both pass between the first rib and clavicle. *D,* CT scan 10 mm lower clearly shows the right subclavian vein (RSV) passing between the first rib and the clavicular head. The axilla is marginated anteriorly by the pectoralis major (PMa) and pectoralis minor (PMi) muscles; posteriorly by the latissimus dorsi (LD), teres major (TMa), and subscapularis (SS) muscles; and medially by the chest wall and serratus anterior (SA) muscle. Other muscles visible at this level and at lower levels (*E* through *H*) include the teres minor (TMi) and infraspinatus (IS), trapezius (T), and rhomboideus major (R).

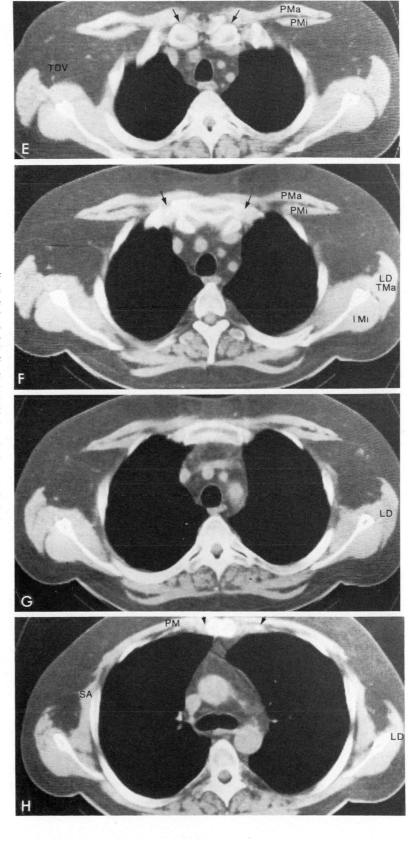

FIGURE 5–4 *Continued* ■ *E,* CT scan at the level of suprasternal notch. The clavicular heads articulate with the posterolateral aspect of the manubrium *(arrows).* The joint space, containing a fibrocartilaginous disc, is sharply defined. The thoracodorsal vessels (TDV), visible at this level and above and below, represent branches of the axillary artery and vein. *F,* CT scan 10 mm below *E* shows the first ribs articulating with the lateral margin of the manubrium at its the widest point *(arrows).* The undersurfaces of the clavicular heads are visible as triangular densities posterior to the manubrium. *G,* CT scan 10 mm below *F* again shows the articulations of the first ribs with the manubrium. The pectoralis major and pectoralis minor muscles appear thinner than at higher levels, and their sternal and costal origins are seen. The axillary space remains sharply defined. *H,* CT scan 30 mm below *G* shows that the sternal body in cross section is much smaller than the manubrium. Incompletely calcified costal cartilages *(arrows)* lie lateral to the manubrium. The pectoral muscles (PM) are now closely applied to the anterior chest wall. The serratus anterior (SA) muscle marginates the medial axilla.

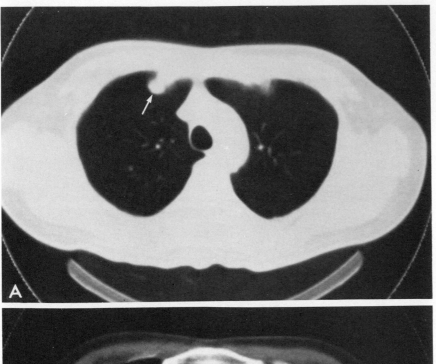

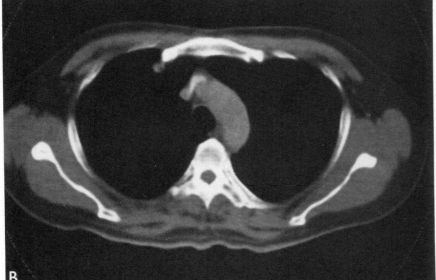

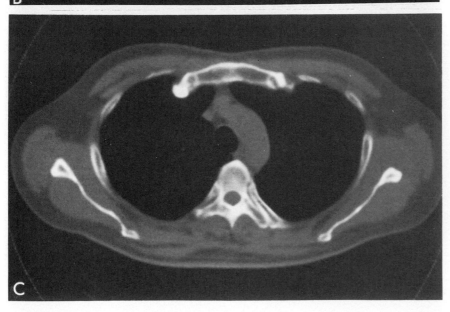

FIGURE 5–5 ■ First rib bony spur mimicking a lung nodule. *A,* CT scan at the level of the articulation of the first rib and manubrium suggests the presence of a right anterior lung nodule *(arrow). B,* CT scan at the same level, at mediastinal window settings, shows the "nodule" of tissue density in relationship to the manubrium. Its density is a result of volume averaging with the lung. C, CT scan at a slightly higher level shows the calcific density of the spur. Although often symmetric, the spur in this patient is present only on the right.

diagnosis (Fig. 5–6). In such cases CT can define the extent of the tumor and the degree of involvement of the chest wall and underlying pleura, lung, or mediastinum.[18]

Metastasis of malignant tumors to the sternum is common and more frequent than primary tumors. Primary tumors of the sternum occur slightly more often in the manubrium than in the sternal body, whereas the xiphoid process is rarely affected. Most primary sternal tumors are chondrosarcomas or myelomas. Because benign sternal tumors are very rare, tumors of the sternum should be considered malignant until proven otherwise.

Evaluation of the sternoclavicular joints and sternum by conventional radiographs is difficult. CT eliminates many of the problems of conventional

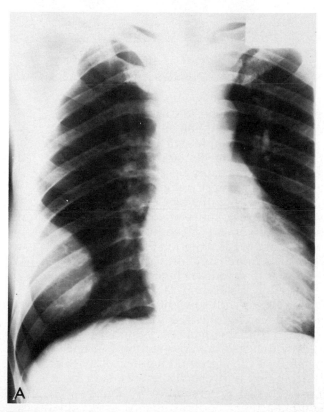

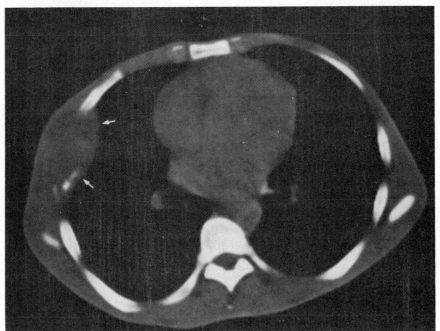

FIGURE 5–6 ■ Lymphoma with rib destruction. *A,* Frontal chest radiograph in a young man shows a well-defined mass in the right hemithorax. The adjacent rib is destroyed. *B,* CT scan shows rib destruction and an extrapleural mass *(arrows).* The sharp definition of the mass suggests it is limited by the pleura and is not invading the lung. Biopsy revealed lymphoma.

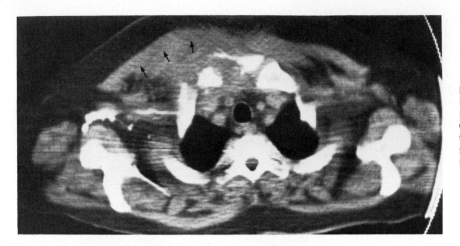

FIGURE 5–7 ■ Sternoclavicular joint osteomyelitis in a diabetic man with a staphylococcal infection of the foot and a right chest wall mass. CT scan shows bone destruction and erosion at the right sternoclavicular joint. An associated soft tissue mass has displaced the right pectoralis major muscle (arrows) anteriorly.

tomography, takes less time, is easier for the patient, and provides superior anatomic information.[9, 12, 13] In general, if plain radiographs fail to resolve a diagnostic problem regarding the sternum or sternoclavicular joints, CT is indicated.

Destouet and colleagues[13] reviewed the CT findings in 12 patients with pathologic conditions involving the sternoclavicular joints or sternum. Six cases of sternoclavicular joint dislocations attributable to trauma were diagnosed. Anterior dislocation of the clavicular head is more common than posterior dislocation, is easier to diagnose clinically, and is easier to treat. Posterior dislocation is more difficult to diagnose clinically or with conventional radiographic techniques and carries the risk of fatal injury to underlying mediastinal structures. Posterior dislocations are easily detected on cross-sectional images.

Osteomyelitis of the sternum and sternoclavicular joints is uncommon and usually follows surgery or radiotherapy. It also occurs in drug abusers and patients with bacterial endocarditis or mediastinal infections.[9, 10, 13] Osteoporosis, periosteal reaction, and bone erosion are seen more easily with CT than with conventional radiography (Fig. 5–7). Thin sections (5 mm or 1.5 mm) can help demonstrate these subtle abnormalities.

Two of the 12 patients studied by Destouet and associates[13] had malignant lesions (lymphoma and metastatic prostatic carcinoma) that caused sternal destruction. CT scans also revealed bony sclerosis and the soft tissue extent of the lesions. Similar findings have been reported by Stark and Jaramillo[9] and Hatfield and co-workers.[10]

Soft tissue lesions of the chest wall are rare and are usually evident clinically; however, CT can be of value in demonstrating involvement of the adjacent bones or intrathoracic structures (Fig. 5–8). Within the superior thorax, soft tissue sarcomas can extend anteriorly under the pectoralis muscles or posteriorly under the subscapularis muscle.[18] Such lesions can be very difficult to palpate, and CT scans often show that their extent is much greater than suspected clinically. This information is important to the surgeon.

The most common soft tissue tumors of the chest wall are lipomas, some of which are dumbbell-shaped, having both an intrathoracic and an extrathoracic component (Fig. 5–9).[19] Liposarcomas are the most frequent malignant tumors.[17, 18] Other lesions involving the chest wall are desmoids, fibrosarcomas, hemangiomas, nerve sheath tumors, rhabdomyosarcomas, and metastases.

Lipomas of the chest wall are invariably benign and do not require treatment unless they are large. When they are transmural, projecting both within

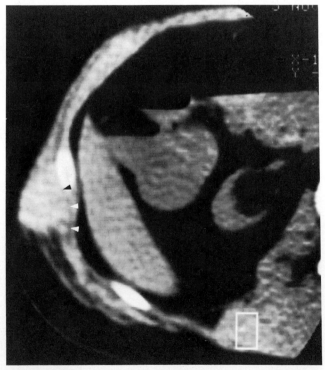

FIGURE 5–8 ■ Chest wall metastasis in a 35-year-old man with a pelvic angiosarcoma and a painful right chest wall mass. Detailed view from a CT scan of the lower right chest wall shows a soft tissue mass. A thin plane of fat (arrowheads) separates the mass from the underlying intercostal muscle, indicating the mass arises within soft tissues external to the thoracic cage, probably within the serratus anterior muscle. Biopsy revealed metastatic angiosarcoma.

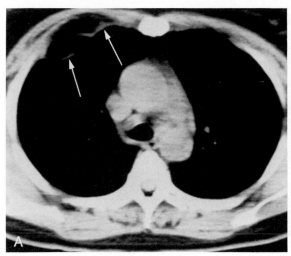
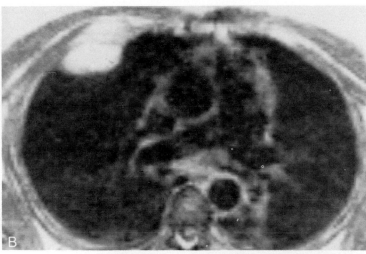

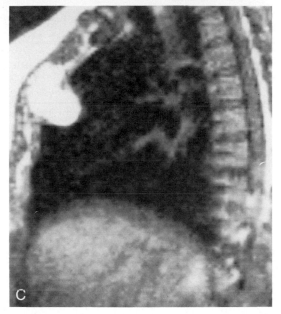

FIGURE 5–9 ■ Transthoracic lipoma in a young adult male. *A*, CT scan shows a low-density mass *(arrows)* in the right anterior chest wall. Mediastinal adenopathy is unrelated. *B*, T1-weighted MR scan at the same level shows the lipoma is of the same intensity as fat and invaginates the lung. *C*, Oblique sagittal MR demonstrates both the intra- and extrathoracic components of the lipoma.

and outside of the thoracic cage, they may be visible on chest radiographs as an extrapleural mass. Both CT and MR show the lesion as a well-demonstrated soft tissue mass with the imaging characteristics of fat (see Fig. 5–9).[20] CT or MR sometimes can help differentiate between a lipoma and liposarcoma, as the latter demonstrates inhomogeneous nonfatty elements.

Desmoid tumors of the chest wall are invasive, requiring excision and radiation therapy for control of local recurrence. Determination of their precise extent is useful in planning surgery but is often difficult with CT.[21–23] Differentiation between the tumor and surrounding muscle is frequently not possible with CT. MR imaging is probably the favored imaging modality for these tumors. With MR, a desmoid may demonstrate low signal intensity on both T1- and T2-weighted sequences.

Chest wall involvement by lymphoma occurs in about 1.5 per cent of patients and may influence the treatment protocol.[24, 25] It most frequently reflects direct extension from the mediastinum. MR is con-

siderably better than CT for detecting chest wall extension from lymphoma. In our experience, MR can detect chest wall infiltration by lymphoma not shown on CT. MR also may show more extensive chest wall invasion than suspected from CT.

Infections of the chest wall are uncommon and usually secondary to osteomyelitis of the shoulder girdle, ribs, spine, or sternum. Less frequently, an empyema can extend into the chest wall.[20] Tuberculosis and several fungal infections, including actinomycosis, blastomycosis, and coccidioidomycosis, can involve the chest wall.[26] Actinomycosis classically extends from the lung to involve the pleura, chest wall muscles, and bones. Infection can be surmised from CT when a soft tissue mass is in continuity with a bony lesion that demonstrates a mixed osteolytic and osteoblastic response. The mass shows an ill-defined margin with inhomogeneous areas of abscess and liquefaction. On MR, chest wall infections are isointense with skeletal muscle on T1- and hyperintense on T2-weighted images.[262] The presence of a subjacent empyema makes the diagnosis almost

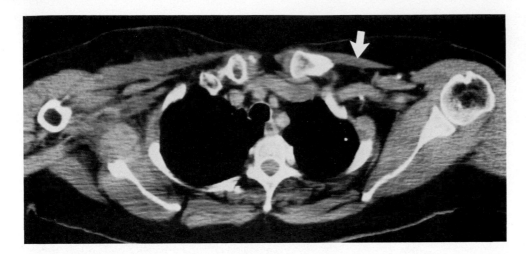

FIGURE 5–10 ■ Left modified radical mastectomy. A typical modified radical mastectomy consists of removal of the breast and pectoralis minor muscle and an axillary lymph node dissection, but the precise techniques vary among surgeons. In this patient, the left pectoralis major muscle *(arrow)* is visible, but the minor pectoralis has been removed. Clips in the left axilla indicate that a node dissection was performed. (From Shea WJ, de Geer G, Webb WR: Radiology 162:157–161, 1987. Reproduced with permission.)

certain.[27] CT or ultrasound can be used to guide aspiration of the area for culture. In addition to the usual cultures, aspirated specimens should be collected under anaerobic conditions. The microbiology laboratory should also be informed of a suspected actinomycosis infection, as this requires special culture media.

Median sternotomy for surgery on the coronary vessels, heart, mediastinum, and lungs is performed at a rate of more than one million times per year in North America. The complication of osteomyelitis of the sternum occurs in less than 3 per cent of instances but can be a diagnostic dilemma and a therapeutic problem.[28] Detection of focal extension of the infection into the prevascular tissues or of a more diffuse mediastinitis is important in planning the type of drainage and extent of debridement that will be required. Following median sternotomy, gas should be resorbed from the retrosternal tissues within 1 week. The edema and hematoma that can occur should also diminish over several weeks. CT is the best method for detecting and localizing a retrosternal abscess.[29, 30] The presence of air in the retrosternal tissues, together with a mass, is highly suspicious for an abscess. CT may show continuity of the fluid collection to a draining sinus through the sternotomy site. Acute mediastinitis shows diffuse widening and replacement of mediastinal fat by higher density inflammatory tissue. Diagnostic aspiration is frequently required for confirmation of infection. Artifacts from sternal wires make MR less useful than CT for evaluation of sternal infections.

MASTECTOMY

Radical mastectomy produces easily recognized alterations in axillary anatomy that have been reviewed in detail.[31] At present, however, the trend is toward more conservative treatment of breast cancer using simple or modified radical mastectomy. The CT findings after these procedures are varied and have also been described.[32]

A radical mastectomy consists of complete removal of the breast tissue and pectoralis major and minor muscles and extensive axillary lymph node dissection. In a study by Shea and colleagues of patients who had undergone this procedure, the chest wall thickness was routinely less than 15 mm, with no subcutaneous fat visible at the site of the operation.[31] Although most of the pectoralis muscles had been removed, residual pectoralis major muscle, which should not be misinterpreted as recurrent tumor, was occasionally identified at its sternal or costal attachment. Congenital absence of the pectoral mus-

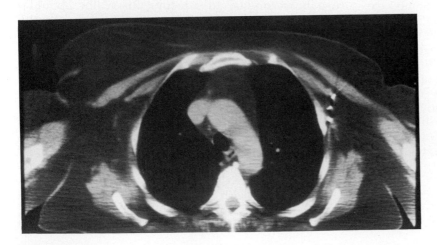

FIGURE 5–11 ■ Simple mastectomy. The left breast has been removed, but the underlying pectoralis muscles are intact. A left axillary lymph node dissection has also been performed. A simple mastectomy with a node dissection is called a *total mastectomy*. (From Shea WJ, de Geer G, Webb WR: Radiology 162:157–161, 1987. Reproduced with permission.)

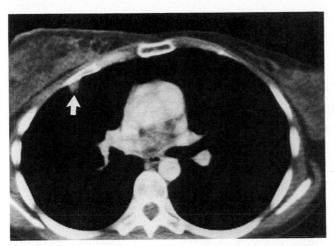

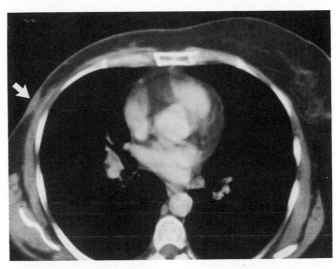

FIGURE 5–12 ■ Segmental right mastectomy and radiation. On the right, residual breast tissue is present. Skin thickening anteriorly on the right and edema of the breast are the results of radiation therapy. Note that the right breast appears full compared with the normal ptotic left breast. The density within the anterior right lung (arrow) represents radiation lung injury. (From Shea WJ, de Geer G, Webb WR: Radiology 162:157–161, 1987. Reproduced with permission.)

FIGURE 5–13 ■ Recurrent breast carcinoma in the skin following right modified radical mastectomy. The focal skin thickening (arrow) is the site of recurrence. (From Shea WJ, de Geer G, Webb WR: Radiology 162:162–164, 1987. Reproduced with permission.)

cles has a similar appearance, but the breast tissue is still present.

A typical modified radical mastectomy consists of removal of the breast and pectoralis minor muscle and an axillary lymph node dissection (Fig. 5–10). The precise techniques for this procedure can vary among surgeons, and a discussion with the surgeon concerning the procedure performed is advisable before interpreting the CT scans. In patients who have undergone a modified radical mastectomy, chest wall thickness is variable, as is the amount of pectoralis minor muscle remaining. Without careful clinical correlation, it is sometimes difficult to distinguish, on CT scans, postsurgical changes from tumor recurrence. This is especially a problem when the patient has difficulty elevating both arms symmetrically for the CT examination. With the arms raised, asymmetry of the pectoralis muscles is accentuated, and the scans are even more difficult to interpret. It is therefore best to obtain scans with the patient's arms at her sides.

A simple mastectomy consists of removal of only breast tissue; the underlying musculature remains intact (Fig. 5–11). Residual breast tissue remains when segmental or partial mastectomy is performed.

Radiation therapy combined with surgery can result in skin thickening (between 5 and 10 mm) in the first 3 months after treatment. CT scans also may reveal wispy strands of soft tissue density within the subcutaneous fat that are no longer visible 6 months after radiation treatment (Fig. 5–12).[33]

CT can detect unsuspected local chest wall recurrence in women treated for breast cancer, and it can be used for needle localization in preparation for biopsy of a suspicious abnormality.[33–35] Shea and co-workers[33] studied 15 patients with recurrent tumor, seven of whom had focal skin thickening (Fig. 5–13)

greater than 1 cm in depth and two of whom had focal soft tissue masses within the subcutaneous tissue. In eight patients, the contour or inhomogeneity of the residual pectoral muscle suggested recurrence (Fig. 5–14). In their study, postsurgical scarring or residual muscle mimicked and could not be differentiated from recurrent tumor. Enlargement of interpectoral lymph nodes between the major and minor pectoral muscles must also be appreciated.[35]

SECONDARY CHEST WALL LESIONS

Direct invasion of the chest wall by a peripheral bronchogenic carcinoma is common and was seen in 9 per cent of 110 patients with unresectable tumors studied by Napoli and colleagues.[36] Similarly, Hodgkin's disease can involve structures of the chest wall

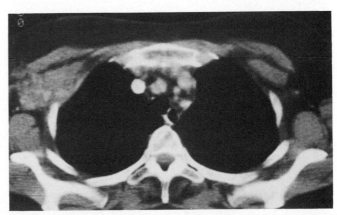

FIGURE 5–14 ■ Breast cancer recurrence involving the pectoralis minor muscle. Following a simple mastectomy, a large inhomogeneous mass is seen in the right axilla. The posterior margin of the pectoralis minor muscle is obliterated. (From Shea WJ, de Geer G, Webb WR: Radiology 162:162–164, 1987. Reproduced with permission.)

by direct invasion from the mediastinum or lung in a small percentage of cases.[37, 38] Malignant mesothelioma is a less common tumor that also can invade the chest wall.[39]

Care must be taken in diagnosing chest wall invasion on the basis of CT appearances. Tumors can abut the visceral pleura without invading the pleura or chest wall. In addition, central bronchogenic carcinoma obstructing a bronchus frequently has a peripheral consolidation that mimics a subpleural mass. After thoracotomy or open biopsy, edema and hematoma in the chest wall can be mistaken for tumor invasion. Reliable findings of chest wall invasion include bone destruction and a discrete extrapleural mass (Fig. 5–15). Such lesions are readily accessible to biopsy guided by CT.

Several pulmonary infections can involve the chest wall by direct extension.[40] These include actinomycosis, nocardiosis, and tuberculosis (Fig. 5–16). If the chest wall disease is associated with adjacent pulmonary consolidation rather than a mass, infection rather than neoplasm may be suggested.

SUPERIOR SULCUS TUMORS

Invasive tumors arising in the superior pulmonary sulcus produce the characteristic clinical findings of Horner's syndrome, and shoulder and arm pain; this presentation is termed *Pancoast's syndrome*.[41] In the past, tumors of the superior sulcus carried a very poor prognosis, but radiation followed by resection of the upper lung lobe, chest wall, and adjacent structures has resulted in 5-year survival rates of 30 per cent.[42, 43] In patients being considered for this combined therapy, CT scans can provide information on the anatomic extent of tumor spread that is useful in planning both the radiation therapy and the surgical approach to the tumor.[44–48]

Extension of tumor posteriorly or laterally from the lung apex involves the chest wall and axillary nerves. Although chest wall invasion does not preclude resection, extensive chest wall and bone involvement make surgical resection difficult, and the prognosis for patients with extensive chest wall disease is poor. Invasion of tumor posteromedially involves the ribs or vertebral bodies. This occurs in one third to one

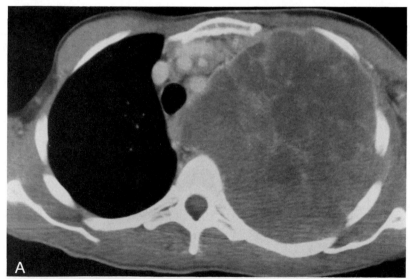

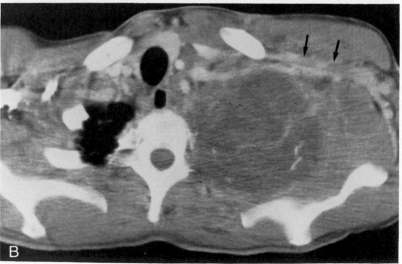

FIGURE 5–15 ■ Chest wall invasion by bronchogenic carcinoma. *A*, CT scan at the level of the manubrium demonstrates a large left upper lobe necrotic bronchogenic carcinoma filling the left hemithorax. *B*, Two centimeters higher, tumor infiltrates the chest wall. The pectoral muscles *(arrows)* are displaced anteriorly and laterally. The ribs, normally visible at this level, are destroyed.

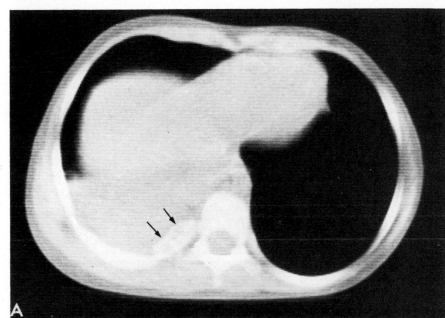

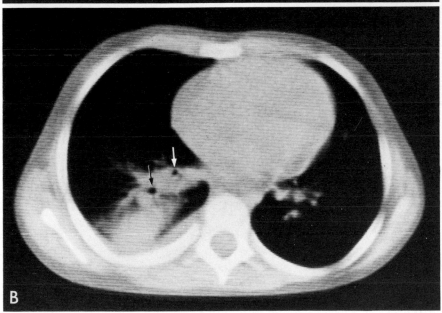

FIGURE 5–16 ■ Actinomycosis of the lung and chest wall in a young girl with low-grade fever and a right posterior chest wall mass. *A,* CT scan shows thickening of soft tissues of the posterior chest wall with destruction and periostitis of a medial rib *(arrows)* and dense lower lobe consolidation. *B,* CT scan at a higher level shows air in bronchi *(arrows)* within consolidated lung and a small pleural effusion. Surgery revealed a large lung abscess from which actinomycosis was cultured. (From Webb WR, Sagel SS: AJR 139:1008, © 1982, American Roentgen Ray Society. Reproduced with permission.)

half of cases and can usually be seen on CT (Figs. 5–2, 5–15, and 5–17).[44] Anterior and medial extension of tumor can involve the esophagus, trachea, and brachiocephalic vessels. Invasion of these structures usually precludes resection. In patients with superior sulcus tumors, as with other bronchogenic carcinomas, the detection of mediastinal invasion by CT can be difficult and has diagnostic limitations.

The better contrast resolution of MR can demonstrate extension of superior sulcus tumors into the lower neck.[46] The relationship of tumor to the vessels and nerves that course over the cupula of the lung is especially well demonstrated (see Fig. 5–3).[46–48] MR techniques using surface coils also can provide excellent morphologic detail. Images in the coronal,

sagittal, or orthogonal plane can assist in determining the extent of chest wall invasion (Fig. 5–18).

Axillary Space

Anatomy

As usually defined, the axilla is bordered by the fascial coverings of the following muscles: anteriorly, the pectoralis major and pectoralis minor; posteriorly, the latissimus dorsi, teres major, and subscapularis; medially, the chest wall and serratus anterior; and laterally, the coracobrachialis and biceps.[14, 49] These are the appropriate boundaries for patients with their arms at their sides (Fig. 5–19A through C). Usually,

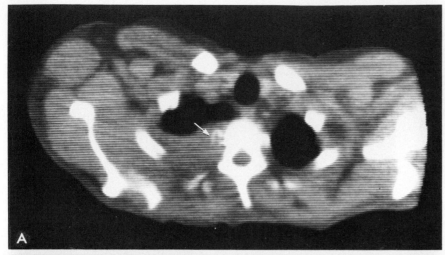

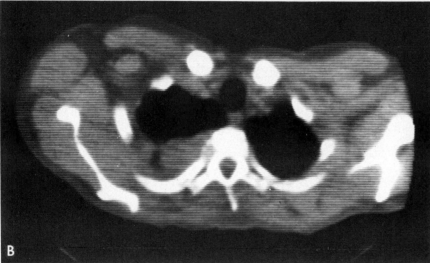

FIGURE 5–17 ■ Pancoast's tumor in a 37-year-old man with right shoulder pain and apical pleural thickening. *A,* CT scan 10 mm above the sternal notch shows a posterior tumor mass and destruction of the medial third rib *(arrow).* *B,* CT scan 10 mm higher again shows destruction of the rib. Biopsy revealed adenocarcinoma. After radiation therapy, an en bloc resection was performed. (From Webb WR, Jeffrey RB, Godwin JD: J Comput Assist Tomogr 5:361, 1981. Reproduced with permission.)

however, patients are scanned with their arms above their heads so that the arm and its musculature no longer form the lateral margin of the axillary space and the axilla is open laterally (see Fig. 5–19D through *F*). On CT scans, the apex, or cephalic extent, of the axilla is best defined by the level at which the pectoralis minor muscle crosses from anterior to posterior above the axillary space and inserts into the coracoid process of the scapula (see Fig. 5–4A).

The axilla contains the axillary artery and vein, branches of the brachial plexus, some branches of the intercostal nerves, and a large number of lymph nodes, all surrounded by fat.[15] The axillary vessels and the brachial plexus extend laterally, near the apex of the axilla, close to the pectoralis minor muscle. They are continued within the fibrous axillary sheath, which is continuous with the deep cervical fascia above the first rib. In general, the axillary vein lies below and anterior to the axillary artery, whereas the brachial plexus is largely above and posterior to the artery.[45, 50] Although two vessels usually can be seen on CT within the axilla (see Fig.

5–4B through *D*), in many normal individuals it is not possible to distinguish between the artery and vein within the axilla (see Fig. 5–19D).

The subscapular artery and vein are the largest branches of the axillary vessels.[15] They divide after a short course into the thoracodorsal artery and vein medially and the circumflex scapular vessels, branches of which descend along the lateral border of the scapula between the teres major and teres minor muscles. These vessels usually are visible on high-quality CT scans (see Figs. 5–4B and C and 5–19D through *F*).

The axillary lymph nodes, of which there are 20 to 30,[15] normally can be up to about 1 cm in maximum diameter and belong to several groups. A *lateral* group of four to six nodes lies near the undersurface of the axillary vein and drains the arm. An *anterior* or *pectoral* group of four to five nodes lies along the lateral border of the pectoralis minor muscle. Their afferent lymph vessels drain the skin and muscles of the anterior and lateral chest walls and the central and lateral breast. A *posterior* or *subscapular* group of six or seven lymph nodes is situated along the lower margin of the posterior axillary wall, close to a branch of the subscapular artery. They drain the upper back and dorsal part of the neck. A *medial* or *subclavicular* group of 6 to 12 nodes lies posterior to the cranial portion of the pectoralis minor muscle. This group drains a portion of the arm and breast. Last, an *intermediate* or *central* group of three or four large nodes lies deep within the axilla and communicates with all the other node groups. Normal lymph nodes are identified routinely on CT scans of the axilla.

Axillary Abnormalities

LYMPHADENOPATHY

Axillary lymph nodes, usually up to 1 cm but occasionally 1.5 cm in maximum diameter, can be seen in normal patients.[51] Lymph nodes larger than 2 cm in diameter generally are considered abnormal.

Axillary lymphadenopathy is seen most frequently in patients with lymphoma or metastatic carcinoma (Figs. 5–20 through 5–22).[49] Lymph node masses are detected most easily by observing both axillae for asymmetry. Enlarged lymph nodes high within the axilla lie beneath the pectoral muscles and may not be palpable. These nodes can be detected by CT, although the sensitivity and accuracy of diagnosis have not been determined.[17]

BRACHIAL PLEXUS TUMORS

The nerves making up the brachial plexus course through the lower neck in a plane between the scalenus anterior and scalenus medius muscles. Although the brachial plexus often is not visible on CT scans as a discrete structure, brachial plexus tumors can often be demonstrated.[18, 50] Tumor involving the brachial plexus is diagnosed when CT shows a mass

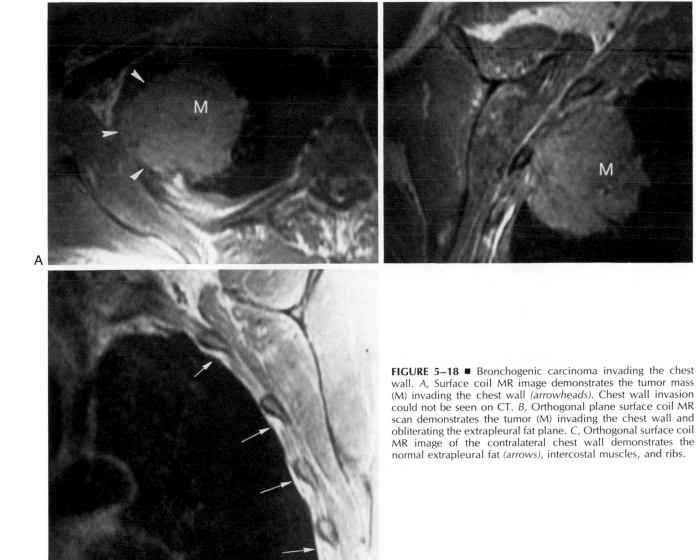

FIGURE 5–18 ■ Bronchogenic carcinoma invading the chest wall. *A,* Surface coil MR image demonstrates the tumor mass (M) invading the chest wall *(arrowheads).* Chest wall invasion could not be seen on CT. *B,* Orthogonal plane surface coil MR scan demonstrates the tumor (M) invading the chest wall and obliterating the extrapleural fat plane. *C,* Orthogonal surface coil MR image of the contralateral chest wall demonstrates the normal extrapleural fat *(arrows),* intercostal muscles, and ribs.

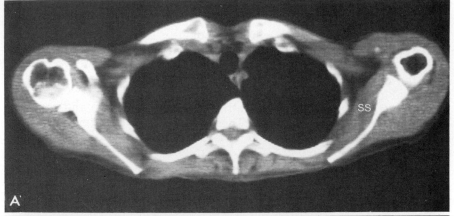

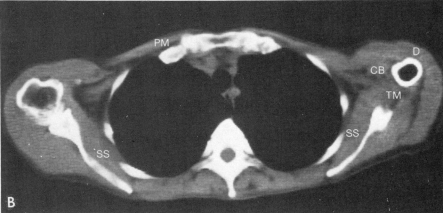

FIGURE 5–19 ■ Normal right axillary anatomy in a woman who had undergone a left radical mastectomy. CT scans were obtained with her arms at her sides (A through C) and raised above her head (D through F). A through C, With the arms positioned at the sides, the axilla is marginated anteriorly by the pectoralis major and pectoralis minor (PM) muscles, posteriorly by the subscapularis (SS) and teres major (TM) muscles, and laterally by the coracobrachialis and biceps (CB) muscles. On the left, the great bulk of the pectoral muscles has been removed surgically. The large deltoid muscle (D) is visible laterally. Axillary vessels are clearly visible. D through F, With the patient's arms positioned above her head, the appearance of the axilla is altered. Scan levels of D through F correspond to those of A through C, respectively. The pectoral muscles (PM) appear thicker, and the clavicle is elevated. The axillary vessels (AV) have a more horizontal course and are more easily seen. The axilla is open laterally. On the left side, the axilla is open anteriorly, because the pectoralis muscle is absent.

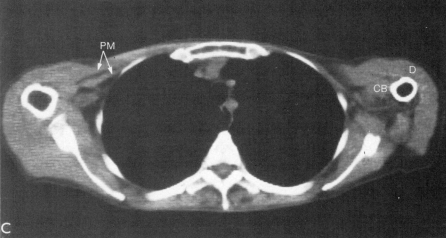

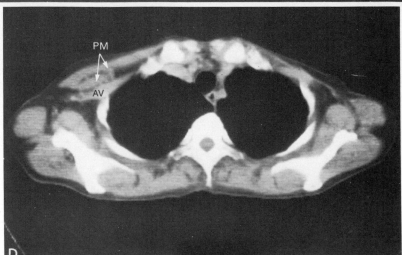

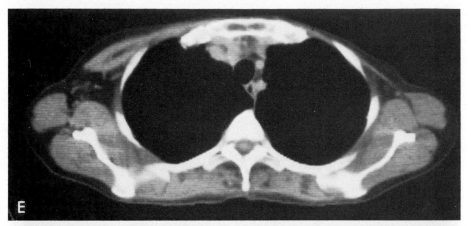

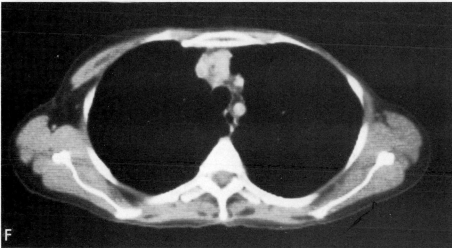

FIGURE 5–19 *Continued*

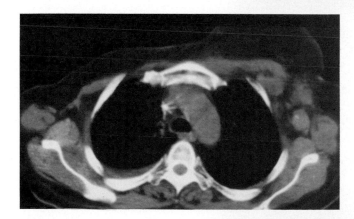

FIGURE 5–20 ■ Right breast cancer metastasis to left axillary nodes. A right modified radical mastectomy has been performed. A right pleural effusion is seen. (From Shea WJ, de Geer G, Webb WR: Radiology 162:162–164, 1987. Reproduced with permission.)

FIGURE 5–21 ■ Lymphoma with mediastinal and axillary adenopathy in a young man with Hodgkin's disease. CT scan shows right mediastinal lymph node enlargement and multiple enlarged left axillary lymph nodes *(arrowheads)*. The right axilla is normal.

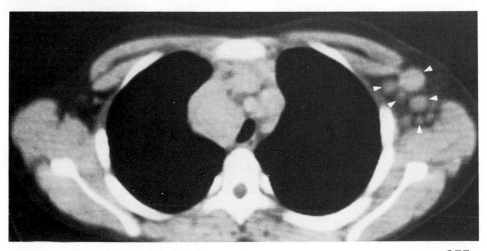

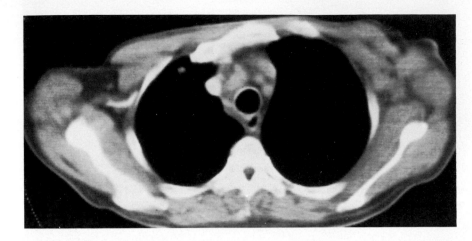

FIGURE 5–22 ■ Nasopharyngeal carcinoma with axillary metastases. CT scan shows several large, clinically palpable lymph nodes within the left axilla.

along the course of the brachial nerves and the clinical picture is compatible with brachial plexopathy (Fig. 5–23). A brachial plexus lesion also can be suggested when the fat plane that normally separates the scalenus anterior and scalenus medius muscles is obliterated or asymmetric when both sides are compared.[33]

Because of its excellent contrast resolution and multiplanar imaging capabilities, MR can identify many brachial plexus lesions (Fig. 5–24).[52–55] Although a detailed study comparing CT with MR has

not been performed, MR descriptions of normal and abnormal brachial plexus anatomy suggest that this method could be superior to CT in imaging this anatomically complex area.

On MR images, the nerves of the brachial plexus are best distinguished from vessels and muscles using T1-weighted images.[53] The nerves appear similar in intensity to muscle on both T1- and T2-weighted imaging sequences, but nerves can be identified because they are surrounded by fat in most locations. Centrally the nerve roots are best demon-

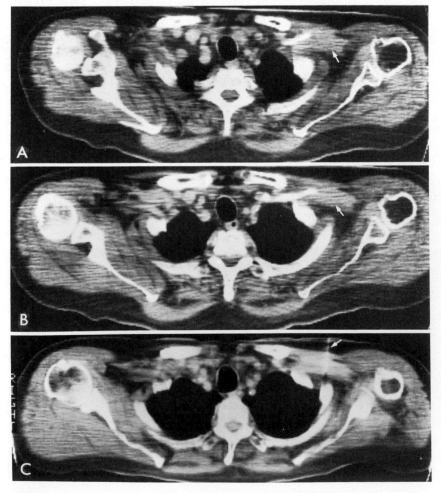

FIGURE 5–23 ■ Metastatic tumor involving the brachial plexus 10 years after a left radical mastectomy for breast carcinoma. The patient noticed a mass in her left supraclavicular fossa with symptoms of left brachial plexopathy. *A* and *B,* CT scans show a mass *(arrows)* posterior to the opacified axillary vein in the position of the brachial plexus. *C,* CT-guided needle biopsy revealed metastatic carcinoma. Arrow indicates needle tract.

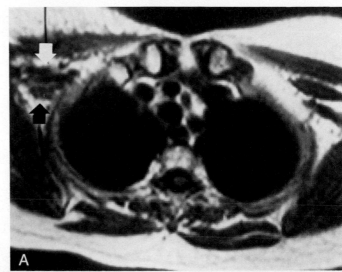

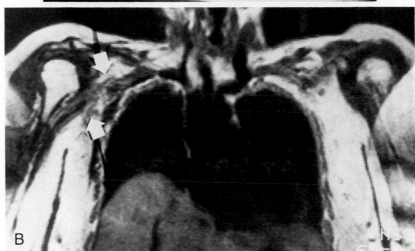

FIGURE 5–24 ■ MR scan of a brachial plexus tumor. A, T1-weighted MR scan shows an ill-defined mass in the right axilla surrounding the axillary nerves. B, On the coronal image, the mass encases the axillary vessels and nerves.

strated in the coronal plane and can be identified in the sagittal and transaxial planes as well. More laterally, sagittal images allow the nerves to be distinguished from the scalenus muscles and the subclavian artery in cross section.

Castagno and Shuman studied 47 patients who were suspected of having brachial plexus involvement by tumor.[52] In 22 patients who had symptoms suggesting brachial plexus lesions, MR determined correctly whether the plexus was surrounded by tumor. In 25 patients who had no neurologic signs or symptoms, MR identified tumor in the vicinity of, but not involving, the brachial plexus.

AXILLARY VEIN OCCLUSION

Occlusion of the axillary vein most frequently occurs as a result of thrombosis or compression by tumor. The condition can be recognized on CT scans after contrast material is injected into an ipsilateral arm vein. Findings include nonopacification of the vein or partial opacification with contrast material outlining a thrombus (Fig. 5–25). Venous collaterals that are not seen normally become visible in the axilla and chest wall. However, the axillary vein can fail to

opacify when a more central venous obstruction is present, causing stasis of blood in the axillary vein. Small veins in the chest wall sometimes do opacify in the absence of venous obstruction, especially when the injection is made into a small arm vein or during a Valsalva maneuver.

SUBTRAPEZIAL SPACE

When a patient's arms are raised above the head, an artifactual space becomes visible beneath the trapezius muscle at the level of the upper thoracic and lower cervical vertebrae (see Fig. 5–4A and B). This compartment has been termed the *subtrapezial space.*[56] Anteriorly and superiorly it is continuous with the posterior triangle of the neck, and anteriorly and inferiorly it is continuous with the apex of the axilla. The subtrapezial space contains lymph nodes belonging to the deep cervical chain; when these nodes are enlarged, they can be seen on CT scans.[56] The levator scapulae and anterior serratus muscles, however, do traverse the subtrapezial space and can cause confusion in the interpretation of CT scans by mimicking lymphadenopathy. The levator scapulae originates from the transverse processes of the upper

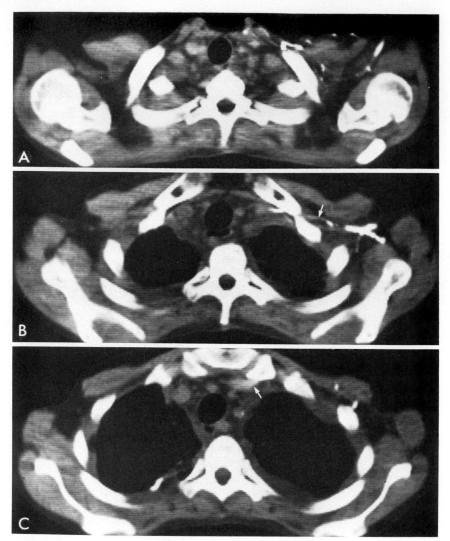

FIGURE 5–25 ■ Axillary vein occlusion. Three CT scans after a bolus injection of contrast material into the left arm vein show axillary vein occlusion. *A,* Numerous small collateral veins are visible within the axilla and anterior chest wall and neck. *B,* At a lower level, the axillary vein is densely opacified laterally but is incompletely seen medially as it passes between the first rib and the clavicle. The contrast seen medially *(arrow)* may be outlining an intraluminal clot. *C,* The left brachiocephalic vein *(arrow)* is only faintly opacified by contrast medium. With normal flow, this vein would be more densely opacified after an injection of contrast medium.

four cervical vertebrae and inserts into the medial border of the scapula. If the muscle is traced on serial CT scans, it is seen to cross the subtrapezial space in a superomedial to inferolateral direction. A portion of the anterior serratus muscle can also be seen in the subtrapezial space and has a somewhat triangular outline. Symmetry of these muscles usually allows differentiation from adenopathy.

Breast

Soft tissues of the breasts can easily be seen on CT scans of female patients in the supine position. Localized breasts masses occasionally are visible, but their CT appearance usually is nonspecific.[57] Breast masses detected incidentally on CT images generally should be evaluated by physical examination and conventional mammography (Fig. 5–26). Early interest in using CT for the diagnosis of breast masses has not been sustained, and CT has proved less valuable for this purpose than other imaging techniques.[57–59]

Breast Carcinoma

CT has not become an established technique for the routine evaluation of patients with breast cancer. However, CT can aid the planning of radiation therapy by providing an accurate measurement of chest wall thickness and by detecting internal mammary lymph node metastases.[18, 60, 61]

Metastases to the internal mammary lymph node chain have been found in one third of patients undergoing extended radical mastectomy for clinically resectable tumors. Internal mammary node metastases are more frequent in patients with tumors in the central or medial portion of the breast.[60] Because internal mammary node metastases are common, irradiating the internal mammary lymph node chain significantly improves local control of tumor and survival in patients treated by radical mastectomy.

Accurate knowledge of the location of the internal mammary lymph nodes is important in planning radiotherapy to ensure that these nodes are irradiated and normal tissues are spared. The internal mammary lymph nodes lie in the upper intercostal spaces

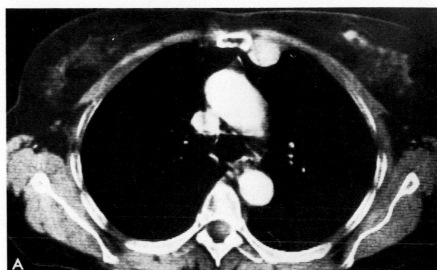

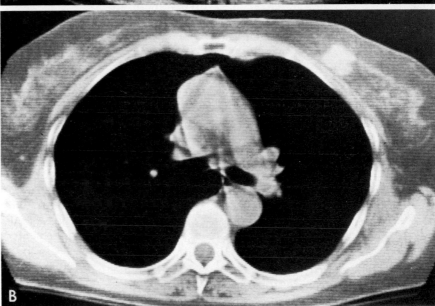

FIGURE 5–26 ■ Breast carcinoma with internal mammary lymphadenopathy seen as a small retrosternal mass on a routine chest radiograph. *A*, CT scan shows enlargement of a left internal mammary lymph node and a breast mass. *B*, CT scan at a lower level shows the left breast mass more clearly. Needle biopsies of the left breast mass revealed adenocarcinoma.

lateral to the sternum and are separated from the pleura only by the endothoracic fascia. Their depth depends on chest wall thickness and is therefore variable. However, CT allows direct measurement of chest wall thickness from the skin to pleura,[60] permitting a treatment volume appropriate for irradiating these nodes but sparing the lung. Munzenrider and associates[60] recommended that a CT determination of chest wall thickness be made in breast cancer patients considered for electron beam therapy (as dose distribution varies significantly with depth), in patients treated with tangential radiation, and in patients who are obese or have intact breasts.

CT can show evidence of internal mammary lymph node and anterior mediastinal lymph node metastases not detected with other radiographic methods (Fig. 5–27).[18, 60, 61] Generally, normal internal mammary lymph nodes are not visible on CT scans, and any visible node is considered abnormal (see Fig. 5–26A). Gouliamos and associates[18] found CT evidence of internal mammary lymph node metastases in 9 of

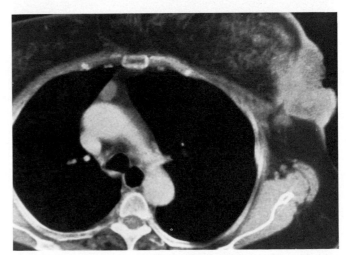

FIGURE 5–27 ■ Anterior mediastinal lymph node metastases from breast carcinoma. CT scan demonstrates a large left fungating breast carcinoma. A 2-cm anterior mediastinal lymph node metastasis is seen that was not visible on chest radiographs.

64 patients with breast carcinoma. Meyer and Munzenrider[61] used CT to detect internal mammary lymphadenopathy in 18 patients with locally recurrent breast carcinoma. In 12 of the patients, lymph node enlargement occurred only on the side of the previously treated carcinoma, and in six it was bilateral. Visible lymph nodes were 7 mm to 2.6 cm in diameter. In only 5 of the 18 patients were plain radiographic abnormalities visible prospectively. In four patients, CT showed sternal destruction by tumor that was not suspected from conventional radiographs.

In addition to detecting internal mammary lymph node metastases in patients with carcinoma of the breast, CT can be used to diagnose axillary lymph node enlargement and metastases to the chest wall or sternum. Gouliamos and colleagues[18] found axillary lymph node enlargement in 21 of 64 patients with breast carcinoma, chest wall involvement in five, and sternal destruction in one.

The CT appearances of augmentation mammoplasty implants are quite characteristic (Figs. 5–28 and 5–29). The homogeneous water density implants normally are situated immediately beneath the skin and are distinctly demarcated from the surrounding breast tissue. Strands of higher density may traverse the implant, and long-standing implants may demonstrate calcification of their walls.

MR of the breast is being investigated actively but is not generally available or used for clinical diagnosis.[62-65] The normal breast demonstrates high signal intensity from fat and low signal intensity from ductal tissue, connective tissue, and vessels on both T1- and T2-weighted images. Normal glands and periglandular fibrous elements cannot be distinguished on MR, and both are slightly more intense than muscle. The patterns of normal breast parenchyma are similar to those described for mammography. Calcifications are not observed on MR images.

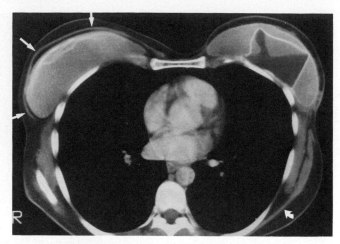

FIGURE 5–29 ■ Bilateral breast prostheses after modified radical mastectomies. On the right, a latissimus dorsi flap *(arrows)* was used to maintain the position of the prosthesis. On the left, the latissimus dorsi *(curved arrow)* is visible in normal position. (From Shea WJ, de Geer G, Webb WR: Radiology 162:157–161, 1987. Reproduced with permission.)

The proliferation of fibrous tissue with ductal dilatation observed in fibrocystic disease of the breast appears on MR as an excess of low-intensity regions on T1- and T2-weighted images. MR may distinguish focal areas of fibrosis from breast carcinoma by these imaging characteristics. Cysts appear on MR imaging as well-defined and well-marginated masses that on T2-weighted images are uniformly very high in signal intensity.

Noncalcified fibroadenomas are well defined and homogeneous and of low signal intensity on T1-weighted images. With T2-weighting, they may have either high or low signal intensity. Calcified fibroadenomas frequently appear heterogeneous and are of low intensity on both T1- and T2-weighted images.

The majority of breast carcinomas more than 2 cm in diameter are demonstrated on MR images. On T1-weighted images they are of low signal intensity and are lobulated or nodular spiculated masses. Dash and colleagues,[62] in their study of 112 women, identified 18 of 21 breast cancers with MR. On T2-weighted images, breast cancers may show low or high signal intensity approaching that of fat. The role of paramagnetic contrast agents in defining breast carcinomas remains unclear. The diagnosis of breast cancer with MR is based on the tumor's morphology and imaging characteristics. Discrimination between benign and malignant tissues on the basis of relaxation parameters has not been established.

Turner and associates[66] conclude that MR is less accurate than mammography for detecting breast carcinoma. MR may, however, have a limited role for evaluating well-defined masses whose cystic nature remains indeterminate after ultrasonography. These authors suggest that gadolinium-DPTA may assist in assessing dense breasts or in differentiating neoplasm from scar tissue. MR spectroscopy awaits further evaluation.

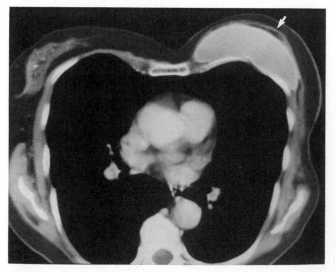

FIGURE 5–28 ■ Left breast prosthesis after simple mastectomy. A thin strip of residual pectoralis major muscle *(arrow)* covers the prosthesis. (From Shea WJ, de Geer G, Webb WR: Radiology 162:157–161, 1987. Reproduced with permission.)

Pleurae

Anatomy

Although the visceral and parietal pleural layers cannot be seen on conventional CT scans, a knowledge of their anatomy and relationships often permits a reliable diagnosis of pleural disease to be made.

COSTAL PLEURA

The combined thickness of the visceral and parietal pleurae surrounding the lung and the pleural space between them is approximately 0.2 to 0.4 mm (Fig. 5–30). The parietal pleura measures about 0.1 mm; the visceral pleura is anatomically similar but somewhat thicker.[67, 68] The width of the pleural space, determined from studies of frozen thoraces, is 10 to 20 nm.

External to the parietal pleura, the thoracic cavity is lined by the fibroelastic endothoracic fascia, which is about 0.25 mm thick. It covers the intercostal muscles and intervening ribs, blends with the perichondrium and periosteum of the costal cartilages and sternum anteriorly, and posteriorly is continuous with the prevertebral fascia covering the vertebral bodies and intervertebral disks (see Fig. 5–30).[69, 70] The parietal pleura is separated from the endothoracic fascia by a layer of loose areolar connective tissue that averages 0.25 mm in thickness in most locations[67, 68] but that can be markedly thickened over the posterolateral ribs, resulting in extrapleural fat pads several millimeters thick.[71, 72]

External to the endothoracic fascia are a layer of fatty connective tissue and three intercostal muscles.[73, 74] The innermost intercostal muscle passes between the internal surfaces of adjacent ribs and is relatively thin (see Fig. 5–30). It is separated from the inner and external intercostal muscles by the space containing the intercostal vessels and nerve. Although the innermost intercostal muscles are incomplete in the anterior and posterior thorax, the transverse thoracic and subcostal muscles can occupy the same relative plane and are considered by some anatomists to be parts of the innermost intercostal muscle.[75] Anteriorly, the transverse thoracic muscle consists of four or five slips that arise from the xiphoid process and lower sternum, passing superolaterally to insert into the second to sixth costal

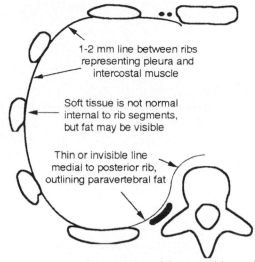

FIGURE 5–31 ■ HRCT characteristics of the normal lung–chest wall interface.

cartilages.[69, 70, 73, 74] The internal mammary vessels lie external to the transverse thoracic muscle. Posteriorly, the subcostal muscles are thin bands of muscle that extend from the inner aspect of the angle of the lower ribs, crossing one or two ribs and intercostal spaces to the inner aspect of a rib below. These structures are best seen using HRCT techniques with narrow collimation. On CT with 1-cm collimation, volume averaging diminishes resolution, and these muscles are poorly seen.

On HRCT in normal patients, a 1- to 2-mm-thick line of soft tissue density visible in the anterolateral and posterolateral intercostal spaces at the point of contact between lung and chest wall represents the combined thicknesses of visceral and parietal pleurae, the fluid-filled pleural space, endothoracic fascia, and innermost intercostal muscle (Figs. 5–31 and 5–32)[75a]. Although the pleura and endothoracic fascia pass internal to the ribs, they are not frequently visible in this location on HRCT unless abnormally thickened.

The ribs are oriented obliquely relative to the plane of a CT scan, with each CT section typically traversing the upper edge, midportion, and lower edge of separate ribs. With either 1-cm collimation or HRCT, a soft tissue density stripe 1 to 2 mm wide, representing primarily the innermost intercostal muscle, can be seen internal to the tapering edges of upper and lower rib segments. This stripe can be distinguished from pleural thickening, because it is continuous with the normal innermost intercostal muscle in the adjacent interspaces. This normal stripe is usually not seen internal to the midportion of the rib; only its edges are visible (see Fig. 5–32). However, when a rib segment is nearly horizontal, as is common posteriorly, and the scan contains only a part of the upper or lower rib margin, then the normal stripe can be seen internal to the entire length of the rib edge, mimicking pleural thickening. The visible rib edge at this site will appear thinner than at other levels.

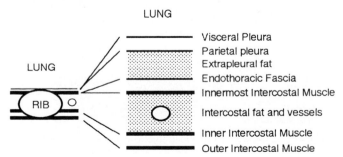

FIGURE 5–30 ■ Schema of soft tissue planes at the lung–chest wall interface. In most individuals, the visceral and parietal pleura, extrapleural fat, endothoracic fascia, and innermost intercostal muscle all make up a 1- to 2-mm linear stripe between the ribs.

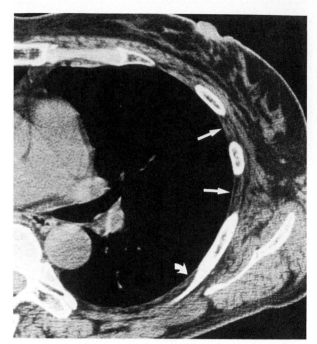

FIGURE 5–32 ■ HRCT scan of the normal lung–chest wall interface. A 1- to 2-mm-thick line of soft tissue density visible in the lateral intercostal spaces *(straight arrows)* represents the combined thickness of visceral and parietal pleurae, the fluid-filled pleural space, endothoracic fascia, and innermost intercostal muscle. Although the pleura and endothoracic fascia pass internal to the ribs, they are not visible in this location. When a rib segment is nearly horizontal, as it is posteriorly, and the scan plane traverses only a part of the lower rib margin, the normal 1- to 2-mm stripe can be seen internal to a part of the rib *(curved arrow)*, sometimes mimicking pleural thickening. (From Im J-G, Webb WR, Rosen A, Gamsu G: Radiology 171:125–131, 1989. Reproduced with permission.)

Normal soft tissue can be seen on HRCT internal to a rib in several locations. A layer of extrapleural fatty connective tissue located between the parietal pleura and endothoracic fascia is thicker next to the lateral ribs than at other sites.[71, 72] It is most abundant over the fourth to eighth ribs and can produce fat pads several millimeters thick that can extend into the intercostal spaces. In normal persons, these costal fat pads are usually difficult to recognize using the usual mediastinal window width of about 500 H but are seen more readily with extended window settings (1500 to 2000 H).

Anteriorly, at the level of the heart and adjacent to the lower sternum or xiphoid process, the transversus thoracis muscle is nearly always visible internal to the ends of ribs or costal cartilages (Figs. 5–32 and 5–33). Posteriorly, at the same level, a 1- to 2-mm-thick line representing the subcostalis muscle is sometimes seen internal to one or more ribs (see Fig. 5–33). In contrast to pleural thickening, the transversus thoracis and subcostal muscles are smooth, uniform in thickness, and symmetric bilaterally.

Paravertebrally the innermost intercostal muscle is absent, and the pleura and endothoracic fascia combine to produce a thinner line than that seen laterally (Figs. 5–31 and 5–34). In some normal individuals, however, the paravertebral line appears thicker than expected and probably represents segments of inter-

costal vessels lying within the scan plane (Fig. 5–35). The diagnosis of pleural thickening requires that this region appear uniformly thickened on multiple sections. Thickened pleura also is distinguishable from underlying vessels when separated by an intervening fat plane.

INTRAPULMONARY FISSURES

Because they are thin and oblique relative to the plane of the scan, the normal major fissures are not seen routinely on CT images obtained with 1-cm collimation. However, the position of each major fissure can be inferred from the position of a relatively avascular plane of lung 2 to 3 cm wide accompanying and paralleling the fissure. In 10 to 20 per cent of patients the major fissures are demonstrated on CT scans with 1-cm collimation as a thin line, although low window levels and narrow window widths may be required to see them. In some patients, a ground-glass band of density is seen in the avascular area that surrounds the major fissure, probably reflecting volume averaging of the fissure itself.[76] On thin-collimation scans, the major fissures are almost always recognizable as thin white lines (Fig. 5–36). Normal collections of fat extending into the

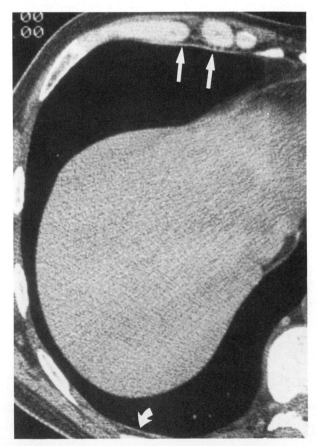

FIGURE 5–33 ■ Normal transversus thoracic and subcostalis muscles. Anteriorly, at the level of the heart, the transversus thoracic muscle *(straight arrows)* is nearly always visible internal to the ends of ribs or costal cartilages. Posteriorly, at the same level, a 1- to 2-mm-thick line is sometimes seen internal to one or more ribs, representing the subcostalis muscle *(curved arrow)*.

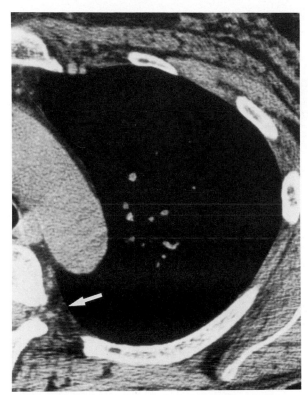

FIGURE 5–34 ■ Normal paravertebral region. HRCT scan shows that in the paravertebral area, the innermost intercostal muscle is absent, and pleura and endothoracic fascia combine to produce a line *(arrow)* thinner than that seen laterally.

inferior aspects of the major fissures at the diaphragmatic surface can simulate fissural pleural thickening or effusion but will be low in density at mediastinal window settings.

The minor fissure usually is invisible, but its plane can also be inferred from the position of the avascular area between the right upper lobe vessels above and the middle lobe vessels below. The avascular plane of lucency, reflecting the position of the minor fissure, is visible in 52 to 100 per cent of patients.[76–79] On HRCT scans the minor fissure can be seen as a white line of varying sharpness and thickness, depending on its orientation. Because the minor fissure often is concave caudally, it can be seen in two locations or can appear to be ring shaped in the plane of the scan, with the middle lobe between the fissure lines or in the center of the ring and the upper lobe anterior and lateral to the fissure.

In patients with an azygos lobe, the four layers of the mesoazygos, or azygos fissure, are visible above the level of the displaced azygos vein.[80] The azygos fissure is C shaped and convex laterally, beginning anteriorly at the right brachiocephalic vein and ending posteriorly at the right anterolateral surface of the vertebral body (Fig. 5–37). Other accessory fissures, most commonly the inferior accessory fissure, are seen occasionally on CT.[81] They are not generally significant in diagnosis, and distinguishing an accessory fissure from a parenchymal scar may sometimes be difficult.

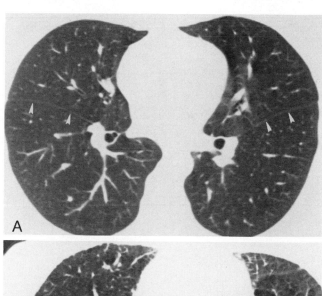

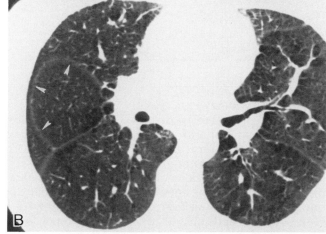

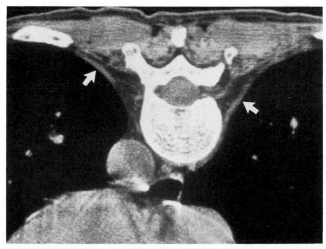

FIGURE 5–35 ■ Normal intercostal veins. Prone HRCT scan shows that in some normal patients, the paravertebral line appears thicker than expected because of segments of intercostal veins *(arrows)* lying adjacent to the pleural surface. (From Im J-G, Webb WR, Rosen A, Gamsu G: Radiology 171:125–131, 1989. Reproduced with permission.)

FIGURE 5–36 ■ Normal fissures. *A,* HRCT scan demonstrates the normal major fissures *(arrowheads)* extending from the costal margins laterally to the hila medially. *B,* HRCT scan in a second patient demonstrates the major and minor fissures. The minor fissure *(arrowheads)* appears as a semicircle. The upper lobe is in front, the lower lobe behind, and the middle lobe within the circle of the minor and major fissures.

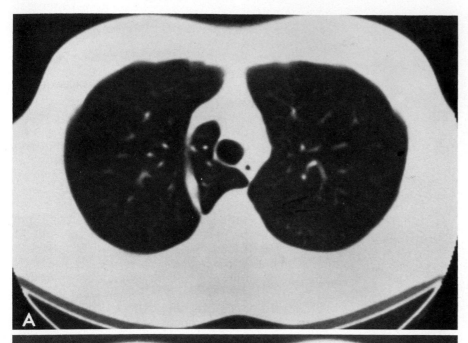

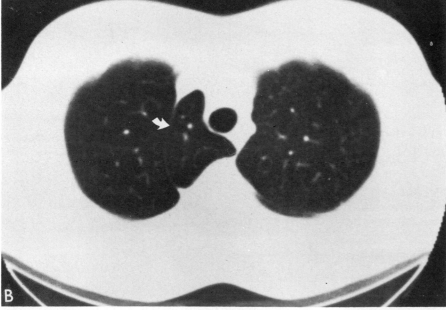

FIGURE 5–37 ■ Azygos lobe and fissure. *A,* CT scan shows the anomalous arch of the azygos vein passing through the right lung. *B,* At a higher level, the azygos fissure *(arrow)* has a **C** shape. (From Speckman JM, Gamsu G, Webb WR: AJR 137:47, © 1981, Am Roentgen Ray Society. Reproduced with permission.)

INFERIOR PULMONARY LIGAMENT

On each side, below the level of the pulmonary hilum, the parietal and visceral pleural layers invaginate the lung to form a fold that extends inferiorly along the mediastinum to end at the level of the diaphragm. The inferior pulmonary ligament anchors the lower lobe to the mediastinum and medial diaphragm.[82] In cross section on CT images viewed at lung window settings, it appears as a small linear density 1 to 2 cm long, pointing laterally into the lung and with its base against the mediastinum (see Chapter 2, Fig. 2–16).[83–85] On both the left and right, it projects laterally from near the esophagus. A similar linear density, seen over several centimeters above the diaphragm and extending laterally from the IVC, is the pleural reflection over the phrenic nerve and not the inferior pulmonary ligament. Pleural effusion or pneumothoraces can be limited and marginated by the inferior pulmonary ligament.[86]

Pleural Abnormalities

PLEURAL FLUID COLLECTIONS

In general, collections of pleural fluid are recognized readily on CT scans of the thorax as arcuate areas of homogeneous density paralleling the chest wall.[1] Small pleural effusions, however, can be difficult to distinguish from pleural thickening. The diagnosis of free-flowing pleural fluid requires a change in patient position from supine to decubitus or prone (Figs. 5–38).[87] Large effusions often extend into the major fissures, displacing the lower lobes medially and posteriorly.

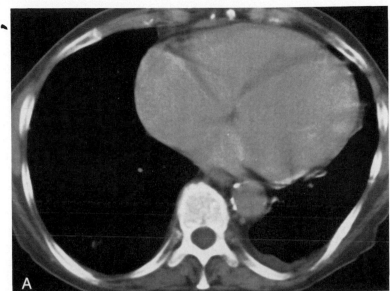

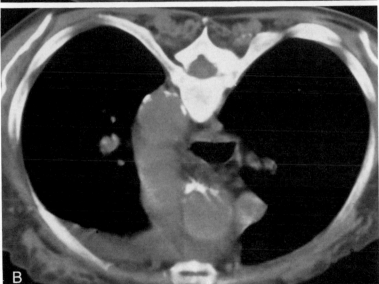

FIGURE 5–38 ■ Pleural effusion. Small free-flowing left pleural effusion demonstrated in supine *(A)* and prone *(B)* CT scans. In the prone position, free-flowing pleural effusion tends to collect in a more cephalic location than in the supine position.

The visceral pleura covers the surface of the lung, and its inferior extent is defined by the inferior extent of lung in the costophrenic angles. The parietal pleura is contiguous with the chest wall and diaphragm and in the costophrenic angles extends well below the level of the lung base.

Thus pleural fluid collections in the costophrenic angles can be seen below the lung base and may mimic collections of fluid in the peritoneal cavity. The parallel curvilinear configuration of the pleural and peritoneal cavities at the level of the perihepatic and perisplenic recesses allows fluid in either cavity to appear as an arcuate or semilunar density displacing liver or spleen away from the adjacent chest wall. The relationship of the fluid collection to the ipsilateral diaphragmatic crus helps to determine its location.[88–92] Pleural fluid collections in the posterior costophrenic angle lie medial and posterior to the diaphragm and cause lateral displacement of the crus (Fig. 5–39). Peritoneal fluid collections are anterior and lateral to the diaphragm; lateral displacement of

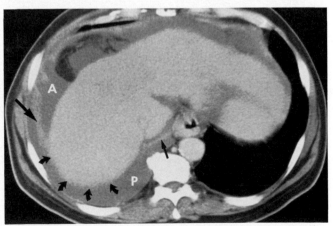

FIGURE 5–39 ■ Ascites and pleural effusion. Pleural fluid (P) is medial and posterior to the right crus *(small arrow)*. Ascites (A) is visible lateral and anterior to the liver; ascites medially and pleural fluid laterally outline the diaphragm *(large arrow)*. The liver edge is ill-defined posteriorly where it contacts pleural fluid *(curved arrows)*. Ascites is not visible at this site, because it is the bare area of the liver.

the crus is not visible. Pleural fluid can also be distinguished from ascites by the sharpness of the interface of the fluid with the liver and spleen.[93] With pleural fluid the interface is hazy, whereas with ascites it is sharp. In patients with both pleural and peritoneal fluid, the diaphragm often can be seen as a uniform, curvilinear structure of muscle density with relatively low-density fluid both anteriorly and posteriorly.

A large pleural effusion will cause the lower lobe to float anteriorly and lose volume. The posterior edge of the lower lobe, when surrounded by fluid both anteriorly and posteriorly, can give the false appearance of the diaphragm, with pleural fluid posteriorly and ascites anteriorly. Sequential scans at more cephalic levels, however, generally allow the correct interpretation to be made. Typically the arcuate density of the atelectatic lower lobe becomes thicker superiorly, is contiguous with the remainder of the lower lobe, and often contains air bronchograms. Unlike the diaphragm, it also tapers laterally and demonstrates sites of interruption.

The specific gravity (density) of pleural fluid obtained at thoracocentesis is helpful in determining the cause of the effusion. Thus high-density or exudative fluid often is associated with infection or neoplasm, whereas low-density or transudative effusion often is the result of congestive heart failure or other diseases that cause a loss of fluid, but not protein, from the pleural capillaries. Although the CT attenuations of the pleural fluid collections might be expected to correlate well with their specific gravities, they cannot be used reliably to predict the specific gravity of the fluid or its cause.[87, 94] Acute or subacute hemothorax can sometimes be inhomogeneous in density, with some areas, particularly dependent regions, having a CT attenuation value greater than that of water.

MR Diagnosis of Pleural Fluid ■ MR has not been shown to be able to characterize pleural fluid. In fact, if a T1-weighted spin-echo sequence is used, the presence of an effusion may be difficult to recognize. On T1-weighted MR images, pleural effusion usually has a low signal intensity similar to that of the adjacent lung (Fig. 5–40). Tscholakoff and colleagues[95] found it difficult to detect effusion on T1-weighted images in 30 per cent of cases. In patients with lung consolidation, it is not unusual to find that an effusion has considerably less signal intensity than adjacent consolidated lung. On T2-weighted images, a significant increase in signal intensity from an effusion is typical, making the effusion much more easily recognized. With this technique, however, effusion may be difficult to differentiate from consolidated lung. With gradient-echo MR imaging, pleural effusion may also be intense, making for confusion with flowing blood.[95a]

In general, exudates, transudates, and sanguineous effusions cannot be distinguished from each other reliably by MR. However, hemothorax of more

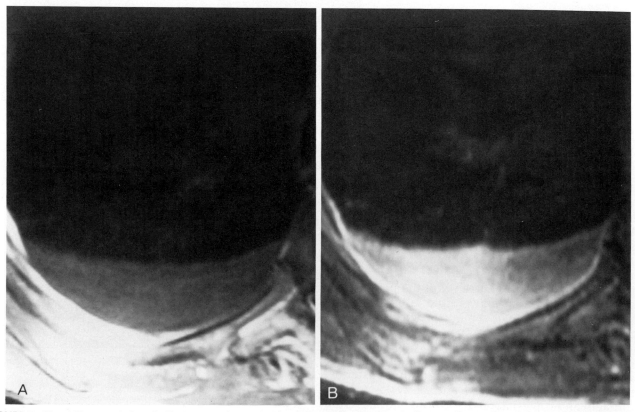

FIGURE 5–40 ■ MR scan of pleural effusion. On the T1-weighted image (A), the pleural effusion is lower than muscle in signal intensity. On the T2-weighted image (B), the pleural effusion shows a marked increase in signal intensity.

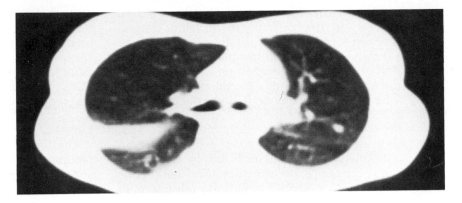

FIGURE 5–41 ■ Pleural fluid causing thickening of the right major fissure. The CT scan shows pleural fluid localized to the right major fissure. The fluid appears as a triangular density based peripherally with its apex directed toward the hilum. The lower lobe is compressed posteriorly and medially.

than several days' duration can sometimes be differentiated from other kinds of fluid collections because of its high signal intensity on T1- and T2-weighted images.[95] Although MR might be expected to distinguish fluid collections with different concentrations of protein, fluid motion resulting from respiration and cardiac pulsation significantly affects the signal intensity and makes this determination difficult. In experimental studies, pleural fluid collections show an absolute increase in signal strength from first to second echo images (a "negative" T2 value) in the presence of motion-related spin dephasing.[96]

FISSURAL FLUID

A focal or loculated collection of pleural fluid in a major or minor fissure can have a confusing appear-

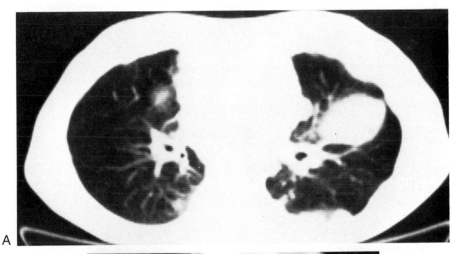

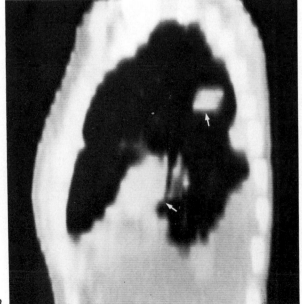

FIGURE 5–42 ■ Loculated pleural fluid in the left major fissure in a patient with lymphoma. A, CT scan shows a lenticular collection of pleural fluid in the inferior left major fissure. B, A sagittal reconstruction shows the pleural fluid in the posterior costophrenic angle and in the left major fissure (arrows).

ance on CT and can be misinterpreted as a parenchymal mass. In the case of an effusion, careful analysis of sequential images usually reveals that the opaque density conforms to the plane of the fissure (Figs. 5–41 and 5–42). If, in addition, the attenuation of the density suggests fluid, the diagnosis becomes likely. The edges of a fissural fluid collection may taper to conform to the fissure, forming a "beak," especially when imaged with thinly collimated scans. Correlation of the scans with plain radiographs can help, particularly for fluid localized in the minor fissure. The presence of loculated fluid collections suggests but does not always indicate adhesions of the pleural surfaces of the fissure.

PARAPNEUMONIC EFFUSIONS

Pleural fluid can accumulate in patients with pneumonia, even when the pleural space is uninfected.

This is termed a *parapneumonic effusion* and probably results from increased permeability of the visceral pleura. Distinguishing pleural effusion from adjacent consolidated lung may be difficult unless contrast material is injected, resulting in opacification of the lung. The pleural fluid remains low in density, whereas the consolidated lung increases in density.

EMPYEMA

The term *empyema* is used to describe a purulent pleural effusion resulting from infection of the pleural space. Empyema usually is diagnosed by thoracentesis. Culture of material aspirated from the pleural space generally reveals the causative organisms. Most empyemas are caused by *Staphylococcus aureus* or gram-negative enteric bacilli or occur in association with mixed anaerobic and aerobic infections.

With conventional radiographic techniques, em-

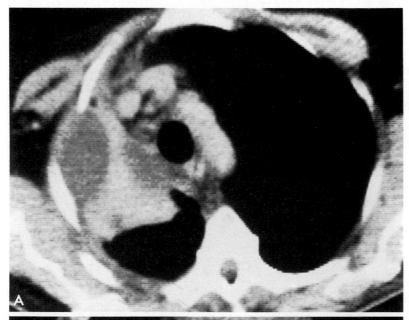
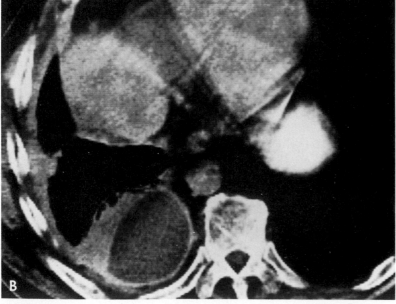

FIGURE 5–43 ■ Empyema in two patients. CT scans show typical features of an empyema without bronchial communication. *A,* After right upper lobe lobectomy, the CT scan demonstrates a lentiform empyema with contrast enhancement of the wall. Pleural fluid is present posteriorly. The lung parenchyma around the empyema shows consolidation. *B,* CT scan shows a right lower empyema with a uniform, low-density center and a wall of uniform thickness.

pyemas may be difficult or impossible to differentiate from peripheral lung abscesses abutting the chest wall. This distinction can be an important one to make, because empyemas usually are treated by tube thoracostomy and systemic antibiotics, whereas most lung abscesses require appropriate systemic antibiotics and postural drainage.[2]

Baber and co-workers[2] reported the differences between empyemas and peripheral lung abscesses as shown by CT—features that have been confirmed by others.[97, 98] Typically an empyema has a regular shape and is round or elliptical in cross section (Fig. 5–43). The edge of the lesion is sharply demarcated from the adjacent lung (Fig. 5–44). An empyema tends to form an obtuse angle with the adjacent lung parenchyma and may be longer in craniocaudal than lateral dimension. When a bronchopleural fistula is present or when air is introduced into the empyema at thoracentesis, its inner margin usually appears smooth and its wall is of uniform thickness (Fig. 5–45). Lung abscesses, on the other hand, are irregularly shaped and often contain multiple loculated collections of air and fluid (see Fig. 5–45). Their inner surfaces often are irregular and ragged, and their outer edges are poorly defined because of adjacent pulmonary parenchymal consolidation. Peripherally situated lung abscesses also tend to form an acute angle with the adjacent costal margin. In some cases, empyema cavities, unlike lung abscess cavities, will change shape when the patient moves from the supine to the prone or decubitus position.

When an abscess or empyema does not contain air and is homogeneously opaque on plain radiographs, contrast-enhanced CT scans can demonstrate the wall of the lesion and suggest its fluid-filled nature (Figs. 5–43, 5–44, and 5–46).[2] The walls of both empyemas and abscesses can demonstrate contrast enhancement but not their fluid content. The walls of an empyema are the visceral and parietal pleural surfaces that, after infusion of contrast material, are split

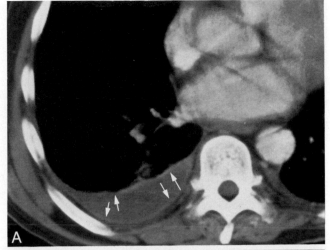

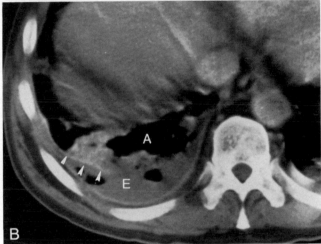

FIGURE 5–45 ■ Lung abscess and adjacent empyema. *A*, CT scan of the right lower thorax demonstrates pleural fluid collection with enhancing parietal and visceral pleurae *(arrows)*. *B*, CT scan 4 cm caudal to *A* shows an abscess cavity (A) within the lung and an empyema cavity (E) containing fluid and air. The enhancing visceral pleura *(arrowheads)* is deficient at the interface between the abscess cavity and the empyema.

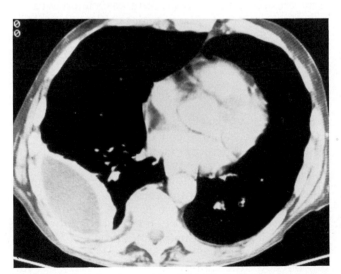

FIGURE 5–44 ■ Empyema. After intravenous injection of contrast material, CT scan shows marked enhancement of both the visceral and parietal pleura constituting the empyema wall.

apart by the fluid collection.[98] Empyemas also compress and displace the lung, acting like a space-occupying mass, whereas lung abscesses destroy the involved lung.

The differentiation of pleural and parenchymal processes is frequently impossible from conventional radiographs. Thus CT provides important information in many patients with pleuroparenchymal disease. Pugatch and colleagues[87] studied 75 patients who had complex pleural processes or combinations of pleural and parenchymal disease. In 21 patients (28 per cent), CT provided unique information that altered the diagnosis or management of these patients. In 30 patients (40 per cent), CT clarified the location of the pleural disease but did not alter management. In another study of patients with lung abscess or empyema,[98] CT provided information not obtained from plain radiographs in 47 per cent of patients and better defined the extent of the process in an additional 34 per cent.

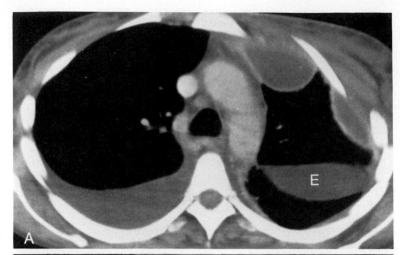

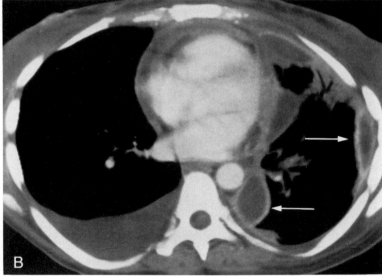

FIGURE 5–46 ■ Multiple loculated pleural effusions with an empyema. *A*, CT scan at the level of the aortic arch demonstrates bilateral pleural effusions. The effusion on the right is free flowing, and the one on the left is loculated at multiple sites. Effusion (E) is present in the left major fissure. *B*, CT scan at a level of the heart again shows the free-flowing right pleural effusion. On the left side, two empyema cavities *(arrows)* are visible laterally and paraspinously. Lung consolidation with air bronchograms is seen in the lingula.

Waite and colleagues[98a] described the CT changes in the parietal pleura and extrapleural tissues suggestive of an infection. The findings were thickening of the parietal pleural and extrapleural subcostal tissues, enhancement of the parietal pleural tissues with intravascular contrast material, and increased density of the extrapleural fat. Some or all of these findings were found with malignant effusions but not with transudative effusions. We think that thickening of the extrapleural soft tissues is a manifestation of a chronic retractile process in the lungs and is seen with chronic lung fibrosis, as well as with pleural fibrosis.

Organizing Empyema ■ In patients with empyema, and especially tuberculous empyema, ingrowth of fibroblasts can result in pleural fibrosis and the development of chronic pleural thickening.[99, 100] CT may show the thickened pleural peel, which can cause lung restriction and decreased lung volume. Frequently a thickened layer of extrapleural fat is visible separating the parietal pleura and inner chest wall. Calcification, which typically is focal in its early stages, may become extensive.

Dense pleural thickening, even with calcification, does not indicate that the pleural disease is inactive.

Loculated fluid collections resulting from active infection may be seen on CT within the thickened pleura. Hulnick and co-workers[99] studied ten patients with chronic pleural thickening associated with tuberculosis, nine of whom had calcification. CT detected focal collections of pleural fluid, indicating active infection in six patients. In some patients the chest wall can also be involved with the chronic pleural process.

THORACOSTOMY TUBES

Infected pleural fluid collections often become loculated, and difficulties may be encountered with drainage by thoracostomy tubes. Chest tube position can be difficult to evaluate on conventional radiographs, whereas CT scans can show the position of the tube accurately. CT is indicated to evaluate thoracostomy tube position when the tube is functioning poorly. On CT scans, malpositioned chest tubes can lie within a fissure; within a loculated fluid collection; or outside the empyema (Fig. 5–47).[101] van-Sonnenberg and colleagues[102] described eight patients with empyema who did not improve because of chest tube malposition; in these patients the em-

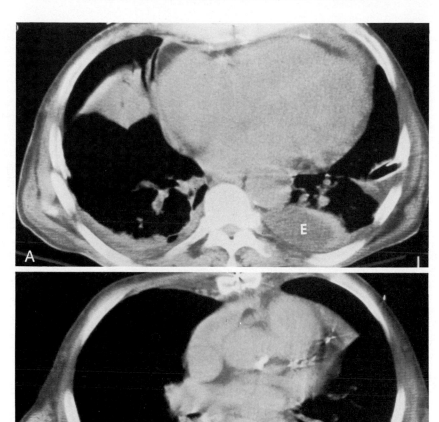

FIGURE 5–47 ■ CT evaluation of thoracostomy tube position. *A,* CT scan shows the thoracostomy tube in the major fissure and not in the empyema cavity (E). *B,* Several centimeters cephalad, the thoracostomy tube is clearly in the major fissure anterior to the consolidated lung and not in the empyema. This empyema was not successfully drained by the tube.

pyema was drained successfully using CT-guided percutaneous catheter placement. After drainage, the empyema cavity typically is obliterated; the pleural thickening usually resolves or leaves only a small plaquelike area of thickening.[102a] Occasionally an empyema cavity remains open and may even contain air in the absence of infection. In these cases extensive pleural fibrosis or other abnormality prevents resorption of the space.

MINIMAL PLEURAL THICKENING

Large pleural lesions such as empyemas or fibrosis are readily recognized on CT. Minimal pleural abnormalities, either fluid or fibrosis, can be more difficult to detect on CT with conventional 1-cm collimation. Typically, on conventional CT, pleural thickening or fluid is evident from a soft tissue density internal to a rib segment. Normal extrapleural fat pads can be present in the same location, particularly in the inferior posterolateral thorax, and may not always be distinguishable from higher density fibrosis because of volume averaging.

The excellent spatial resolution at the lung–chest wall interface provided by HRCT permits the detection of minimal pleural thickening (Fig. 5–48). In a group of patients with mild pleural thickening stud-

ied by the authors, the abnormal pleura was visible as a discrete, thin, irregular or smooth linear density usually separated from the underlying rib (Fig. 5–49) or intercostal or subcostalis muscle (Fig. 5–50) or in a paravertebral location (Fig. 5–51) by extrapleural

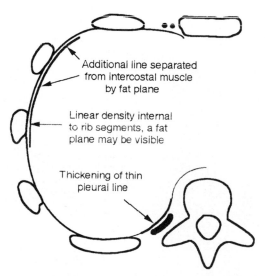

Additional line separated from intercostal muscle by fat plane

Linear density internal to rib segments, a fat plane may be visible

Thickening of thin pleural line

FIGURE 5–48 ■ Schema of HRCT findings in pleural thickening.

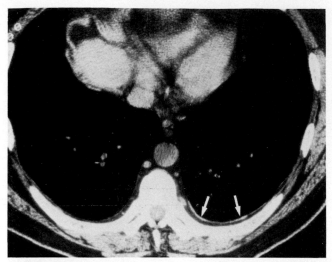

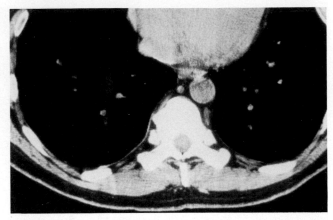

FIGURE 5–51 ■ Asbestos-related pleural thickening. HRCT scan shows a pleural plaque along the right paravertebral line. The left side is normal.

FIGURE 5–49 ■ Asbestos-related pleural thickening. HRCT scan shows left pleural plaques (arrows) as white lines internal to the rib and, in this instance, separated from the rib by a layer of extrapleural fat.

fat 1 to 4 mm in thickness. This fat layer is seen more clearly when pleural thickening is present than in normal persons, perhaps because it is outlined by the thickened pleura. An alternative explanation is that there is thickening of this layer similar to that occurring with a chronic or organizing empyema.[99, 100] This fat layer, along with mildly thickened overlying pleura, can be seen using conventional CT with 1-cm collimation, but its appearance is less easily appreciated than with HRCT.

ASBESTOS-RELATED PLEURAL DISEASE

Pleural thickening occurs commonly in patients with occupational asbestos exposure. CT can detect and characterize this abnormality.[1] Although pleural thickening and plaques can frequently be seen on plain radiographs, CT is more sensitive in detecting pleural disease in almost all situations. Of 36 patients

with asbestos exposure studied by Katz and Kreel,[103] abnormal pleural thickening was detected in 27 with CT, whereas only 24 had evidence of pleural thickening on plain radiographs. In the 27 patients with pleural disease, CT showed more extensive involvement in 15, whereas in three patients, the disease was judged more extensive on plain radiographs.

Asbestos-related pleural abnormalities have a typical appearance on CT. Early pleural disease is discontinuous; plaques of thickened pleura are visible adjacent to the inner surfaces of ribs or vertebral bodies, and the intervening pleura is normal (see Figs. 5–49 through 5–51).[103] These pleural plaques can be distinguished from normal extrapleural soft tissues by their location, configuration, and density.[87, 104] In patients with extensive disease, pleural thickening can be concentric. Calcification of pleural plaques was evident on CT scans in nine of the 27 patients with abnormal pleural thickening studied by Katz and Kreel,[103] whereas it was visible on plain radiographs in only six. HRCT can also detect and diagnose pleural plaques and thickening related to

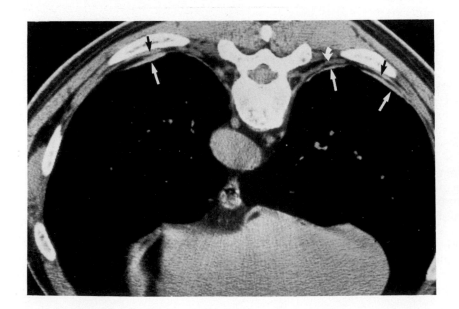

FIGURE 5–50 ■ Asbestos-related pleural plaques. Prone HRCT scan shows pleural plaques (straight white arrows) separated by a layer of extrapleural fat from an intercostal vein (curved white arrow) and subcostalis muscles (black arrows).

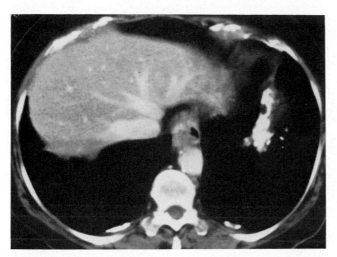

FIGURE 5–52 ■ Calcified pleural plaques. CT scan at the level of the diaphragm demonstrates calcification within plaques along both posterior costal margins and over the left hemidiaphragm.

asbestos exposure.[105, 106] HRCT demonstrates abnormalities of the pleura with greater frequency than chest radiographs or conventional CT. Aberle and colleagues[107] studied the detection of pleural plaques and calcification with conventional radiographs, conventional CT, and HRCT in 100 patients occupationally exposed to asbestos. Although HRCT was obtained only at selected levels, it was more sensitive in detecting plaques than the other two modalities. Plaques were identified in 64 persons with HRCT, in 56 with conventional CT, and in 49 with chest radiographs. Similarly, calcification was identified with HRCT in 20 subjects, with conventional CT in 16, and with chest radiographs in 13. Diffuse pleural thickening, which is probably the result of prior asbestos-related benign pleural effusion,[108] was found by Aberle and co-workers[107] in 7 of the 100 patients. These authors defined thickening as a sheet of thickened pleura at least 5 cm in lateral dimension and 8 cm in craniocaudal dimension.

The diaphragmatic pleura is commonly involved in patients with asbestos-related pleural disease (Fig. 5–52). Katz and Kreel[103] found diaphragmatic pleural irregularities on the CT scans in 11 of 27 patients with abnormal pleural thickening. However, the diaphragm lies roughly in the plane of the scan, and the detection of uncalcified pleural plaques on the diaphragmatic surface can be difficult. In some patients, diaphragmatic pleural plaques are visible deep in the posterior costophrenic angle, below the lung base. Mediastinal pleural plaques have been considered unusual in patients with asbestos-related pleural disease but are visible on CT scans in 40 per cent of patients, almost exclusively over the heart.[103] In some patients, areas of abnormal pleura are associated with "transpulmonary bands," which presumably represent areas of pulmonary parenchymal and pleural scarring. Paravertebral pleural thickening is common and was seen in all but one (97 per cent) of Katz and Kreel's 36 patients with pleural disease.[103]

Although unusual, pleural thickening can involve a fissure and result in a localized intrapulmonary plaque. The CT appearance may simulate that of a lung nodule, but the plain radiograph will demonstrate that the plaque is within a fissure.[109]

Lynch and colleagues[110] demonstrated that fissural pleural plaques could be identified with HRCT; these investigators found such plaques in 6 of 260 occupationally exposed asbestos workers. The precise relationship of the plaque to the fissure was readily identified on HRCT, making the diagnosis certain.

MALIGNANT MESOTHELIOMA

Diffuse mesothelioma is a highly malignant, progressive neoplasm with an extremely poor prognosis. It is characterized morphologically by gross and nodular pleural thickening. Hemorrhagic pleural effusion often occurs and may obscure the underlying pleural disease on chest radiographs. Malignant mesothelioma spreads most commonly by local infiltration of the pleura, although hematogenous pulmonary and distant metastases can occur. In most patients, malignant mesothelioma is related to asbestos exposure, and although it is rare in the general population, the incidence in asbestos workers is 5 to 7 per cent.

Malignant mesothelioma can be difficult to diagnose. Symptoms generally are nonspecific but usually include dyspnea and chest pain. Chest radiographs usually show a pleural effusion, which can be loculated and irregular; alternatively, nodular pleural thickening may be evident. In 20 per cent of patients, radiographic findings of asbestosis or asbestos-related pleural abnormalities are evident. Open biopsy is usually necessary to diagnose malignant mesothelioma, as cytologic studies of pleural fluid or needle biopsy of the pleura can yield misleading results.[39]

In patients with malignant mesothelioma, CT can expedite the initial diagnosis and define the extent of tumor.[1] Irregular pleural thickening is usually present and is most pronounced at the lung bases but can involve the entire hemithorax (Fig. 5–53).[111] Tumor extension into the mediastinum is not uncommon, and tumor spread to the opposite hemithorax via the posterior mediastinum does occur.[39] Pleural fluid accumulations usually can be distinguished from mesothelioma when the latter has a lobulated contour. We have seen instances of low-density pleural tumor deposits from mesotheliomas that mimic pleural fluid. CT scans with the patient in the prone or decubitus position help show the underlying mesothelioma. Enhancement of the tumor after infusion of contrast medium also can help differentiate it from adjacent fluid collections.

Another CT feature of malignant mesothelioma is thickening of the fissures, particularly their inferior portions, from tumor, pleural effusion, or both.[111] Comparing mesothelioma and asbestos pleural disease, Rabinowitz and co-workers[112] found that nodular thickening of the fissures, ipsilateral volume loss of the hemithorax, and pleural effusion were sugges-

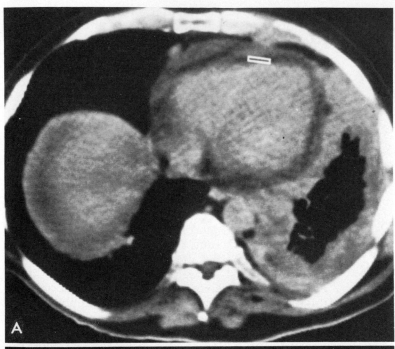

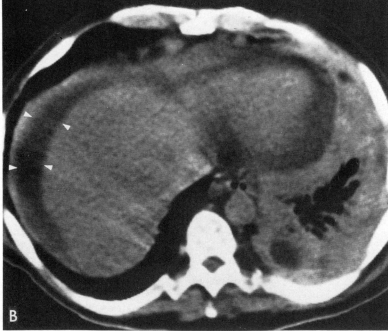

FIGURE 5–53 ■ Malignant mesothelioma. *A* and *B,* CT scans show encasement of the left lower lobe by a thick, irregular pleural rind that consists of tumor. (Tumor also extended into the upper abdomen.) The fluid density separating the right hemidiaphragm from the liver is ascites *(arrowheads).*

tive of mesothelioma. Kawashima and Libshitz[111a] found fissural pleural thickening in 43 of 50 patients with malignant mesothelioma. In patients with advanced asbestos-related pleural disease, large pleural plaques can superficially resemble malignant mesothelioma, but involvement of the fissures is uncommon and pleural plaques tend to be more dense.

Although pleural mesothelioma is visible most frequently along the lateral chest wall, mediastinal pleural thickening, sometimes with adjacent mediastinal adenopathy or invasion, also can be present. The abnormal hemithorax can appear contracted and fixed, with little change in size during inspiration.[111] Pulmonary nodules frequently are hematogenous metastases. Diaphragmatic involvement by tumor is frequent but may be difficult to demonstrate on CT.[113]

BENIGN MESOTHELIOMA

Benign mesothelioma (pleural fibroma) is an uncommon tumor usually detected incidentally on chest radiographs. This tumor can be associated with hypoglycemia and hypertrophic pulmonary osteoarthropathy. It usually arises from the visceral pleura and therefore can be within a fissure, but more commonly it involves the costal pleural surface. On CT scans, these lesions demonstrate findings analogous to those seen on plain radiographs. Specifically, they are solitary, smooth, sharply defined, often

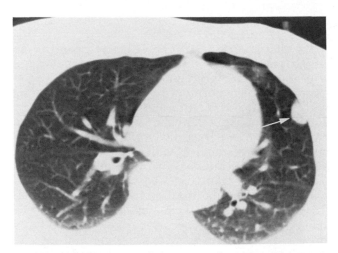

FIGURE 5–54 ■ Benign mesothelioma. A well-circumscribed, peripheral, pleural-based mass is demonstrated on the left side *(arrow)*. The patient is undergoing a biopsy, and the hub of a needle is visible anteriorly. A small pneumothorax is present.

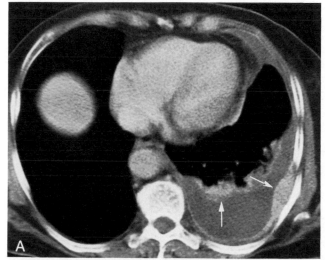

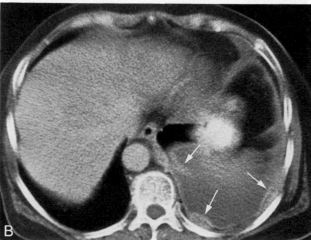

FIGURE 5–55 ■ Pleural metastasis from breast carcinoma. *A* and *B,* CT scans at two levels demonstrate a moderately large left pleural effusion. Parietal pleural masses *(arrows)* represent metastatic deposits.

large lesions contacting a pleural surface (Fig. 5–54).[114] Usually they are homogeneous on CT scans, but necrosis can result in a multicystic appearance. Although pleural abnormalities generally form obtuse angles at their point of contact with the chest wall, benign mesotheliomas typically show acute angles with slightly tapered pleural thickening adjacent to the mass. This thickening may reflect a small amount of fluid accumulating in the pleural space at the point where the visceral and parietal pleural surfaces are separated by the mass. A similar "beak" or "thorn" sign often is visible on plain radiographs in patients with a benign fissural mesothelioma.

METASTASES

In patients with intrathoracic or extrathoracic tumors, metastases to the pleura can cause nodular pleural thickening and pleural effusion.[1, 115] Usually pleural effusion masks the underlying pleural mass, but occasionally the lesion can be seen on CT images (Fig. 5–55). For example, in patients with a malignant thymoma that has metastasized to the pleura, pleural effusion often is lacking, and the pleural metastases are visible.[1, 115, 116] These usually are discrete and form obtuse angles at their junctions with the chest wall. Flat subpleural masses can occur in patients with lymphoma, and CT is particularly valuable in their detection.[37, 111]

With contrast infusion, pleural metastases, regardless of their origin, often increase in CT density relative to the adjacent effusion and then become evident. In many cases of pleural metastasis, focal, discrete pleural masses are not found; instead the appearance is of irregular pleural thickening indistinguishable from malignant mesothelioma (Fig. 5–56).

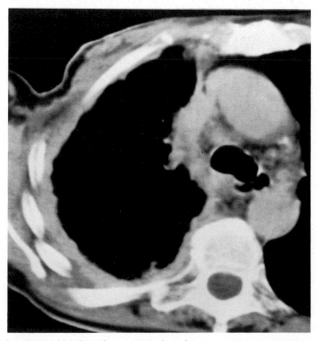

FIGURE 5–56 ■ Pleural metastasis from breast carcinoma. Concentric nodular thickening of the right costal and mediastinal pleura is from a primary breast carcinoma and mimics a malignant mesothelioma.

Diaphragm

Anatomy

The diaphragm is a dome-shaped muscular sheet that separates the thoracic cavity from the abdomen. Its periphery consists of muscle fibers that originate from the circumference of the thoracic cage, converge, and insert into a fibrous central tendon. These muscle fibers can be grouped according to their origin: lumbar, sternal, and costal.

The lumbar fibers arise from the diaphragmatic crura and from two aponeurotic arches on each side, called the *medial* and *lateral lumbocostal arches*.[14] The right and left diaphragmatic crura (Fig. 5–57) are tendinous structures that arise inferiorly from the anterior surfaces of the upper lumbar vertebral bodies and intervening disks and are continuous with the anterior longitudinal ligament of the spine.[117] The crura ascend anterior to the spine on each side of the aorta and then pass medially and anteriorly, joining the muscular diaphragm anterior to the aorta to form the aortic hiatus. The right crus, which is larger and longer than the left, arises from the first three lumbar vertebral levels; the left crus arises from the first two lumbar segments.[117]

The aortic hiatus and the anterior crura are invariably demonstrated by CT.[118, 119] CT scans at caudal levels show the individual crura as discrete oval or round structures posterolateral to the aorta and anterior to the vertebral column. The larger and longer right crus has a greater cross-sectional diameter than

the left and is visible at lower levels (see Chapter 2, Figs. 2–17 and 2–18).

The diaphragmatic crura can be mistaken for enlarged lymph nodes or masses because of their round appearance; paraaortic lymph nodes can indeed be seen in a similar position.[117, 120] However, on contiguous CT scans, the crura merge gradually with the diaphragm at more cephalic levels, which differentiates them from paraaortic lymph nodes. The thickness of the crura also varies with lung volume, increasing in thickness at full inspiration when compared with expiration.[120]

The medial lumbocostal arch is a tendinous arch that arises medially from the ipsilateral crus and the side of the first or second lumbar vertebral body.[14] It crosses anterior to the psoas muscle and attaches laterally to the transverse process of the first or second lumbar vertebra. On CT scans, the position of the medial lumbocostal arch can be inferred from the position of the psoas muscle. At this level, the diaphragm is discontinuous, and the psoas muscle separates the crus medially from the posterior leaf of the diaphragm laterally. The lateral lumbocostal arch crosses the anterior surface of the quadratus lumborum and is attached medially to the transverse process of the first lumbar vertebra and laterally to the twelfth rib.

Caudal to the domes of the diaphragm, segments of the posteromedial diaphragm on either side often are outlined by abdominal fat, allowing them to be demonstrated as discrete structures. On the right, fat

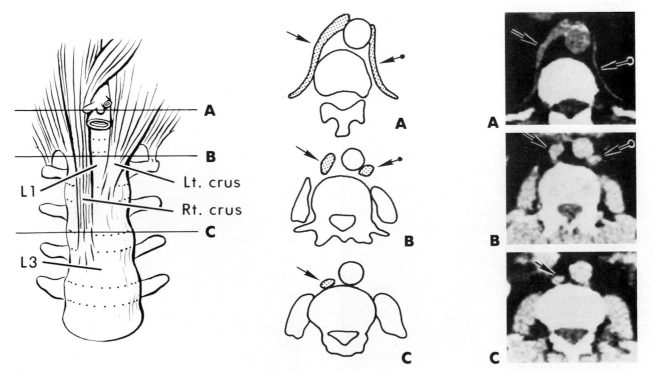

FIGURE 5–57 ■ Diaphragmatic crura. *A,* The diaphragmatic crura ascend along the anterior aspect of the spine on each side of the aorta, joining anterior to the aorta to form the aortic hiatus. *B* and *C,* The right crus is longer and larger than the left crus and extends to a lower level. The characteristic position of the crura on each side of the aorta allows them to be distinguished from abnormalities in the region. (From Callen PW, Filly RA, Korobkin M: Radiology 126:413, 1978. Reproduced with permission.)

outlining the medial hemidiaphragm defines the most cephalic extent of the posterior pararenal space. Naidich and colleagues[118] identified fat in this region in 62 of 75 patients (83 per cent). On the left, the visibility of this fat layer is less consistent, probably because of variations in the size and shape of the spleen.

The crura are somewhat variable in thickness and appearance. In approximately half of normal patients, the crura appear thicker than the posterolateral diaphragm, with a smooth, gradual transition between the two. However, in approximately one fourth of normal patients, the crura are atrophic and no thicker than the lateral diaphragm. The crura can appear somewhat lobulated or nodular, particularly on the right side, and the transition between the crura and the posterior diaphragm can be relatively abrupt, or there may be a discontinuity between the crura and diaphragm.

The diaphragm generally is considered to have two hemispheric domes formed by the right and left lateral leaflets attached to the central diaphragmatic tendon. However, a third dome consisting of the middle leaflet and the central tendon is present anteriorly and medially.[121] The middle leaflet lies below the inferior surface of the heart and blends partially with the parietal pericardium. Anteriorly it is attached to the xiphoid process of the sternum and the costal cartilages. The xiphoid and costal cartilages form an inverted V- or U-shaped arch when viewed from the front, and the anterior diaphragm assumes a similar shape. The cephalic extent and shape of the anterior diaphragmatic dome varies with body habitus, and although this structure is visible on CT in most subjects, its appearance varies. The anterior diaphragm most often appears as a smooth or slightly wavy linear density outlined by fat on either side, concave posteriorly, and continuous across the midline. Typically it is seen at about the level of the xiphoid process. The anterior diaphragm commonly appears discontinuous anteriorly, with the right and left diaphragmatic leaves diverging to insert onto the right and left costal cartilages. As the plane of scan moves cephalad to the xiphoid process, the right and left leaves gradually converge.

An understanding of the anatomy of the anterior portion of the diaphragm is essential in correctly diagnosing Morgagni's hernia. The presence of bowel anterior to the heart can suggest the existence of a hernia, but if the bowel loop is surrounded by diaphragm, with the apex of the arch at the level of the xiphoid process, no hernia is present.[121] If bowel extends above the xiphoid process and is not marginated by muscle laterally or superiorly, then a hernia is present.

The sternal portion of the diaphragm arises from the dorsum of the xiphoid process, whereas the costal part arises from the inner surfaces of the cartilage and bony surfaces of the inferior six ribs.[14] Because of the transverse axial plane of the image, the central portion of the diaphragm is not a distinct structure,

and its position can be inferred only by the position of the lung base and upper abdominal organs. As the more peripheral portions of the diaphragm descend toward their sternal and costal origins, the posterior and lateral portions of the diaphragm become visible adjacent to retroperitoneal fat. Where the diaphragm is contiguous with the liver or spleen, it cannot usually be delineated by CT unless thin-collimation CT is used and a subdiaphragmatic fat layer is present.

Caskey and colleagues[122] used CT to study the morphologic changes that occur in the diaphragm with age. They found that the thickness of diaphragmatic crura is about 5 mm and does not change with age. However, the width of the esophageal hiatus increases significantly in both men and women. In addition, diaphragmatic defects seen posteriorly increased markedly with age, from being rare in younger patients to being found in more than 50 per cent of patients over the age of 70. Localized herniation of retroperitoneal fat could be seen through the larger discontinuities in the diaphragm. Focal nodularity and irregularity of the posterior diaphragm also appeared after the fourth decade and increased in frequency in subsequent decades.

OPENINGS IN THE DIAPHRAGM

The diaphragm is perforated by several openings that allow structures to pass from the thorax to the abdomen.[14] The aortic hiatus is posterior and lies at the level of the twelfth thoracic vertebra. It is bounded posteriorly by the vertebral body and anteriorly by the crura. Through it pass the aorta, the azygos and hemizygous veins, the thoracic duct, intercostal arteries, and splanchnic nerves. The esophageal hiatus is situated more anteriorly, in the muscular portion of the diaphragm at the level of the tenth thoracic vertebra. Through it pass the esophagus, the vagus nerves, and small blood vessels.[14] The foramen of the inferior vena cava pierces the fibrous central tendon of the diaphragm anterior and to the right of the esophageal hiatus.

Of these three structures, the aortic hiatus is defined most readily. On CT scans, the esophageal foramen is visible as an opening at the junction of the esophagus and stomach. The foramen of the inferior vena cava must be inferred from the position of the inferior vena cava. The foramina of Morgagni and of Bochdalek are not visible on CT scans in normal patients.

Diaphragmatic Abnormalities

HERNIAS

Abdominal or retroperitoneal contents can herniate into the chest through congenital or acquired areas of weakness in the diaphragm or through traumatic diaphragmatic ruptures. Hernias of the stomach through the esophageal hiatus are the most common.

Hernias through the foramen of Bochdalek were previously thought to be uncommon in adults; how-

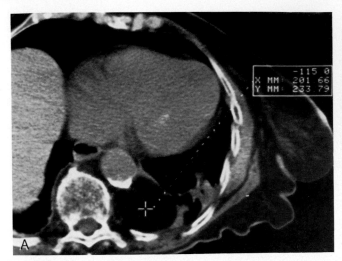
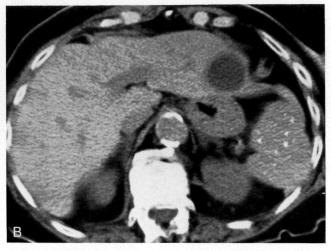

FIGURE 5–58 ■ Left Bochdalek's hernia. *A*, CT scan of the left lower thorax demonstrates a large fat-containing structure in the posterior costal phrenic angle. The left crus of the diaphragm is absent. *B*, Two centimeters inferiorly, the top of the left kidney is visible, protruding into the hernia. Both adrenal glands are visible. Splenic calcifications are from prior histoplasmosis. A metastasis is present in the left lobe of the liver.

ever, CT has shown that small Bochdalek defects may occur in as many as 6 per cent of old individuals (Fig. 5–58).[112] This is also the most common type of diaphragmatic hernia in infants.[123] Most are left sided, and although they are often located in the posterolateral diaphragm, they can occur anywhere along the posterior costodiaphragmatic margin.[124] Bochdalek hernias in adults usually contain retroperitoneal fat (see Fig. 5–58) or a kidney. A rare diaphragmatic hernia involves the medial hemidiaphragm, through which the kidney and stomach can herniate (Fig. 5–59).

Parasternal hernias through the foramen of Morgagni are rare, constituting less than 10 per cent of all diaphragmatic hernias.[123, 125] Morgagni's foramen is bounded by sternal slips of the diaphragm medially and by fibers arising from the seventh costal cartilage laterally. Normally it provides a pathway for the internal mammary vessels. Most Morgagni's hernias occur on the right and, in contrast to Bochdalek hernias, usually contain an extension of the peritoneal sac. Their contents can include omentum, liver, or bowel (Fig. 5–60).[125]

Diaphragmatic rupture can result from penetrating or nonpenetrating trauma to the abdomen or thorax.[126] Traumatic hernias, however, account for only a small percentage of all diaphragmatic hernias. In the majority of cases, the left hemidiaphragm is

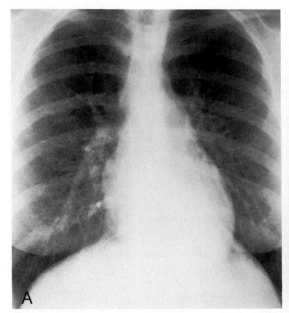
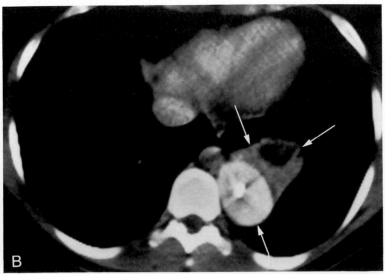

FIGURE 5–59 ■ Intrathoracic kidney and stomach in a young woman with vague chest pain. *A*, Chest radiograph demonstrates a retrocardiac mass contiguous with the left hemidiaphragm. *B*, CT scan through the lower thorax after injection of intravascular contrast material shows that the left kidney and stomach *(arrows)* have herniated through a medial diaphragmatic defect into the left lower hemithorax. (Courtesy of Colleen Bergen, MD, Palo Alto, CA).

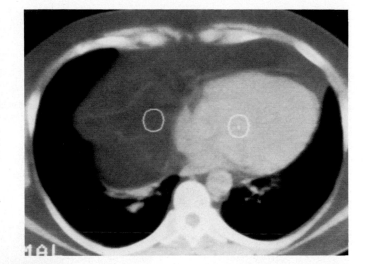

FIGURE 5–60 ■ Morgagni's hernia. CT scan through the lower thorax demonstrates a large right pericardial mass consisting of the liver herniating through a large defect in the foramen of Morgagni. Vessels are seen within the liver after injection of intravascular contrast material.

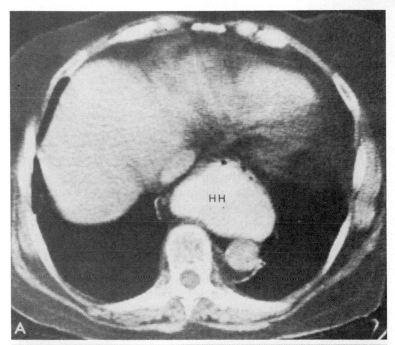

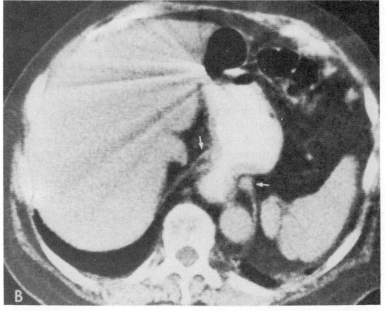

FIGURE 5–61 ■ Hiatal hernia. *A,* CT scan after oral administration of contrast material shows a large opacified hiatal hernia (HH) in the lower mediastinum. *B,* At a lower level, the hernia is shown passing through the esophageal hiatus *(arrows)* to connect with the remainder of the stomach.

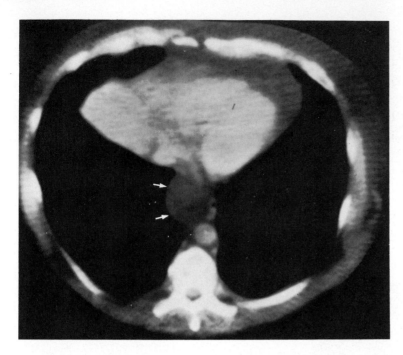

FIGURE 5–62 ■ Paraesophageal hernia. CT scan near the diaphragm shows a fatty mass in the mediastinum *(arrows)*, displacing the esophagus to the left. At surgery, a paraesophageal hernia consisting of omentum was found.

affected, with ruptures of the central or posterior diaphragm being the most frequent.[126] Omentum, stomach, small or large intestine, spleen, or kidney may all herniate through the diaphragmatic rent.

CT scans sometimes show herniation of abdominal contents into the chest through one of the diaphragmatic foramina. However, the anatomic boundaries of these foramina often are difficult to recognize, and it may not be possible to diagnose a hernia with certainty.[127] Knowledge of the normal positions of the foramina is essential in making the correct diagnosis. A mediastinal hiatal hernia can be diagnosed when the hernia opacifies with oral contrast material or contains both air and liquid and has an air-fluid level on the supine image (Fig. 5–61). Contiguity of a hiatal hernia, with the esophagus above and the stomach below, and its relationship to the esophageal hiatus also assist in diagnosis. Paraesophageal hernias of omental (Fig. 5–62) or extraperitoneal fat may not be distinguishable from a mediastinal lipoma.

In one reported instance, CT assisted in the diagnosis of traumatic rupture of the diaphragm.[126] In this case, CT scans showed an interruption in the cross-sectional image of the diaphragm that indicated a congenital or acquired traumatic defect. However, traumatic rupture of the diaphragm is more usually diagnosed from conventional radiographs.[128, 129]

DIAPHRAGMATIC EVENTRATION

Local eventration of the right hemidiaphragm and superior displacement of the liver can be confused radiographically with a peripheral pulmonary or pleural mass. CT scans after infusion of contrast medium can demonstrate opacification of normal intrahepatic vessels in the apparent mass; this opacification identifies it as normal liver.[130] In addition, scans reformatted in the coronal plane can show that the "mass" has the same density as liver.

The coronal display of MR images and the distinctive imaging features of the liver allow this modality to clearly demonstrate an elevated diaphragm with subphrenic hepatic structures.

TUMORS OF THE DIAPHRAGM

Tumors of the diaphragm are rare.[131] Primary benign tumors and primary malignant tumors occur with nearly equal frequency. The most common benign lesions include lipomas, fibromas, neurogenic cysts, and mesothelial or bronchogenic cysts. Primary malignant tumors generally are of fibrous origin, such as fibrosarcoma. Both benign and malignant primary tumors appear radiographically as extrapleural masses.

Most metastatic neoplasms involve the diaphragm by direct extension. Examples of such tumors are carcinomas of the lung, stomach, pancreas, kidney, adrenal gland, and colon and primary or secondary liver tumors. An invasive tumor can be a well-defined extrapleural mass, or it can produce pleural effusion or pulmonary invasion. Radiographically visible hematogenous metastases to the diaphragm are very rare.

The radiographic appearance of a diaphragmatic tumor is nonspecific; most patients with an apparent diaphragmatic mass have a local eventration, a diaphragmatic hernia, or a pleural or pulmonary parenchymal lesion abutting the diaphragm. These conditions can be suggested by CT, which thus helps exclude the possibility of a diaphragmatic tumor.

References

1. Kreel L: Computed tomography of the lung and pleura. Semin Roentgenol 13:213, 1978.
2. Baber CE, Hedlund LW, Oddson TA, Putman CE: Differen-

tiating empyemas and peripheral pulmonary abscesses. The value of computed tomography. Radiology 135:755, 1980.

3. van Waes PFGM, Zonneveld FW: Direct coronal body computed tomography. J Comput Assist Tomogr 6:58, 1982.

4. Webb WR, Jensen BG, Gamsu G, Sollitto R, Moore EH: Coronal magnetic resonance imaging of the chest: normal and abnormal. Radiology 153:729, 1984.

5. Webb WR, Jensen BG, Gamsu G, Sollitto R, Moore EH: Sagittal MR imaging of the chest: normal and abnormal. J Comput Assist Tomogr 9:471, 1985.

6. Mayo JR, Webb WR, Gould R, Stein MG, Bass I, et al: High-resolution CT of the lungs: an optimal approach. Radiology 163:507, 1987.

7. Goldberg RP, Carter BL: Absence of thoracic osteophytosis in the area adjacent to the aorta: computed tomography demonstration. J Comput Assist Tomogr 2:173, 1978.

8. Paling MR, Dwyer A: The first rib as the cause of a "pulmonary nodule" on chest computed tomography. J Comput Assist Tomogr 4:847, 1980.

9. Stark P, Jaramillo D: CT of the sternum. AJR 147:72, 1986.

10. Hatfield MK, Gross BH, Glazer GM, Martel W: Computed tomography of the sternum and its articulation. Skeletal Radiol 11:197, 1984.

11. Stark P, Watkins GE, Hildebrandt-Stark HE, Dunbar RD: Episternal ossicles. Radiology 165:143, 1987.

12. Goodman LR, Teplick SK, Kay H: Computed tomography of the sternum. AJR 141:219, 1983.

13. Destouet JM, Gilula LA, Murphy WA, Sagel SS: Computed tomography of the sternoclavicular joint and sternum. Radiology 138:123, 1981.

14. Soteropoulos GC, Cigtay OS, Schellinger D: Pectus excavatum deformities simulating mediastinal masses. J Comput Assist Tomogr 3:596, 1979.

15. Gray H. In Goss CM (ed): Anatomy of the Human Body. Philadelphia, Lea & Febiger, 1966, pp 416–418, 448–461, 455–456, 614–618, 752–754.

16. Omell GH, Anderson LS, Bramson RJ: Chest wall tumors. Radiol Clin North Am 11:197, 1973.

17. Franken EA Jr, Smith JA, Smith WL: Tumors of the chest wall in infants and children. Pediatr Radiol 6:13, 1977.

18. Gouliamos AD, Carter BL, Emami B: Computed tomography of the chest wall. Radiology 134:433, 1980.

19. Faer MJ, Burnam RE, Beck CL: Transmural thoracic lipoma: demonstration by computed tomography. AJR 130:161, 1978.

20. Weschler RJ, Steiner RM: Cross-sectional imaging of the chest wall. J Thorac Imaging 4:29, 1989.

21. Hudson TM, Vandergriend RA, Springfield DS, Hawkins IF Jr, Spanier SS, et al: Aggressive fibromatosis: evaluation by computed tomography and angiography. Radiology 150:495, 1984.

22. Rubenstein WA, Gray G, Auh TH, Honig CL, Thorbjarnarson B, et al: CT of fibrous tissues and tumors with sonographic correlation. AJR 147:1067, 1986.

23. Francis IR, Dorovini-Zis K, Glazer GM, Lloyd RV, Amendola MA, Martel W: The fibromatosis: CT-pathologic correlation. AJR 147:1063, 1986.

24. Press GA, Glazer HS, Wasserman TH, Aronberg DJ, Lee JKT, Sagel SS: Thoracic wall involvement by Hodgkin disease and non-Hodgkin lymphoma: CT evaluation. Radiology 157:195, 1985.

25. Meyer JE, Linggood RM, Lindfors KK, McLoud TC, Stomper PC: Impact of thoracic computed tomography on radiation therapy planning in Hodgkin's disease. J Comput Assist Tomogr 8:892, 1984.

26. Palmer PES: Pulmonary tuberculosis—usual and unusual radiographic presentations. Semin Roentgenol 14:204, 1979.

26a. Sharif HS, Clark DC, Aabed MY, Aideyan OA, Haddad MC, Mattsson TA: MR imaging of thoracic and abdominal wall infections: comparison with other imaging procedures. AJR 154:989, 1990.

27. Bhatt GM, Austin HM: CT demonstration of empyema necessitatis. J Comput Assist Tomogr 9:1108, 1985.

28. Weber LD, Peters RW: Delayed chest wall complications of median sternotomy. South Med J 79:723, 1986.

29. Goodman LR, Kay HR, Teplick SK, Mundth ED: Complica-

tions of median sternotomy: computed tomographic evaluation. AJR 141:225, 1983.

30. Rosenthal DI, Johnson RD, Oot RF: Evaluation of postoperative osteomyelitis of the sternum using tomography and computerized tomography. J Can Assoc Radiol 35:24, 1984.

31. Shea WJ, de Geer G, Webb WR: Chest wall after mastectomy. I. CT appearance of normal postoperative anatomy, postirradiation changes, and optimal scanning techniques. Radiology 162:157, 1987.

32. Hellman S, Harris JR: Breast cancer: considerations in local and regional treatment. Radiology 164:593, 1986.

33. Shea WJ, de Geer G, Webb WR: Chest wall after mastectomy. II. CT appearance of tumor recurrence. Radiology 162:162, 1987.

34. Lindfors KK, Meyer JE, Busse PM, Kopans DB, Munzenrider JE, Sawicka JM: CT evaluation of local and regional breast cancer recurrence. AJR 145:833, 1985.

35. Holbert BL, Holbert JM, Libschitz HI: CT of interpectoral lymph nodes. AJR 149:687, 1987.

36. Napoli LD, Hansen HH, Muggia FM, Twigg HL: The incidence of osseous involvement in lung cancer, with special reference to the development of osteoblastic changes. Radiology 108:17, 1977.

37. Ellert J, Kreel L: The role of computed tomography in the initial staging and subsequent management of the lymphomas. J Comput Assist Tomogr 4:368, 1980.

38. Press GA, Glazer HS, Wasserman TH, Aronberg DJ, Lee JKT, Sagel SS: Thoracic wall involvement by Hodgkin disease and non-Hodgkin lymphoma: CT evaluation. Radiology 157:195, 1985.

39. Alexander E, Clark RA, Colley DP, Mitchell SE: CT of malignant pleural mesothelioma. AJR 137:287, 1981.

40. Webb WR, Sagel SS: Actinomycosis involving the chest wall: CT findings. AJR 139:1007, 1982.

41. Hepper NGG, Herskovic T, Witten DM, Mulder DW, Woolner LB: Thoracic inlet tumors. Ann Intern Med 64:979, 1966.

42. Paulsen DL: Carcinomas in the superior pulmonary sulcus. J Thorac Cardiovasc Surg 70:1095, 1975.

43. Miller JI, Mansour KA, Hatcher CR Jr: Carcinoma of the superior pulmonary sulcus. Ann Thorac Surg 28:44, 1979.

44. Webb WR, Jeffrey RB, Godwin JD: Thoracic computed tomography in superior sulcus tumors. J Comput Assist Tomogr 5:361, 1981.

45. O'Connell RS, McLoud TC, Wilkins EW: Superior sulcus tumor: radiographic diagnosis and workup. AJR 140:25, 1983.

46. Heelan RT, Demas BE, Bains M, Martini N, Burt M, et al: Advantage of coronal MR imaging in the evaluation of superior sulcus tumors. Radiology 165P:22, 1987.

47. Haggar AM, Pearlberg JL, Froelich JW, Hearshen DO, Beute GH, et al: Chest wall invasion by carcinoma of the lung. Detection by MR imaging. AJR 148:1075, 1987.

48. Musset D, Grenier P, Carette MF, Frija G, Hauuy MP, et al: Primary lung cancer staging: prospective comparative study of MR imaging with CT. Radiology 160:607, 1986.

49. Fishman EK, Zinreich ES, Jacobs CG, Rostock RA, Siegelman SS: CT of the axilla: normal anatomy and pathology. Radiographics 6:475, 1986.

50. Gebarski KS, Glazer GM, Gebarski SS: Brachial plexus: anatomic, radiologic, and pathologic correlation using computed tomography. J Comput Assist Tomogr 6:1058, 1982.

51. Kalisher L: Xeroradiography of axillary lymph node disease. Radiology 115:67, 1975.

52. Castagno AA, Shuman WP: MR imaging in clinically suspected brachial plexus tumor. AJR 149:1496, 1987.

53. Blair DN, Rapoport S, Sostman HD, Blair OC: Normal brachial plexus: MR imaging. Radiology 165:763, 1987.

54. Kellman GM, Kneeland JB, Middleton WD, Cates JD, Pech P, et al: MR imaging of the supraclavicular region: normal anatomy. AJR 148:77, 1987.

55. Kneeland JB, Kellman GM, Middleton WD, Cates JD, Jesmanowicz A, et al: Diagnosis of diseases of the supraclavicular region by use of MR imaging. AJR 148:1149, 1987.

56. Thomson JS, Kreel L: The subtrapezial space. J Comput Assist Tomogr 3:355, 1979.

57. McLeod RA, Grisvold JJ, Stephens DH, Beabout JW, Sheedy

PF: Computed tomography of soft tissues and breast. Semin Roentgenol 13:267, 1978.

58. Grisvold JJ, Reese DF, Karsell PR: Computed tomographic mammography (CTM). AJR 133:1143, 1979.
59. Chang CHJ, Nesbit DE, Fisher DR, Fritz SL, Dwyer SJ III, et al: Computed tomographic mammography using a conventional body scanner. AJR 138:553, 1982.
60. Munzenrider JE, Tchakarova I, Castro M, Carter B: Computerized body tomography in breast cancer: I. Internal mammary nodes and radiation treatment planning. Cancer 43:137, 1979.
61. Meyer JE, Munzenrider JE: Computed tomographic demonstration of internal mammary lymph node metastasis in patients with locally recurrent breast carcinoma. Radiology 139:661, 1981.
62. Dash N, Lupetin AR, Daffner RH, Deeb ZL, Sefczek RJ, Schapiro RL: Magnetic resonance imaging in the diagnosis of breast disease. AJR 146:119, 1986.
63. El Yousef SJ, Duchesneau RH: Magnetic resonance imaging of the human breast: a phase I trial. Radiol Clin North Am 22:859, 1984.
64. El Yousef SJ, O'Connell DM, Duchesneau RH, Smith MJ, Hubay CA, Guyton SP: Benign and malignant breast disease: magnetic resonance and radiofrequency pulse sequences. AJR 145:1, 1985.
65. McSweeney MB, Small WC, Cerny V, Sewell W, Powell RW, Goldstein JH: Magnetic resonance imaging in the diagnosis of breast disease: use of transverse relaxation times. Radiology 153:741, 1984.
66. Turner DA, Alcorn FS, Adler YT: Nuclear magnetic resonance in the diagnosis of breast cancer. Radiol Clin North Am 26:673, 1988.
67. Policard A, Galy P: La Plevre. Paris, Masson, 1942, pp 23–33.
68. Bernaudin J-F, Fleury J: Anatomy of the blood and lymphatic circulation of the pleural serosa. In Chretien J, Bignon J, Hirsch A (eds): The Pleura in Health and Disease. New York, Marcel Dekker, 1985, pp 101–124.
69. Woodburne RT: Essentials of Human Anatomy, 6th ed. New York, Oxford University Press, 1978, pp 310–312.
70. Gray H: In Goss CM (ed): Anatomy of the Human Body, 28th ed. Philadelphia, Lea & Febiger, 1966, pp 379–380, 413–415.
71. Vix VA: Extrapleural costal fat. Radiology 112:563, 1974.
72. Sargent EN, Boswell WD Jr, Ralls PW, Markovitz A: Subpleural fat pads in patients exposed to asbestos: distinction from non-calcified pleural plaques. Radiology 152:273, 1984.
73. Moore KL: Clinically Oriented Anatomy. Baltimore, Williams & Wilkins, 1980, pp 23–26.
74. Thorek P: Anatomy in Surgery, 3rd ed. New York, Springer-Verlag, 1985, pp 260–263.
75. Smith JK, Murphy TR, Blair JSG, Lowor KG: Regional Anatomy Illustrated. New York, Churchill Livingstone 1983, pp 130–135.
75a. Im JG, Webb WR, Rosen A, Gamsu G: Costal pleura: appearances at high-resolution CT. Radiology 171:125, 1989.
76. Marks BW, Kuhns LR: Identification of the pleural fissures with computed tomography. Radiology 143:139, 1982.
77. Frija J, Schmit P, Katz M, Vadrot D, Laval-Jeantet M: Computed tomography of the pulmonary fissures: normal anatomy. J Comput Assist Tomogr 6:1069, 1982.
78. Proto AV, Ball JB Jr: Computed tomography of the major and minor fissures. AJR 140:439, 1983.
79. Goodman LR, Golkow RS, Steiner RM, Teplick SK, Haskin ME, et al: The right midlung window: a potential source of error in computed tomography of the lung. Radiology 143:135, 1982.
80. Speckman JM, Gamsu G, Webb WR: Alterations in CT mediastinal anatomy produced by an azygos lobe. AJR 137:47, 1981.
81. Godwin JD, Tarver RD: Accessory fissures of the lung. AJR 144:39, 1985.
82. Rabinowitz JG, Wolf BS: Roentgen significance of the pulmonary ligament. Radiology 87:1013, 1966.

83. Rost RC Jr, Proto AV: Inferior pulmonary ligament: computed tomographic appearance. Radiology 148:479, 1983.
84. Cooper C, Moss AA, Buy J-N, Stark DD: CT appearance of the normal inferior pulmonary ligament. AJR 141:237, 1983.
85. Godwin JJ, Vock P, Osborne DR: CT of the pulmonary ligament. AJR 141:231, 1983.
86. Godwin JJ, Merten DF, Baker ME: Paramediastinal pneumatocele: alternative explanations to gas in the pulmonary ligament. AJR 145:525, 1985.
87. Pugatch RD, Faling LJ, Robbins AH, Snider GL: Differentiation of pleural and pulmonary lesions using computed tomography. J Comput Assist Tomogr 2:601, 1978.
88. Dwyer A: The displaced crus: a sign for distinguishing between pleural fluid and ascites on computed tomography. J Comput Assist Tomogr 2:598, 1978.
89. Halvorsen RA, Fedyshin PJ, Korobkin M, Thompson WM: CT differentiation of pleural effusion from ascites. An evaluation of four signs using blinded analysis of 52 cases. Invest Radiol 21:391, 1986.
90. Federle MP, Mark AS, Guillaumin ES: CT of subpulmonic pleural effusions and atelectasis: criteria for differentiation from subphrenic fluid. AJR 146:685, 1986.
91. Halvorsen RA, Foster WL Jr, Fedyshin PJ, Thompson WM, Korobkin M: Ascites or pleural effusion? CT differentiation: four useful criteria. Radiographics 6:135, 1986.
92. Naidich DP, Megibow AJ, Hilton S, Hulnick DH, Siegelman SS: Computed tomography of the diaphragm: peridiaphragmatic fluid localization. J Comput Assist Tomogr 7:641, 1983.
93. Teplick JG, Teplick SK, Goodman L, Haskin ME: The interface sign: a computed tomographic sign distinguishing pleural and intra-abdominal fluid. Radiology 144:359, 1982.
94. Vock P, Effman EL, Hedlund LW, Lischko MM, Putman CE: Analysis of the density of pleural fluid analogs by computed tomography. Invest Radiol 19:10, 1984.
95. Tscholakoff D, Sechtem U, de Geer G, Schmidt H, Higgins CB: Evaluation of pleural and pericardial effusions by magnetic resonance imaging. Eur J Radiol 7:169, 1987.
95a. Wallner B, Edelman RR, Finn JP, Mattle HP: Bright pleural effusion and ascites on gradient-echo MR images: a potential source of confusion in vascular MR studies. AJR 155:1237, 1990.
96. Ehman RL, McNamara MT, Brasch RC, Felmlee JP, Gray JE, Higgins CB: Influence of physiologic motion on the appearance of tissue in MR images. Radiology 159:777, 1986.
97. Williford ME, Hidalgo H, Putman CE, Korobkin M, Ram PC: Computed tomography of pleural disease. AJR 140:909, 1983.
98. Stark DD, Federle MP, Goodman PC, Podrasky AE, Webb WR: Differentiating lung abscess and empyema: radiography and computed tomography. AJR 141:163, 1983.
98a. Waite RJ, Carbonneau RJ, Balikian JP, Umali CB, Pezzella AT, Nash G: Parietal pleural changes in empyema: appearances at CT. Radiology 175:145, 1990.
99. Hulnick DH, Naidich DP, McCauley DI: Pleural tuberculosis evaluated by computed tomography. Radiology 149:759, 1983.
100. Schmitt WGH, Hubener KH, Rucker HC: Pleural calcification with persistent effusion. Radiology 149:633, 1983.
101. Stark DD, Federle MP, Goodman PC: CT and radiographic assessment of tube thoracostomy. AJR 141:253, 1983.
102. vanSonnenberg E, Nakamoto SK, Mueller PR, Casola G, Neff CC, et al: CT- and ultrasound-guided catheter drainage of empyemas after chest-tube failure. Radiology 151:349, 1984.
102a. Neff CC, vanSonnenberg E, Lawson DW, Patton AS: CT follow-up of empyemas: pleural peels resolve after percutaneous catheter drainage. Radiology 176:195, 1990.
103. Katz D, Kreel L: Computed tomography in pulmonary asbestosis. Clin Radiol 30:207, 1979.
104. Sargent EN, Boswell WD Jr, Ralls PW, Markovitz A: Subpleural fat pads in patients exposed to asbestosis: distinction from non-calcified pleural plaques. Radiology 152:273, 1984.
105. Aberle DR, Gamsu G, Ray CS, Feuerstein IM: Asbestos-related pleural and parenchymal fibrosis: detection with high-resolution CT. Radiology 166:729, 1988.
106. Friedman AC, Fiel SB, Fisher MS, Radecki PD, Lev-Toaff AS,

Caroline DF: Asbestosis-related pleural disease and asbestosis: a comparison of CT and chest radiography. AJR 150:269, 1988.

107. Aberle DR, Gamsu G, Ray CH: High-resolution CT of benign asbestos-related diseases: clinical and radiographic correlation. AJR 151:883, 1988.

108. McLoud TC, Woods BO, Carrington CB, Epler GB, Gaensler EA: Diffuse pleural thickening in an asbestos-exposed population: prevalence and causes. AJR 144:9, 1985.

109. Webb WR, Cooper C, Gamsu G: Interlobar pleural plaque mimicking a lung nodule in a patient with asbestos exposure. J Comput Assist Tomogr 7:135, 1983.

110. Lynch DA, Gamsu G, Ray CS, Aberle DR: Asbestos-related focal lung masses: manifestations on conventional and high-resolution CT scans. Radiology 169:603, 1988.

111. Kreel L: Computed tomography in mesothelioma. Semin Oncol 8:302, 1981.

111a. Kawashima A, Libshitz HI: Malignant pleural mesothelioma: CT manifestations in 50 cases. AJR 155:965, 1990.

112. Rabinowitz JG, Efremidis SC, Cohen B, Dan S, Efremidis A, et al: A comparative study of mesothelioma and asbestosis using computed tomography and conventional chest radiography. Radiology 144:453, 1982.

113. Law MR, Gregor A, Husband JE, Kerr IH: Computed tomography in the assessment of malignant mesothelioma of the pleura. Clin Radiol 33:67, 1982.

114. Dedrick CG, McLoud TC, Shepard J-AO, Shipley RT: Computed tomography of localized pleural mesothelioma. AJR 144:275, 1985.

115. Brown LR, Muhm JR, Gray JE: Radiographic detection of thymoma. AJR 134:1181, 1980.

116. Baron RL, Lee JKT, Sagel SS, Levitt RG: Computed tomography of the abnormal thymus. Radiology 142:127, 1982.

117. Callen PW, Filly RA, Korobkin M: Computed tomographic evaluation of the diaphragmatic crura. Radiology 126:413, 1978.

118. Naidich DP, Megibow AJ, Ross CR, Beranbaum ER, Siegelman SS: Computed tomography of the diaphragm: normal anatomy and variants. J Comput Assist Tomogr 7:633, 1983.

119. Panicek DM, Benson CB, Gottlieb RH, Heitzman ER: The diaphragm: anatomic, pathologic, and radiologic considerations. Radiographics 8:385, 1988.

120. Williamson BRJ, Gouse JC, Rohrer DG, Teates CD: Variation in the thickness of the diaphragmatic crura with respiration. Radiology 163:683, 1987.

121. Gale EM: Anterior diaphragm: variations in the CT appearance. Radiology 161:635, 1986.

122. Caskey CI, Zerhouni EA, Fishman EK, Rahmouni AD: Aging of the diaphragm: a CT study. Radiology 171:385, 1989.

123. Reed JO, Lang EF: Diaphragmatic hernia in infancy. AJR 82:437, 1959.

124. Gale EM: Bochdalek hernia: prevalence and CT characteristics. Radiology 156:449, 1985.

125. Betts RA: Subcostosternal diaphragmatic hernia with report of five cases. AJR 75:269, 1956.

126. Heiberg E, Wolverson MK, Hurd RN, Jagannadharao B, Sundaram M: CT recognition of traumatic rupture of the diaphragm. AJR 135:369, 1980.

127. Rohlfing BM, Korobkin M, Hall AD: Computed tomography of intrathoracic omental herniation and other mediastinal fatty masses. J Comput Assist Tomogr 1:181, 1977.

128. Schulman A, Fataar S: CT in diaphragmatic rupture? Letter. AJR 136:1256, 1981.

129. Heiberg E, Sundaram M, Wolverson MK: CT in diaphragmatic rupture? Letter. AJR 136:1256, 1981.

130. Rubenstein ZJ, Solomon A: CT findings in partial eventration of the right diaphragm. J Comput Assist Tomogr 5:719, 1981.

131. Anderson LS, Forrest JV: Tumors of the diaphragm. AJR 119:259, 1973.

CHAPTER 6

HEART AND PERICARDIUM

CHARLES B. HIGGINS

For more than 30 years definitive diagnosis of diseases of the heart and pericardium has depended on cardiac catheterization. Angiography has remained the major imaging technique for the diagnosis and assessment of the severity of heart disease, even though it has substantial limitations for both cardiac and pericardial diseases. Although new imaging techniques that are noninvasive and provide new insights into diagnosis usually are readily accepted, reliance on cardiac catheterization and angiography for definitive diagnosis of heart disease has persisted. This is partly because the diagnosis of cardiac conditions necessitates both accurate morphology assessment and also quantitative evaluation of function. Echocardiography was not regarded as definitive for more than 15 years after its introduction into clinical medicine. Even though it is now being accepted for some diseases, most patients still undergo cardiac catheterization and angiography before cardiac surgery. Although this approach is valid for evaluation of coronary artery disease, it no longer has a rational basis for the evaluation of many nonischemic cardiac and pericardial diseases.

Even though the tomographic imaging techniques of computed tomography (CT) and magnetic resonance (MR) imaging have become primary tests for diagnosis in almost all organs of the body, cardiac disease remains the exception to this general practice. CT and MR had clear limitations for cardiac evalua-

tion during their early development, because they required seconds to minutes to produce images, and initially they were inadequate for precisely depicting the anatomy of the constantly beating heart. They also lacked the sampling frequency necessary to evaluate cardiac function. On early CT scanners, gating techniques were difficult to employ and lengthened the examination time inordinately. CT and MR did not become capable of adequately evaluating the heart until the early 1980s. Because of these technologic limitations during their early years, these techniques have had less impact on the diagnosis of diseases of the heart and pericardium than on diagnosis of diseases in other regions of the body.

These limitations for the most part have been overcome, and nearly all cardiac diagnostic evaluations are now moving toward the use of noninvasive techniques. Echocardiography is increasingly displacing cardiac catheterization and angiography for the diagnosis of many cardiac diseases, with the exception of obstructive coronary disease. Although echocardiography will remain the preeminent noninvasive cardiac diagnostic technique for a period of time, it is likely that the diagnostic capabilities and advantages of fast (cine-) CT and MR will become recognized in the near future. This chapter describes the capabilities and clinical applications of CT and MR for the diagnosis of diseases of the heart and pericardium. These imaging techniques can not only identify morphologic abnormalities, but also assess cardiac function. Consequently this chapter discusses anatomic diagnosis and quantitative and qualitative assessment of cardiac function.

Techniques for Examination

Computed Tomography

Standard CT with 2- to 5-second scan times has not gained widespread acceptance for cardiac evaluation. Cardiac motion and, to a lesser extent, respiratory motion significantly degrade image quality because of the long scan time needed for standard CT in relation to the cardiac cycle. The ability to obtain only one slice at a time is a major drawback of CT for cardiac purposes. A further disadvantage of CT imaging in assessing cardiac function is the need for intravascular contrast medium; standard ionic contrast media can have important effects on cardiac performance and regional myocardial blood flow.

CT scanning of the heart usually requires modification of standard CT techniques used in other parts of the body. Standard CT techniques, as described in earlier chapters, are usually adequate for the evaluation of pericardial disease and patency of coronary arterial bypass grafts. Assessment of cardiac function and precise definition of intracardiac anatomy requires either electrocardiographic (ECG) gating of conventional CT scanners or, preferably, the use of a millisecond scanner (cine-CT).

ECG-GATED COMPUTED TOMOGRAPHY

Electrocardiographically gated CT is one method of overcoming the problem of cardiac motion and is critical in obtaining quantitative dimensions of the heart and functional information such as ejection fractions.[1, 2] It can also measure wall thickening during the cardiac cycle.[3] Gated CT scanning is more complicated than standard CT scanning. To obtain a reconstructed image of a stationary object by conventional CT, a nearly full complement of angular radiographic data must be obtained over the scanning cycle from 0° to 360° without significant gaps in the angular data set.[3] Multiple scans are required to obtain the necessary angular data to reconstruct a gated image of the heart.

Two gating techniques that have been used are retrospective and prospective gating (Fig. 6–1).[1] With retrospective gating, the CT scan data and the ECG are recorded simultaneously, but the ECG signal does not guide the CT acquisition. Subsequently the image is reconstructed from data obtained within a selected time or "biologic" window, bracketing the desired portion of the ECG signal, such as the QRS complex at end-diastole.

Prospective ECG gating uses preselection of a fraction of the RR interval to be monitored (Fig. 6–1). The biologic window width sets the fraction of the cardiac cycle to be represented by each image. Prospective gating ensures the even distribution of

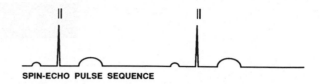

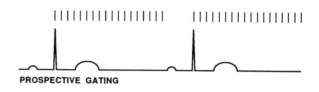

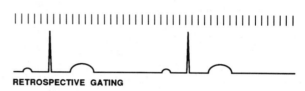

FIGURE 6–1 ■ Diagram of the x-ray exposure or MR pulse sequence in relation to the ECG for prospective and retrospective ECG gating. For prospective gating, the series of CT x-ray exposures or MR pulse sequences is initiated by the R wave of the ECG. For retrospective gating the exposures and pulse sequences occur continuously while the ECG is recorded simultaneously. The imaging data are later segregated into specified segments of the cardiac cycle.

R waves throughout the scanning cycle in the minimal number of scans. This is accomplished by firing the x-ray tube at the appropriate time relative to the R wave on the ECG input such that one of the following R waves falls in the largest gap in the already acquired angular x-ray data. In most studies, the width of the biologic window is set at 10 per cent of the RR interval. With the heart rate at 100 beats per minute, each frame represents 60 ms. With the biologic window set at 10 per cent of the RR interval, approximately eight scanner rotations are required to obtain a full complement of gated angular radiographic data, requiring approximately 45 seconds of breath holding. This period of apnea makes the procedure unrealistic for many patients with cardiac diseases.

CINE–COMPUTED TOMOGRAPHY

Electronic scanning methods used in the fast CT scanner (cine-CT) allow a complete cardiac image to be obtained in real time without ECG gating.[4] The exposure time of each scan is 50 ms. The fast CT scanner is not limited by inertia associated with moving mechanical parts, as in a conventional CT scanner. It uses a focused electron beam that is swept across four cadmium tungstate target arcs in succession (Fig. 6–2). Each of the four arcs generates a fan beam of x-ray photons that pass from beneath the patient to a bank of detectors arranged in a semicircle above the patient.

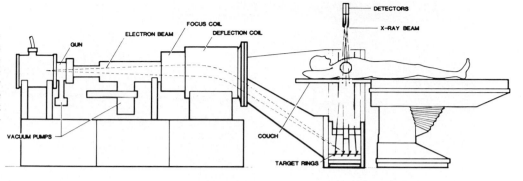

FIGURE 6–2 ■ Diagram of a cine-CT scanner. The scanner employs a focused electron beam magnetically deflected onto tungsten targets. The targets emit an x-ray beam that projects through the subject and is registered by a bank of detectors arranged in a semicircle.

The cine-CT scanner can be operated in three different modes. The *cine mode* is used to assess global and regional myocardial function. The scans are obtained with an exposure time of 50 ms at a rate of 17 scans per second. The *flow mode* is used for blood flow analysis and employs a series of 10 to 20 successive scans in which each of the 50-ms exposures is electrocardiographically triggered at a specific phase of the cardiac cycle of successive heart beats. Triggering can be set to occur after every second, third, or later R wave. From the series of CT scans, time-density curves can be constructed for specific regions of interest within a cardiac chamber or the myocardium to provide an estimate of transit time or perfusion. The third mode is the *volume mode,* in which eight scans are obtained using all four target areas. These eight transverse scans can often encompass the entire left ventricular chamber and thereby provide an estimate of left ventricular volume and myocardial mass. In patients with left ventricular enlargement, eight levels covering 8 cm do not encompass the entire left ventricle, and two separate acquisitions may be required.

Magnetic Resonance Imaging

The technique used for MR imaging of the heart depends on the primary goal of the procedure. For anatomic abnormalities ECG-gated spin-echo techniques provide static images with high signal-to-noise ratios. For cardiac contractile function, cine MR techniques are used.[5] These techniques use narrow flip angles (less than 90°) and gradient-refocused echoes. Because the repetition time (TR) and echo delay time (TE) values are approximately 20 to 30 ms and 10 to 15 ms, respectively, the cardiac cycle can be divided into more than 30 time frames. By lacing these together in a cinematic format, tomograms of the beating heart are obtained.

The imaging plane used for a study also depends on the information desired. For purely anatomic information, imaging in a transverse, sagittal, or coronal plane can be used (Fig. 6–3). For measurements of cardiac dimensions such as the diameter of the ventricle and ventricular wall thickness or for derivation of functional parameters, imaging in the plane perpendicular to the cardiac long axis, known as the *cardiac short axis*, is indicated.[6] The long axis

of the left ventricle is a plane that transects the middle of the aortic valve and the apex of the left ventricle, and the short axis plane is perpendicular to the long axis. Obtaining short-axis images generally requires a two-step angulation of the slice-selective gradient relative to the orthogonal axis of the body and consequently increases the total imaging time.

The blood pool has a unique signal on both spin-echo and gradient-refocused images. The blood pool on the ECG-gated spin-echo images generally is a signal void that provides high contrast between intracardiac blood and the myocardial wall (Figs. 6–4 and 6–5). On the other hand, the blood pool produces a very bright signal when a gradient-refocused technique is used (Fig. 6–6). This also results in a high degree of contrast between intracardiac blood and myocardial wall. Abnormal flow patterns cause intraluminal bright signal within the signal void on spin-echo images and a focal signal void within the high-intensity blood pool on gradient-refocused images.

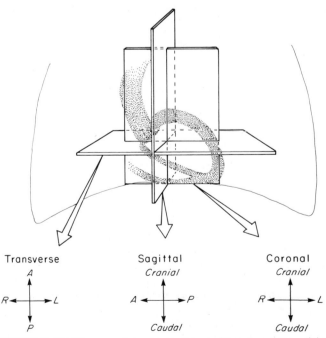

FIGURE 6–3 ■ Diagram of standard orthogonal imaging planes of the heart for MR.

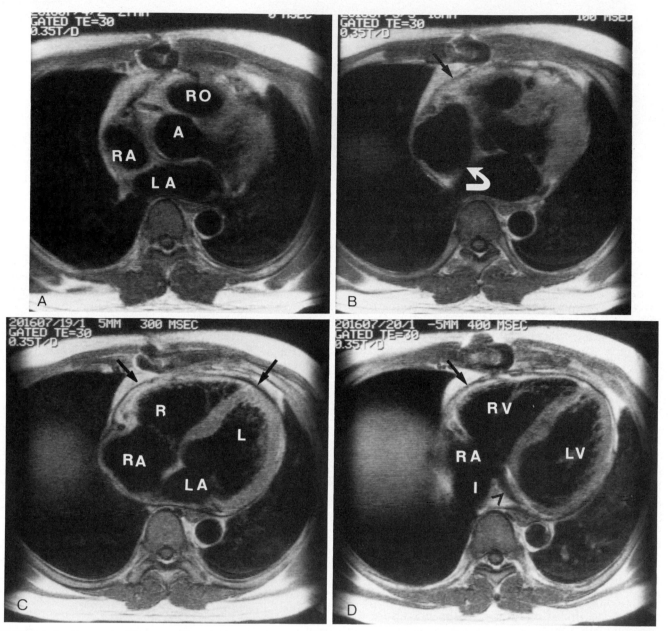

FIGURE 6–4 ■ Transverse MR images from the base to the apex of the heart. *A,* Level of aortic valve. *B,* Level of the left ventricular outflow tract. *C,* Level of middle of left ventricle. *D,* Level of junction of inferior vena cava and coronary sinus with the right atrium. A = Base of aorta; I = inferior vena cava ostium; L = left ventricle; LA = left atrium; LV = left ventricle; R = right ventricle; RA = right atrium; RO = right ventricular outflow tract; RV = body of right ventricle; arrowhead = coronary sinus; black arrows = pericardium; white arrow = atrial septum.

Heart

Anatomy

The heart begins in embryologic life as a simple tube that subsequently becomes folded and coiled on itself so that eventually it has the shape of a blunt cone with an apex and a base. The apex of the heart lies in a caudal and ventral position, pointing to the left.[7] Although its position changes continually during life, the apex in the adult remains close to the left fifth intercostal space approximately 8 cm from the midsternal line.

The heart is overlapped by an extension of the pleura and lungs and the anterior thoracic wall. The base of the heart forms the base of the blunt cone, facing to the right, cranial and also dorsal. The base comprises primarily the left atrium but also part of the right atrium and a small part of the proximal portion of the great vessels. The diaphragmatic surface of the heart lies against the diaphragm and comprises the two ventricles. The coronary sulcus marks the plane of the atrioventricular groove.

The left ventricle and a small part of the left atrial appendage form the left border of the heart. The right atrium is larger than the left atrium and has a capacity of approximately 60 mL in the adult; its

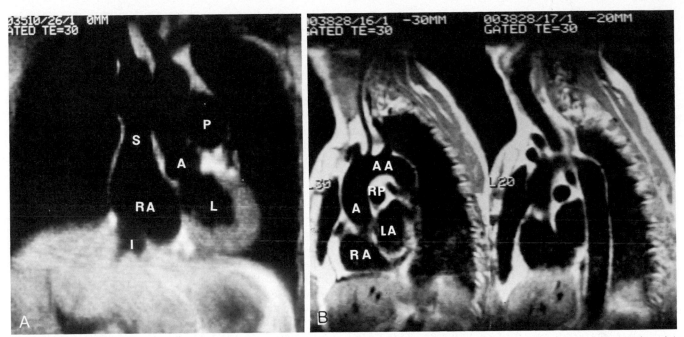

FIGURE 6–5 ■ Coronal *(A)* and oblique sagittal *(B)* imaging planes on MRI. A = Aorta; AA = aortic arch; I = inferior vena cava; L = left ventricle; LA = left atrium; P = pulmonary artery; R = right ventricle; RA = right atrium; RP = right pulmonary artery; S = superior vena cava.

walls are about 2 mm thick. The right atrial cavity consists of two parts: a principal cavity and an appendage or auricle. The right atrial appendage is shaped like the ear of a dog and is a blind pouch extending cranially between the superior vena cava and the right ventricle. Muscular bundles, termed *musculi pectinati* because they resemble the teeth of a comb, compose the internal surface of the atrium.

The superior vena cava opens into the cranial and posterior part of the right atrium. Its orifice directs blood toward the atrioventricular opening. The inferior vena cava opens into the most caudal part of the right atrium near the interatrial septum and its orifice is larger than the superior vena caval opening.

The coronary sinus enters the right atrium between the inferior vena cava and the atrioventricular opening. It is responsible for returning blood from the heart itself.

The left ventricular chamber is an ellipsoid sphere surrounded by muscular walls 8 to 11 mm thick, which is three times thicker than those of the right ventricle. The left ventricle has two walls: a medial wall (the ventricular septum), which is shared with the right ventricle, and a lateral wall. Both walls are concave toward the cavity. The septum is triangular in shape, with its base located at the level of the aortic valve. The left ventricle is entirely muscular except for the small membranous septum located just

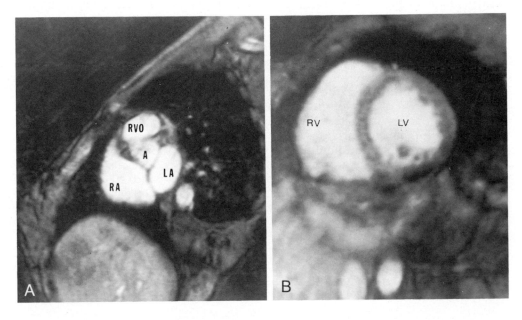

FIGURE 6–6 ■ Gradient-refocused short-axis MR images at the left of the atria *(A)* and ventricles *(B)*. A = Aorta; LA = left atrium; LV = left ventricle; RA = right atrium; RVO = right ventricular outflow tract.

below the right and posterior aortic cusps. The upper third of the septum has a smooth endocardial surface. The other two thirds of the septum and the remainder of the ventricular walls are ridged by interlacing muscles, the trabeculae carneae.[8] The ventricular wall, exclusive of the septum, is often referred to as the *free wall of the left ventricle*. Although the left ventricle composes the lower left lateral cardiac border in the frontal chest radiograph, the major portion of its external surface is actually posterolateral. The right ventricle occupies most of the ventral or sternocostal surface of the heart, anteriorly and to the right of the midline. The right ventricular chamber is triangular and located anteriorly and toward the right of the heart. The pulmonary conus, which is the outflow tract of the right ventricle, swings to the left of the midline.

The aortic valve is located at the apex of the outflow tract of the left ventricle. It is a tricuspid valve with the posterior leaflet contiguous with the anterior leaflet of the mitral valve. The outflow tract of the left ventricle is irregular but changes to a roughly triangular shape at the sinus of Valsalva. The aortic valve is situated at the triangular sinus of Valsalva and immediately caudal to the circular aortic root. The valve lies in a plane anterior to the left atrium, with the right atrium on the right and the right ventricle and infundibulum on the left.

The mitral valve is located alongside the aortic valve and has two leaflets. The anteroseptal leaflet, the larger and more mobile of the mitral leaflets, is suspended like a curtain diagonally from the top of the posteromedial septum across the ventricular cavity to the anterolateral ventricular wall, separating the left ventricular cavity into an inflow and an outflow tract. The inflow tract, which is funnel shaped, is formed by the mitral anulus and by both mitral leaflets and their chordae tendineae. It directs blood from the left atrium inferiorly, anteriorly, and to the left. The outflow tract is formed by the inferior surface of the anteroseptal mitral valve leaflet the ventricular septum, and the free left ventricular wall. It lies at right angles to the inflow tract and directs blood from the apex superiorly and to the right. The anteromedial mitral leaflet is continuous with supporting tissues of the noncoronary aortic cusps that lie above it. The posterior leaflet, although much shallower in depth than the anterior leaflet, is attached over two thirds of the mitral anulus. The papillary muscles, located below the anterolateral and posteromedial commissures, arise from the junction of the apical and middle thirds of the ventricular wall. Chordae tendineae are strong chords of fibrous tissue that pass from the papillary muscles to the leaflets of the mitral valve. The tricuspid valve is oriented vertically, separating the right atrium from the right ventricle.

Various anatomic structures on the surface of the heart can be demonstrated on CT and MR images. The atrioventricular grooves on both the right and the left form indentations along the heart borders.

The right coronary artery and circumflex coronary artery lie in the right and left atrioventricular grooves, respectively. The left anterior descending coronary artery arises from the left coronary artery and courses along the left anterior surface of the heart over the ventricular septum. The left descending coronary artery is commonly surrounded by fat, and its proximal segment is frequently demonstrated on scans.

The standard tomographic imaging plane is transverse (perpendicular) to the long axis of the body. The standard orthogonal planes, especially the transverse plane, are adequate for most anatomic observations. Because the heart lies within the chest at about a 45° angle to the sagittal plane, the transverse plane transects the heart obliquely relative to the long axis of the ventricle (see Fig. 6–3). The coronal and sagittal planes likewise transect the heart obliquely. Imaging planes that transect the heart either parallel or perpendicular to the long axis of the left ventricle are preferred (see Fig. 6–6). For the precise measurement of wall thickness and perhaps some other dimensional measurements, the short axis plane has advantages. The patient can be rotated to obtain sections approximating the left anterior and right anterior oblique views (see Fig. 6–5B).

Images in any plane can be achieved with MR. Angulation of the cine-CT table allows one to somewhat approximate the long and short axis planes with this modality. However, this is not possible in all patients, and success depends on body habitus and size. Because intracardiac anatomy is depicted more vividly with MR and all images in planes can be acquired precisely using MR, the anatomic features of the heart and pericardium at the various tomographic levels are described here using gated spin-echo MR images. The transverse plane is standard for both CT and MR, and emphasis will be placed on the anatomy in this plane.

Transverse images at the base of the heart demonstrate the muscle of the right ventricular outflow tract anteriorly (see Fig. 6–4A). Immediately behind the right ventricular outflow tract is the base of the aortic valve, or the sinus of Valsalva, and farther posteriorly is the left atrium. Images at this level provide a general idea of the size of the left atrium and right ventricular outflow tract. In the normal person the anteroposterior (AP) dimension of the left atrium is no more than 1.5 times the AP diameter of the base of the aorta.

Proceeding caudally, the next transverse image shows the left ventricular outflow tract and the undersurface of the aortic valve (see Fig. 6–4B). This level also reveals a major portion of the atrial septum and frequently the moderator band of the right ventricle. The right ventricle can be distinguished from the left ventricle by several anatomic characteristics, including the presence of muscle between the tricuspid valve and the pulmonic valve; the presence of the moderator band, coursing between the septum and the free wall of the right ventricle; the heavier internal trabeculations; and the absence of distinct papillary muscles. In addition, the tricuspid valve is positioned ventral to the mitral valve. Recognition of these characteristic differences between the right and left ventricles is important in situations in which their positions are unreliable, such as complex cardiovascular anomalies, dextrocardia, and isomere syndromes.

Tomographic images through the middle of the ventricles demonstrate their internal topography (see Fig. 6–4C). At this level the coronary vessels are frequently shown coursing in the right atrioventricular groove. The various components of the ventricular septum and atrial septum are also demonstrated at this level.

As the ventricles are transected further caudally, the sections no longer include the left atrium and contain only the most inferior portion of the right atrium (see Fig. 6–4D). At the inferior portion of the right atrium is the junction of the inferior vena cava and coronary sinus with the right atrium. On images in the transverse plane the anterior apical region of the left ventricular myocardium is thinner than the other regions of the left ventricle in many individuals. On spin-echo images the myocardium usually is discriminated clearly from the intracardiac blood pool, and there is sharp delineation of both the epi- and endocardial borders of the myocardium. At all levels, the pericardium and contents occur as a thin line of low signal intensity. This line is highlighted by pericardial fat externally and epicardial fat internally.

The coronal plane can be useful in certain instances (see Fig. 6–5A), such as for abnormalities involving the diaphragmatic surface of the left ventricle. In transverse images the diaphragmatic surface of the heart is parallel to the imaging plane and cannot be evaluated adequately. However, the diaphragmatic surface is demonstrated in its entirety using the coronal imaging plane. The coronal imaging plane also demonstrates the connection of the superior and inferior venae cavae with the right atrium.

The sagittal plane is used infrequently for imaging the heart and pericardium, even though it can readily demonstrate the heart and the extent of the pericardium along the great vessels. The superior pericardial recesses are displayed in both sagittal and transverse planes.

An oblique sagittal view of the heart can be obtained by elevating the patient's right side 20° to 30° and imaging in the sagittal plane (see Fig. 6–5B). It also can demonstrate the ascending and transverse thoracic aorta and the origin of the arch vessels. It also shows the inlet, outlet, and trabecular portions of the ventricular septum to good effect.

The long axis of the left ventricle generally can be determined from the coronal view, and then, by double angulation of the slice-selective gradient, the short-axis view perpendicular to the long axis can be obtained. Short-axis views through the base of the heart demonstrate the atria without the ventricles on the same image (see Fig. 6–6A). Short-axis views through the ventricles demonstrate the right and left

ventricle without the atria or atrioventricular valves on the same images (see Fig. 6–6B). This isolation of the ventricles from their atrioventricular and semilunar valves and from the atria may be a disadvantage when assessing valvular abnormalities or attempting to determine whether an abnormal MR flow signal within the ventricle is originating from a semilunar or atrioventricular valve. Moreover, the short-axis view can distort the anatomic relationships between the heart and surrounding organs.

Pathology

ANATOMIC DIAGNOSIS: COMPUTED TOMOGRAPHY
Ischemic Heart Disease ■ Ischemic heart disease, also known as *coronary artery disease,* is the prime killer of men older than 35 years and of all adults older than 40 years in the United States. Each year at least 1.2 million Americans sustain their first heart attack; of these, at least one third die within a month. Only 50 per cent of surviving patients can be completely rehabilitated. Thus coronary artery disease is perhaps the most urgent medical problem of our time.[9]

Stenosis, or obstruction of one or more coronary arteries, jeopardizes the blood supply to regions of the myocardial wall. The process ultimately results in progressive ischemic damage and replacement of viable heart muscle by connective tissue. Damage may follow an acute episode of myocardial infarction, or it may develop insidiously. The patient's prognosis is related to the extent of the damaged myocardium, which may be as much as one third of the entire heart.

The tissue changes caused by ischemia are poorly detected by presently available diagnostic techniques. Perhaps the best available procedure for determining myocardial blood flow is the thallium scan. Unfortunately the images produced by this procedure (showing the distribution of radioactive tracer in the heart wall) are of low resolution and can only estimate relative myocardial perfusion.

The established noninvasive modalities of echocardiography and isotope imaging have contributed greatly to the routine management of patients with ischemic heart disease but have not yet significantly reduced the need for cardiac catheterization, mainly because these techniques are unable to provide the necessary structural and functional information obtained by angiocardiography. CT and MR can provide most of this structural and functional information and in the future may become able to measure myocardial blood flow.

The site, size, and complications of myocardial infarctions have been revealed by standard CT and cine-CT. CT scans have displayed the extent of wall thinning of the left ventricle in patients with previous infarctions.[1, 2, 10] CT also has shown the presence of and differentiated between true and false aneurysms of the left ventricle. The distinguishing features of false aneurysms on CT include the small ostium between the left ventricular cavity and the aneurysm; the posterior site; and the large volume of the aneurysm projecting beyond the left ventricular contour.

Left ventricular aneurysm formation is an important complication of acute myocardial infarction and occurs in 12 to 15 per cent of cases.[11, 12] Most aneurysms are chronic and form slowly. The patient becomes symptomatic weeks or months after the acute infarction, exhibiting chronic congestive heart failure or episodes of peripheral emboli.

The anterolateral wall of the left ventricle and interventricular septum usually are involved. During ventricular systole, the aneurysm expands as blood is forced into it from the functional part of the ventricle. The ejection fraction falls, and cardiac output diminishes. During ventricular diastole, the blood in the aneurysm is added to the atrial blood entering the ventricle and results in an increase in resting ventricular volume. The benefits from excision of a ventricular aneurysm are controversial. Systemic embolism, chronic heart failure, and persistent arrhythmia generally are considered indications for surgery.[13] Detection of chronic aneurysm is thus important. CT scanning is a simple, noninvasive method for detecting and studying ventricular aneurysm.[2, 14]

Quantitation of regional myocardial wall thickening is an effective method for evaluating regional myocardial contractility during or after ischemia. Gated CT in an animal model of regional ischemia has identified the sites of ischemia by the loss of wall thickening during cardiac contraction.[10] A number of patients with documented coronary artery disease and myocardial infarction have been evaluated by cine-CT to define regional contraction abnormalities.[15] Regional wall thickening and inward motion were studied, and an absence or decrease in wall thickening during systole was indicative of a regional contraction abnormality caused by the previous ischemic event (Fig. 6–7). The presence and the site of regional contraction abnormalities defined by cine-CT had a 91 per cent correlation with wall motion abnormalities demonstrated by left ventriculography and with critical coronary artery stenoses shown by coronary arteriography.[10]

Intracardiac Thrombus ■ The ability to define the internal and external margins of the myocardium is a significant advantage of CT scanning over angiography. After myocardial infarction and open heart surgery, mural thrombi develop within the left ventricular cavity in 20 to 60 per cent of patients.[16, 17] After intravenous contrast medium infusion, the ventricular cavity and the myocardial wall opacify with contrast material. Mural thrombus does not change its CT density after contrast medium infusion and is readily seen as a nonenhancing mass within the heart chamber (Fig. 6–8).[18, 19] Computed tomography and two-dimensional echocardiography have been found to be equally accurate in identifying left ventricular mural thrombus.[15] Tomada and colleagues[20] have shown CT to have greater accuracy than two-dimen-

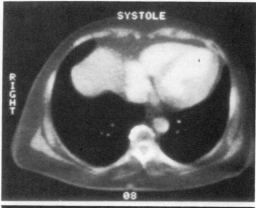
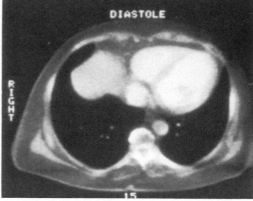

FIGURE 6–7 ■ Cine-CT scans at end-systole (top) and end-diastole (bottom) in a patient with a prior anteroseptal myocardial infarction. The infarcted wall is thinner than the remainder of the left ventricle and shows no wall thickening during systole.

sional echocardiography in demonstrating thrombus in the left atrium, especially thrombus situated on the lateral atrial wall and in the atrial appendage.

Coronary Artery Bypass Grafts ■ Approximately 100,000 patients undergo coronary artery bypass graft surgery annually in the United States.[21] The operation bypasses sites of proximal coronary artery stenosis and restores blood flow to the myocardium. Recurrence of symptoms after surgery is common and can result from progressive stenosis of the coronary arteries or from closure of the bypass grafts. Before dynamic CT scanning became available, angiography by selective catheterization of the bypass graft was the only reliable method for demonstrating graft patency.

Both conventional CT (nongated) and cine-CT have accurately demonstrated patency of coronary artery bypass grafts.[1, 22–25] A multicenter prospective study using cine-CT has shown a greater than 90 per cent accuracy of CT for this purpose, with validation of CT findings by coronary angiography.[22] The accuracy of CT has been better for grafts to the left anterior descending and right coronary arteries than for grafts to the circumflex coronary artery. The optimal CT scan level is free of metallic clips and is situated at approximately the level of the pulmonary artery bifurcation. The site of the bypass graft on contrast-enhanced CT scans can be related to a clock viewed

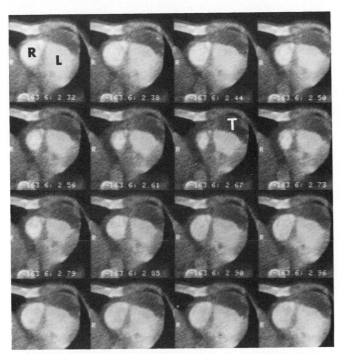

FIGURE 6–8 ■ Left ventricular aneurysm and mural thrombus. Cine-CT scans at 17 scans/sec in a patient with left ventricular aneurysm and mural thrombus (T). Images are from end-diastole of one heart beat *(upper left)* through systole *(middle two horizontal panels)* to the next diastolic period *(lower horizontal panels)*. Scans demonstrate systolic thickening of the posterolateral wall but absence of thickening in the septum and anterolateral wall. L = Left ventricle; R = right ventricle.

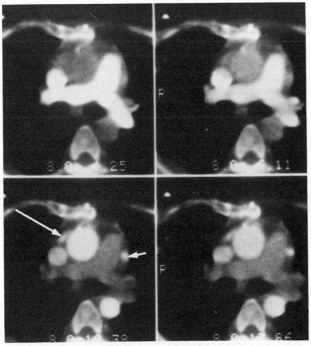

FIGURE 6–9 ■ Coronary artery bypass graft. Cine-CT scans from successive heart beats during passage of contrast medium through the central circulation. Upper panels show opacification of the pulmonary artery. Lower panels show opacification of the aorta and aortocoronary vein grafts to the right coronary artery *(long arrow)* and a branch of the circumflex coronary artery *(short arrow)*.

from the feet looking upward. The grafts to the right coronary artery are situated between the 9 and 11 o'clock positions (Fig. 6–9). The grafts to the left anterior descending artery are situated between the 12 and 2 o'clock positions, whereas the graft to the circumflex system is located between the 2 and 4 o'clock positions. Diagnostic confidence is enhanced by imaging the grafts at two adjacent anatomic levels and by showing contrast enhancement of the graft coincident with aortic opacification. Dynamic CT scanning using multiple sequential CT scans at the same level after peripheral intravenous injections of 20 to 30 mL of contrast medium demonstrates opacification and washout of contrast material from the grafts.[23, 25] Sequential CT scans obtained during the opacification and clearance of contrast medium from the grafts can be used to generate radiographic attenuation-versus-time curves from regions of interest over the grafts and can roughly assess the adequacy of blood flow in the graft. The CT density in the graft rises as the bolus of contrast medium arrives and then falls slowly during the washout phase. The rise in CT density typically takes 2 to 3 seconds and the fall approximately 10 seconds. Contrast bolus lengths of 5 to 10 seconds are typical, and only a small amount of diffusion occurs from the vascular space on the first pass of a bolus. Both internal mammary artery–to–coronary artery grafts and saphenous vein aortocoronary bypass grafts can be demonstrated accurately.

Cardiomyopathy ■ Cardiomyopathy can be defined as a disease of the myocardium not caused by abnormality of the coronary arteries.[26] Cardiomyopathies are classified both functionally and etiologically (Table 6–1), and both classifications are of practical value. The disease can be difficult to diagnose clinically, and conventional radiographic studies frequently do not assist in diagnosis. Obstructive cardiomyopathy is characterized by an asymmetric increase in the muscle mass of the ventricles. The left ventricular cavity is small and heavily trabeculated. CT scans can demonstrate the distribution and severity of the asymmetric hypertrophy of the left ventricle (Fig. 6–10).

Cine-CT also can assess the severity of dilated or congestive cardiomyopathy by measuring ventricular

TABLE 6–1 ■ **Classification of Cardiomyopathy**

Functional
  Hypertrophic
  Congestive
  Restrictive
Etiologic
  Primary: enzyme deficiencies, genetic influences
  Secondary
  Viral infection
  Neurogenic (e.g., Friedreich's ataxia)
  Infiltration (e.g., amyloid)
  Toxic (e.g., alcohol)
  Metabolic (e.g., diabetes mellitus)
  Connective tissue disease (e.g., lupus erythematosus, scleroderma)

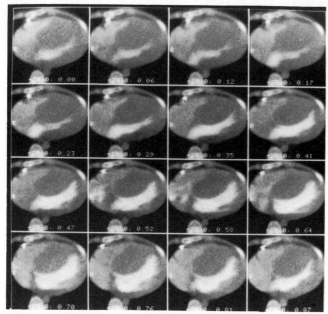

FIGURE 6–10 ■ Hypertrophic cardiomyopathy. Cine-CT scans at 17 scans/sec in a patient with hypertrophic cardiomyopathy of the asymmetric septal variety. Images from systole (upper left) to diastole (lower left) and into the next systole (lower right) demonstrate marked hypertrophy of the ventriclar septum. (Courtesy of Bruce Brundage, MD, Chicago, IL.)

volumes and ejection fractions. It can document changes in ejection fraction or volumes in response to therapy and can monitor the progress of the myocardial dysfunction quantitatively over time.

Neoplasm ■ Cardiac neoplasms can be primary or metastatic. Primary neoplasms are rare, occurring in fewer than 1 in 1000 autopsies.[27] Atrial myxomas account for about 50 per cent of primary neoplasms[28, 29] and can be difficult to diagnose, because they can simulate a variety of other cardiac or noncardiac diseases. Other primary cardiac neoplasms are rhabdomyoma, fibroma, lipoma, angioma, papilloma, teratoma, and sarcoma.[30, 31] Cardiac myxomas arise in the left atrium in 75 per cent of instances, in the right atrium in 20 per cent, and at other sites in 5 per cent.

The most frequent cardiac tumor in children is the rhabdomyoma, which occurs sporadically and also as part of the syndrome of tuberous sclerosis. The tumor frequently is small and wholly contained within the myocardial wall; consequently it may not be detectable by CT. It is one of the important causes of ventricular arrhythmias in young children.

Metastatic tumor to the heart is 20 to 50 times more common than primary tumor, although fewer than 10 per cent are diagnosed while the patient is still alive.[31, 32] The most common tumors to spread hematogenously to the heart are melanoma, breast carcinoma, lymphoma, and lung carcinoma.[31, 32] Alternative modes of spread to the heart are direct invasion through the pericardium and tumor growth along the great veins into the heart. Intraluminal metastases to the right side of the heart are seen with soft tissue and bony sarcomas, choriocarcinoma, melanoma, and carcinoid tumors.

Contrast-enhanced CT has been effective for demonstrating masses adjacent to the heart and masses within the cardiac chamber.[1] Because metastatic tumors are 40 to 50 times more frequent than primary cardiac tumors, most masses are encountered in patients with a known primary tumor.

Intracardiac tumors are recognized as filling defects projecting into the contrast-enhanced blood pool of a cardiac chamber (Fig. 6–11).[2, 33–35] Intramural tumors may not be discernible on CT unless they cause a focal alteration of wall thickness or contour, or display differential contrast enhancement relative to the myocardium. The CT appearance of myxoma is characterized by its atrial situation and attachment to the atrial septum by a stalk. A lipoma or lipomatous degeneration of the atrial septum is recognized by increased thickness and sometimes by distortion of the atrial septum by tissue of fat density. In general, the location and extent of cardiac tumors can be demonstrated, as can any additional tumor masses. In one case of a metastatic osteogenic sarcoma, an area of high CT density was found.[34]

The paracardiac location of a tumor can be defined by an intact pericardial line and no pericardial effusion. However, the absence of a pericardial line adjacent to a paracardiac mass does not reliably indicate pericardial penetration or involvement, as the pericardium is not visible in all patients and frequently it is not visible over the left side of the heart.[36]

Congenital Heart Disease ■ Standard and cine-CT have been used to demonstrate congenital cardiac lesions.[37, 38] However, the use of CT in congenital

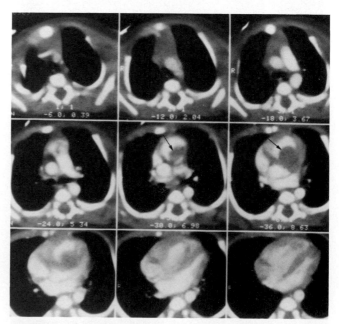

FIGURE 6–11 ■ Right ventricular tumor. Cine-CT scans from above the aortic arch to the middle of the ventricles demonstrate a tumor (arrow) partially obstructing the right ventricular outflow region.

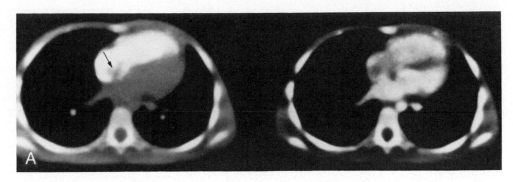

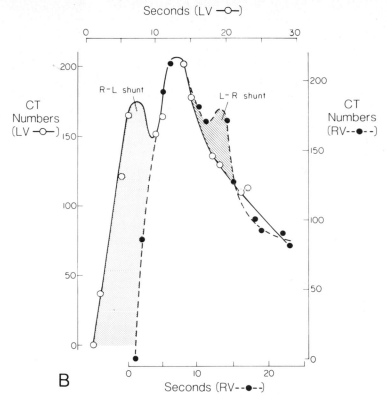

FIGURE 6–12 ■ *A,* Atrial septal defect with bidirection shunting. CT scan was taken during opacification of right ventricle *(left)* and left ventricle *(right).* Unopacified blood passes from the left atrium to the right atrium *(arrow)* during contrast opacification of the right atrium. *B,* Theoretical time-versus-density (CT number) curves for the left ventricle (LV) and right ventricle (RV) for a bidirection shunt at the ventricular level. Superimposition of the peak curves for the RV and LV demonstrate the components of the right-to-left (R L) shunt and the left-to-right (L–R) shunt. (*A,* Courtesy of Jay Eldridge, MD.)

heart disease has been overshadowed by the results of MR. The multiple images available with MR provide a distinct advantage over CT for the depiction of structural features of congenital heart disease. The general application of tomographic techniques in congenital heart disease is described in the section on MR.

Cine-CT after intravascular contrast material infusion can demonstrate blood shunting from one chamber to another in septal defects (Fig. 6–12A). In left-to-right shunts, the shunting of unopacified blood can be recognized during opacification of right-sided cardiac chambers after bolus injection of contrast medium. In right-to-left shunts, the shunting of opacified blood from the right to the left chamber can also be discerned after an intravenous bolus injection of contrast medium. Time-density curves acquired from regions of interest over various cardiac chambers can assess the severity of left-to-right and right-to-left shunts semiquantitatively (Fig. 6–12B).

FUNCTIONAL DIAGNOSIS: COMPUTED TOMOGRAPHY

Fast CT scanners can evaluate cardiac function effectively.[39–43] The acquisition time of 50 ms attained by cine-CT is adequate for quantitating many aspects of cardiac function. Several investigators[39, 42] have verified that the three-dimensional nature of the combined CT images permits precise measurement of chamber volume. Both right and left ventricular volumes can be assessed with equivalent accuracy. Although right ventricular end-diastolic and end-systolic volumes are larger than left ventricular volumes in normal patients, stroke volumes of the two ventricles measured by cine-CT are nearly equal.[39] A disparity in stroke volume between the ventricles is caused by cardiac lesions, such as shunts and valvular regurgitation, that result in volume overload of the ventricle. The precision demonstrated by cine-CT in measuring volumes of both the right and left ventricles and in demonstrating equivalent stroke volumes of the two ventricles indicate that this technique should be reliable for quantitating volume overload lesions.

Sequential images can be acquired during a single heart beat with cine-CT, making it ideal for monitoring the effect of interventions on the right and left ventricles. Cine-CT obtained during the peak effort of supine bicycle exercise can identify an abnormal response in patients with hemodynamically significant coronary arterial stenoses.[40] The abnormal response is characterized by a less than 5 per cent increase in ejection fraction, the elicitation of a regional wall motion abnormality between rest and exercise, or both.[40] Cine-CT also has been able to detect abnormal right ventricular function. It can depict structural and functional cardiac abnormalities in a subset of patients with ventricular arrhythmias originating from a right ventricular focus (J. Abbott, personal communication).

Functional abnormalities at rest and during bicycle exercise in patients with chronic lung disease have been detected using cine-CT.[44] Cine-CT performed at rest in patients with severe pulmonary arterial hypertension shows dilated right-sided chambers and loss or reversal of the normal curvature of the ventricular septum (Fig. 6–13). A dilated inferior vena cava is indicative of tricuspid regurgitation. Tomographic images of normal patients show that the septal curvature is convex toward the right ventricle during systole. The ejection fraction and stroke volume of the right ventricle may not be reduced, even in the presence of severe pulmonary arterial hypertension and right ventricular heart failure, because of tricuspid regurgitation. The volume of blood regurgitating through the tricuspid valve is the difference between right ventricular and left ventricular stroke volumes. Thus the stroke volume may be

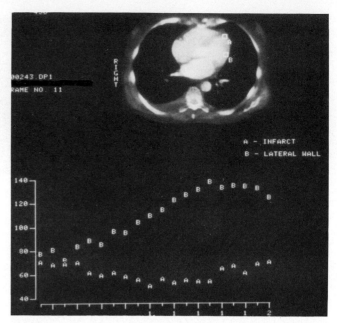

FIGURE 6–14 ■ Regional myocardial perfusion by cine-CT. Regions-of-interest cursors from infarcted (A) and normal (B) myocardium are placed on sequential CT scans during the passage of contrast medium through the myocardium. The time-density curve shows enhancement of the normal and no enhancement of the infarcted myocardium.

maintained with tricuspid regurgitation while the forward stroke volume is reduced. The left ventricular stroke volume must be equivalent to the forward right ventricular stroke volume. The level of exercise achieved by many patients with severe lung disease and pulmonary arterial hypertension is submaximal, and most patients display an abnormal cardiac response consisting of an increase in right ventricular end-diastolic volume, a less than 5 per cent increase in ejection fraction of the left or both ventricles, and an increase in tricuspid regurgitation. Cine-CT during a single heart beat is an effective technique for the evaluation of ventricular function during peak exercise.

Cine-CT also has been proposed for measuring regional myocardial perfusion at rest and during interventions that increase myocardial blood flow, such as exercise and the administration of vasodilator drugs.[43] Perfusion is estimated by monitoring regional myocardial CT density values over time on scans exposed sequentially during peak opacification and washout of contrast medium (Fig. 6–14). The study simulates the thallium perfusion study obtained at rest and during exercise, but with a greater degree of spatial resolution.

ANATOMIC DIAGNOSIS: MAGNETIC RESONANCE IMAGING

The advantages of MR over CT for imaging of the heart are (1) the clear delineation of the endocardial and epicardial margins of the cardiac walls; (2) the clear depiction of internal cardiac morphology, including normal trabecular structures, intraluminal tumors, and thrombi; and (3) the direct demonstra-

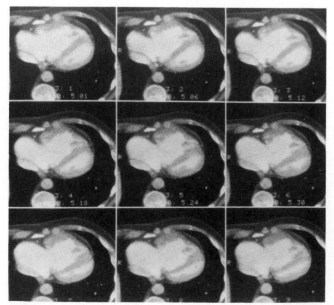

FIGURE 6–13 ■ Chronic lung disease. Cine-CT from diastole *(upper left)* to systole *(lower right)* in a patient with pulmonary arterial hypertension from chronic lung disease. The ventricular septum is bowed toward the left ventricle in systole, the reverse of the normal.

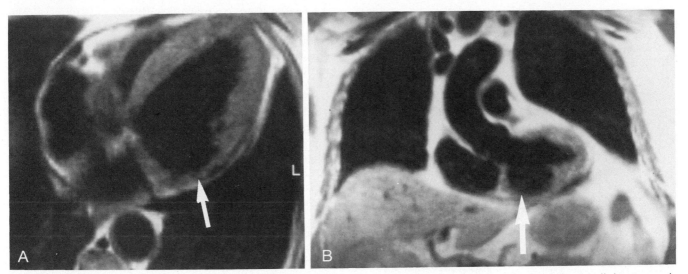

FIGURE 6–15 ■ Posteroinferior myocardial infarction. Transverse *(A)* and coronal *(B)* ECG-gated spin-echo images show wall thinning at the site of infarction *(arrow).*

tion of the pericardium, intrapericardial fluid, and paracardiac masses. Several investigations have been directed toward the evaluation of ischemic heart disease with MR.[45–48] The clinical indications for MR being developed include evaluation of diseases afflicting the myocardial walls, pericardial disease, cardiac and paracardiac masses, and some aspects of congenital heart disease. MR may also be effective for the diagnosis of abnormalities of the thoracic aorta, such as aneurysm and dissection, and some abnormalities of the central pulmonary arteries, such as chronic thromboembolic disease.

Ischemic Heart Disease ■ MR can show the extent of myocardial loss after an acute myocardial infarction and also the complications of infarction, such as ventricular aneurysms and mural thrombus.[46–48] Studies in animals[45] and in humans[47] have demonstrated that acute infarctions are readily visualized on MR images as regions of increased MR signal intensity.[49, 50] The MR signal intensity on spin-echo images increases with an increase in hydrogen (spin) density and with shortening of T1 and lengthening of T2 relaxation times. Acutely infarcted myocardium is edematous and results in an increase in hydrogen density and prolongation of T1 and T2 relaxation times.[45, 51] The tissue contrast between normal and infarcted myocardium is increased on the second echo image (TE = 56 to 60 ms) compared with the first echo image (TE = 28 to 30 ms). The second echo image accentuates the T2 difference between normal and edematous myocardium.

Sites of old myocardial infarction can be detected on MR images as regions of wall thinning (Fig. 6–15).[46, 48] The transition between normal myocardial wall thickness and wall thinning is distinctive and makes possible an estimate of the extent of the left ventricle involved by the prior infarction.[52]

McNamarra and Higgins[48] found that in some patients with remote infarction the residual myocardial wall was sufficiently thick to allow measurement of MR signal intensity. In these cases, signal intensity of the infarcted region was decreased compared with normal myocardium. In contradistinction to acute infarctions, the T2 relaxation times were prolonged relative to those for normal myocardium. The current concepts of the relationship between histology and relaxation times in acute and chronic myocardial infarctions are summarized in Table 6–2.

Complications of myocardial infarctions can be demonstrated on MR images. Gated MR images displayed regions of extreme wall thinning and bulging of segments of the left ventricle in patients with myocardial aneurysms. These MR findings have been correlated with left ventriculography and echocardiography.[46] The MR image can demonstrate the ostium of the aneurysm, and a small ostium, compared with the diameter of the aneurysm, suggests a false aneurysm (Fig. 6–16). Mural thrombi have also been shown projecting into the signal void within the left ventricular chamber.

An unfulfilled goal of MR in ischemic heart disease is to reliably detect ischemic but uninfarcted myocardium (known as *jeopardized myocardium*). Paramagnetic contrast agents have been used to outline the jeopardy region after acute coronary occlusion in animals.[53–55] Contrast media have also been used to distinguish between occlusive and reperfused myocardial infarctions.[51] Imaging of nuclei other than protons[56, 57] and MR spectroscopy[58] may be novel methods for studying reversible myocardial ischemia.

TABLE 6–2 ■ **The Relationship Between Histology and Relaxation Times in Acute and Chronic Myocardial Infarction**

	ACUTE INFARCTION	CHRONIC INFARCTION
Signal intensity (compared with normal myocardium)	Increased	Decreased
T2 relaxation time	Increased	Decreased
Pathology	Edema	Fibrosis

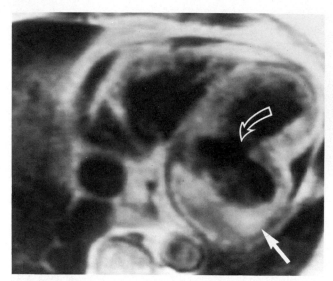

FIGURE 6–16 ■ Left ventricular false aneurysm. ECG-gated MR shows the aneurysm posteriorly *(solid arrow)*, arising from the posteroinferior left ventricular wall. A narrow ostium *(open arrow)* connects the aneurysm with the LV chamber.

Cardiomyopathy ■ MR provides sharp delineation of the left ventricular wall and is excellent for evaluating the presence and severity of cardiomyopathies. Higgins and co-workers[59] have shown that MR can accurately define the extent, location, and severity of left ventricular hypertrophy in hypertrophic cardiomyopathy. In many patients, the hypertrophy is present only in the outflow septum of the left ventricle. In some the entire septum is hypertrophied, and in still others hypertrophy may extend from the septum into the free wall or apex. Magnetic resonance imaging has been particularly useful in defining the variant forms of idiopathic hypertrophic cardiomyopathy. These patterns of muscle hypertrophy in cardiomyopathy, shown by MR, have correlated well with two-dimensional echocardiographic findings.[59] Often the resolution of MR is superior to that of echocardiography, and in particular, it more clearly defines the endocardial and epicardial borders of the left ventricular wall. Moreover, the larger field of view of MR may be useful in depicting the overall extent of hypertrophy. MR also has been shown to be effective for measuring left ventricular mass.[60]

MR demonstrates dilatation of the cardiac chambers characteristic of congestive cardiomyopathy. It has shown that ischemic cardiomyopathy can usually be recognized by the presence of disproportionate wall thinning in one or more regions of the left ventricle. Idiopathic congestive cardiomyopathy usually is characterized by normal wall thickness or mild generalized wall thinning. Cine-MR has been used to quantitate left ventricular volumes, ejection fraction, and mass. Cine-MR measurements show a considerable increase in left ventricular mass but a reduced mass–to–end-diastolic volume ratio.[61]

Measurements of MR relaxation times in groups of patients with hypertrophic and congestive cardiomyopathies have shown no significant difference in relaxation times compared with normal subjects. Tissue characterization by relaxation times is considered crude at present. It may become more specific as additional quantitative parameters of magnetic resonance are further developed for imaging.

Neoplasm ■ MR can demonstrate intracardiac masses within the signal void of the cardiac chambers.[62–64] The absence of MR signal from blood in motion within the cardiac chambers provides contrast for imaging the mass (Fig. 6–17). MR also can detect direct extension or tumor metastasis to the heart.[65] An intracavitary tumor on MR must be differentiated from thrombi, normal structures, and intracavitary signal generated from stasis of blood flow in a chamber. The signal from stasis of flow increases dramatically on second spin-echo images (TE = 56 to 60 ms) compared with first spin-echo images (TE = 28 to 30 ms). Moreover, the signal from blood stasis varies or appears only at certain phases of the cardiac cycle. Normal intravascular signal usually occurs within the ventricles in late diastole and within the atrium in systole.[66] Consequently it is usually possible to distinguish between blood stasis and tumor by obtaining images acquired at different phases of the cardiac cycle.

Differentiation between the signal caused by slow blood flow and an intracardiac mass can be done using cine-MR. With this technique the blood pool has high intensity and outlines the mass, which produces low or medium intensity. MR also is effective for showing intracardiac thrombus in any chamber. Using spin-echo techniques, the MR signal intensity of thrombus can vary from high to low depending on the age of the thrombus. Because tumor can also produce a wide range of signal intensities on spin-echo images, tumor cannot always be distinguished from intracardiac thrombus using

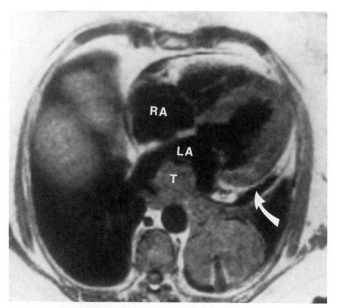

FIGURE 6–17 ■ Tumor in the left atrium. Tumor (T) extends through the pericardium, causing pericardial effusion *(arrow)*, and then into the left atrium (LA). RA = Right atrium.

this technique. On the other hand, the two can usually be distinguished using the cine-MR sequence. The cine MR is a version of the gradient-echo sequence, which is extremely sensitive to loss of signal caused by magnetic susceptibility effects. Components of thrombus, such as iron in various forms and deoxyhemoglobin, exert strong magnetic susceptibility effects. Consequently thrombus has very low signal (less than skeletal muscle), whereas tumor causes medium signal (higher than skeletal muscle) (Fig. 6–18).[66a]

Intramural masses produce an increase in thickness of the involved cardiac wall and a contour abnormality of the involved region. The cardiac walls are well delineated on MR images, and MR is effective for the evaluation of intramural masses.[67] Experience with the MR evaluation of cardiac tumors is too limited to judge whether there are consistent differences in intensity between tumor and normal myocardium.

Congenital Heart Disease ■ MR demonstrates internal cardiac anatomy without the use of contrast medium or ionizing radiation. The absence of ionizing radiation is an important consideration in children, because angiography is associated with high radiation doses. MR is effective for the evaluation of a wide variety of congenital cardiac anomalies.[68–71] The tomographic imaging format facilitates definition of congenital lesions such as the components of complex anomalies involving great vessel orientation, the type of bulboventricular loop, and visceroatrial situs. The major indications for MRI in suspected congenital heart disease are the evaluation of thoracic aortic anomalies (see Fig. 6–19); pulmonary arterial abnormalities, especially pulmonary atresia (Fig. 6–20); complex anomalies of the ventricles, especially single ventricle; and postoperative conduits and anastomoses, such as Rastelli and Fontan procedures.

Analysis of complex cardiac relationships is facilitated by obtaining a series of transverse MR images extending from the base of the heart to the superior aspect of the liver. This series of images allows the determination of the type of ventricular loop, the relationship of the atria to the ventricles, the rela-

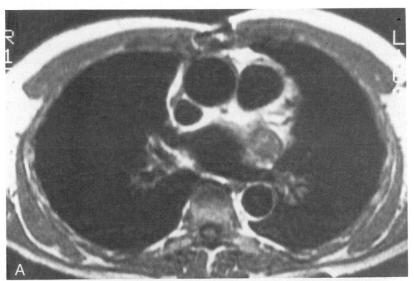

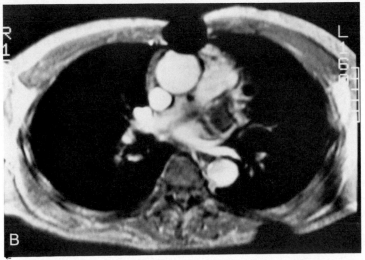

FIGURE 6–18 ■ ECG-gated spin-echo *(A)* and cine-MR *(B)* images of patient with clot in left atrial appendage. The mass in the appendage has low signal intensity on the cine-MR image. This finding is characteristic of a clot.

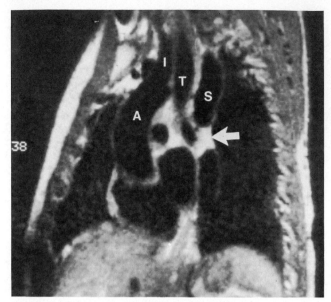

FIGURE 6–19 ■ Interruption of the descending aorta. Atretic segment *(arrow)* separates the aortic arch from the descending aorta. The high signal intensity at the site of discontinuity could represent either fat or thrombus. A = Ascending aorta; I = innominate artery; S = subclavian artery, which is dilated; T = trachea.

tionship of atria to visceral situs, and the atrial connections of the systemic and pulmonary veins.[71]

As Didier and colleagues[71] and Guit and co-workers[72] showed, positional abnormalities of the great vessels are demonstrated clearly on transaxial images. These include anterior and rightward position of the aorta with D-transposition, anterior and leftward position of the aorta with L-transposition of the great vessels, and side-by-side position of the great vessels with double-outlet right ventricle and the single large vessel indicative of truncus arteriosus. Coarctation or interruption of the aorta also is well shown on sagittal or oblique-sagittal images.[73]

MR has consistently demonstrated ventricular septal defects.[69, 71] These include defects of both the inflow (posterior) and outflow (anterior) portions of the septum, which are particularly well shown on transverse images. Even small ventricular septal defects can be identified on transverse images as an abrupt truncation of the septum, compared with the usual appearance, in which the septum is seen to taper smoothly from its muscular into its membranous portion. Delineation of a common ventricle with a rudimentary septum and single ventricle with a hypoplastic inverted right ventricular outflow chamber has been documented on transverse images and is particularly well shown on coronal images.

Atrial septal defects are demonstrated on transverse MR images with high diagnostic accuracy.[74, 75] In the secundum type of atrial septal defect, the cranial portion of the atrial septum is clearly visible, as is the residual septum adjacent to the defect. In contrast, some normal subjects show signal dropout in the central portion of the septum in the region of the fossa ovalis. In septum primum atrial septal

defects, the caudal portion of the atrial septum is absent, and the inflow ventricular septum is truncated in transverse MR images. In patients with atrial septal defects, it also is possible to determine the pattern of drainage of the pulmonary veins, which may be anomalous.

There is still too little clinical experience with MR in congenital heart disease to predict its eventual role in comparison with angiography. However, it appears that MR can define intracardiac, great vessel, and visceral situs inversus at least as well as, and in some instances more definitively than, angiography.

Patients with congenital heart disease usually are evaluated initially with two-dimensional echocardiography, and in many congenital lesions, MR is the secondary diagnostic procedure. In many instances MR provides images with anatomic display equal to that of angiography. Consequently the evaluation of congenital heart disease can be less costly, safer, and at least as precise as angiography when echocardiography is followed by MR imaging. In anomalies of the aortic arch, such as coarctation, MR may become the favored procedure. MR imaging frequently is the most useful study for demonstrating congenital pulmonary arterial abnormalities and for identifying the presence and size of central pulmonary arteries in patients with pulmonary atresia.[70] Likewise, MR can evaluate the status of the pulmonary arteries after central shunt operations.

FUNCTIONAL DIAGNOSIS: MAGNETIC RESONANCE IMAGING

Functional evaluation of the cardiovascular system is now practical with cine-MR.[76, 77] Several reports have described multiphasic or cine-MR imaging for

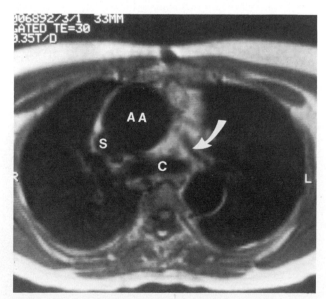

FIGURE 6–20 ■ Pulmonary atresia. Transverse image at level of the tracheal carina shows a hypoplastic left pulmonary artery *(arrow)* and no confluence of the right and left pulmonary arteries. The central right pulmonary artery is absent, as shown by the lack of a vessel between the right main bronchus and the ascending aorta (AA). C = Tracheal carina; S = superior vena cava.

evaluation of abnormal blood flow patterns,[77, 78] left ventricular and right ventricular dimensions and stroke volumes,[60] left ventricular masses,[60] and regional myocardial function.[76]

Cine-MR can achieve a temporal resolution of more than 30 frames per cardiac cycle, providing images at both end-diastole and end-systole (Fig. 6–21). From these images end-diastolic and end-systolic volumes, stroke volume, and ejection fraction can be calculated.[76] Good correlation has been found between left ventricular volumes measured from cine-MR images and volumes measured by two-dimensional echocardiography.[76] The volumes measured from cine-MR in general are smaller than those that have been obtained from traditional angiographic measurements. The advantages of MR imaging for these measurements are that this technique is truly three-dimensional and encompasses the entire cardiac chamber being assessed. In comparison, angiographic measurements depend on geometric assumptions of varying validity, depending on the shape of the chamber.

Functional evaluation in ischemic heart disease is achieved with MR by measuring wall thickening during the cardiac cycle. Pflugfelder and colleagues[79] have shown that in patients with prior myocardial infarction, MR imaging readily distinguishes the site of previous myocardial injury by a diminution or absence of wall thickening during ventricular systole.

The blood pool usually has a homogeneous high signal intensity throughout most of the cardiac cycle on cine MR. A normally occurring exception is a decrease in signal intensity that occurs near the tricuspid and mitral valves as they open during early diastole. A momentary signal loss also may be present behind the tricuspid and mitral valves during

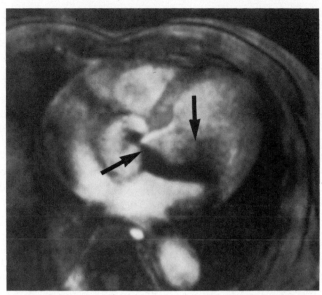

FIGURE 6–22 ■ Aortic regurgitation. Cine-MR image in mid-diastole at a level just beneath the aortic valve. Signal void (arrows) emanating from the aortic valve represents aortic regurgitation.

their rapid closure. Regurgitation through either the atrioventricular or the semilunar valves causes a high-velocity jet that results in a signal void within the relevant chamber that otherwise shows high signal intensity (Figs. 6–22 and 6–23).[5] The appearance of this signal void emanating from the insufficient valve can identify the presence of valvular regurgitation.[5, 76] In aortic regurgitation, the signal void is in the ventricle and is in continuity with the closed aortic valve (see Fig. 6–22), whereas in mitral

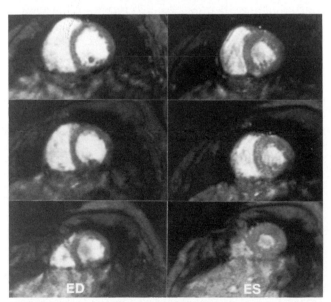

FIGURE 6–21 ■ Normal cine-MR near end-diastole (ED, left panels) and end-systole (ES, right panels). Images at the basal, middle, and apical levels of the ventricles demonstrate thickening of myocardial wall and reduction in ventricular chambers from end-diastole to end-systole.

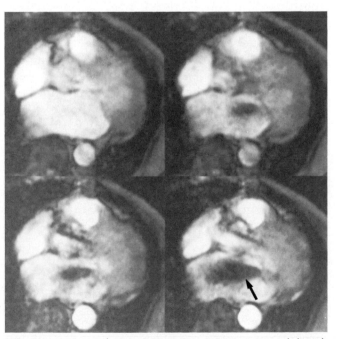

FIGURE 6–23 ■ Mitral regurgitation. Cine-MR images at end-diastole (left upper panel) and at three phases of systole. Signal void (arrow) in the left atrium emanating from the mitral valve represents mitral regurgitation.

regurgitation it is in the atrium and is in continuity with the closed mitral valve (see Fig. 6–23).

Severity of valvular regurgitation is quantitated by measuring the right and left ventricular stroke volumes and then using the values obtained to calculate the regurgitant volume with standard formulas.[76, 80] The ventricular blood pool is measured from the areas of multiple images encompassing the two ventricles at both end-diastole and end-systole. The difference between the volumes is the stroke volume. In the normal patient, the stroke volume for the two ventricles is equal. In the abnormal situation, the stroke volume of the left ventricle exceeds that of the right ventricle by a value equivalent to the regurgitant volume. With quantitative MR, patients with moderate or severe aortic or mitral regurgitation can be distinguished from normal patients and patients with mild regurgitation.[80] Quantitation of regurgitation also can be done from measurements of the dimension of the MR signal void.[76, 81] The volume of the signal void is measured during diastole on multiple MR tomographic images encompassing the recipient chamber. Another method consists of measuring length and width of the base of the regurgitant jet at the point where it arises from the insufficient valve.

Mitral regurgitation can be quantitated from the signal intensity within the left atrium during the systolic phase of the cardiac cycle.[82] Normal persons show a moderate increase in signal intensity within the left atrium during systole. Patients with mitral regurgitation show a distinct decrease in signal intensity within the left atrium during this phase. The magnitude of the decrease in signal intensity in the left atrium seems to bear an approximate relationship to the severity of mitral regurgitation.[82] Cine-MR studies to estimate the severity of regurgitation are encouraging but need to be further evaluated in a large group of patients with normal and abnormal chamber sizes and ventricular function.

More complex measurements of myocardial function also can be achieved with MR.[76] Wall stress of the left ventricle can be estimated from a combination of blood pressure measurements referenced to the carotid pulse and cine-MR images. The end-systolic and peak-systolic wall stresses can be calculated and are markedly elevated in patients with congestive (dilated) cardiomyopathy, when compared with those of normal persons.[76] This approach shows promise for determining the effectiveness of various pharmacologic agents in patients with congestive cardiomyopathies and other cardiac diseases.

Measurements of Blood Flow

Techniques for accurate quantification of blood flow utilize either time-of-flight or phase-shift phenomena.[5, 82a, 82b, 82c] In conventional spin-echo sequences, the effect of blood moving through the acquisition volume and the dephasing effect of motion on protons within flowing blood degrade image quality. However, these effects are exploited in MR angiography to selectively detect flow and suppress signal from stationary tissues. These techniques have been used to demonstrate the carotid vessels, the cerebral circulation, flow within the heart and great vessels (Fig. 6–24), and flow in the peripheral circulation. In the thorax, blood flow has been quantified in the proximal pulmonary vessels, but techniques that utilize gradient-recalled echoes are limited for imaging vessels within the lung parenchyma.

Pericardium

The structure and function of the pericardium have interested physicians for centuries. Hippocrates described the pericardium as a "smooth mantle surrounding the heart and containing a small amount of fluid resembling urine."[83] Some investigators have suggested that the pericardium prevents overdilatation of the heart,[84–86] reduces friction with surrounding structures,[86] facilitates atrial filling,[84] and moderates the pressure-volume relationships of the cardiac chambers.[87] Congenital, neoplastic, infectious, metabolic, traumatic, drug-induced, and primary myocardial diseases can all affect the pericardium.

CT and MR are sensitive noninvasive methods for evaluation of the pericardium both in health and in disease. They can demonstrate the normal pericardium and adjacent cardiac and extracardiac anatomy. Intravenous contrast material delineates vascular structures but is not always necessary for CT evaluation of pericardial diseases.

Anatomy

The pericardium is a two-layered stiff membrane that envelops all four cardiac chambers, as well as the origins of the great vessels. The two layers are separated by a small amount of fluid. The pericardium is divided into two distinct layers, the visceral and parietal pericardium, that become continuous at the attachment to the great vessels and form a closed sac surrounding the heart. The pericardium extends to include the proximal ascending aorta, main pulmonary artery, proximal pulmonary veins, and proximal venae cavae.[88]

The base of the pericardium is attached to the central tendon of the diaphragm. Anteriorly ligaments attach the pericardium to the sternum from the manubrium to the xiphoid. Posteriorly additional ligaments extend to the dorsal spine.

The visceral pericardium is a serous layer of mesothelial cells closely applied to the surface of the heart and epicardial fat. The membrane is thin, and its close apposition to cardiac structures prevents its demonstration on CT or MR images.

The parietal pericardium is a fibrous layer of tissue composed of serosa, fibrosa, and an outer layer of connective tissue containing blood vessels, nerves, and lymphatics. The normal thickness of the parietal

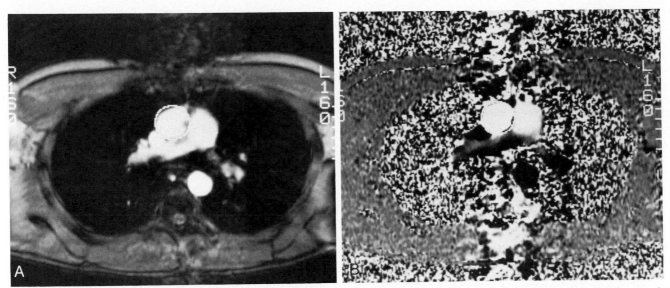

FIGURE 6–24 ■ Magnitude *(A)* and phase *(B)* images through the great arteries using the velocity encoded cine-MRI technique. The signal in the vessels on the phase image is directly proportional to blood flow velocity. Note that the shade of signal is dark in the descending aorta and bright in the ascending aorta. These diametric shades are an indication of flow in opposite directions; flow in the ascending aorta has caudocranial direction and in the descending aorta has craniocaudal direction.

pericardium is 1 to 4 mm. The visceral pericardium is separated from the parietal pericardium by a thin layer of pericardial fluid.

Portions of the normal pericardium can be demonstrated by CT and MR in almost all persons.[89–91] The inferior, ventral pericardium lies between mediastinal and epicardial fat and is the area usually seen on CT scans and MR images, especially where epicardial fat surrounds the coronary vessels. This part of the pericardium can have slightly thicker areas than the rest of the pericardium.[89]

The normal pericardium is composed primarily of fibrous tissue, which produces little MR signal.[91] Both extrapericardial and subepicardial fat produce an area of high MR signal intensity at the external margin of the heart, resulting in a high degree of contrast between the pericardium and adjacent fat (see Fig. 6–4B through D). The pericardial line is recognized as a thin lucent line surrounding portions of the circumference of the heart, where it is highlighted by adjacent fat. In most normal persons the pericardium is visualized only over the right anterior aspect of the heart.[91] Because pure fluid also produces little or no MR signal, this lucent line is usually composed of normal pericardial fluid, as well as the two layers of pericardium. Pericardial thickness greater than 5 mm on MR is abnormal.

Pathology

CONGENITAL ANOMALIES

Congenital malformations of the pericardium are uncommon. These include defects or absence of portions of the pericardium, cysts, diverticula, and benign teratomas.[92] Defects of the pericardium have been recognized since the sixteenth century. Their cause is obscure, but they may occur secondary to embryologic abnormalities in the vascular supply to the pericardium. Most pericardial defects are partial, and absence of the entire pericardium occurs in only 9 per cent of cases. Approximately 70 per cent of defects are on the left side. In about half of these, the entire left side of the pericardium is absent, and in the other half, the pericardium is partially deficient.[92, 93] Partial defects on the right represent only 4 per cent of cases, whereas diaphragmatic pericardial defects account for 17 per cent.[93]

Approximately one third of patients with pericardial defects have other congenital abnormalities, including atrial septal defect,[94] patent ductus arteriosus,[95] bronchogenic cyst,[96] pulmonary sequestration,[97] mitral stenosis, and tetralogy of Fallot.[93] Patients with cardiac abnormalities can experience atypical chest pain, syncope, and dyspnea. Patients without other congenital abnormalities are usually asymptomatic, and the pericardial defect is found on a routine chest radiograph. Complications include herniation and entrapment of a cardiac chamber, especially an atrial appendage, or compression of a coronary artery.[93]

CT scans readily demonstrate a pericardial defect and may be able to suggest an associated cardiac abnormality. On CT scans, absence of the fibrous parietal pericardium can be noted, as well as the direct contact between lung and cardiac chambers.[89, 98] When absence of the diaphragmatic pericardium is part of a pericardioperitoneal communication, CT scans can show herniation of abdominal organs or fat into the pericardium.[99]

Pericardial cysts and diverticula are uncommon lesions. The majority of pericardial cysts contain clear fluid with a CT density of 0 to 20 Hounsfield units (H). They usually are located at the right cardiophrenic angle. True pericardial cysts contain all layers of the pericardium and do not communicate with the pericardial space. CT scans provide an excellent method for differentiating pericardial cysts from other masses occurring in this region. On CT scans, pericardial cysts are homogeneous and have a thin, smooth wall. Rarely, calcification may occur in the wall of a pericardial cyst.[89, 100, 101] Congenital diverticula of the pericardium are similar to pericardial cysts but communicate with the pericardium. Their CT appearance should be similar.

EFFUSION

The normal pericardial space contains approximately 20 to 30 mL of fluid. This serous fluid is an ultrafiltrate of serum containing 1.7 to 3.5 per cent protein.[84] Venous or lymphatic obstruction of the drainage from the heart will lead to a pericardial effusion that comes from the visceral pericardium.

The CT density of effusions varies depending on the protein, cellular, and fat content of the fluid. Common causes of serous effusions are congestive heart failure, hypoalbuminemia, and thoracic irradiation. Serosanguineous effusions usually arise from trauma (including surgery), neoplasm, acute myocardial infarction, and disorders of coagulation. Chylous effusions are rare but can be seen after injury to the thoracic duct. Exudative effusions are caused by an inflammatory response to infection or neoplasm within the pericardium. Some causes of pleural effusion are cited in Table 6–3.

In the supine patient, a small effusion tends to accumulate posteriorly. A larger effusion forms a layer of fluid that surrounds the heart, displacing the

TABLE 6–3 ■ Causes of Pericarditis and Pericardial Effusion

Infection
  Bacterial
  Tuberculous
  Fungal: histoplasmosis, actinomycosis
  Viral: coxsackie B, influenza
  Parasitic: amebiasis, toxoplasmosis, echinococcosis
Postinjury
  Postmyocardial infarction syndrome: acute myocardial infarction
  Postpericardiotomy
  Posttraumatic: penetrating and nonpenetrating wounds
  Physical: burns, ionizing radiation
Neoplasma
  Lymphoma, leukemia, sarcoma
  Carcinoma: breast, lung
  Mesothelioma
Connective tissue disease
  Lupus erythematosus
  Rheumatic fever
  Rheumatoid arthritis
  Scleroderma
Metabolic
  Uremia
  Hypothyroidism
Drugs
  Procainamide
  Hydralazine
  Psicofuranine
Dissecting aortic aneurysm
Chylopericardium
Idiopathic

parietal pericardium away from the heart. Pericardial effusion is recognized on CT scans as a layer of fluid density between the heart and mediastinal fat, parietal pleura, mediastinal organs, or the lungs. Because the whole chest is scanned by CT, associated abnormalities elsewhere in the mediastinum and lungs can be detected during the same procedure. Pericardial effusion as small as 50 mL of fluid can be detected on CT scans, which makes CT as sensitive as echocardiography.[102, 103] Effusions of 200 mL are required to surround the heart completely.

Most pericardial effusions are of low signal intensity on spin-echo images.[104] On the T1-weighted spin-echo images, bloody effusions are represented by high signal intensity. MR can usually demonstrate pericardial hematomas by their imaging characteristics.

PERICARDITIS AND PERICARDIAL THICKENING

Today pericarditis is most commonly viral, specifically caused by coxsackie viruses. Nontuberculous bacterial pericarditis has become uncommon and usually has a predisposing factor such as trauma, surgery, immunosuppression, or infective endocarditis. Tuberculosis and irradiation both cause pericardial thickening that can lead to constriction. Pericarditis and thickening also can be associated with systemic disease such as renal failure, rheumatoid arthritis, scleroderma, and systemic lupus erythematosus.

The pericardium responds to many inflammatory stimuli by producing varying amounts of fluid, fibrin deposition, and cellular proliferation. For instance, hemopericardium after surgery can resolve without evidence of pericardial thickening or can result in constrictive pericarditis.

CT scanning can assist in the difficult clinical problem of separating constrictive pericarditis from restrictive cardiomyopathy. The clinical signs, symptoms, and hemodynamic findings of these two conditions are virtually indistinguishable. Echocardiography can be helpful if the constriction is secondary to pericardial effusion. However, echocardiography is relatively insensitive in the detection of pericardial thickening. Several reports have suggested that in the correct clinical context, the finding of 5 to 20 mm of pericardial thickening on CT scans is suggestive of pericardial constriction (Fig. 6–25).[89, 90] A normal pericardium, on the other hand, virtually excludes constriction, leading to the presumptive diagnosis of restrictive cardiomyopathy.

The evaluation of possible pericardial constriction should include assessment of the morphology of the ventricles after contrast enhancement. The ventricles are usually seen as compressed, tubular cavities, and the atrioventricular groove is narrowed.[105]

On MR images an increase in thickness of the rim of nonfatty tissue around the myocardium has been observed in the presence of thickened pericardium in patients with constrictive pericarditis (Fig. 6–26).[104, 106] Low MR signal intensity of the thickened

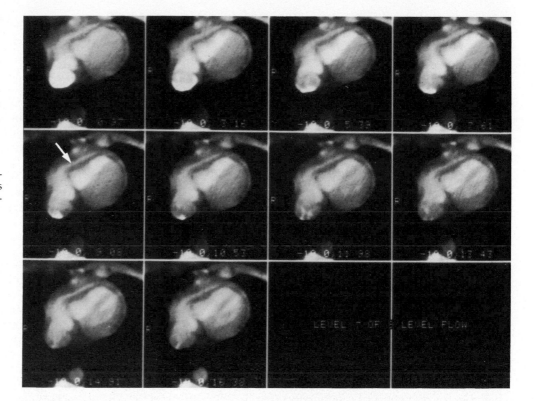

FIGURE 6–25 ■ Constrictive pericarditis. Sequential cine-CT scans show a markedly thickened anterior pericardium *(arrow)*.

pericardium suggests that it is composed mostly of fibrous tissue, as would be expected in chronic constrictive pericarditis. In patients with uremic pericarditis, the MR images demonstrated pericardial effusion and abundant inflammatory exudate on the pericardium. In contradistinction to the normal pericardium, the inflamed pericardium produces a high-

intensity MR signal, as do adhesions between the visceral and parietal pericardium. The signal intensity of the pericardium in these circumstances is greater on images with a longer TE, which is consistent with the long T2 relaxation time observed from other edematous tissues.

Prominent thickening without constriction can be

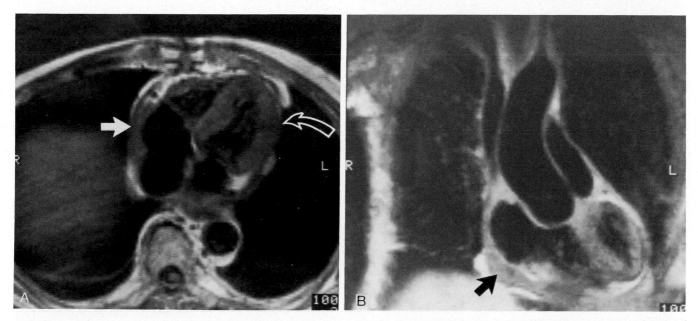

FIGURE 6–26 ■ Two patients with pericardial constriction. Transverse spin-echo image *(A)* shows thickened pericardium over the right side of the heart *(solid arrow)*. The surgical interruption of the pericardium *(open arrow)* on the left side is a pericardial window to relieve recurrent pericardial effusions. Coronal image *(B)* demonstrates markedly thickened pericardium *(arrow)* between the pericardial and subepicardial fat on the right.

seen in several conditions, including the postpericardiotomy and postmyocardial infarction syndromes. These syndromes occur following cardiac surgery and acute myocardial infarction, respectively, and are most likely immune related. The clinical syndrome includes fever, myalgia, and chest pain, and it typically occurs 1 week to 1 year after the initial insult.[107] CT scans of the chest demonstrate prominent pericardial thickening and effusion. Intravenous infusion of contrast material can show enhancement of the thickened pericardium and improve the delineation of pericardial effusion.

CALCIFICATION

Calcification of the pericardium represents the end stage of many inflammatory processes. The most common causes are prior tuberculosis, viral infections, rheumatic fever, and trauma. However, in many instances, no cause can be found. Histologic study of the pericardium rarely provides a specific diagnosis.[108] Calcification can be microscopic or macroscopic and can encircle the entire heart. The presence of pericardial calcification does not indicate impending constriction.

CT scanning—especially cine-CT, with its high-density resolution—is the most sensitive method available for detection of calcification (Fig. 6–27). The cross-sectional tomographic format can localize the site of pericardial calcifications. The significance of pericardial calcification, however, should be determined from the patient's symptoms and physical examination.

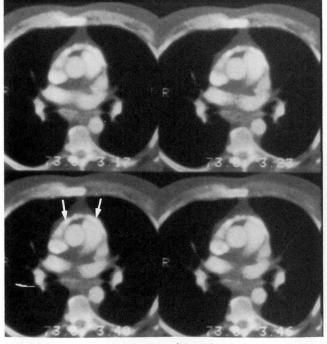

FIGURE 6–27 ■ Constrictive pericarditis with calcification. Contrast-enhanced cine-CT scans show that the pericardium over the base of the heart is thickened and calcified (arrows).

NEOPLASM

Primary neoplasms of the pericardium are exceedingly rare. The differentiation of primary malignant myocardial tumors from pericardial tumors can be extremely difficult, if not impossible, even at autopsy. The most common benign tumors are teratoma, lipoma, fibroma, and angioma. Malignant primary pericardial tumors include mesothelioma and both differentiated and undifferentiated sarcoma.

Metastasis to the pericardium is much more common than primary pericardial neoplasm. Autopsy series have shown that 5 to 10 per cent of patients with cancer have metastases to the pericardium.[32, 109] In many, however, the pericardial deposits are asymptomatic and not detected before death. Metastasis to the pericardium can occur with almost any neoplasm. Lymphoma, leukemia, breast cancer, and lung carcinoma are the most frequent. Melanoma, although an uncommon tumor, has a high frequency of dissemination to the pericardium.

The combination of the excellent density resolution and the tomographic format of CT scans provides a sensitive noninvasive imaging method to localize and characterize neoplasms of the pericardium.

The CT density of malignant pericardial effusion can vary widely depending on the response of the pericardium. Chylous or pseudochylous effusions, with relatively low attenuation values, can be secondary to neoplastic involvement. Transudative effusions have intermediate attenuation values. Exudative or hemorrhagic effusions can have higher values, depending on their protein and cellular contents. Unless pericardial masses are evident, the differentiation of malignant effusion from other causes, such as radiation-induced pericarditis or idiopathic pericarditis, is not possible with CT scanning. In most cases, pericardiocentesis or thoracotomy and biopsy are necessary for definitive diagnosis of pericardial neoplasms.

Pericardial cysts and tumors have been clearly defined by MR.[104, 110] Indeed, the pericardial origin of these masses and whether they are cystic or solid are usually better defined by MR than by other imaging modalities. Because MR defines the low-signal-intensity pericardial layer, it can show the presence of masses of usually high intensity in relationship to the outside or inside of the pericardium (Fig. 6–28).

MR also is useful in evaluating pericardial masses because of its clear delineations of the cardiac walls and cardiac chambers and the direct visualization of the pericardium. MR images allow spatial separation of the various chambers and the various regions of each chamber, such as the septal from the lateral cardiac walls. The large field of view of MR can also show the cardiac chambers in relation to other mediastinal and pulmonary structures.

MR can distinguish between paracardiac and intracardiac masses unequivocally (see Figs. 6–17 and 6–28).[65, 110, 111] It can also determine the extent of mass lesions of the thorax and whether mediastinal, lung, and pericardial tumors extend into the heart (see Fig.

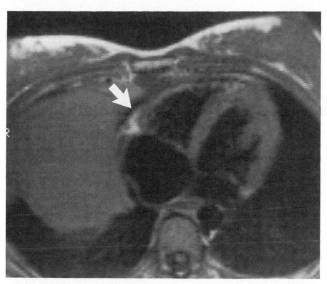

FIGURE 6–28 ■ Paracardiac tumor. Pericardial line *(arrow)* separates the tumor from the right ventricle and right atrium.

6–17). MR can determine the presence and volume of pericardial effusions encountered in association with malignant cardiac tumors. Finally, it can be used to establish the presence of pericardial involvement by tumor as the cause of recurrent pericardial effusions.

The principal clinical complication of primary or metastatic neoplasm of the pericardium is pericardial effusion and tamponade.[112] Both can develop insidiously or catastrophically. The clinical features of pericardial tamponade are similar to those of tumor obstruction of the venae cavae. CT scans after intravenous contrast material infusion frequently separate the two. Although venous obstruction is well demonstrated on CT scans and MR images (see Chapter 5), a large pericardial effusion can likewise be readily shown. The clinical syndrome of cardiac tamponade can also be caused when cardiac restriction results from encasement of the pericardium by tumor. CT and MR scanning is helpful for identifying this type of pericardial involvement.

Comparison of Cardiac Imaging Techniques

Echocardiography remains the preeminent noninvasive cardiac imaging technique. Importantly, it uses portable equipment so that it can be performed on the critically ill patient, in the operating room, and in the coronary care unit. It also enjoys widespread availability and familiarity among cardiac diagnosticians. Echocardiography has the added advantage of high temporal resolution, which is required for the assessment of cardiac function. Echo Doppler and color flow mapping also give enormous capability for the qualitative and quantitative assessment of valvular abnormalities. At present, echocar-

diography is the primary imaging modality and in many instances the choice for imaging of valvular heart disease; cardiomyopathies, especially hypertrophic cardiomyopathies; pericardial effusion; and many types of congenital heart disease. For the foreseeable future it will remain the initial study and, in many instances, the definitive study for the diagnosis of congenital heart disease. The major limitation of echocardiography is that an adequate echocardiogram cannot be obtained in all patients because of differences in body habitus or overly expansive lungs. These problems usually are not present in children, and comprehensive studies can be accomplished in most children with congenital heart disease. CT and especially MR are complementary for the diagnosis of cardiomyopathies, pericardial effusions, and congenital heart disease.

Cine-MR has substantial capability for the quantitation of valvular regurgitation and consequently will have an as yet undefined role in relationship to echocardiography for these lesions. At the present time, MR is used predominantly for thoracic aortic disease; central pulmonary artery abnormalities, especially pulmonary atresia; and complex cardiovascular anomalies involving both the heart and great vessels. It can determine the sizes of the two ventricles in complex lesions and define the extent of the ventricular septum in such lesions. The eventual role of MR and echocardiography used in concert for the full evaluation of congenital heart disease may be substantially greater than for each alone, and these two may replace angiography in many situations.

Nuclear scintigraphy has its primary role in the detection of myocardial ischemia. The thallium study at rest and during exercise or during maximal vasodilatation is used to detect the presence of myocardial ischemia. Although concern remains as to the reliability of these studies, they continue to be the cornerstone for detection of myocardial ischemia in both initially symptomatic and postoperative patients.

The role of MR and CT in ischemic heart disease is primarily in the assessment of the patient with a previous myocardial infarction. Neither of these methods has been reliable for the initial detection of ischemic heart disease. Although there is interest in the use of cine-CT for identifying coronary arterial calcification in asymptomatic persons, the interpretation of this finding and the manner in which it will be used for clinical management remain far from clear. Both cine-CT and MR can identify the consequences of previous myocardial infarctions, such as the amount of muscle that has been lost by a previous infarction, the development of ventricular aneurysms, and the presence of mural thrombus.

Positron emission tomography (PET), like CT and MR, is still in a developmental phase. Its eventual role for evaluation of cardiac disease is unclear. However, PET, for the most part, yields information different from that obtained from CT and MR. The major ability of PET is to simultaneously demonstrate perfusion and metabolism of a region of myocardium. This dual observation can define myocardium that has reduced perfusion but continues to have metabolic activity and therefore is considered to be potentially salvageable.

For many cardiac diagnosticians angiography remains the gold standard and the procedure of choice for the definitive diagnosis of most cardiac disease. However, progress is clearly moving in the direction of replacement of angiography with noninvasive imaging techniques. With the exception of obstructive coronary artery disease, there is no cardiac or pericardial abnormality that is not demonstrated by some noninvasive imaging technique equally as well as it is by angiography.

References

1. Higgins CB, Carlsson E, Lipton MJ (eds): CT of the Heart and Great Vessels. Mount Kisco, NY, Futura Publishing, 1983, pp 167–168.
2. Lackner K, Thurn P: Computed tomography of the heart: ECG gated and continuous scans. Radiology 140:413, 1981.
3. Mattrey RF, Higgins CB: Detection of regional myocardium dysfunction during ischemia with computerized tomography. Documentation and basis. Invest Radiol 17:329, 1982.
4. Lipton MJ, Higgins CB, Farmer D, Boyd DP: Cardiac imaging with a high-speed cine-CT scanner: preliminary results. Radiology 152:579, 1984.
5. Sechtem U, Pflugfelder PW, White RD, Gould RG, Holt W, et al: Cine MRI: potential for the evaluation of cardiovascular function. AJR 148:239, 1987.
6. Dinsmore RE, Wismer GL, Levine RA, Leurne RA, Ikada RD, Brady TJ: Magnetic resonance imaging of the heart: positioning and gradient angle selection for optimal imaging planes. AJR 143:1135, 1984.
7. Gray H. In Goss (ed): Anatomy of the Human Body, 28th ed. Philadelphia, Lea & Febiger, 1966, p 543.
8. Silverman ME, Schlant RC. In Hurst JW, Logue RB, Schlant RC, Wenger NK (eds): The Heart, 4th ed. New York, Mc-Graw-Hill, 1978, pp 19–32.
9. Braunwald ED: Protection of the ischemic myocardium. Circulation 53(suppl I):1, 1976.
10. Farmer DW, Lipton MJ, Higgins CB, Ringertz H, Dean P, et al: In vivo assessment of left ventricular wall and chamber dynamics during transient myocardial ischemia using cine CT. Am J Cardiol 55:560, 1985.
11. Abrams DL, Edelist A, Luria MH, Miller AJ: Ventricular aneurysm: a reappraisal based on a study of sixty-five consecutive autopsied cases. Circulation 27:164, 1963.
12. Schlicter J, Hellerstein HK, Katz LN: Aneurysm of the heart. Medicine 33:43, 1954.
13. Gay WA Jr, Ebert PA. In Norman JC, Lawrence EP (eds): Coronary Artery Medicine and Surgery: Concepts and Controversies. New York, Appleton-Century-Crofts, 1975, pp 659–661.
14. Herfkens RJ, Goldstein J, Lipton MJ, Schiller NB, Ports TA, Brundage BH: Evaluation of left ventricular aneurysms with contrast enhanced computed tomography and two dimensional echocardiography. Abstract. Invest Radiol 17:S10, 1982.
15. Lipton MJ, Farmer DW, Killebrew E, Bouchard A, Dean PB, et al: Evaluation of regional myocardial function with fast CT in patients with prior myocardial infarction. Radiology 157:735, 1985.
16. DeMaria AN, Bommer W, Neumann A, Grehl T, Weinart L, et al: Left ventricular thrombi identified by cross-sectional echocardiography. Ann Intern Med 90:14, 1979.
17. Hurst JW, King SP. In Hurst JW, Logue RB, Schlant RC, Wenger NK (eds): The Heart, 4th ed. New York, McGraw-Hill, 1978, pp 1129–1130.
18. Goldstein JA, Lipton MJ, Schiller NB, Ports TA, Brundage BH: Evaluation of intracardiac thrombi with contrast enhanced computed tomography and echocardiography. Am J Cardiol 49:972, 1982.
19. Godwin JD, Herfkens RJ, Skioldebrand CG, Brundage BH, Schiller NB, Lipton MJ: Detection of intraventricular thrombi by computed tomography. Radiology 138:717, 1981.
20. Tomada H, Hoshai M, Furuya H, Kuribayashi S, Ootaki M, et al: Evaluation of intracardiac thrombus with computed tomography. Am J Cardiol 51:843, 1983.
21. Anderson RP: The prognosis of patients with coronary artery disease after coronary bypass operations. Time-related progress of 532 patients with disabling angina pectoris. Circulation 50:274, 1974.
22. Sanford W, Brundage B, McMillan R, Chomka EV, Lipton MJ, et al: Sensitivity and specificity of assessing coronary bypass graft patency with ultrafast computed tomography: results of a multicenter study. J Am Coll Cardiol 12:1, 1988.
23. Brundage BH, Lipton MJ, Herfkens RJ, Berninger WH, Redington RW, et al: Detection of patent coronary bypass grafts by computed tomography: a preliminary report. Circulation 61:826, 1980.
24. Moncada R, Salinas M, Churchill R, Love L, Reynes C, et al: Patency of saphenous aortocoronary bypass grafts demonstrated by computed tomography. N Engl J Med 303:503, 1980.
25. Daniel WG, Dohring W, Lichtler PR, Stender HS: Noninvasive assessment of aortocoronary bypass graft patency by computed tomography. Lancet 1:1023, 1980.
26. Goodwin JF: Clarification of the cardiomyopathies. Mod Concepts Cardiovasc Dis 41:41, 1972.
27. Abrams HL, Adams DF, Grant HA: The radiology of tumors of the heart. Radiol Clin North Am 9:299, 1971.
28. Meller J, Teichholz LE, Pichard AD, Matta R, Litwak R, et al: Left ventricular myxoma: echocardiographic diagnosis and review of the literature. Am J Med 63:816, 1977.
29. O'Neil M Jr, Grehl T, Hurley E: Cardial myxomas: a clinical diagnostic challenge. Am J Surg 138:68, 1979.
30. Prichard RW: Tumors of the heart: review of the subject and report of one hundred and fifty cases. Arch Pathol 51:98, 1951.
31. Wenger NK. In Hurst JW (ed): The Heart, Arteries, and Veins. New York, McGraw-Hill, 1978, pp 1668–1682.
32. Hanfling SM: Metastatic cancer to the heart: review of the literature and report of 127 cases. Circulation 24:474, 1960.
33. Huggins TJ, Huggins MJ, Schnapf DJ, Brott WH, Sinnott RC, Shawl FA: Left atrial myxoma: computed tomography as a diagnostic modality. J Comput Assist Tomogr 4:253, 1980.
34. Dunnick NR, Seibert K, Dramer HR Jr: Cardiac metastasis from osteosarcoma. J Comput Assist Tomogr 5:253, 1981.
35. Hidalgo H, Korobkin M, Sbreiman RS, Kisslo JR: CT of intracardiac tumor. AJR 137:608, 1981.
36. Moncada R, Baker M, Salinas M, Demos T, Churchill R, et al: Diagnostic role of computed tomography in pericardial heart disease. Am Heart J 103:263, 1982.
37. Farmer DW, Lipton MJ, Webb WR, Ringertz H, Higgins CB: Computed tomography in congenital heart disease. J Comput Assist Tomogr 8:677, 1984.
38. Eldredge WJ, Flicker S, Steiner RM. In Pohost G, Higgins CB, Morganroth J, Richie J, Schelbert H (eds): New Concepts in Cardiac Imaging. Chicago, Year Book Medical, 1987, pp 265–290.
39. Feiring AJ, Rumberger JA, Reiter SJ, Skorton DJ, Collins SM, et al: Determination of left ventricular mass in dogs with rapid-acquisition cardiac computed tomographic scanning. Circulation 72:1355, 1985.
40. Caputo GR, Lipton MJ. In Pohost GM, Higgins CB, Morganroth J, Ritchie JL, Schelbert HR (eds): New Concepts in Cardiac Imaging. Chicago, Year Book Medical, 1988, pp 231–257.
41. Fiering AJ, Rumberger JA, Skorton DJ, Rees M, Marcus ML: Sectional and segmental variability in left ventricular function: experimental and clinical studies using ultrafast computed tomography. J Am Coll Cardiol 12:415, 1988.
42. Garrett J, Lanzer P, Jaschke W, Botvinick E, Sievers R, et al:

Quantitation of cardiac output by cine CT. Am J Cardiol 56:657, 1985.

43. Gould RG, Lipton MJ, McNamara MT, Sievers RE, Koshold S, Higgins CB: Measurement of regional myocardial flow in dogs using ultrafast CT. Invest Radiol 23:348, 1988.

44. Himelman RB, Abbott JA, Lipton MJ, Schiller NB: Cine computed tomography compared with echocardiography in the evaluation of cardiac function in emphysema. Am J Cardiac Imaging 2:283, 1988.

45. Pflugfelder PW, Wisenberg G, Prato FS, Carroll SE, Turner KL: Early detection of canine myocardial infarction by magnetic resonance imaging in vivo. Circulation 71:587, 1985.

46. Higgins CB, Lanzer P, Stark D, Botvinick E, Schiller NB, et al: Nuclear magnetic resonance imaging in chronic ischemic heart disease in man. Circulation 69:523, 1984.

47. McNamara MT, Higgins CB, Schechtmann N, Botvinick E, Amparo EG, Chatterjee K: Detection and characterization of acute myocardial infarctions in man using gated magnetic resonance imaging. Circulation 71:717, 1985.

48. McNamara MT, Higgins CB: Magnetic resonance imaging and characterization of chronic myocardial infarction. AJR 146:315, 1986.

49. Filipchuk NG, Peshock RM, Malloy CR, Corbett JR, Rehr RB, et al: Detection and localization of recent myocardial infarction by magnetic resonance imaging. Am J Cardiol 58:214, 1986.

50. Fisher MR, McNamara MT, Higgins CB: Acute myocardial infarction: MR evaluation in 25 patients. AJR 248:247, 1987.

51. Saeed M, Wagner S, Wendland MF, Derugin N, Finkbeiner WE, Higgins CB: MRI distinction between occlusive and reperfused myocardial infarcts: Differentiation with Mn DPDP–enhanced, MR imaging. Radiology 172:59, 1989.

52. Akins EW, Hill JA, Sievers KW, Conti CR: Assessment of left ventricular wall thickness in healed myocardial infarction by magnetic resonance imaging. Am J Cardiol 59:42, 1987.

53. Brown JJ, Higgins CB: Myocardial contrast agents for magnetic resonance imaging. AJR 151:239, 1988.

54. Runge VM, Clanton JA, Wehr CJ, Partain CL, James AE: Gated magnetic resonance imaging of acute myocardial ischemia in dogs: application of multiecho techniques and contrast enhancement with Gd-DTPA. Magn Reson Imaging 3:255, 1985.

55. Rehr RB, Peshock RM, Malloy Cr, Killer AM, Parkey RW, et al: Improved in vivo magnetic resonance imaging of acute myocardial infarction after intravenous paramagnetic contrast agent administration. Am J Cardiol 57:864, 1986.

56. Cannon PJ, Maudsley AS, Hilal SK, Simon HB, Cassidy F: Sodium nuclear magnetic resonance imaging of myocardial tissue of dogs after coronary artery occlusion and reperfusion. J Am Coll Cardiol 7:573, 1986.

57. Nunnally RL, Babcock BB, Horner SD, Peshock RM: Fluorine-19 NMR spectroscopy and imaging investigations of myocardial perfusion and cardiac function. Magn Reson Imaging 3:399, 1985.

58. Bottomly PA, Herfkens RJ, Smith LS, Bruzzamano S, Blinder R, et al: Noninvasive detection and monitoring of regional myocardial ischemia in situ using depth-resolved P-31 NMR spectroscopy. Proc Natl Acad Sci USA 82:8747, 1985.

59. Higgins CB, Byrd BF III, Stark D, McNamara MT, Lanzer P, et al: Magnetic resonance imaging of hypertrophic cardiomyopathy. Am J Cardiol 55:1121, 1985.

60. Keller AM, Peshock RM, Malloy CT, Buja LM, Nunnally R, et al: In vivo measurement of myocardial mass using nuclear magnetic resonance imaging. J Am Coll Cardiol 8:113, 1986.

61. Buser PT, Auffermann W, Holt WW, Wagner S, Kircher B, et al: Noninvasive evaluation of the global left ventricular function using cine MR imaging. J Am Coll Cardiol 13:1294, 1989.

62. Applegate PM, Tajik AJ, Julsrud PR, Miller RA: Two-dimensional echocardiographic and magnetic resonance imaging observations in massive lipomatous hypertrophy of the atrial septum. Am J Cardiol 59:489, 1987.

63. Conces DJ, Vix VA, Klatte EC: Gated MR imaging of left atrial myxomas. Radiology 156:445, 1985.

64. Go R, O'Donnell JK, Underwood DA, Feiglin DH, Salcedo EE, et al: Comparison of gated cardiac MRI and 2D echocardiography of intracardiac neoplasms. AJR 145:21, 1985.

65. Brown JJ, Barakos JA, Higgins CB: Magnetic resonance imaging of cardiac and paracardiac masses. Thorac Radiol 4:58, 1989.

66. von Schulthess GK, Fisher MR, Crooks LE, Higgins CB: The nature of intracardiac signal on gated NMR images in normals and patients with abnormal left ventricular function. Radiology 156:125, 1985.

66a. Seelos KC, Caputo GR, Hricak H, Higgins CB: Differentiation of tumor versus non-tumor thrombus using sequential gradient echo imaging (cine MRI). Abstract of the American Roentgen Ray Society 1990 Annual Meeting, May 1990.

67. Freedberg RS, Krozon I, Runnancik WM, Liebeskind D: The contribution of magnetic resonance imaging to the evaluation of intracardiac tumors diagnosed by echocardiography. Circulation 77:96, 1988.

68. Fletcher BD, Jacobstein MD, Nelson AD, Riemenschneider TA, Alfidi RJ: Gated magnetic resonance imaging of congenital malformations. Radiology 150:137, 1984.

69. Higgins CB, Byrd BF III, Farmer D, Osaki L, Silverman NH, Cheitlin MD: Magnetic resonance imaging in patients with congenital heart disease. Circulation 70:851, 1984.

70. Sommerhoff BK, Sechtem UP, Higgins CB: Evaluation of pulmonary blood supply by nuclear magnetic resonance imaging in patients with pulmonary atresia. J Am Coll Cardiol 11:166, 1988.

71. Didier D, Higgins CB, Fisher M, Osaki L, Silverman N, Cheitlin M: Congenital heart disease: gated MR imaging in 72 patients. Radiology 158:227, 1986.

72. Guit GL, Bluemm R, Rohmer J, Wenink AC, Chin JG, et al: Levotransposition of the aorta: identification of segmental cardiac anatomy using MR imaging. Radiology 161:673, 1986.

73. Fletcher BD, Jacobstein MD: MRI of congenital abnormalities of the great arteries. AJR 146:941, 1986.

74. Diethelm L, Dery R, Lipton MJ, Higgins CB: Atrial level shunts: sensitivity and specificity of MR in diagnosis. Radiology 162:181, 1987.

75. Sommerhoff BA, Diethelm L, Teitel DF, Sommerhoff CP, Higgins CB: Magnetic resonance imaging of congenital heart disease: sensitivity and specificity using receiver operator characteristic curve analysis. Am Heart J 118:155, 1989.

76. Higgins CB, Holt W, Pflugfelder P, Sechtem U: Functional evaluation of the heart with magnetic resonance imaging. Magn Reson Med 6:121, 1988.

77. Fisher MR, von Schulthess GK, Higgins CB: Quantitation of regional left ventricular wall thickness using rotated gated magnetic resonance imaging. AJR 145:27, 1985.

78. von Schulthess GD, Fisher MR, Higgins CB: Detection of abnormal pulmonary flow pattern by magnetic resonance imaging in pulmonary arterial hypertension. Ann Intern Med 103:317, 1985.

79. Pflugfelder PW, Sechtem UP, White RD, Higgins CB: Quantification of regional myocardial function by rapid (cine) magnetic resonance imaging. AJR 150:523, 1988.

80. Sechtem U, Pflugfelder PW, Cassidy MM, White RD, Cheitlin MD, et al: Mitral or aortic regurgitation: quantification of regurgitant volumes with cine MR imaging. Radiology 167:425, 1988.

81. Wagner S, Auffermann W, Buser P, Lim TH, Kircher B, et al: Diagnostic accuracy and estimation of the severity of valvular regurgitation from the signal void on cine MR. Am Heart J 118:760, 1989.

82. Pflugfelder PW, Sechtem UP, White RD, Cassidy MM, Schiller NB, Higgins CB: Noninvasive evaluation of mitral regurgitation by analysis of left atrial signal loss in cine magnetic resonance. Am Heart J 117:1113, 1989.

82a. Firmin DN, Nagler GL, Klipstein RH, Underwood SR, Rees RSO, Longmore DB: In vivo validation of MR velocity mapping. J Comput Assist Tomogr 11:751, 1987.

82b. Kondo C, Caputo GR, Semelka R, Higgins CB: Right and left ventricular stroke volume measurements with velocity encoded cine NMR imaging. In vitro and in vivo validation. AJR, 1991 (in press).

82c. Walker MF, Souza SP, Dumoulin CL: Quantitative flow measurement in phase contrast MR angiography. J Comput Assist Tomogr 12:304, 1988.

83. Spodick DH: Medical history of the pericardium. Am J Cardiol 26:447, 1970.

84. Holt JP: The normal pericardium. Am J Cardiol 26:455, 1970.

85. Bartle SH, Herman JH, Cavo JW, Moore RA, Costenbader JM: Effect of the pericardium or left ventricular volume and function in acute hypervolemia. Cardiovasc Res 3:284, 1961.

86. Shabetai R, Mangiarde L, Bhargava V, Ross J Jr, Higgins CB: The pericardium and cardiac function. Prog Cardiovasc Dis 22:107, 1979.

87. Mursky I, Ramkin JS: The effects of geometry, elasticity and external pressures on the diastolic pressure-volume and stiffness-stress relations: how important is the pericardium? Circ Res 44:601, 1979.

88. Shabetai R: The Pericardium. New York, Grune & Stratton, 1981, pp 1–3.

89. Moncada R, Baker M, Salinas M, Demos T, Churchill R, et al: Diagnostic role of computed tomography in pericardial heart disease: congenital defects, thickening, neoplasms and effusions. Am Heart J 103:263, 1982.

90. Doppman JL, Reinmuller R, Nissner J, Cyan J, Bolte HD, et al: Computed tomography in constrictive pericarditis. J Comput Assist Tomogr 5:1, 1981.

91. Sechtem U, Tscholakoff D, Higgins CB: MRI of the normal pericardium. AJR 147:239, 1986.

92. Edwards JE: Congenital malformations of the heart and great vessels. In Gould SE (ed): Pathology of the Heart and Blood Vessels, 3rd ed. Springfield, IL, Charles C Thomas, 1968, pp 376–378.

93. Nassar WK. In Reddy PS, Leon DF, Shaver JA (eds): Pericardial Disease. New York, Raven Press, 1982, pp 93–111.

94. Tabakin BS, Hanson JS, Tampas JP, Caldwell EJ: Congenital absence of left pericardium. AJR 94:122, 1965.

95. Schuster B, Alejandrino S, Yavuz F, Imm CW: Congenital pericardial defect: report of a patient with an associated patent ductus arteriosus. Am J Dis Child 110:199, 1965.

96. Mukerjee S: Congenital partial left pericardial defect with bronchogenic cyst. Thorax 19:176, 1964.

97. Nassar WK: Congenital absence of the left pericardium. Am J Cardiol 26:466, 1970.

98. Baum RS, MacDonald IL, Wise DJ, Lenkei SC: Computed tomography of absent left pericardium. Radiology 135:127, 1980.

99. Larrieu AJ, Wiener I, Alexander R, Wolma FJ: Pericardiodiaphragmatic hernia. Am J Surg 139:436, 1980.

100. Pugatch RD, Braver JH, Robbins AH, Faling LJ: CT diagnosis of pericardial cysts. AJR 131:515, 1978.

101. Rogers CI, Seymour Q, Brock GJ: Atypical pericardial cyst location: the valve of computed tomography. J Comput Assist Tomogr 4:683, 1980.

102. Wong BYS, Kyo RL, McArthur R: Diagnosis of pericardial effusion by CT. Chest 81:177, 1982.

103. Tomada H, Hoshiai M, Furuyu H, Oeda Y, Matsumoto S, et al: Evaluation of pericardial effusion with computed tomography. Am Heart J 99:701, 1980.

104. Sechtem U, Tscholakoff D, Higgins CB: MRI of the abnormal pericardium. AJR 147:245, 1986.

105. Reinmuller R, Seiderer M, Doliva R, Kemkes V, Lissner J: Pericardial and congestive heart failure with CT- and MR-imaging. Ann Radiol 29:95, 1986.

106. Soulen RL, Stark DD, Higgins CB: Magnetic resonance imaging of constrictive pericardial heart disease. Am J Cardiol 55:480, 1985.

107. Engle ME, Klein AA, Hepner S, Ehlers KH: The postpericardiotomy and other similar syndromes. Cardiovasc Clin 7:211, 1976.

108. Shapiro JH, Jacobson HG, Rubenstein BM, Poppel MH, Schwedel JB: Calcifications of the Heart. Springfield, IL, Charles C Thomas, 1963, p 198.

109. Deloach JF, Haynes JW: Secondary tumors of the heart and pericardium: review of the subject and report of 137 cases. Arch Intern Med 91:224, 1953.

110. Amparo EG, Higgins CB, Farmer K, Gamsu G, McNamara M: Gated magnetic resonance imaging (MRI) of cardiac and paracardiac masses. AJR 143:1151, 1984.

111. Winkler M, Higgins B: Suspected intracardiac masses: evaluation with MR imaging. Radiology 165:117, 1987.

112. Posner MR, Cohen GI, Srarin AT: Pericardial disease in patients with cancer: the differentiation of malignant from idiopathic and radiation-induced pericarditis. Am J Med 71:407, 1981.

CHAPTER 7

TRAUMA

PIERRE SCHNYDER • *GORDON GAMSU* • *AXEL ESSINGER* •
BERTRAND DUVOISIN

Trauma is the third leading cause of death in industrialized countries such as the United States and the leading cause of death in children and young adults.[1, 2] Chest trauma accounts for mortality in approximately one third of patients. In 50 per cent of the remaining cases, chest injuries contribute significantly to patient mortality.[2] In industrialized countries, most blunt trauma to the chest is the result of motor vehicle accidents.[3] Other important causes are assaults, falls from a height, and work-related injuries. The immediate outcome of the patient with chest trauma is determined by the severity of the injury, the time required to transport the patient to an appropriately equipped hospital, and the availability of a medical team capable of providing emergency treatment at the scene of the accident.[1] Significant improvements in patient transport, including the use of helicopters, and telecommunications with the emergency team have markedly enhanced survival of critically injured patients. Specialized trauma centers capable of lifesaving measures by a specialized medical team are important features of modern trauma care. Also important are the immediate availability of advanced diagnostic techniques such as computed tomography (CT), angiography, and interventional radiology.[4] The mortality rate for blunt chest trauma in patients alive at admission to an emergency facility, is between 4 and 12 per cent.[5] For patients with multiple organ involvement, the mortality rate rises to 30 to 35 per cent.

The value of CT in evaluating neurologic and abdominal injuries is well established, whereas its role in thoracic trauma is only now becoming appreciated.[6-8] Several studies have described the CT findings in specific thoracic injuries, although studies large enough to determine the diagnostic efficacy of CT in chest trauma are yet to be undertaken.[7, 9]

Techniques

The basic imaging equipment for assessment of a patient with thoracic trauma has been the conventional portable chest radiographic unit. Virtually all emergency rooms are equipped with such units. Most emergency rooms also have mobile ultrasound. In the thorax, this is used primarily to detect the presence of pleural or pericardial effusion and trauma to the ascending aorta. Many large trauma centers have angiographic capabilities for immediate assessment of the thoracic vessels. In addition, interventional procedures can be performed without having to transport the patient to a separate radiologic facility.

CT scanning is a major technological improvement of the last decade for assessment of the traumatized patient. Its frequent use in head and abdominal injuries has clearly established its place for trauma evaluation. CT is usually unnecessary for minor chest wall injuries, and it should not be undertaken until the patient's general medical condition has been stabilized. CT protocols for the trauma patient should be modified to obtain maximum information in a minimum of time.[8, 10]

In patients suspected of having mediastinal vascular injuries, the CT examination should be obtained only following intravenous injection of contrast material. CT scans can be limited to the upper mediastinum at the level of the aortic arch, and to the lower mediastinum through the level of the heart. Ten to fifteen scans are sufficient to cover these areas. In patients suspected of having bronchial or lung injury, conventional 8- or 10-mm-thick sections should be obtained at 20- or 25-mm intervals. The examination is performed in less than 10 minutes, and about 15 scans are obtained. The CT scans should be correlated with chest radiographs and the CT projection images to ensure that all sites of potential abnormality have been evaluated.

Image quality is frequently adversely affected by streak artifacts induced by the metallic components of life-support equipment and endogastric and endotracheal tubes. The patient's arms frequently cannot be positioned above the head and must be placed along the sides. Although often degraded, the images are still sufficient to make a correct diagnosis. Removal of supportive equipment is frequently not feasible or required. Angulation of the CT gantry can be used to minimize streak artifacts from appliances fixed to the patient's skin. Medical personnel frequently must be in attendance during scanning and should be trained to tend to patients within the CT gantry. They should also be responsible for coordinating ventilation with the CT exposures to minimize motion artifacts in patients receiving artificial ventilation. Manual ventilation can be used to maintain full inspiration during scanning and improve imaging of the lungs.

Pathology

Chest Wall

BLUNT TRAUMA

Trauma to the chest wall is the most common chest injury and occurs in about 40 per cent of all patients admitted with torso injuries. Most of these injuries are minor, such as rib fractures, costochondral separation, fracture of the clavicle, and fracture of the sternum. For the overwhelming majority of injuries a combination of physical examination and radiographs is sufficient to define their nature and extent. Laceration of the veins and arteries of the chest wall from rib fractures can result in large soft tissue hematomas not detected on chest radiographs but readily seen on CT.[11] Trauma to the subclavian vessels over the apex of the lung can produce an extrapleural accumulation of blood or "pleura cap" that on supine chest radiographs mimics a large hemothorax.[12] CT readily distinguishes between an extrapleural collection of blood over the apex of the

lung and a hemothorax. Apical extrapleural hematomas can extend into the superior mediastinum. In this situation, CT, a thoracic aortogram, or both may be needed to exclude aortic or great vessel injury.[13, 14] Contusion of the subclavian vessels can produce thrombosis without laceration of the vessels. When clinically suspected, this diagnosis requires angiographic confirmation.

Rib fractures are frequently not identified from portable frontal chest radiographs. In one report, up to 50 per cent of rib fractures were not visible.[15] Careful scrutiny of CT scans may assist in identifying rib fractures. Fractures of the first and second ribs are of special importance and are frequently unaccompanied by fractures of other ribs.[13, 16] They usually result from blunt trauma by a directed narrow object or, more often, are indicative of a major impact to the thorax that can be associated with laceration of the distal trachea or main bronchus or major vascular injury. Thoracic CT should be considered in all patients with fractures of the first and second ribs.

Stretching of an upper limb in abduction is a common occurrence in motorcycle accidents and can lead to scapulothoracic dislocation.[17, 18] Injury to the vascular and nerve supplies of the upper limb is common and usually occurs in combination. When clinical evidence of damage to one is present, investigation should be carried out to determine whether injury to both has occurred. Conventional chest radiographs can show indirect signs of injury, such as lateral displacement of the scapula and separation of the acromioclavicular joint. CT can demonstrate fractures, hematomas within the soft tissue, extrapleural extension of the hematoma, and displacement and compression of the subclavian vessels. An emergency arteriogram is indicated prior to surgery.

Gas within the soft tissues of the thorax is more readily displayed with CT than with conventional radiographs.[19, 20] With blunt trauma, it usually occurs from laceration of the parietal and visceral pleura and will be present with an associated pneumothorax. The gas collections are generally located between the intercostal muscles, along the muscular planes of the chest wall, and within the subcutaneous tissues. Extensive subcutaneous emphysema can make the radiographic detection of an underlying pneumothorax difficult. CT readily identifies the pneumothorax in this situation.

Sternal fractures are the result of direct trauma, usually from steering wheel and seat belt injuries. Fractures of the sternum are being reported with increasing frequency and constitute 5 to 10 per cent of all thoracic injuries.[15] Sternal fractures can result in a large anterior mediastinal hematoma from laceration of the internal mammary vessels. They may also be associated with vascular, mediastinal, or cardiac injuries.[11] The most common associated visceral injury is myocardial contusion, which can lead to significant arrhythmias and hemodynamic instability. CT is the method of choice for displaying sternal fractures and the adjacent hematoma. CT can demonstrate the fracture line even when it lies transversely, parallel to the plane of the CT scan. Sternoclavicular dislocation with posterior clavicular displacement is another injury that is perhaps best visualized with CT.[21]

Large hematomas around the scapula are caused by three specific fractures secondary to major direct trauma: fractures of the scapula, particularly comminuted fractures involving the glenoid fossa and coracoid process; fractures of the first rib and clavicle with or without laceration of the axillary vessels and their branches; and comminuted fracture-dislocations of the head of the humerus. Conventional radiographs frequently do not provide precise evaluation of these fractures. Additional information within a short time frame can be obtained with CT. Glenoid or coracoid process fractures may require surgical stabilization when the fracture elements are separated. CT can help in defining the extent of displacement of these fractures.[22]

PENETRATING TRAUMA

Diagnoses of open chest wounds is usually obvious, and CT is seldom required to assist in the diagnosis. In addition to the wound and pain, the patient may experience signs of ventilatory insufficiency if a large pneumothorax is present. Noise from the site of the open wound increases with inspiration and expiration. Bloody froth may escape from the open wound during expiration. CT can be used to precisely locate metallic foreign bodies following penetrating chest injuries. Adler and Rosenberger[23] studied two cases demonstrating the ability of CT to establish the precise intrathoracic position of a bullet fragment and shrapnel fragment and to assist in determining whether surgical removal was necessary.

Pleura

PNEUMOTHORAX

Pneumothorax is the second most common injury following blunt chest trauma, occurring in up to 40 per cent of patients.[24] Pneumothorax usually indicates disruption of the visceral pleura and is most commonly secondary to rib fractures. Following blunt compression injury to the thorax, pneumothorax can occur without rib fractures or evidence of predisposing cause (Fig. 7–1). A large pneumothorax with atelectasis of the underlying lung and ipsilateral shift of the mediastinum will be obvious on supine conventional radiographs. A small pneumothorax may be more difficult to identify on supine radiographs. In the supine position, a pneumothorax tends to collect in the anteroinferior costodiaphragmatic angle and in the subpulmonic space between the lower lobe and the diaphragm.[25]

CT is the most sensitive method for detecting a small pneumothorax in the supine position.[26, 27] Occult pneumothoraxes are probably more common than previously thought. Tocino and colleagues[26] demonstrated 11 incidental occult pneumothoraxes in 15 patients undergoing CT scanning for head injuries. As a general rule, any patient undergoing

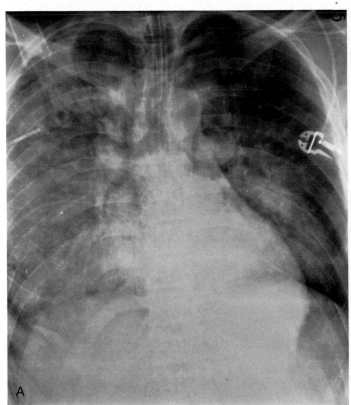

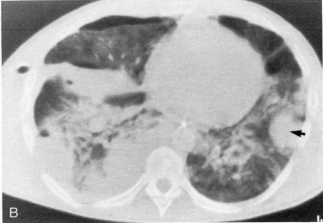

FIGURE 7–1 ■ Pneumothorax and lung contusion following a fall from 45 feet. *A,* Chest radiograph demonstrates bilateral patchy and diffuse lung consolidation. *B,* CT scan shows a small right pneumothorax and patchy consolidation in both lungs. A right hemothorax is also seen posteriorly. An area of contusion *(arrow)* is visible in the left lung.

CT scanning for major trauma should have an image obtained through the lower hemithorax to detect a small pneumothorax. In the clinical circumstances of major trauma, patients may be candidates for emergency surgery or mechanical ventilation. In these circumstances, prophylactic thoracostomy tubes are usually required. In fact, in the study by Tocino and colleagues,[26] 9 of the 11 patients with small pneumothoraces required prophylactic thoracostomy tube insertion.

CT may also help in distinguishing among the causes of confusing air collections adjacent to the mediastinum.[28] Paramediastinal blebs can be distinguished from a medial pneumothorax, air in the inferior pulmonary ligament, and localized pneumopericardium.

PLEURAL EFFUSION

Traumatic pleural effusions are composed of blood, transudate, exudate, or chyle, or a mixture of these fluids. Hemothorax usually occurs from tears of the intercostal, diaphragmatic, mediastinal, or pulmonary veins. Massive hemothorax from arterial bleeding is invariably clinically evident; the patient presents with shock, ventilatory embarrassment, and a large pleural collection on chest radiographs. Emergency tube thoracostomy is normally required. Transudative effusions can be observed without rib fractures or hemothoraces. They can occur with acute lung atelectasis or can be subsequent to vigorous resuscitation with overhydration of the patient. Chylothorax is most common on the left side following laceration of the thoracic duct at the level of its superior arch. The usual cause is direct trauma to the left thoracic inlet, often with an associated fracture of the medial end of the left clavicle.[29]

Pleural effusions of less than 100 to 200 mL cannot be detected on supine chest radiographs (see Fig. 7–1). Most small pleural fluid collections do not require emergency therapeutic intervention, especially in the seriously injured patient. However, changes in their size need to be followed, and they may require sampling to determine their cause. The CT density of a fluid collection may suggest its origin. Fresh hematomas can have a CT density between 50 and 90 H, transudates between 10 and 20 H, and chylothoraces between 0 and − 10 H. These figures are only suggestive of the cause of pleural effusion, and thoracentesis is invariably required for a precise diagnosis.

Lung Parenchyma

CT will demonstrate one or more sites of parenchymal opacification in the overwhelming majority of patients with severe blunt chest trauma.[8] In most of these patients the chest radiographs will be normal. Parenchymal opacification from blunt injury can result from numerous causes. The most common are atelectasis; aspiration of gastric content, blood, or foreign material; pulmonary contusion; pulmonary hemorrhage; focal pulmonary edema; and pulmonary laceration. In most circumstances, neither CT nor conventional chest radiographs can distinguish among these causes of diffuse lung density.

Pulmonary contusion is generally accepted as the primary lung injury following blunt chest trauma.[30, 31] It may occur in as many as 70 per cent of patients after significant blunt chest trauma. Pulmonary contusion implies injury with bleeding into the air spaces and interstitium of the lung but without major disruption of lung architecture.[32] The presence of blood in the lung can cause reactive edema that additionally fills the interstitium and alveoli spaces of the lung. Pulmonary contusion is usually caused by a compression injury adjacent to the site of chest wall injury. The chest wall injury often manifests as a rib fracture or chest wall hematoma.

The radiographic appearance of a pulmonary contusion is variable and ranges from small, patchy, ill-defined areas of consolidation without segmental distribution to large areas of dense parenchymal consolidation. Radiographic abnormalities usually appear within 4 to 6 hours, and the initial radiograph of the contused lung may appear normal. CT is more sensitive than chest radiographs in detecting sites of pulmonary contusion, as well as associated rib fractures or chest wall hematomas.[8, 33] The CT appearance is one of localized, ill-defined areas of hazy ground-glass density or consolidation, usually with a peripheral distribution in the lung (Fig. 7–2). Most lung contusions start resolving within 72 hours and clear in 10 to 14 days without CT or radiographic residue.[8]

Lung laceration is a more severe form of lung injury than pulmonary contusion. Pulmonary laceration implies disruption of the lung architecture with the development of a space containing blood (hematoma) or air (traumatic lung cyst). Radiographically, pulmonary laceration manifests as a circumscribed area of lung density containing air, fluid, or both (Fig. 7–3). Pulmonary laceration can be from penetrating or blunt injury. With penetrating lung injury, the laceration has a configuration conforming to the track of the course of the penetrating injury. In blunt trauma, a laceration initially may be obscured by surrounding pulmonary contusion. Identification of the hematoma or air space within contused lung can be difficult when the contusion is larger than the hematoma or cyst. A concomitant large hemothorax may also obscure the laceration (Fig. 7–4). CT scanning is considerably more sensitive than radiographs in detecting lung lacerations, especially when a fluid level is associated with the laceration. Wagner and co-workers[33] believe that lung laceration is not uncommon. They assert that it is the fundamental component of parenchymal lung injury in pulmonary contusion, hematoma, or traumatic lung cyst, as well as the cause of most cavities in areas of pulmonary contusion. They found that CT scans demonstrated 99 lung lacerations in 85 patients with chest trauma who had an area of

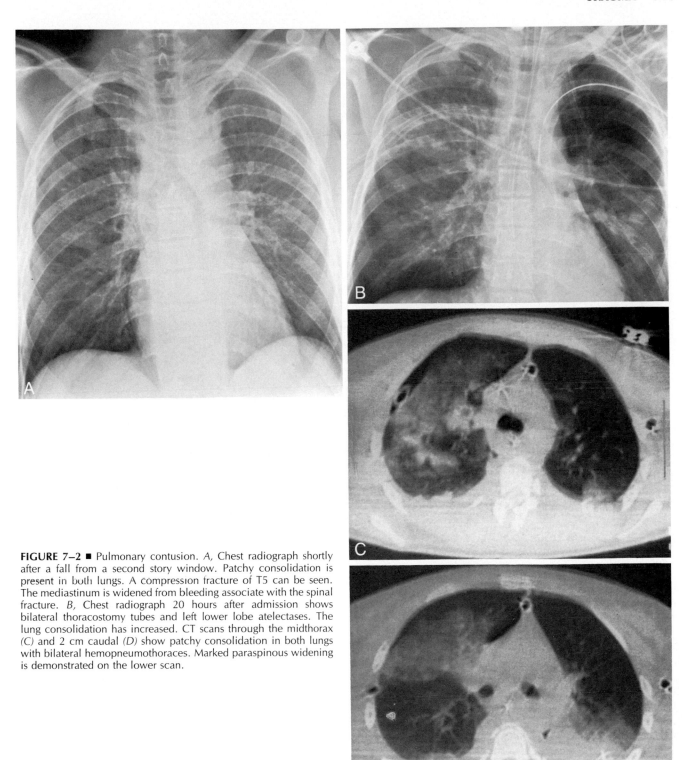

FIGURE 7-2 ■ Pulmonary contusion. *A,* Chest radiograph shortly after a fall from a second story window. Patchy consolidation is present in both lungs. A compression fracture of T5 can be seen. The mediastinum is widened from bleeding associate with the spinal fracture. *B,* Chest radiograph 20 hours after admission shows bilateral thoracostomy tubes and left lower lobe atelectases. The lung consolidation has increased. CT scans through the midthorax *(C)* and 2 cm caudal *(D)* show patchy consolidation in both lungs with bilateral hemopneumothoraces. Marked paraspinous widening is demonstrated on the lower scan.

density on chest radiographs consistent with pulmonary contusion. They described the typical CT appearances of laceration as an air-fluid level in an intraparenchymal cavity; an air space with a linear, nonsegmental configuration within the lung paren-

chyma; or a small peripheral cavity or linear lucency close to the site of a rib fracture, usually associated with a pneumothorax. They also found a paravertebral location to many of their lung lacerations, leading them to postulate that blunt trauma may cause a

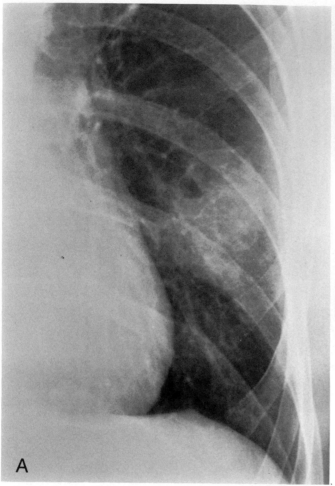

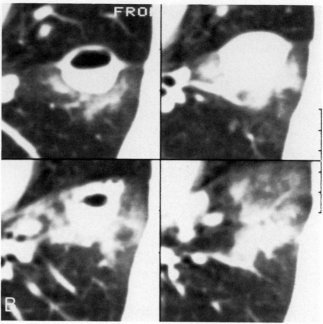

FIGURE 7–3 ■ Pulmonary laceration 3 days after a motor vehicle accident causing left chest trauma. *A,* Chest radiograph shows a circumscribed density in the left lung with a small air-fluid level. *B,* Serial CT scans from superior to inferior demonstrate a well-defined lung mass containing an air-fluid level. Adjacent scans show surrounding patchy consolidation of lung contusion.

sheering injury of the lower lobe across a vertebral body.

The appearances of a cavity several days to 1 week following blunt trauma can be from (1) liquefaction and excavation of a parenchymal hematoma, (2) infection and abscess formation in a site of contusion, (3) abscess formation from aspiration or infection, or (4) clearing of blood around and in a parenchymal laceration.

Pulmonary lacerations normally resolve in weeks to months, or they can become infected.[34] In most instances they resolve without leaving a visible radiographic or CT abnormality but may give rise to a posttraumatic pneumatocele.[35]

Acute traumatic pneumatocele is a thin-walled cystic space resulting from disruption of alveolar walls from a compression injury. It frequently is subpleural and appears in the first hours following trauma.[35] Pulmonary pneumatoceles are a potential cause of pneumothorax, especially in patients undergoing mechanical ventilation requiring high peak-inspiratory pressures or positive end-expiratory pressure. Any patient demonstrating thin-walled subpleural cystic spaces and who is being mechanically ventilated should be considered for prophylactic thoracostomy drainage tubes or carefully monitored for development of a tension pneumothorax.

Both obstructive and nonobstructive atelectases, particularly of the lower lobes, are frequent complications of blunt chest trauma. They can be caused by one or several potential contributing factors. Pain from chest wall injury leads to reduced inspiratory effort, coughing, and movement. Aspiration of foreign material or bronchial wall injury can lead to bronchial obstruction. Edema and blood in the alveolar spaces can produce multiple peripheral endobronchial plugs with airway obstruction. The radiographic features vary from small subsegmental areas of atelectasis to segmental or lobar consolidation. Atelectasis of portions of lung frequently accompanies lung contusion (Fig. 7–5). The CT patterns of lung atelectasis have been described in Chapter 1. CT is more sensitive than chest radiographs in detecting both small and large areas of atelectasis in the immobilized traumatized patient. The presence on CT of a branching pattern of crowded air bronchograms within an area of lung density indicates nonobstructive atelectasis.

Mediastinum

Mediastinal injuries can be from penetrating or blunt trauma. Penetrating injuries from gunshot and stab wounds are most commonly to the heart, coro-

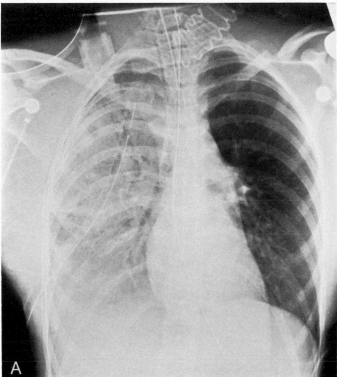

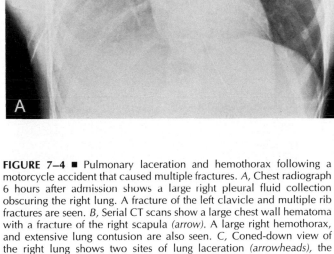

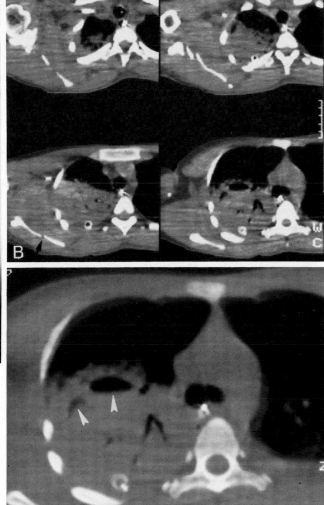

FIGURE 7–4 ■ Pulmonary laceration and hemothorax following a motorcycle accident that caused multiple fractures. *A,* Chest radiograph 6 hours after admission shows a large right pleural fluid collection obscuring the right lung. A fracture of the left clavicle and multiple rib fractures are seen. *B,* Serial CT scans show a large chest wall hematoma with a fracture of the right scapula *(arrow).* A large right hemothorax, and extensive lung contusion are also seen. *C,* Coned-down view of the right lung shows two sites of lung laceration *(arrowheads),* the anterior one containing an air-fluid level. Although air bronchograms are present, no atelectasis has occurred. The posterior chest tube is in good position.

nary arteries, and ascending aorta, resulting in early exsanguination and death.[36] Lesser injuries to these structures may allow the patient to survive until arrival in an emergency care facility. Blunt injuries to the mediastinum include compression injury with or without sternal fractures, deceleration injury to the major arterial vessels, and penetration of mediastinal structures from rib or costochondral fractures. Blunt trauma can result in injury to mediastinal veins and arteries, the trachea and bronchial tree, and, uncommonly, the esophagus.

MEDIASTINAL VESSELS

Blunt injury of the thoracic aorta is frequently lethal. Parmley and colleagues,[37] in an autopsy study, found that 85 per cent of patients with aortic disruption died before arriving at a hospital. Injuries to the ascending aorta are virtually always fatal. Even patients arriving alive at an emergency facility have a high mortality, with 60 per cent dying within the first week. In those who initially survive, the mech-

anism of aortic disruption is thought to be a deceleration injury with sheering of adjacent aortic segments. Eighty-five per cent of these injuries occur at the aortic isthmus, which is the junction between the more fixed distal aortic arch and more mobile descending aorta. With incomplete transection of the aorta, aortic adventitial continuity is maintained, leading to the development of an unstable false aneurysm. These focal disruptions of the aortic wall can enlarge and rupture or can persist as a chronic, calcified pseudoaneurysm that can still rupture.[38] In the acute phase they require prompt diagnosis and surgical repair.

Vertical deceleration injuries of the aorta, caused by falls from a height, most frequently involve the ascending aorta or the aortic arch at the site of origin of the innominate artery. Multiple aortic tears can occur in up to 20 per cent of patients.[37, 39]

The clinical presentation of blunt trauma to the aorta varies from severe cardiovascular compromise to remarkably benign. Up to one half of patients do

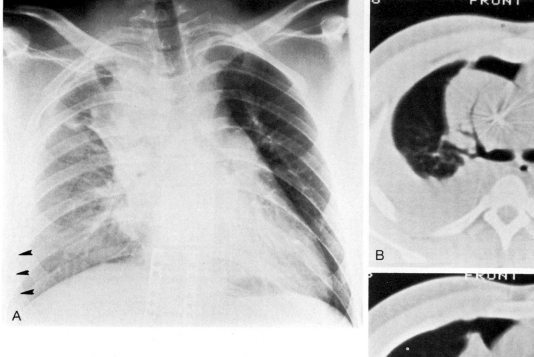

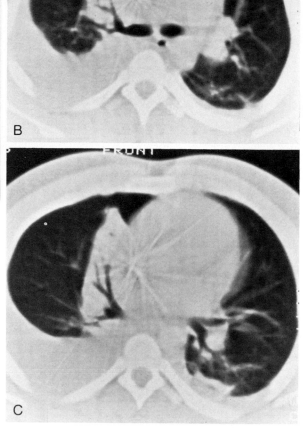

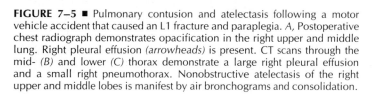

FIGURE 7–5 ■ Pulmonary contusion and atelectasis following a motor vehicle accident that caused an L1 fracture and paraplegia. A, Postoperative chest radiograph demonstrates opacification in the right upper and middle lung. Right pleural effusion *(arrowheads)* is present. CT scans through the mid- *(B)* and lower *(C)* thorax demonstrate a large right pleural effusion and a small right pneumothorax. Nonobstructive atelectasis of the right upper and middle lobes is manifest by air bronchograms and consolidation.

not show evidence of external injury. Hypotension and shock may be evident, and patients may complain of retrosternal or intrascapular pain. A difference in blood pressure between upper and lower extremities may be found in up to one third of patients.

The chest radiographic findings are frequently nonspecific and may include mediastinal widening or alteration in contour; obscuration of the area of the aortic arch, which is evidence of mediastinal hematoma; left pleural effusion; and left lung atelectasis.[12, 40, 41] A left apical pleural cap, deviation of the trachea or esophagus to the right, depression of the left main stem bronchus, and widening of the paravertebral stripes are all indications of mediastinal bleeding and hematoma but are not specific for aortic injury. Fracture of the first and second ribs, sternal fractures, and pulmonary contusion are all indications of massive injury to the thorax, even though they, too, are not specific for an aortic or great vessel injury.[42] Less than 20 per cent of patients with clinical

and radiographic findings suggestive of aortic trauma have angiographic confirmation of an aortic tear.

CT with the intravenous injection of contrast material can distinguish unrelated causes of mediastinal widening from a mediastinal hematoma following vascular injury. Heiberg and colleagues[43] used CT to study ten patients with suspected thoracic aortic injury. They found a multiplicity of CT findings in the four patients with incomplete aortic tear or transection. The findings included a visible false aneurysm that opacified with contrast material, a linear lucency within the opacified aortic lumen indicative of the torn edge of the aortic intima and media, marginal irregularity of the opacified aortic lumen, a mass adjacent to the aorta indicative of periaortic or intramural aortic hematoma, and evidence of aortic dissection. The CT features of a false aneurysm consisted of a focal increase in caliber of the aortic lumen or a saccular outpouching of the aortic wall and deformity of the opacified aortic lumen.

Sanchez and colleagues[44] have shown that in traumatized patients with suspected aortic injury, CT can show an alternative cause of an apparent wide superior mediastinum, obviating the need for angiography. These benign causes of mediastinal widening included focal deposits of fat, a persistent left SVC, hemiazygos continuation of the IVC, and a right aortic arch with or without an aberrant left subclavian artery. A paravertebral pleural effusion on a supine radiograph can also mimic mediastinal widening or widening of the left paraspinal line. In patients with CT findings indicating an aortic injury, an aortogram is usually needed to confirm the diagnosis prior to surgical repair. If CT provides an alternative cause for the mediastinal widening, angiography can be avoided. Available experience is insufficient to determine whether a normal CT of the aorta can exclude all aortic injuries and obviate the need for aortography. Investigation of the clinically unstable patient with suspected aortic injury should not include CT, and the more conclusive arteriogram should be undertaken immediately (Fig. 7–6).[45]

TRACHEA AND BRONCHI

Traumatic disruption of the tracheobronchial tree usually occurs in the lower third of the trachea or main stem bronchi and only with severe trauma, as manifest by multiple rib or sternal fractures.[46] The clinical presentation often includes hemoptysis, airway obstruction, tension pneumothorax, and subcutaneous emphysema. The chest radiograph classically shows pneumomediastinum and pneumothorax. Failure of the lung to collapse in the presence of a large pneumothorax may be indicative of bronchial mucosal hematoma with bronchial obstruction and a tear of the bronchial wall. Alternatively, with complete transection of the hilar bronchus and a large pneumothorax, the lung falls to a dependent position in the hemithorax, producing the so-called "falling lung" sign. CT may demonstrate a subtle pneumomediastinum in the midmediastinal compartment that is not evident from chest radiographs.[47] With tracheal tears, CT may demonstrate malposition of the tip of an endotracheal tube, with protrusion beyond the tracheal lumen or overdistention of an endotracheal balloon cuff, both indicating discontinuity of the tracheal wall.[9] Urgent bronchoscopy is required for confirmation of suspected tracheal or bronchial injury.

HEART AND PERICARDIUM

Traumatic wounds to the heart, whether caused by open or blunt injuries, have a mortality rate of approximately 50 per cent. The spectrum of traumatic injuries to the heart and pericardium ranges from the inconsequential to the immediately fatal. Blunt cardiac injury can occur from one or a combination of several mechanisms. Direct force to the pericardium, compression of the heart between the sternum and the vertebral column, differential deceleration, or rapid increase in intracardiac volume due to abdominal compression can all result in cardiac injury. Most blunt cardiac injuries are the result of motor vehicle accidents. In fatal injuries, rupture of one or more of the cardiac chambers occurs in two thirds of instances, and multiple organ injury occurs in 50 per cent.[48]

Myocardial contusion is the most frequent result of blunt trauma to the heart. The right ventricle,

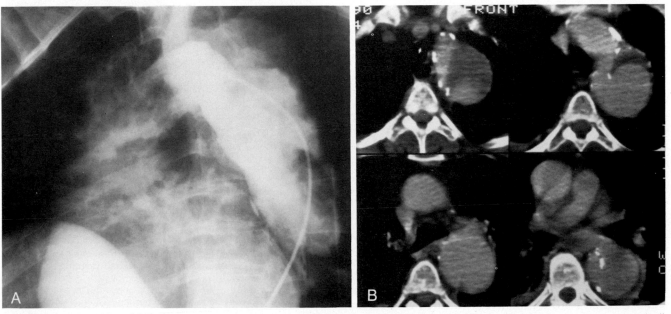

FIGURE 7–6 ■ Traumatic rupture of the aorta in a 70-year-old woman following a deceleration accident. A chest radiograph showed a markedly widened mediastinum. *A,* Thoracic aortic angiogram shows an angiographic catheter with its tip in the false channel of a traumatic dissection. The catheter could not be advanced beyond the midaortic arch. Both true and false lumens of the aorta are opacified. *B,* CT scan following the angiogram shows the partially clotted false aneurysm *(upper panels)* and aortic dissection *(bottom panels).*

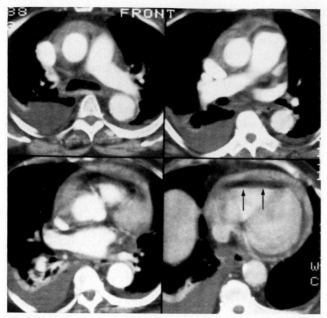

FIGURE 7–7 ■ Hemopericardium and hemothorax after an airplane accident that caused cardiogenic shock. An echocardiogram was suggestive of cardiac tamponade. Serial CT scans show a large hemopericardium with a fat–soft tissue level *(arrows)*, anteriorly. High-density (60 to 80 H) blood extends into the superior pericardial recesses around the aortic root. A large right hemothorax is causing compression atelectasis of the right lower lobe.

anteriorly located, is more liable to damage than the other cardiac chambers. In addition to myocardial contusion and rupture, cardiac injuries include damage to the pulmonary arteries, valvular incompetence, traumatic interventricular septal defects, and pericardial bleeding.[48, 49]

Cardiac tamponade resulting from hemopericardium is unusual with nonpenetrating chest trauma, unless it is associated with aortic rupture, coronary artery laceration, or mediastinal hemorrhage (Fig. 7–7). Small pericardial hematomas without clinical or functional significance are not uncommon and may be seen as an incidental finding on CT examination of the injured thorax.

CT is not indicated in patients with suspected cardiac injury who manifest right or left ventricular dysfunction or cardiogenic shock. An emergency echocardiogram should be obtained to detect significant pericardial fluid that may require urgent drainage. Later evaluation of the myocardium with a detailed echocardiogram and isotope studies can be undertaken to predict possible long-term sequelae, such as the development of scar tissue and dyskinetic segments and possible future arrythmias.

MEDIASTINAL HEMATOMA

Focal or diffuse bleeding into the mediastinum is common following compression injuries of the thorax. Concomitant sternal fractures may be present. Bleeding into the mediastinum can be from rupture of mediastinal veins or arteries. In the absence of significant damage to the aortic or coronary vessels, venous bleeding is most likely. Clinical evi-

dence of continued bleeding without apparent cause should lead to careful angiographic evaluation of the internal mammary and intercostal arteries and their branches.

In patients with mediastinal bleeding, CT can demonstrate focal accumulation of blood or diffuse bleeding in the mediastinum. Bleeding will show focal soft tissue densities or diffuse replacement of mediastinal fat density by soft tissue density (Fig. 7–8). The mediastinal tissue planes between adjacent organs will be disrupted. CT only rarely shows the site of bleeding, even after infusion of a bolus of contrast material. The site of the accumulation of blood within

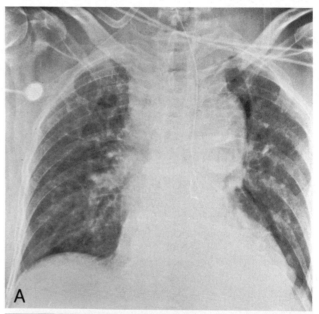

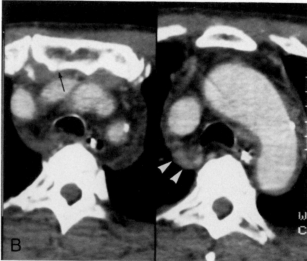

FIGURE 7–8 ■ Mediastinal hematoma from mediastinal venous bleeding. *A,* Chest radiograph shows marked widening of the upper mediastinum without obscuration of the aortic arch. A paramediastinal air collection on the left represents a pneumothorax in the supine patient. *B,* CT scans through the upper mediastinum show a dilated aorta, a fracture of the manubrium *(arrow)*, and obliteration of tissue planes. An aortogram did not show an aortic tear. At necropsy, a lacerated azygous arch was found. In retrospect, irregularity in the region of the azygous vein *(arrowheads)* may have been significant.

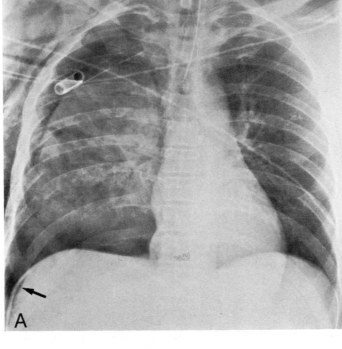
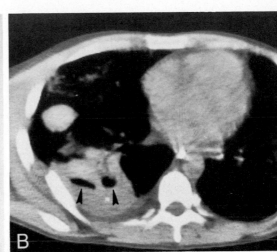
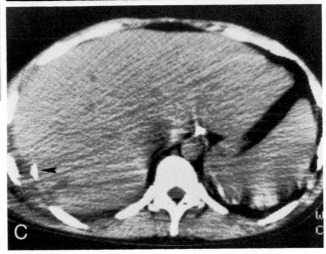

FIGURE 7–9 ■ Perforated diaphragm following a motor vehicle accident that caused multiple fractures and a perforated right hemidiaphragm. *A,* Chest radiograph demonstrates a right clavicle fracture, multiple right rib fractures, a large pneumothorax, and air beneath the right hemidiaphragm *(arrow). B,* CT scan through the lower thorax shows two sites of lung laceration *(arrowheads)* with a large area of contusion around them. A small pleural effusion is present. *C,* CT scan through the liver shows a rib segment *(arrowhead)* that had perforated the diaphragm.

the mediastinum may provide an indirect indication of the bleeding site.

Diaphragm

Diaphragmatic tear or rupture is more commonly caused by abdominal trauma than by chest injury.[50-52] Both penetrating wounds and blunt trauma to the lower chest and upper abdomen can cause diaphragmatic disruption. Most commonly, the cause of blunt diaphragmatic rupture is an abrupt increase in pressure as a result of compression of the upper abdomen and lower anterior thorax. Internal injury to the diaphragm can also be from fractures of the lower thoracic ribs (Fig. 7–9). With blunt trauma the diaphragm most frequently ruptures at the junction of its central fibrous tendon and muscular peripheral portions. The posterior and posterolateral diaphragmatic segments are those most commonly involved. The left hemidiaphragm is more commonly involved than the right, with a ratio of 2:1.[53, 54] Earlier studies gave a 90 to 95 per cent predominance of left-sided rupture, an overestimate because of the difficulty in diagnosing right hemidiaphragmatic injuries.[55] Small lacerations of the diaphragm may enlarge over time, and a delay of months or years in diagnosis is not

uncommon. With laceration of the left hemidiaphragm, a loop of bowel, omentum, part of the stomach, or spleen can herniate into the thorax. With tears of the right hemidiaphragm, the right lobe of the liver is the offending organ.

Conventional radiographs disclose an apparent elevation of the hemidiaphragm with large lacerations. A mass or pseudomass is frequently visible at the lung base.[52, 56] A specific diagnosis of diaphragmatic rupture can be made when gas-containing bowel loops are clearly demonstrated above the level of the hemidiaphragm. A concomitant pleural effusion or hemothorax can obscure the precise location of the underlying diaphragm and its laceration. When a pneumothorax is present, air may enter the abdominal cavity through the traumatized parietal pleura, diaphragm, and peritoneum. The conventional chest radiograph is abnormal in most patients with diaphragmatic rupture and strongly suggests the diagnosis in about 50 per cent of instances.[52, 56, 57] Occasionally an inserted nasogastric tube can be seen passing through the esophageal hiatus and then coursing superiorly to the expected position of the left lower lung.

Several reports have discussed the use of CT for imaging lacerations of the left hemidiaphragm.[30, 56, 58]

CT can detect the defect in the diaphragm, the bowel loops protruding into the thorax, and the site at which the loops are narrowed as they pass through the defect. Laceration of the right hemidiaphragm is more difficult to demonstrate with CT, because the diaphragm and liver are of similar density, and it can be difficult to separate the two.[58a]

Ultrasonograms using appropriate transducers are the best and simplest method of demonstrating diaphragmatic lacerations.[59, 60] The diaphragm is readily displayed as an echogenic structure. Pleural effusions, which are commonly present, allow for demonstration of the diaphragm and its site of discontinuity. The quality of the ultrasound examination may be compromised in patients with a pneumothorax or with distended bowel. Mirvis and colleagues[61] have described a single case in which MR was used to evaluate the left hemidiaphragm for possible rupture. Transaxial, sagittal, and coronal images confirmed herniation of the colon through a tear in the anterior diaphragm.

Indications for CT in Thoracic Trauma

Modern imaging technology, including CT and ultrasound, is applied to the acutely traumatized patient. CT is an established important modality for imaging of abdominal trauma, and this has led to its more frequent use in the patient with thoracic trauma. CT can assist in the evaluation of patients with suspected injuries to the chest wall, sternum, scapula, and other components of the thoracic cage. Detection of small pneumothoraces may have definite clinical importance in the patient being considered for ventilatory support or general anesthesia. In the clinically stable patient with suspected damage to the great vessels, CT can exclude benign causes of mediastinal widening and demonstrate features that strongly suggest aortic disruption. The CT finding of hemorrhage within the mediastinum is invariably an indication for aortography. CT can detect and assess sites of injury to the lungs, including pulmonary contusion and laceration.

Additional studies to define the sensitivity and specificity for the CT detection of injuries to the diaphragm and the aorta are warranted. With the proliferation of CT scanners and their availability and proximity to emergency facilities, the increasing use of CT in imaging of the injured patient can be anticipated. Appropriate efficacy studies are definitely needed to further define the clinical circumstances in which CT will be of major benefit.

References

1. Baxt WG, Moody P: The impact of a rotorcraft aero-medical emergency care service on trauma mortality. JAMA 249:3047, 1982.
2. Blair E, Topuzulu C, Deane RS. Major blunt chest trauma. In Current Problems in Surgery. Chicago, Year Book Medical, 1969.
3. Federle MP: CT: a major innovation in care of trauma victims. Diagn Imaging 3:58, 1987.
4. McCort JJ: Improving results of trauma care: The contribution of radiology. President's address at the Radiological Society of North America, 72nd Scientific Assembly and Meeting, Chicago, IL, December 1, 1986.
5. Davis SJ, Bryson BL, Thompson JS, Anderson JC: The role of computed tomography in blunt trauma. Nebr Med J 70:3, 1985.
6. Zimmerman RA, Bilaniuk LT, Gennarelli T, Bruce D, Dolinskas C, Uzzell B: Cranial computed tomography in diagnosis and management of acute head trauma. AJR 131:127, 1978.
7. Tocino I, Miller MH, Frederick PR, Bahr AL, Thomas F: CT detection of occult pneumothorax in head trauma. AJR 143:987, 1984.
8. Tocino I, Miller MH: Computed tomography in blunt chest trauma. J Thorac Imaging 2:45, 1987.
9. Tocino IM: Role of CT in chest trauma. Radiology 2:164, 1990.
10. Toombs BD: Acute chest trauma. In Toombs BD, Sandler CM, Computed Tomography in Trauma. Philadelphia; WB Saunders, 1987.
11. Somogyi JW, Finucane BT: Traumatic and iatrogenic changes in the pleura and mediastinum. In Murphy CH, Murphy MR (eds): Radiology for Anesthesia and Critical Care. Edinburgh, Churchill Livingstone, 1987.
12. Simeone JF, Minagi H, Putnam CE: Traumatic disruption of the thoracic aorta: significance of the left apical extrapleural cap. Radiology 117:265, 1975.
13. Fisher RG, Ward RE, Ben-Menachem Y, Mattox KL, Flynn TC: Arteriography and the fractured first rib: too much for too little? AJR 138:1059, 1982.
14. Barica TC, Livoni JP: Indications for angiography in blunt thoracic trauma. Radiology 147:15, 1983.
15. Trunkey DD, Lewis FR: Chest trauma. Surg Clin North Am 60:1541, 1980.
16. Livoni JP, Barcia TC: Fracture of the first and second rib: incidence of vascular injury relative to type of fracture. Radiology 145:31, 1982.
17. Rubenstein JD, Ebrahein NA, Kellam JF: Traumatic scapulothoracic dissociation. Radiology 157:297, 1985.
18. Oreck SL, Burgess A, Levine AM: Traumatic lateral displacement of the scapula: a radiographic sign of neurovascular disruption. J Bone Joint Surg 66A:758, 1984.
19. Goodman PC: CT of chest trauma. In Federle MP, Brant-Zawadzki M (eds): Computed Tomography in the Evaluation of Trauma. 2d ed. Baltimore, Williams & Wilkins, 1986, p. 168.
20. Kattan KR: What to look for in rib fractures and how. JAMA 243:262, 1980.
21. Levinsohn EM, Bunnell WP, Yuan HA: Computed tomography in the diagnosis of the sternoclavicular joint. Clin Orthop 140:12, 1979.
22. Neer CS, Rockwood CA Jr: Fractures and dislocations of the shoulder. In Rockwood CA Jr, Green DP (eds): Fractures. Philadelphia, JB Lippincott, 1975, p 585.
23. Adler OB, Rosenberger A: Localization of metallic foreign bodies in the chest by computed tomography. J Comput Assis Tomogr 6:955, 1982.
24. Dougall AM, Paul ME, Finley RJ, Holliday RL, Coles JG, Duff JH: Chest trauma: current morbidity and mortality. J Trauma 17:547, 1985.
25. Tocino IM: Pneumothorax in the supine patient. Radiographic anatomy. Radiographics 5:557, 1985.
26. Tocino I, Miller MH, Frederick PR, Bahr AL, Thomas F: CT detection of occult pneumothorax in head trauma. AJR 143:987, 1984.
27. Wall S, Federle MF, Jeffrey RB, Brett CM: CT diagnosis of unsuspected pneumothorax after blunt abdominal trauma. AJR 141:919, 1983.
28. Godwin JD, Merten DF, Baker ME: Paramediastinal pneumatocele: alternative explanations to gas in the pulmonary ligament. AJR 145:525, 1985.
29. MacFarlan JR, Holman CW: Chylothorax. Am Rev Resp Dis 105:287, 1972.
30. Toombs BD, Sandler CM, Lester RG: Computed tomography of chest trauma. Radiology 140:733, 1981.

31. Stevens E, Templeton AW: Traumatic nonpenetrating lung contusion. Radiology 85:247, 1985.
32. Shackford SR: Blunt chest trauma: the intensivist's perspective. J Intensive Care Med 1:125, 1986.
33. Wagner RB, Crawford WO Jr, Schimpf PP: Classification of parenchyma injuries of the lung. Radiology 167:77, 1988.
34. Crawford WO Jr: Pulmonary injury in thoracic and non-thoracic trauma. Radiol Clin North Am 11:527, 1973.
35. Ganske JG, Dennis DL, Vanderveer JB Jr: Traumatic lung cyst: case report and literature review. J Trauma 21:493, 1981.
36. Symbas PN, Sehdeva JS: Penetrating wounds of the thoracic aorta. Ann Surg 171:441, 1970.
37. Parmley LF, Mattengly TW, Manion WC, Jahnke EJ: Nonpenetrating traumatic injury of the aorta. Circulation 17:1086, 1958.
38. Fleming AW, Green DC: Traumatic aneurysms of the thoracic aorta. Ann Thorac Surg 18:91, 1974.
39. Greendyke RM: Traumatic rupture of the aorta: special reference to automobile accidents. JAMA 195:119, 1966.
40. Tisnado J, Tsai FY, Als A, Roach JF: A new radiographic sign of acute traumatic rupture of the thoracic aorta: displacement of the nasogastric tube to the right. Radiology 125:603, 1977.
41. Stark P: Traumatic rupture of the thoracic aorta: a review. CRC Crit Rev Diagn Imaging 21:229, 1984.
42. Seltzer SE, D'Orsi C, Kirschner R, DeWeese JA: Traumatic aortic rupture plain radiographic findings. AJR 137:1011, 1981.
43. Heiberg E, Wolverson MK, Sundaram M, Shields JB: CT in aortic trauma. AJR 140:1119, 1983.
44. Sanchez FW, Greer CF, Thomason DM, Vijie I: Hemiazygous continuation of a left inferior vena cava: misleading radiographic findings in chest trauma. Cardiovasc Interven Radiol (W Ger) 8:140, 1985.
45. Mirvis SE, Pais SO, Gens DR: Thoracic aorta rupture: advantages of intraarterial digital subtraction angiography. AJR 146:987, 1986.
46. Deslauries J: Major injuries: bronchial rupture. In Grillo HC, Eschapasse H (eds): International Trends in General Thoracic Surgery, Vol 2. Major Challenges. Philadelphia, WB Saunders, 1987, p 246.
47. Rollins RJ, Tocino IM: Early radiographic signs of tracheal rupture. AJR 148:695, 1987.
48. Parmley LF, Manion WC, Mattingly TW: Nonpenetrating traumatic injury of the heart. Circulation 18:371, 1958.
49. Dow RW: Myocardial rupture caused by trauma. Surgery 91:246, 1982.
50. Orringer MB, Kirsch MM: Traumatic rupture of the diaphragm. In Kirsch MM, Sloan H (eds): Blunt Chest Trauma. General Principles of Management. Boston, Little, Brown, 1977.
51. Brooks JK: Blunt traumatic rupture of the diaphragm. Ann Thorac Surg 26:199, 1978.
52. Wiencek RG, Wilson RF, Steiger Z: Acute injuries of the diaphragm: an analysis of 165 cases. J Thorac Cardiovasc Surg 92:989, 1986.
53. Brown GL, Richardson JD: Traumatic diaphragmatic hernia: a continuing challenge. Ann Thorac Surg 39:170, 1985.
54. Beal SL, McKennan M: Blunt diaphragm rupture: a morbid injury. Arch Surg 26:199, 1978.
55. Ramstrim S, Alsen S: Diaphragmatic rupture following abdominal injuries. Acta Chir Scand 107:304, 1954.
56. Heiber E, Wolverson MK, Hurd RN, Jagannadharao B, Sundaram M: Case report. CT recognition of traumatic rupture of the diaphragm. AJR 135:369, 1980.
57. Ball T, McCrory R, Smith JO, Clements JL Jr: Traumatic diaphragmatic hernia: errors in diagnosis. AJR 138:633, 1982.
58. Adamthwaite DN, Snyders DC, Mirwis J: Traumatic pericardiophrenic hernia: a report of 3 cases. Br J Surg 70:117, 1983.
58a. Gelman R, Mirvis SE, Gens D: Diaphragmatic rupture due to blunt trauma: sensitivity of plain chest radiographs. AJR 156:51, 1991.
59. Rao KG, Woodlief RM: Grey scale ultrasonic demonstration of ruptured right hemidiaphragm. Br J Radiol 53:812, 1980.
60. Ammann AM, Brewer WH, Maull KI, Walsh JW: Traumatic rupture of the diaphragm: real-time sonographic diagnosis. AJR 140:915, 1983.
61. Mirvis SE, Keramati B, Buckman R, Rodriguez A: MR imaging of traumatic diaphragmatic rupture. J Comput Assist Tomogr 12:147, 1988.

CHAPTER 8

INTERVENTIONAL TECHNIQUES

JEFFREY S. KLEIN

Interventional procedures are now commonly performed for pulmonary, pleural, and mediastinal disorders. This chapter describes the use of computed tomography (CT) for percutaneous transthoracic needle biopsy of pulmonary nodules and masses and for the percutaneous drainage of intrathoracic fluid collections.

Percutaneous Transthoracic Needle Biopsy

First described in 1888, transthoracic needle biopsy (TNB) is a diagnostic procedure performed by radiologists and pulmonologists to evaluate focal chest disease. Advances in imaging technology and interventional techniques, the development of small-gauge needles capable of providing histologic specimens, and the emergence of cytopathology as a subspecialty have made TNB a safe, rapid, and accurate diagnostic test.

At our institution, the majority of transthoracic biopsies are performed using CT guidance. This is primarily because of the ready availability of CT as compared with biplane or C-arm fluoroscopy and the preference of the radiologists who routinely perform this procedure. An additional benefit of CT-guided biopsy is that it can be performed immediately following indeterminate CT nodule densitometry,

thereby making optimal use of CT time and expediting diagnosis. Patients with suspected bronchogenic carcinoma or metastatic disease are often anxious, and a rapid diagnosis after detection of an intrathoracic mass cannot be overemphasized.

Indications and Patient Selection

Most patients referred for TNB have been evaluated by a pulmonologist or thoracic surgeon after referral by a primary care physician for an intrathoracic mass. These patients are usually in one of the categories listed in Table 8–1.

TNB should be performed by physicians who have extensive experience with the technique and access to the imaging modalities required to perform the procedure. The availability of expert cytopathologists is critical to the proper handling and interpretation

TABLE 8–1 ■ Indications for Transthoracic Needle Biopsy of the Thorax

1. A new or enlarging solitary pulmonary nodule or mass
2. An undiagnosed mediastinal mass
3. A hilar mass when bronchoscopy is nondiagnostic
4. An intra- or extrathoracic malignancy and a hilar, mediastinal, or parenchymal mass/adenopathy requiring staging
5. Focal or multifocal parenchymal consolidation when an infectious organism has not been isolated
6. Suspected lymphangitic carcinomatosis or opportunistic pneumonia when bronchoscopy is nondiagnostic

TABLE 8–2 ■ Relative Contraindications to TNB

1. Moderate or severe obstructive lung disease (FEV$_1$ <1.0 L)
2. Patient on positive end-expiratory pressure (PEEP) ventilation
3. Bullae in the vicinity of the lesion undergoing biopsy
4. Bleeding diathesis (prothrombin time >3 sec over control or platelet count <100,000)
5. Possible echinococcal cyst
6. Possible pulmonary arteriovenous malformation
7. Patient uncooperative or unable to maintain constant position (e.g., prone)
8. Intractable cough
9. Prior pneumonectomy
10. Pulmonary hypertension

of the aspirated specimens. A close rapport between operator and radiology technician facilitates accurate localization of the lesion and shortens the duration of the procedure, thereby limiting patient discomfort and reducing the incidence of complications.

Contraindications

There are no absolute contraindications to TNB of the chest. However, several preexisting conditions significantly increase the complication rate from TNB. Chronic obstructive pulmonary disease (COPD) is the most common condition encountered as a risk factor for TNB-related pneumothorax and the rare entity of air embolism. When any of the other recognized risk factors are present (Table 8–2), an attempt is made to correct them (e.g., platelet transfusion for thrombocytopenia), or alternative methods of diagnosis are considered.

Prebiopsy Imaging and Testing

In addition to having frontal and lateral chest radiographs, most patients referred for TNB undergo contrast-enhanced chest CT to characterize the focal abnormality and assess the hila and mediastinum. When CT demonstrates a hypervascular lesion (e.g., metastatic renal cell carcinoma), the risks of hemorrhage must be weighed against the information obtainable from TNB. If a specific diagnosis (e.g., calcified granuloma, hamartoma, anteriovenous malformation, bronchogenic cyst) cannot be made by CT and there is no endobronchial or mediastinal lesion accessible to bronchoscopic biopsy, the patient usually proceeds to TNB. When performed for suspected bronchogenic carcinoma, the chest CT should continue caudally through the upper abdomen to screen for metastatic involvement of the liver, spleen, and adrenal glands. This is important, because patients with a chest lesion suggestive of a primary neoplasm and a liver or adrenal mass are often best diagnosed and staged by biopsy of the abdominal lesion.

A CT is also useful in planning a safe approach to a lesion that will be biopsied using biplane fluoroscopy or ultrasound for localization. For example, lesions that are visible in only one plane on radiographs or fluoroscopy can be localized on CT and the depth from the needle entry site measured to facilitate fluoroscopic biopsy.[1] Masses that are seen on CT to involve the chest wall or pleura or demonstrate a broad area of contact with the pleura may undergo biopsy using real-time ultrasound. Biopsies can be safely performed on these peripheral masses using cutting needles that provide specimens suitable for histology.

We advocate that all patients have a blood coagulation profile, including a platelet count, prothrombin time, and partial thromboplastin time. Those with central lesions in whom intravenous contrast might be used to facilitate a CT-guided biopsy may require renal function tests (blood urea nitrogen and serum creatinine). Pulmonary function tests, although somewhat useful in predicting a patient's risk of developing a pneumothorax, are not routinely performed prior to TNB.

Frontal and lateral chest radiographs are obtained immediately prior to performing CT-directed TNB. This baseline examination aids in the detection of postbiopsy pneumothorax and hemorrhage. Rarely, the preprocedure films show that the lesion has regressed or disappeared, obviating the need for biopsy.

Informed Consent and Arrangements with Pathology

Nearly 85 per cent of TNBs performed at our institution are done as outpatient procedures, and consent is obtained just prior to the biopsy on the morning of the patient's arrival at the hospital. Usually the referring physician has had a preliminary discussion of the procedure with the patient and has instructed the patient not to eat for at least 6 hours before the procedure. Prior to the procedure, the physician performing the biopsy should explain to the patient the details of TNB, including specific risks and benefits of the procedure and alternative methods of diagnosis (including the option of no further procedures or tests). The patient should be given the opportunity to ask questions regarding the procedure prior to giving consent.

The cytopathologist is consulted well before the procedure is to begin. This is important, because at many medical centers one person is responsible for all fine-needle aspiration biopsies performed on a given day, and arrangements must be made to have a microscope at the biopsy site for immediate determination of the adequacy of the aspirated specimen. Especially important are a history of malignancy, prior biopsies, or surgery (and whether these were performed at the same institution) and the most likely origin of the lesion under investigation. For instance, if metastatic breast carcinoma is a possibility, the cytopathologist may bring liquid nitrogen to the biopsy area so that the specimen can be processed for estrogen receptors. Similarly, a refrigerated plastic fixative (1 per cent paraformaldehyde) is needed for cell surface marker studies of lymphoma cells.

CT-Directed TNB

Biplane fluoroscopy, CT, and ultrasound can all be used to guide TNB. The size, position, and visibility of the lesion; the patient's ability to cooperate; the availability of the equipment; and the preference of the physician performing the procedure are all factors to consider when deciding which modality to use. Most radiologists perform the majority of biopsies under fluoroscopy, because it is familiar to most operating physicians, is readily available, and provides real-time visualization during needle placement and sampling of the lesion. An immediate assessment for a large pneumothorax can be made while the patient remains on the fluoroscopy table, and if necessary, a small-bore chest tube can be placed.

Recently several investigators have reported the use of ultrasound to guide TNB.[2, 3] The chest wall and diaphragm provide the only acoustic windows, and ultrasound is limited to masses that are apical, juxtadiaphragmatic, next to the chest wall, and in the anterior mediastinum.[2] Real-time imaging allows biopsy of juxtadiaphragmatic lesions that move with respiration. Puncture of the lesion can be visualized, certifying accurate sampling. The detection of cystic areas within a mass can prevent sampling of a necrotic area that lacks viable cells needed to make a diagnosis. Additional advantages of ultrasound include transducers with adapters that allow accurate needle placement; the ability to localize vascular structures, the portable nature of many ultrasound units, and the absence of ionizing radiation. Disad-

TABLE 8–3 ■ Advantages and Disadvantages of CT-Directed TNB

Advantages
1. Nodule densitometry and biopsy can be performed at one appointment
2. Biopsy of nodules not seen on fluoroscopy or seen in only one plane
3. Direct visualization of intervening bullae and vessels
4. Contrast enhancement distinguishes central masses from postobstructive pneumonitis
5. Confirmation of position of needle tip within mass (small, peripheral, or cavitary lesions)

Disadvantages
1. Longer length of procedure
2. Lack of real-time capability (increased number of pleural punctures)
3. Higher incidence of pneumothorax

vantages include the inability to image and sample lesions not contiguous with the chest wall or diaphragm, a lack of familiarity with the modality by most physicians performing TNB, and the bulkiness of the linear array probe with its puncture unit, making intercostal scanning difficult.[3]

The advantages and disadvantages of CT-directed TNB are shown in Table 8–3. The ability to biopsy a nodule immediately following indeterminate nodule densitometry is a major advantage of CT. CT is most often used when a lesion is visible in only one plane on radiographs or fluoroscopy (Fig. 8–1). In this situation, CT can be used to measure the depth of the lesion for subsequent fluoroscopic biopsy. Alternatively, the entire procedure can be performed using CT. CT is also used to perform biopsies on

FIGURE 8–1 ■ *A*, Coned-down view of the right lung in a 72-year-old asymptomatic man demonstrates an 8-mm nodule in the right midlung not seen on the lateral radiograph. *B*, CT scan through the nodule immediately following TNB shows the needle tract opacified by the blood patch administered on removal of the outer coaxial needle. Cytologic examination revealed a fibroma, which has remained stable for two years.

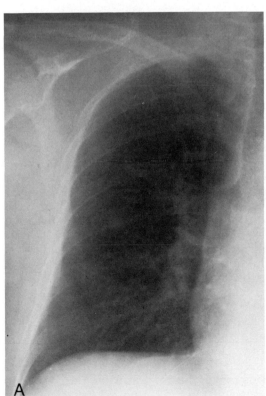
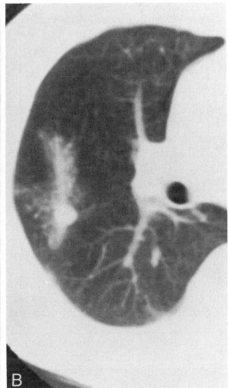

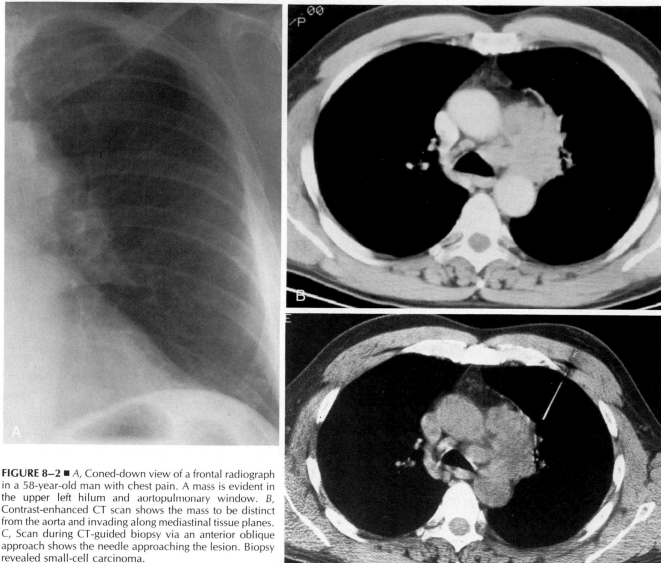

FIGURE 8–2 ■ *A*, Coned-down view of a frontal radiograph in a 58-year-old man with chest pain. A mass is evident in the upper left hilum and aortopulmonary window. *B*, Contrast-enhanced CT scan shows the mass to be distinct from the aorta and invading along mediastinal tissue planes. *C*, Scan during CT-guided biopsy via an anterior oblique approach shows the needle approaching the lesion. Biopsy revealed small-cell carcinoma.

small or peripheral subpleural lesions not visible on fluoroscopy. In patients with bullae, small apical lung masses in proximity to the subclavian vessels, or small central lesions abutting major vascular structures, CT allows planning of the biopsy tract and a safe passage for the biopsy. For similar reasons, lesions around the hilum or in the mediastinum should undergo biopsy with the aid of CT (Fig. 8–2).[4] TNB in patients with central masses and postobstructive pneumonitis should employ contrast-enhanced CT to distinguish between the hypovascular central mass and the enhancing consolidated lung, thereby facilitating biopsy of the mass. The transaxial images of CT allow accurate localization of the tip of the biopsy needle, ensuring that the lesion has been sampled. This is important when malignant cells are not recovered from the aspirate and the cytopathologist is trying to diagnose benign disease. Biopsies of cavitary masses are best obtained using CT localization so that the needle may be directed toward

viable tumor within the wall of the cavity and sampling of the central cavity can be avoided.

Biopsies performed under CT generally take longer than those performed under fluoroscopy or ultrasound guidance. This is because of the time required for repeated image acquisition and reconstruction and the time required to reposition and repuncture the lung for accurate needle tip placement within small lesions. A higher incidence of pneumothorax from CT-directed TNB has been attributed to the longer length of CT-guided procedures and the greater number of pleural punctures required for needle positioning.

Biopsy Needles

A wide array of needles can be used for TNB. Initially, large-bore (12- to 16-gauge) needles designed for use in other parts of the body and capable of obtaining large tissue samples were used in the 1960s and 1970s. These needles caused a relatively high rate of bleeding and pneumothorax and limited the appeal of TNB. The emergence of cytopathology as a subspecialty and the development of small-gauge (18- to 22-gauge) needles capable of providing both histologic and cytologic material in a majority of cases have made TNB a widely accepted procedure that is associated with a high diagnostic yield and a low complication rate.

The biopsy needles used are generally of two types: aspirating needles (e.g., spinal and Chiba needles) and cutting needles (Fig. 8–3). The latter may have a circumferential cutting tip (Greene needle), a receptacle slot just proximal to the tip (Westcott needle), or an inner receptacle combined with an outer guillotine type cutting sheath (Tru-Cut needle). Most of these needles are available in diameters ranging from 16 to 22 gauge. They may be introduced alone, in tandem with a localizing thin needle, or coaxially through a parent needle. Thin needles alone create a smaller hole in the lung and pleura, thereby minimizing the risk of bleeding or pneumothorax. Of course, this benefit holds true only if adequate material is obtained on the first pass, and thus the experience of the operator and cytopathologist and the size, nature, and position of the mass become important. For example, the diagnosis of lymphoreticular malignancies (such as lymphoma) and of benign lesions (such as hamartomas) can be difficult from cytologic specimens. Although many investigators report a greater than 50 per cent recovery of histologic specimens with the use of 22-gauge cutting needles, this has not been our experience. When it is necessary to obtain a specimen for histologic evaluation, we use a larger cutting needle alone or in tandem with a thinner needle, or we obtain a tissue specimen on withdrawal of the outer coaxial needle. For biopsy of rib or vertebral lesions, we use a 17-gauge E-Z-EM threaded bone biopsy needle (Fig. 8–4). When the lesion on which the biopsy is to be performed provides a large window (usually large mediastinal, pleural, or chest wall masses), a cutting needle (e.g., Tru-Cut) can be safely used initially and provides the best specimen. Similarly, when expert cytopathologists are not available, it may be advisable to attempt a core biopsy for histologic material.

Technique

The gowned patient is brought to the CT scanner and placed in the supine, prone, or, uncommonly, decubitus position, depending on the approach to be used. The patients' arms are raised above their head whenever possible. Generally we choose the shortest vertical path that affords a reasonable window to the lesion and avoids traversing bullae or vessels. Angulation of the CT gantry can assist in gaining access to the best biopsy path. As discussed previously, prebiopsy CT provides valuable information in choosing the appropriate needle pathway. Costello and colleagues[5] described the use of a stereotactic device for CT-directed biopsy that allows biopsy off the vertical or axial plane and reduces the number of manipulations necessary to place the needle within the lesion.

The lesion for biopsy is localized with CT images obtained at functional residual capacity (the lung volume at the end of a normal expiration). The appropriate level is chosen, and the computerized grid on the selected slice is used to determine a skin entry site (Fig. 8–5A). The distance from the midpoint of the grid (which corresponds to the midpoint of the field of view and is shown by the gantry laser light on the patient) to the desired skin entry site is measured on the CT viewing screen. The depth from the skin surface to the outer edge of the lesion is also measured (see Fig. 8–5A). This site can then be marked with a radiopaque marker and a scan obtained to check its position (see Fig. 8–5B). Care must be taken to choose an entry site that allows safe introduction of the biopsy needle(s) over the superior surface of a rib. The site is marked and the patient removed from the gantry. The biopsy area is thoroughly cleansed with a suitable antiseptic solution and anesthesia obtained with lidocaine solution injected intradermally and subcutaneously. It is important to adequately anesthetize the pleura. A small stab incision is made to aid introduction of the needle.

In patients undergoing TNB for an intrapulmonary nodule, we employ a coaxial technique. The patient is instructed to suspend respiration at the same lung

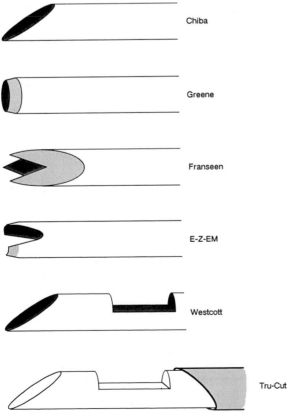

Chiba

Greene

Franseen

E-Z-EM

Westcott

Tru-Cut

FIGURE 8–3 ■ Needles commonly used for TNB.

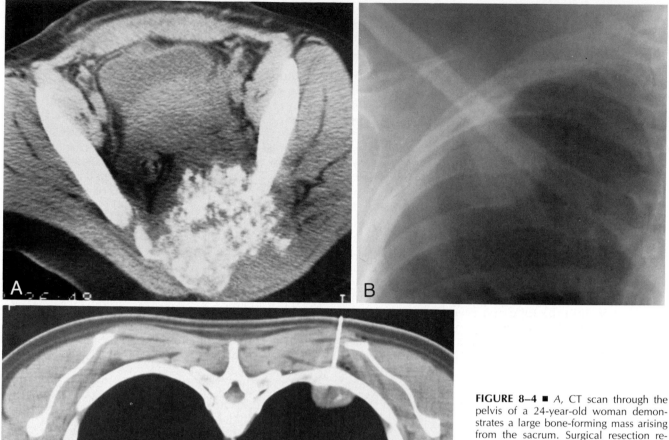

FIGURE 8–4 ■ *A*, CT scan through the pelvis of a 24-year-old woman demonstrates a large bone-forming mass arising from the sacrum. Surgical resection revealed a chondrosarcoma. *B*, Coned-down view of the right upper thorax 2 months after surgery shows an extrapulmonary mass and a sclerotic right posterior fourth rib. *C*, Scan during biopsy of the rib using a 17-gauge bone biopsy needle. The specimen obtained revealed metastatic chondrosarcoma.

volume when a needle is being introduced or manipulated or when the stylet is removed and the needle open to the atmosphere. A 19-gauge Greene needle is placed through the incision to a predetermined depth with its tip at the edge of the mass. The position of the needle tip is checked by obtaining 5-mm collimation scans at three levels encompassing the anticipated position of the needle (see Fig. 8–5C). Once the needle is optimally positioned, the patient is instructed to hold her or his breath as the stylet is removed, and a 22-gauge Greene or Chiba needle with an attached syringe is placed through the outer needle into the lesion. The operator often can feel the increased resistance as the fine needle pierces the lesion. A tissue sample is obtained by creating suction and piercing the lesion repeatedly with a series of rapid, short, up-and-down and

rotatory motions. Suction is then discontinued and the biopsy needle removed, with care taken to occlude the lumen of the outer needle immediately on removal of the thin needle. The syringe and attached needle are carefully handed to the cytopathologist, who ejects the aspirated material onto prepared slides. Any visible tissue fragments are isolated and placed in preservative. The aspirate is smeared onto the slides and is immediately fixed. The slides are stained and examined under a portable microscope.

The decision to perform additional biopsies depends on whether the cytopathologist is confident in making a diagnosis with the available material. If, after four to seven aspirations, the cytopathologist is unable to make a diagnosis of malignancy and the operator can document accurate placement of the biopsy needle within the mass, we either place an

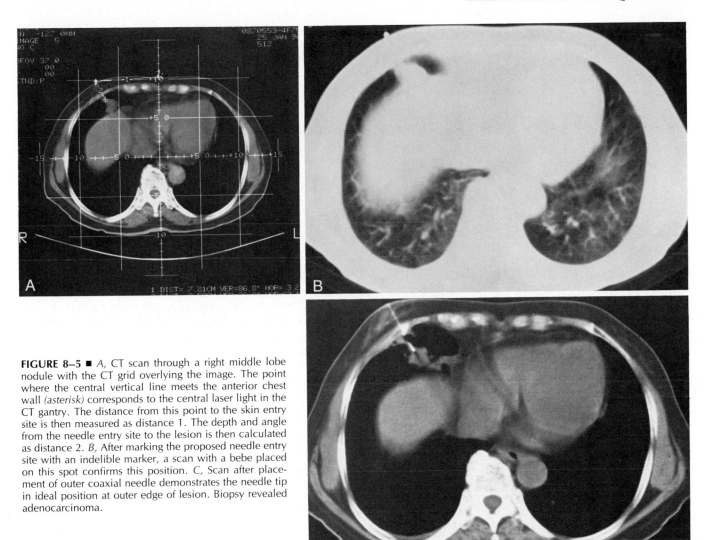

FIGURE 8–5 ■ *A,* CT scan through a right middle lobe nodule with the CT grid overlying the image. The point where the central vertical line meets the anterior chest wall *(asterisk)* corresponds to the central laser light in the CT gantry. The distance from this point to the skin entry site is then measured as distance 1. The depth and angle from the needle entry site to the lesion is then calculated as distance 2. *B,* After marking the proposed needle entry site with an indelible marker, a scan with a bebe placed on this spot confirms this position. *C,* Scan after placement of outer coaxial needle demonstrates the needle tip in ideal position at outer edge of lesion. Biopsy revealed adenocarcinoma.

18- or 19-gauge cutting needle into the lesion in tandem with the indwelling needle or attempt a core biopsy with the outer coaxial needle as it is withdrawn. The use of an outer coaxial needle with a circumferential cutting tip allows for sampling of core tissue when necessary. In patients in whom malignancy has not been confirmed, additional aspirates are sent to the microbiology department for appropriate bacterial, fungal, and mycobacterial stains and cultures.

If malignancy is confirmed, the outer needle is withdrawn during suspended respiration while 10 mL of autologous blood clot is injected to create a blood patch and obliterate the needle tract, possibly reducing the incidence of postbiopsy pneumothorax, although this has been difficult to prove[52] (see Fig. 8–1B). A blood patch is not necessary when a large mediastinal, peripheral, or chest wall lesion undergoes biopsy and no normal lung is traversed. Using the outer needle to obtain tissue eliminates the ability to administer a blood patch while withdrawing this needle.

Immediate Postprocedure Care

After completion of the biopsy, a single scan is obtained through the lower thorax on expiration to check for bleeding (Fig. 8–6) or a pneumothorax (Fig. 8–7). A large or symptomatic pneumothorax should be treated by immediate percutaneous placement of an 18- or 16- gauge angiocath through the biopsy site into the pleural space and evacuation of the pneumothorax. If there is no pneumothorax, the patient is moved onto a stretcher and carefully positioned prone or supine so that the biopsy site is dependent. This may reduce the incidence of postbiopsy pneumothorax and prevent transbronchial spread of biopsy-induced intraparenchymal hemorrhage.[6]

Stable patients may be transferred to a ward for further monitoring or held in the radiology department if a suitable observation area is available. All patients remain with the biopsy site dependent for 3 hours. A nurse monitors the patient's vital signs and breath sounds every 15 minutes for the first hour and every 30 minutes thereafter. The patient is ques-

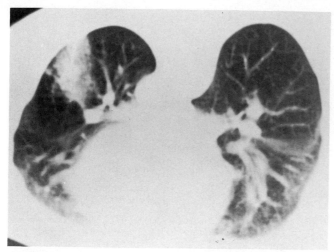

FIGURE 8–6 ■ CT scan during biopsy of a right lower lobe nodule via a posterior approach with the patient prone shows segmental air space consolidation representing intraalveolar hemorrhage.

tioned for chest pain or shortness of breath. Clinical suspicion of a new or enlarging pneumothorax requires an immediate chest radiograph. A routine upright expiratory radiograph is obtained 3 to 4 hours after the biopsy. If there is no pneumothorax or only a small stable pneumothorax in an asymptomatic patient, the patient may be safely discharged to home. This policy is based on the results of a retrospective review of 673 TNBs of the thorax by Perlmutt and colleagues,[7] who found that 98 per cent of all pneumothoraces and 100 per cent of pneumothoraces requiring intervention (i.e., chest tube drainage) were detected within 1 hour of the biopsy. The patient is asked to avoid straining and physical exertion until the following morning and is instructed to proceed

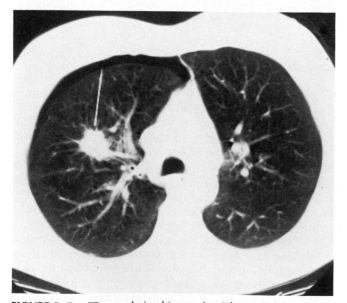

FIGURE 8–7 ■ CT scan during biopsy of a right upper lobe mass in a patient with severe emphysema. The 19-gauge needle is in good position adjacent to the mass. A pneumothorax, evident anteriorly, required percutaneous catheter evacuation because of dyspnea that worsened during the procedure.

immediately to an emergency room should he or she develop any pleuritic chest pain, hemoptysis, or shortness of breath.

Complications and Their Treatment

The most common complications from TNB are pneumothorax and hemoptysis. The reported incidence of pneumothorax ranges from 0[2, 8] to 61 per cent,[4] with most large series reporting an incidence of 5 to 30 per cent.[3, 5, 7, 9–26] Perhaps more important than the overall pneumothorax rate is the percentage of biopsy patients requiring treatment of pneumothorax with chest tube drainage, generally reported as 0 to 15 per cent.[3, 5, 7, 9–26]

Variables that are associated with a higher incidence of pneumothorax include increasing depth of the lesion,[27, 28] decreasing size of the lesion, advanced age, obstructive airway disease,[29, 30] arterial hypoxemia,[30] intractable coughing, increased outer diameter of biopsy needle, the use of cutting needles or biopsy guns for core biopsies in contrast to smaller aspirating needles for cytology,[31] increased number of times the pleura is traversed, increased duration of the procedure, cavitary lesions, and inexperience of the person performing the biopsy. The recognition of factors associated with a higher rate of TNB-induced pneumothorax is important, because it allows recognition of patients at greater risk for a pneumothorax and allows some of these factors to be corrected (e.g., the administration of bronchodilators or antitussives) or to seek alternative initial methods of diagnosis, such as bronchoscopy. Quon and colleagues,[30] in a retrospective study of 308 chest biopsies, each consisting of an average of three passes with a 22-gauge needle, found that severe airway obstruction (forced expiratory volume in 1 second/forced vital capacity [FEV_1/FVC] < 60 per cent predicted) and severe arterial hypoxemia (PaO_2 < 59 mm Hg) were associated with a significantly higher incidence of biopsy-induced pneumothorax but were not associated with an increased incidence of hemorrhage. Similarly, Miller and colleagues[29] found that the prebiopsy identification of airway obstruction (FEV_1 < 70 per cent predicted), decreased lesion size, and increased lesion depth from the skin surface were all related to an increased incidence of pneumothorax, whereas age, sex, presence of restrictive lung disease, and the number of needle passes were not significant factors. In a prospective study, Poe and colleagues[27] conclude that the depth of the lesion and total lung capacity were the only factors associated with a significant increase in the risk of biopsy-related pneumothorax. From these data, Poe and colleagues devised a formula to calculate the probability of pneumothorax according to the depth of the lesion. Even though pulmonary function studies may help in predicting a pneumothorax, we do not advocate their routine use as a screening procedure before TNB.

A higher rate of pneumothorax has also been

reported when TNB is performed under CT guidance.[4, 32] This has been attributed to the needle remaining in position longer with CT-directed biopsies when compared with fluoroscopy, and because smaller, more central lesions are chosen for CT-directed biopsies. Other conditions with higher pneumothorax rates include opportunistic pneumonia,[33] lymphangitic carcinomatosis,[34] and mechanical ventilation.[35]

In addition to the prebiopsy assessment of patients undergoing TNB, other measures can reduce the pneumothorax rate. Clearly, thin (19-gauge or less) needles should be used whenever feasible. CT, used either to guide a subsequent fluoroscopic biopsy or as the prime modality, can aid in choosing a short approach crossing the fewest pleural surfaces and avoiding bullae. VanSonnenberg and colleagues[36] described a novel technique in which CT is used to guide the placement of a 23-gauge needle within small hilar, mediastinal, or central pulmonary lesions. The hub of the 23-gauge needle is removed, a 19-gauge needle is then slid over the 23-gauge needle, and one or multiple passes are made coaxially through the 19-gauge needle with a 22-gauge needle. This technique presumably makes the biopsy of such lesions safer.

Several investigators have studied specific techniques to reduce the incidence of biopsy-related pneumothorax. Skupin and colleagues[35] examined the pneumothorax rate in 16 anesthetized dogs on whom biopsies were performed using a coaxial technique while being ventilated with 10 cm H_2O of positive end-expiratory pressure (PEEP). In seven of the eight dogs in which the needle was removed after biopsy, a pneumothorax developed. Only two of eight dogs injected with 0.5 mL of isobutyl-2-cyanoacrylate via the 20-gauge outer needle developed a pneumothorax. Berger and Smith[37] performed a case-control study in which one group of patients was placed biopsy-side down in the decubitus position after biopsy, and the other group of patients (the control group) remained supine. They concluded that both the rate of postbiopsy pneumothorax and the percentage of patients requiring treatment for pneumothorax were no different between the two groups. Bourgouin and co-workers[38] prospectively studied the effect of injecting a 10-mL blood patch during withdrawal of the outer coaxial needle on the incidence of postbiopsy pneumothorax. They concluded that the use of a blood patch did not significantly reduce the pneumothorax rate.

A small pneumothorax should be managed conservatively with monitoring of vital signs, administration of nasal oxygen, and follow-up radiographs to confirm stability. A large or symptomatic pneumothorax requires immediate evacuation. We place an 18- or a 16-gauge angiocath into the pleural space through the biopsy and withdraw the pneumothorax using a large volume syringe, a three-way stopcock, and connecting tubing. If this maneuver is unsuccessful and the pneumothorax recurs, it should be treated by placement of a percutaneous small-bore drainage catheter connected to water seal or a Heimlich valve.

Hemoptysis is the second most common complication of TNB. Fine needles for aspiration and biopsy have reduced the incidence of significant bleeding and hemoptysis to between 1 and 10 per cent, with most series reporting an incidence of less than 5 per cent. Caution should be exercised in biopsy of mediastinal masses and vascular pulmonary lesions, such as metastases from renal cell carcinoma, because major intrathoracic hemorrhage and death have been reported rarely in such cases.[39] It is imperative that all patients considered for TNB have a preprocedure coagulation profile performed, with measures taken to correct any abnormalities. In the absence of a bleeding diathesis, hemoptysis is almost always self-limiting. The patient should be reassured and placed biopsy-site down to prevent the transbronchial aspiration of blood.

Vasovagal reactions, pericarditis, and malignant seeding of the biopsy tract[40] have all been reported but are exceedingly rare.

Several cases of systemic arterial air embolism leading to myocardial infarction, stroke, or death have been reported following TNB.[41-44] Aberle and colleagues[41] described a case of fatal systemic arterial air embolism after TNB of a lesion that subsequently proved to be a lung abscess, and several cases of nonfatal air embolism have been reported.[42, 43] The mortality rate from TNB is 0.02 per cent, and as little as 0.5 mL of air is sufficient to induce coronary ischemia and fatal arrhythmias.[41] The mechanism of systemic arterial air embolism is presumed to be either air entry through the needle directly into a pulmonary vein or the iatrogenic formation of a broncho- or alveolovenous fistula from the introduced needle. The pressure gradient from airway to vein is increased by coughing, deep inspiration that precedes coughing, and positive pressure ventilation. Once the signs and symptoms of air embolus (hypotension, acute loss of consciousness, seizures, multifocal neurologic deficits, arrhythmias) are recognized, the patient should be placed either in the left lateral decubitus position or Trendelenburg's position to prevent any residual air within the left atrium from embolizing to the head. Blood pressure and ventilatory support must be provided, and 100 per cent oxygen must be administered to promote the resorption of air bubbles. Immediate transfer to a hyperbaric unit should be arranged.

Results of TNB

Accumulated experience with imaging-guided fine-needle aspiration biopsy and the widespread availability of expert cytopathologists have made TNB extremely accurate for the diagnosis of intrathoracic malignancy, with an overall sensitivity of 82 to 97 per cent in most series.[2, 4, 8–11, 13, 17, 21, 24, 25, 32, 45] Stanley and colleagues,[10] using a 22- or 23-gauge Chiba needle yielding cytologic specimens only, reported a

97 per cent sensitivity for malignancy. Khouri and colleagues[9] reported a sensitivity of 95 per cent for malignancy using cytology and histology. Other investigators[11, 26] have shown that cytologic and histologic specimens can increase the yield for malignancy above that achieved by cytologic specimens alone. This is particularly important in the diagnosis of lymphoma, which has a yield in cytology on the order of 65 to 75 per cent, considerably lower than the yield for other intrathoracic malignancies.[46] When lymphoma is a prime diagnostic consideration, an attempt to obtain a histologic specimen should be considered.

Although cytologic specimens obtained with TNB are very accurate for diagnosing intrathoracic malignancy, their ability to differentiate among the different cell types of bronchogenic carcinoma is less well established. A retrospective comparison of the preoperative cell typing from TNB and the final pathologic cell typing in 38 resected malignancies[13] showed that only 65 per cent of the malignancies were correctly typed preoperatively. A similar study by Thornbury and colleagues[47] showed agreement between the results of TNB-obtained cytologic specimens and subsequent resected specimens in 81 per cent of instances. The greatest difficulty is with poorly differentiated squamous cell carcinoma and adenocarcinoma. The requirement for differentiation between cell types is more of theoretic than practical importance, because patient management decisions are affected only by the ability to distinguish small-cell from non–small-cell bronchogenic carcinoma, a differentiation that can be made cytologically in the vast majority of instances. Even this latter differentiation is not always of clinical importance, as patients with small, localized small-cell carcinoma can benefit from surgical resection.[48] Of the 312 patients correctly diagnosed with malignancy by Stanley and colleagues,[10] no patient was judged to have been treated inappropriately because of an incorrect preoperative cell typing from TNB.

A shortcoming of TNB is the difficulty in making specific benign diagnoses from cytologic specimens. Although Khouri and colleagues[9] reported a specificity of 88 per cent for diagnosing benign lesions with a combination of cytology and histology, only 77 per cent of those were specific diagnoses. Similarly, Stanley and colleagues,[10] using cytology only, reported a 97 per cent specificity, with 48 per cent of those being specific diagnoses. In other series, the specificity for benign disease has been as low as 16 per cent.[49] The difficulty in making a specific benign diagnosis is multifactorial. Among these are sampling errors of a malignant lesion, failure to send aspirated specimens for appropriate stains and cultures, and the difficulty in making a benign diagnosis from cytologic findings alone. Cytopathologic diagnoses that are specific for benign disease (thus yielding a negative predictive value of 100 per cent) include tuberculosis, hamartoma, abscess, lipoma, lipoid pneumonia, histoplasmosis, actinomycosis, scar,

cryptococcosis, pseudotumor, and cyst.[50] A diagnosis of benign disease can confidently exclude malignancy and reduce the number of negative thoracotomies by as much as 55 per cent.[15] The key to increasing the yield on benign lesions is repeat sampling or biopsy if necessary, expert cytopathology, and the use of larger cutting needles that provide histologic specimens when repeated aspirations of a lesion through accurately placed needles fail to demonstrate evidence of malignancy. In 42 patients, 75 per cent of whom had mediastinal or pleural-based lesions, Goralnik and colleagues[26] demonstrated an increased yield in the specific diagnosis of benign lesions (from 22 to 55 per cent) when a Tru-Cut needle was used to obtain histologic specimens as compared with an aspirating needle yielding only cytologic specimens. Greene and colleagues[11] have shown that small circumferentially beveled cutting needles can provide histologic specimens in 72 per cent of cases and can aid in diagnosing specific benign lesions. Hamper and colleagues[23] correctly diagnosed 12 of 14 pulmonary hamartomas; histology alone was diagnostic in 11 of the 12, whereas cytology alone was diagnostic in only five. When unable to make a cytologic diagnosis of malignancy with a 22-gauge aspirating needle, one can attempt a tissue sample with a cutting needle or by aspirating with the outer coaxial needle before it is withdrawn. Biopsy can be safely performed on large mediastinal or pleural-based lesions using a cutting needle.

Follow-up

Every patient undergoing TNB should schedule a follow-up visit with the referring clinician to discuss the results of the biopsy. If tuberculosis is a prime diagnostic possibility prior to the biopsy, the referring physician should allow the appropriate interval for these cultures to grow (Fig. 8–8). Patients with specific benign infectious diagnoses should receive antibiotics when appropriate and be followed radiographically for improvement or resolution. Patients shown to have primary or metastatic malignancy should have appropriate surgery, radiation therapy, or chemotherapy. Patients in whom TNB yields a nonspecific benign diagnosis or an inadequate specimen should be considered for repeat biopsy or have the lesion removed. The need for repeat biopsy is not uncommon and was necessary in 13 per cent of 650 patients who underwent biopsy by Khouri and colleagues.[9] If the unsuccessful biopsy was performed under fluoroscopy, we usually repeat the biopsy using CT guidance. CT can verify that the biopsy needle is in the lesion and allows sampling of different areas within the lesion so that a necrotic or inflammatory portion of a malignancy is not preferentially sampled. Furthermore, contrast-enhanced CT can help distinguish a central mass from postobstructive atelectasis or pneumonitis, again permitting accurate sampling of the lesion.

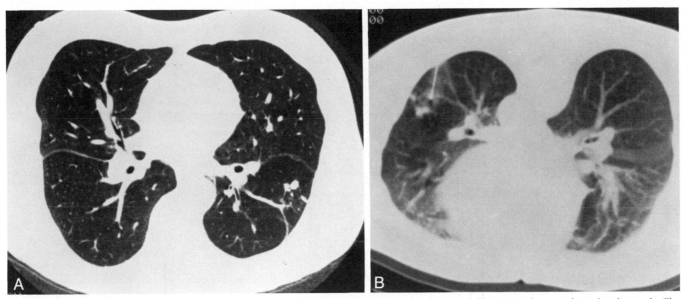

FIGURE 8–8 ■ *A*, High-resolution CT scan in a patient with a nodular density in the left lower lobe seen only on a frontal radiograph. The density is composed of several adjacent nodular densities. *B*, CT scan during biopsy shows the needle within the nodules. Culture of the aspirated material grew *Mycobacterium gordonii*.

Percutaneous Catheter Drainage of Intrathoracic Fluid Collections

The treatment of intrathoracic fluid collections using imaging-guided percutaneous catheter drainage (PCD) was developed in the 1980s. Ultrasound and CT can localize intrathoracic fluid collections accurately, and advances in catheter design and interventional techniques have made PCD possible. Initially referrals to the radiologist for PCD were limited to patients who had failed pleural drainage with large-bore thoracostomy tubes and in whom open surgical drainage was either contraindicated or refused by the patient.[51] More recently, PCD has been used as the initial therapy for empyemas and pneumothoraces and is being used more frequently for the treatment of mediastinal fluid collections[52] and lung abscesses.[53] Radiologists skilled in interventional techniques have a high success and a low complication rate. Reduced patient discomfort from the small-diameter catheters used has led to widespread acceptance of the technique by clinicians.

Indications

The indications for percutaneous aspiration and drainage of intrathoracic fluid collections are shown in Table 8–4. One of the most common referrals for PCD is for the symptomatic relief and sclerosis of malignant pleural effusion. Known or suspected empyema, mediastinal fluid collections, and lung abscess also can be aspirated and drained percutaneously. Noninfected, nonmalignant transudative pleural effusions are managed with small-diameter catheters when diuresis and fluid restriction have failed to achieve their resolution.

There are no absolute contraindications to PCD, although the presence of coagulopathy or thrombocytopenia are relative contraindications. In such patients, the administration of blood products and platelets immediately before the procedure can minimize the risk of bleeding.

Imaging for Drainage

Computed tomography,[51, 52, 54–56] ultrasound,[51, 54–58] fluoroscopy,[59] or any combination of the three can be used to guide entry into the fluid collection. The choice of imaging procedure depends on the patient's condition, the availability and logistics of the various modalities, and the preference of the radiologist performing the procedure. Interventions in the pleural space may be performed with equal safety using any of these modalities. Patients with large, free-flowing pleural effusions can undergo catheter drainage without imaging guidance (Fig. 8–9). In patients with smaller effusions or loculated collections (i.e., following unsuccessful pleurodesis), CT or ultrasound is used to guide aspiration and drain-

---

TABLE 8–4 ■ **Indications for Percutaneous Drainage of Intrathoracic Fluid Collections**

1. Drainage and subsequent sclerosis of symptomatic free-flowing effusions, most commonly malignant pleural effusions
2. Loculated or free-flowing empyema, especially in patients failing thoracostomy tube drainage
3. Mediastinal abscess in critically ill patients who are not candidates for immediate surgical drainage
4. Management of large serous effusions secondary to ascites or liver failure
5. Lung abscess in a patient failing medical therapy who is not a candidate for surgical resection

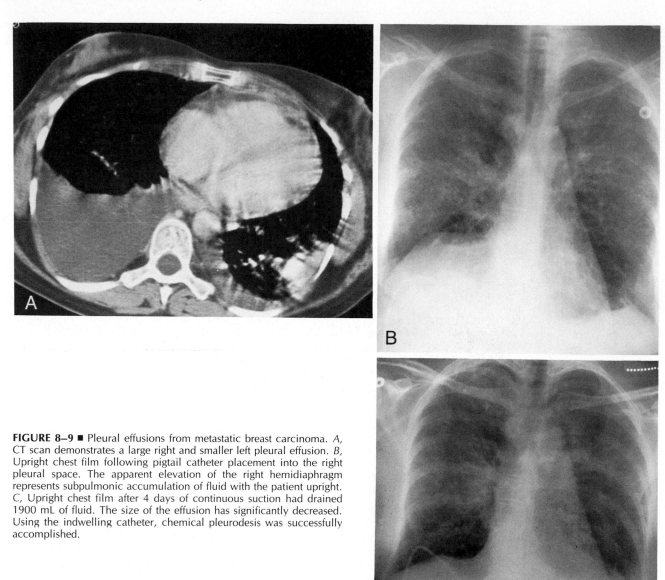

FIGURE 8–9 ■ Pleural effusions from metastatic breast carcinoma. *A,* CT scan demonstrates a large right and smaller left pleural effusion. *B,* Upright chest film following pigtail catheter placement into the right pleural space. The apparent elevation of the right hemidiaphragm represents subpulmonic accumulation of fluid with the patient upright. *C,* Upright chest film after 4 days of continuous suction had drained 1900 mL of fluid. The size of the effusion has significantly decreased. Using the indwelling catheter, chemical pleurodesis was successfully accomplished.

age of the fluid collections. Both CT and ultrasound are excellent in demonstrating the presence of loculation, although ultrasound is more sensitive in showing fine septations within large loculated collections. CT is the method of choice for known or suspected collections in the mediastinum or lung parenchyma, because precise visualization of the path traversed by the aspirating needle and drainage catheter is critical. An additional advantage of CT-directed drainage is the ability to visualize the entire thorax and accurately assess the size and location of all fluid collections. This helps determine the number of catheters necessary and serves as a baseline for follow-up studies to assess adequacy of drainage. When CT is used for localization of a collection that subsequently will be aspirated and drained under

fluoroscopy or ultrasound, the skin is marked with indelible ink at an appropriate entry site at the upper margin of the closest rib with the patient at end-expiration. The distance from the skin entry site to the center of the collection should then be measured and recorded.

Technique

The technique used for the CT-directed PCD of intrathoracic fluid collections is the same as that used for abdominal and pelvic abscesses. A fully sterile technique is used, with the physicians gowned, masked, and wearing sterile gloves. Prior to aspiration and drainage of a fluid collection, an appropriate skin entry site is chosen from the CT images

(Fig. 8–10). The area around the entry site is washed with an iodine solution and draped with sterile cloths. A 1 per cent solution of lidocaine is liberally injected, particularly to the periosteum of the rib and parietal pleura, which are heavily innervated. After a small stab incision is made, the subcutaneous tissues are spread with a forceps to ease subsequent catheter introduction.

A 20- or 22-gauge needle is then inserted to a predetermined depth during breath holding at end-expiration. Five to 10 mL of fluid are aspirated from the collection and examined grossly. If no fluid can be aspirated, the position of the needle tip is verified by obtaining a CT image at the level of needle entry at the skin. If the needle is adequately positioned and no fluid can be aspirated, a larger gauge needle should be inserted in tandem to aspirate thick or semisolid material. If frank pus is aspirated, one should proceed directly with drainage. If it is unclear from gross inspection whether the fluid obtained represents an empyema or abscess, then the speci-

men should be stained with Gram's stain immediately. The finding of bacteria or white cells on Gram's stain should lead to percutaneous drainage. The aspiration of clear fluid that yields nothing on Gram's stain does not require catheter drainage. These collections should be aspirated as completely as possible and the needle removed. If a question still remains as to the presence of an infected collection, a catheter should be inserted. The results of culture, fluid pH, cell differential, and chemistry studies show whether long-term drainage is necessary. The material should also undergo cytologic evaluation, especially in lung abscesses, as necrotic tumors can be secondarily infected.

At this point, a drainage catheter can be placed by direct trocar insertion, particularly when the collection is large and peripheral. Alternatively, a Seldinger technique may be employed. With this method, a puncture is made with an 18- or 19-gauge Teflon sheath needle, usually in tandem with the smaller needle already in place from the aspiration. Proper

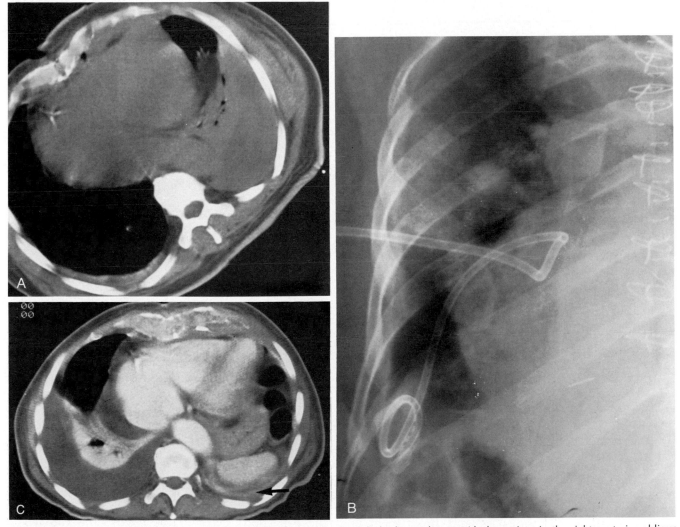

FIGURE 8–10 ■ CT-guided drainage of fluid collections. *A,* CT scan through the lower thorax with the patient in the right posterior oblique position shows a skin marker over a left posterolateral fluid collection. *B,* Coned-down view of the indwelling no. 10 French Cope loop catheter coiled in the fluid collection. Cultures grew *Aspergillus* organisms. *C,* Contrast-enhanced CT 5 weeks after drainage shows opposed, enhancing pleural layers *(arrow)* in the region of the previous collection.

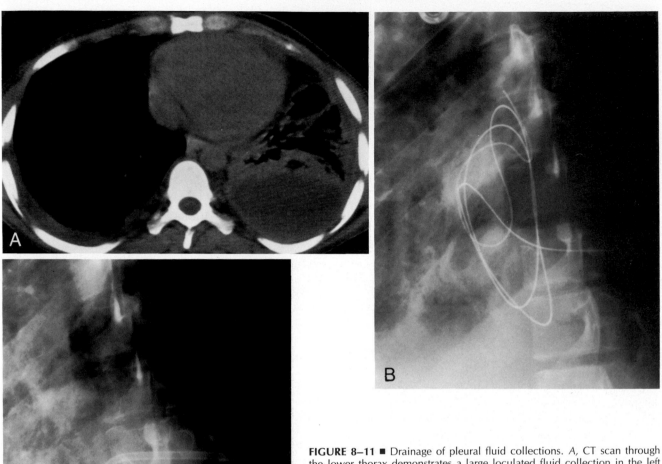

FIGURE 8–11 ■ Drainage of pleural fluid collections. *A,* CT scan through the lower thorax demonstrates a large loculated fluid collection in the left posterior thorax. Note the convex anterior surface of the collection, which displaces the consolidated and collapsed left lower lobe anteriorly. *B,* A lateral film obtained during empyema drainage. A long segment of floppy guide wire is coiled within the empyema cavity. *C,* Following dilatation of the tract, a Cope type catheter is placed into the collection.

location of the needle tip is confirmed by aspiration. It is important not to evacuate the collection completely at this point, because complete evacuation makes the placement of a guide wire and drainage catheter more difficult. The drainage can then proceed on the CT table in a blind fashion. The narrow CT table and lack of real-time visualization of the guide wire and catheter paths make catheter placement in the CT gantry less than ideal. CT scans through the collection can be used after each manipulation to check guide wire and catheter position, but this is cumbersome, time consuming, and often compromises the sterile field. Alternatively, most radiologists complete the drainage procedure under fluoroscopic guidance. In this situation, the Teflon sheath is affixed to the skin, and the patient is carefully moved to a fluoroscopy suite. A floppy-tipped guide wire is placed through the sheath and a long segment coiled in the collection (Fig. 8–11*A,*

B). The sheath is then removed, and angiographic dilators are used to dilate the tract to the diameter of the drainage catheter. The drainage catheter should contain a single lumen with multiple large side holes and have either a pigtail or curved tip for retention within the cavity (see Fig. 8–11*C*). For serous collections, a no. 8- to no. 10 French catheter is adequate, whereas a no. 12 to no. 14 French or larger catheter must be used for adequate drainage of thick pus. Catheters specifically designed for empyema drainage have been developed.[57] These are no. 12 French catheters with multiple large side holes and a gently curved tip to encompass the abscess or empyema cavity (Fig. 8–12). The catheter with its inner stiffening cannula is introduced over the guide wire into the collection. Once in the cavity, the catheter is advanced off its cannula and coiled within the cavity. Some manipulation may be necessary to ensure that all the side holes are within the cavity and that some

Cope type loop nephrostomy catheter

VanSonnenberg empyema catheter

FIGURE 8–12 ■ Catheters used for pleural fluid and empyema drainage.

are in a dependent position to aid drainage. This may require that a long segment of the catheter be coiled in the cavity.

Once properly positioned, the catheter should be fixed to the skin by taping the catheter and suturing through the tape and by affixing Stomadhesive or an ostomy cover to the skin. Infected collections should be drained as completely as possible. Large (>1500 mL), chronic, noninfected fluid collections should be drained more slowly, generally over 24 to 48 hours, to avoid the development of reexpansion pulmonary edema.[59] Before the catheter is attached to suction, non-ionic contrast material can be instilled to exclude a fistulous communication with a bronchus, the esophagus, or a subphrenic abscess. Dilute nonionic contrast should be used to avoid the development of pulmonary edema should a bronchopleural fistula be present. The catheter is attached to a Pleur-evac device, and suction pressure of −20 cm H_2O is applied. All connections are secured with tape, and petrolatum gauze is placed around the catheter entry site.

Immediately following catheter placement for drainage of infected collections, a repeat CT scan is performed so that additional catheters can be placed to drain any remaining collections.[60]

Management and Follow-up

Each patient with an indwelling drainage catheter is monitored daily as to condition, catheter maintenance, and drainage-related complications. The patient's general condition, along with recorded temperatures, white blood cell (WBC) counts, and culture results, should be checked. The daily amount and character of the drainage fluid should be noted. The catheter site should be examined for signs of infection or hematoma and the catheter flushed at least twice daily with 10 mL of normal saline. If fluid is seen leaking around the catheter, the catheter may be occluded or broken or may have been inadvertently withdrawn into the skin tract. These possibilities can be checked by fluoroscopy and a sinogram and measures taken to correct the problem.

Progress in empyema drainage may be monitored by chest radiographs, CT (Fig. 8–13A), or ultrasound, whereas mediastinal collections are best followed by CT. The mean duration of empyema drainage is approximately 7 days and ranges from 24 hours to 3 weeks. Alternatively, serial sinograms can be performed. If the patient fails to improve after initial drainage, repeat ultrasound or CT scans can be performed to seek undrained collections. At this point the decision can be made whether to reposition the catheter, place additional drains, exchange the catheter for a larger one to promote drainage, instill urokinase, or perform surgical drainage.[60a] When drainage becomes less than 10 mL in 24 hours, the patient shows clinical improvement (no fever, normal WBC count), and there is radiographic resolution of the collection (see Fig. 8–13B), the catheter(s) may be removed.[60]

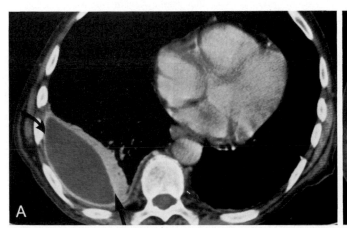
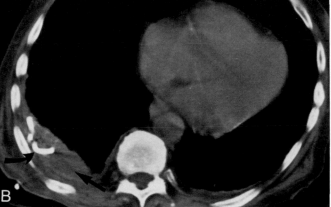

FIGURE 8–13 ■ *A,* Contrast-enhanced CT scan in a patient with persistent fever following treatment for right lower lobe pneumonia. A lenticular fluid collection with enhancing visceral *(straight arrow)* and parietal *(curved arrow)* pleurae is seen posterolateral to atelectatic right lower lobe. *B,* CT scan obtained 1 week after initial catheter placement. The collection has significantly decreased in size, with a small amount of fluid *(straight arrow)* remaining about the tip of the catheter *(curved arrow).* Because drainage had stopped and the patient was afebrile, the catheter was removed.

Free-flowing pleural effusions are most easily followed with upright and decubitus chest radiographs. In patients with chronic effusions unresponsive to medical therapy, sclerosing agents can be administered through the indwelling catheter once the effusion has been sufficiently drained to allow for pleural symphysis.

Results

Successful treatment of an empyema or mediastinal or lung abscess is defined as clinical improvement with radiographic resolution of the collection without further need for thoracostomy tube or surgical intervention. Success rates for empyema drainage range from 60 to 90 per cent in most reported series.[51, 54–61] The chronicity of the pleural process is the most important factor influencing outcome. Patients with chronic empyemas in the organizing stage generally respond poorly to closed drainage, because pleural fibrosis prevents apposition of visceral and parietal pleural surfaces.[54–57] These patients often require open drainage with rib resection or decortication. Other reasons for unsuccessful catheter drainage include pleural metastases, interstitial pulmonary fibrosis, and lymphangitic carcinomatosis, all of which prevent the lung expansion necessary to obliterate the pleural space. In the few small series of patients reported to have undergone percutaneous mediastinal or lung abscess drainage, successful drainage was accomplished in 80 to 100 per cent.[52, 53]

Complications

Complications related to PCD are rare, with most large series reporting a zero per cent major complication rate.[54, 57, 59, 62, 63] Minor complications relate to the interventional procedures themselves (e.g., vasovagal reactions) and to the catheter (e.g., kinking, fracture, leakage, inadvertent removal). Other rarer complications include pneumothorax, bleeding, subcutaneous emphysema, lung laceration, inadvertent subdiaphragmatic placement of the catheter, and infection of sterile fluid collections.[56] In one series of 18 patients, a single cardiopulmonary arrest was reported.[55] Too-rapid evacuation of a large (>1500 mL) chronic pleural fluid collection may lead to reexpansion pulmonary edema; thus these collections should be drained gradually over 24 to 48 hours.

References

1. Cohan RH, Newman GE, Braun SD, Dunnick NR: CT assistance for fluoroscopically guided transthoracic needle aspiration biopsy. J Comput Assist Tomogr 8:1093, 1984.
2. Ikezoe J, Sone S, Higashihara T, Morimoto S, Arizawa J, Kuriyama K: Sonographically guided needle biopsy for diagnosis of thoracic lesions. AJR 143:229, 1984.
3. Yang PC, Luh KT, Sheu JC, Kuo SH, Yang SP: Peripheral pulmonary lesions: ultrasonography and ultrasonically guided aspiration biopsy. Radiology 155:451, 1985.
4. Fink I, Gamsu G, Harter LP: CT-guided aspiration biopsy of the thorax. J Comput Assist Tomogr 6:958, 1982.
5. Costello P, Onik G, Cosman E: Computed tomographic-guided stereotaxic biopsy of thoracic lesions. J Thorac Imaging 2:271, 1987.
5a. Herman SJ, Weisbrod GL: Usefulness of the blood patch technique after transthoracic needle aspiration biopsy. Radiology 176:395, 1990.
6. Moore EH, Shepard JO, McLoud TC, Templeton PA, Kosiuk JP: Positional precautions in needle aspiration lung biopsy. Radiology 175:733–735, 1990.
7. Perlmutt LM, Braun SD, Newman GE, Oke EJ, Dunnick NR: Timing of chest film followup after transthoracic needle aspiration. AJR 146:1049, 1986.
8. Wernecke K, Vassallo P, Peters PE, vonBassewitz DB: Mediastinal tumors: biopsy under US guidance. Radiology 172:473, 1989.
9. Khouri NF, Stitik FP, Erozan YS, Gupta PK, Kim WS, et al: Transthoracic needle aspiration biopsy of benign and malignant lung lesions. AJR 144:281, 1985.
10. Stanley JH, Fish GD, Andriole JG, Gobien RP, Betsill WL, et al: Lung lesions: cytologic diagnosis by fine-needle biopsy. Radiology 162:389, 1987.
11. Greene R, Szyfelbein WM, Isler RJ, Stark P, Jantsch H: Supplementary tissue-core histology from fine-needle transthoracic aspiration biopsy. AJR 144:787, 1985.
12. Conces DJ, Schwenk R, Doering PR: Thoracic needle biopsy: improved results utilizing the team approach. Chest 91:813, 1987.
13. Horrigan TP, Bergin KT: Correlation between needle biopsy of lung tumors and histopathologic analysis of resected specimens. Chest 90:638, 1986.
14. Morgenroth A, Pfeuffer HP, Austgen M, Viereck HJ, Tendelenburg F: Six years' experience with perthoracic core needle biopsy of pulmonary lesions. Thorax 44:177, 1989.
15. Linder J, Olsen GA, Johnston WW: Fine-needle aspiration biopsy of the mediastinum. Am J Med 81:1005, 1986.
16. Westcott JL: Direct percutaneous needle aspiration of localized pulmonary lesions: results in 422 patients. Radiology 137:31, 1980.
17. Westcott JL: Percutaneous needle aspiration of hilar and mediastinal masses. Radiology 141:323, 1981.
18. Castellino RA, Blank N: Etiologic diagnosis of focal pulmonary infection in immunocompromised patients by fluoroscopically guided percutaneous needle aspiration. Radiology 132:563, 1979.
19. Adler OB, Rosenberger A, Peleg H: Fine-needle aspiration biopsy of mediastinal masses: evaluation of 136 experiences. AJR 140:893, 1983.
20. Poe RH, Kallay MC: Transthoracic needle biopsy of lung in nonhospitalized patients. Chest 92:676, 1987.
21. Sider L, Davis TM: Hilar masses: evaluation with CT-guided biopsy after negative bronchoscopic examination. Radiology 164:107, 1987.
22. Weisbrod GL, Herman SJ, Tao LC: Preliminary experience with a dual cutting edge needle in thoracic percutaneous fine-needle aspiration biopsy. Radiology 163:75, 1987.
23. Hamper UM, Khouri NF, Stitik FP, Siegelman SS: Pulmonary hamartoma: diagnosis by transthoracic needle-aspiration biopsy. Radiology 155:15, 1985.
24. Wang KP, Kelly SJ, Britt JE: Percutaneous needle aspiration biopsy of chest lesions. Chest 93:993, 1988.
25. Nahman BJ, Van Aman ME, McLemore WE, O'Toole RV: Use of the Rotex needle in percutaneous biopsy of pulmonary malignancy. AJR 145:97, 1985.
26. Goralnik CH, O'Connell DM, El Yousef SJ, Haaga JR: CT-guided cutting-needle biopsies of selected chest lesions. AJR 151:903, 1988.
27. Poe RH, Kallay MC, Wicks CM, Odoroff CL: Predicting risk of pneumothorax in needle biopsy of the lung. Chest 85:232, 1984.
28. Fish GD, Stanley JH, Miller KS, Schabel SI, Sutherland SE: Postbiopsy pneumothorax: estimating the risk by chest radiography and pulmonary function tests. AJR 150:71, 1988.
29. Miller KS, Fish GB, Stanley JH, Schabel SI: Prediction of

pneumothorax rate in percutaneous needle aspiration of the lung. Chest 93:742, 1988.

30. Quon D, Fong TC, Mellor J, Brandschwei FH, Desautels JEL: Pulmonary function testing in predicting complications from percutaneous lung biopsy. J Can Assoc Radiol 39:267, 1988.

31. Perker SH, Hopper KD, Yakes WF, Gibson MD, Ownbey JL, Carter TE: Image-directed percutaneous biopsies with a biopsy gun. Radiology 171:663, 1989.

32. vanSonnenberg E, Casola G, Ho M, Neff CC, Varney RR, et al: Difficult thoracic lesions: CT-guided biopsy experience in 150 cases. Radiology 167:457, 1988.

33. Wallace JM, Batra P, Gong H: Percutaneous needle lung aspiration for diagnosing pneumonitis in the patient with acquired immunodeficiency syndrome (AIDS). Am Rev Respir Dis 131:38, 1985.

34. Weisbrod GL, Stoneman HR, Tao LC: Diagnosis of diffuse malignant infiltration of lung (lymphangitic carcinomatosis) by percutaneous fine-needle aspiration biopsy. J Can Assoc Radiol 36:238, 1985.

35. Skupin A, Gomez F, Husain M, Skupin C, Bigman O: Complications of transthoracic needle biopsy decreased with isobutyl 2-cyanoacrylate: a pilot study. Ann Thorac Surg 43:406, 1987.

36. vanSonnenberg E, Lin AS, Deutsch AL, Mattrey RF: Percutaneous biopsy of difficult mediastinal, hilar, and pulmonary lesions by computed-tomographic guidance and a modified coaxial technique. Radiology 148:300, 1983.

37. Berger R, Smith D: Efficacy of the lateral decubitus position in preventing pneumothorax after needle biopsy of the lung. South Med J 81:1140, 1988.

38. Bourgouin PM, Shepard JO, McLoud TC, Spizarny DL, Dedrick CG: Transthoracic needle aspiration biopsy: evaluation of the blood patch technique. Radiology 166:93, 1988.

39. Milner LB, Ryan K, Gullo J: Fatal intrathoracic hemorrhage after percutaneous aspiration lung biopsy. AJR 132:280, 1979.

40. Muller NL, Bergin CJ, Miller RR, Ostrow DN: Seeding of malignant cells into the needle track after lung and pleural biopsy. J Can Assoc Radiol 37:192, 1986.

41. Aberle DR, Gamsu G, Golden JA: Fatal systemic arterial air embolism following lung needle aspiration. Radiology 165:351, 1987.

42. Tolly TL, Feldmeier JE, Czarnecki D: Air embolism complicating percutaneous lung biopsy. AJR 150:555, 1988.

43. Cianci P, Posin JP, Shimshak RR: Air embolism complicating percutaneous thin needle biopsy of lung. Chest 92:749, 1987.

44. Baker BK, Awwad EE: Computed tomography of fatal cerebral air embolism following percutaneous aspiration biopsy of the lung. J Comput Assist Tomogr 12:1082, 1988.

45. Harter LP, Moss AA, Goldberg HI, Gross BH: CT-guided fine needle aspirations for diagnosis of benign and malignant disease. AJR 140:363, 1983.

46. Westcott JL: Transthoracic needle biopsy of the hilum and mediastinum. J Thorac Imaging 2:41, 1987.

47. Thornbury JR, Burke DP, Naylor B: Transthoracic needle aspiration biopsy: accuracy of cytologic typing of malignant neoplasms. AJR 136:719, 1981.

48. Sorensen HR, Lund C, Alstrup P: Survival in small cell lung carcinoma after surgery. Thorax 41:479, 1986.

49. Winning AJ, McIvor J, Seed WA: Interpretation of negative results in fine needle aspiration of discrete pulmonary lesions. Thorax 41:875, 1986.

50. Gobien RP, Valicenti JF, Paris BS, Daniell C: Thin-needle aspiration biopsy: methods of increasing the accuracy of a negative prediction. Radiology 145:603, 1982.

51. vanSonnenberg E, Nakamoto SK, Mueller PR, Casola G, Neff CC, et al: CT and ultrasound-guided catheter drainage of empyemas after chest-tube failure. Radiology 151:349, 1984.

52. Gobien RP, Stanley JH, Gobien BS, Vujic I, Pass HI: Percutaneous catheter aspiration and drainage of suspected mediastinal abscesses. Radiology 151:69, 1984.

53. Parker LA, Melton JW, Delany DJ: Percutaneous small bore catheter drainage in the management of lung abscesses. Chest 92:213, 1987.

54. Hunnam GR, Flower CDR: Radiologically guided percutaneous catheter drainage of empyemas. Clin Radiol 39:121, 1988.

55. Merriam MA, Cronan JJ, Dorfman GS, Lambiase RE, Haas RA: Radiographically guided percutaneous catheter drainage of pleural fluid collections. AJR 151:1113, 1988.

56. Casola G, vanSonnenberg E, Keightley A, Ho M, Withers C, Lee AS: Pneumothorax: radiologic treatment with small catheters. Radiology 166:89, 1988.

57. Silverman SG, Mueller PR, Saini S, Hahn PF, Simeone JF, et al: Thoracic empyema: management with image-guided catheter drainage. Radiology 169:5, 1988.

58. Reinhold C, Illescas FF, Atri M, Bret PM: Treatment of pleural effusions and pneumothorax with catheters placed percutaneously under imaging guidance. AJR 152:1189, 1989.

59. vanSonnenberg E, Ferrucci JT, Mueller PR, Wittenberg J, Simeone JF: Percutaneous drainage of abscesses and fluid collections: technique, results, and applications. Radiology 142:1, 1982.

60. Stavas J, vanSonnenberg E, Casola G, Wittich GR: Percutaneous drainage of infected and noninfected thoracic fluid collections. J Thorac Imaging 2:80, 1987.

60a. Moulton JS, Moore PT, Mencini RA: Treatment of loculated pleural effusions with transcatheter intracavitary urokinase. AJR 153:941, 1989.

61. Conces DJ Jr, Tarver RD, Gray WC, Pearcy EA: Treatment of pneumothoraces utilizing small caliber chest tubes. Chest 94:55, 1988.

62. O'Moore PV, Mueller PR, Simeone JF, Saini S, Butch RJ, et al: Sonographic guidance in diagnostic and therapeutic interventions in the pleural space. AJR 149:1, 1987.

63. Westcott JL: Percutaneous catheter drainage of pleural effusion and empyema. AJR 144:1189, 1985.

CHAPTER 9

THE LARYNX AND PIRIFORM SINUSES

GORDON GAMSU

Computed tomography (CT) and magnetic resonance (MR) imaging, unique methods for imaging the larynx, have gained widespread application. Before the advent of these techniques, accurate assessment of the deep tissues and cartilages of the larynx could be achieved only by surgical exploration. Laryngoscopy, laryngography, and conventional tomography demonstrate the mucosal surface of the larynx and can suggest abnormalities of the deep structures only indirectly. Numerous studies have shown that CT and MR complement and extend these methods of visualizing the cavity of the larynx.[1-4] In the clinical assessment of patients, CT or MR is usually performed in conjunction with direct or indirect laryngoscopy and cannot compete with laryngoscopy in the evaluation of the laryngeal surface.

Interpretation of CT or MR of the larynx is difficult. Detailed knowledge of laryngeal anatomy and its appearance in the transverse plane is essential. Rigorous attention must be paid to detail when performing the examination. Misdiagnoses can occur if the patient's head is tilted or incorrectly extended. Detection and characterization of pathologic processes in the larynx require careful observation and experience. An understanding of the medical and surgical treatment for various laryngeal diseases and of the potential impact of the results of imaging studies on patient management is also important.

Anatomy

The larynx with its delicate cartilages, finely controlled muscles, and intricate joints and ligaments is a modified sphincteral valve at the entrance to the airway.[5] Suspended from above and continuous with the mobile trachea below, the larynx is capable of considerable vertical movement and rotation. It consists of an articulated cartilaginous skeleton surrounding the laryngeal airway, with many ligaments supporting the cartilages. Numerous muscles control movement of the cartilages, ligaments, and joints. Surrounding the entire larynx is a second group of muscles and ligaments that suspend the larynx from above and stabilize it from below.

Understanding of the MR anatomy of the larynx requires familiarity with the signal intensity of the various laryngeal structures on spin-echo images (Table 9–1). T1-weighted spin-echo images are usually used for imaging the larynx, and the MR ap-

TABLE 9–1 ■ Signal Intensity of Laryngeal Structures on T1-Weighted MR Images

High:	Pre-epiglottic fat
	Submucosal fascia
	Fatty marrow
	Thyroepiglottic ligament
	Mucous glands
Intermediate:	Hyaline cartilage
	Lymphatic tissue
	Aryepiglottic folds
	Positive chemical shift artifacts
Low:	Muscles
	Vocal ligament
	Fibroelastic cartilage
	Ligaments
	Perichondrium
	Tumor mass
Absent/Minimal:	Calcified cartilage
	Airways
	Blood vessels
	Negative chemical shift artifacts

Source: Modified from Teresi LM, Lufkin RB, Hanafee WN: Radiol Clin North Am 27:393, 1989.

pearance will differ with the age of the patient and degree of calcification of the laryngeal skeleton.

Laryngeal Skeleton

Three large single cartilages (thyroid, cricoid, and epiglottic) and three small paired cartilages (arytenoid, corniculate, and cuneiform) constitute the laryngeal skeleton (Fig. 9–1). In men, the larynx measures only 4.4 × 4.3 × 3.6 cm (length, coronal diameter, sagittal diameter); in women, it is about 25 per cent smaller.[6]

THYROID CARTILAGE

The thyroid cartilage is the largest of the laryngeal cartilages and is shaped like the prow of a ship (see Fig. 9–1). It is easily palpable beneath the skin and fascia of the neck. The cartilage is formed by two quadrangular plates or laminae (alae) fused in the midline at an angle of about 90° in the male and 120° in the female. A large V-shaped notch interrupts the superior margin in the midline and projects downward for about one third of the vertical height of the cartilage. The apex of the V projects slightly forward as the laryngeal prominence, or Adam's apple. The superior margin curves down posteriorly and then turns upward to become the superior horns or cornua. The strong thyrohyoid membrane attaches to the superior margin. During swallowing or a Valsalva maneuver, the thyroid cartilage ascends so that the thyroid notch lies within the horseshoe arch of the hyoid bone.

Inferiorly, the rounded posterior borders of the laminae become the inferior thyroid horns, which provide attachment for the longitudinal pharyngeal muscles. The short, thick, inferior thyroid horns have small medial facets for articulation with the cricoid cartilage. The cricothyroid ligaments attach to the midportion of the inferior borders of the laminae, and the cricothyroid muscles attach to the remainder of the inferior border. The thyrohyoid, sternothyroid, and inferior constrictor muscles are obliquely attached to the outer surface of each slightly convex lamina. Thus the thyroid cartilage is stabilized from above, below, and posteriorly by muscle and ligamentous connections.

The inner surfaces of the thyroid laminae near the midline and below the level of the notch have attachments for the three ligaments and two muscles that form the bulk of the internal structures of the larynx. From superior to inferior, they are the thyroepiglottic, ventricular (false cord), and vocal (true cord) ligaments. The thyroepiglottic and thyroarytenoid muscles attach close to these ligaments.

The thyroid cartilage is visibly calcified on CT in most adults older than 30 years.[7] The degree of thyroid calcification varies among patients, but generally it increases with age. The symmetry of calcification of the two laminae varies considerably, as do the inner and outer tables of each lamina. The posterior third of the thyroid cartilage invariably calcifies earlier than the anterior two thirds. Additional sites of dense calcification are the anterior midportion below the thyroid notch and the anterior portion of each lamina above the level of the notch. In older adults, the laminae frequently ossify, and the cavity contains medullary tissue. The appearance of the thyroid laminae on CT depends on the spatial resolution of the scans. High-resolution scans can differentiate between cortex and medulla in most older people.

On MR images in young patients, the thyroid cartilage shows uniform intermediate signal intensity on T2-weighted images, corresponding to the moderately high CT density of hyaline uncalcified cartilage.[8] In most patients older than 30 years, high-intensity foci are seen in the medullary cavity of the inferior horns, along the dorsal thyroid alae, and near the thyroid notch. Linear high-intensity foci are evident beneath the cortex in the medullary cavity of the midportion of the thyroid alae.[9] In most older patients, the thyroid cartilage at the level of the vocal cords shows inhomogeneous foci of high signal intensity on T1-weighted images. The margin of the thyroid cartilage consists of perichondrium when unossified and cortical bone later in life. At high field strengths, perichondrium exhibits a low to intermediate signal intensity, slightly lower than surrounding unossified cartilage. When cortical bone develops, it shows a decrease in signal intensity. At high field strengths fat within the marrow cavity produces a chemical shift artifact, causing a spurious obscuration or exaggeration of the very low intensity cortical rim of the thyroid cartilage.[9] When fat is not adjacent to the cortex of thyroid cartilage, this chemical shift artifact will not be found.

CRICOID CARTILAGE

The "signet ring," or cricoid, cartilage forms the only complete cartilaginous ring in the airway (see Fig. 9–1). It is smaller, thicker, and stronger than the

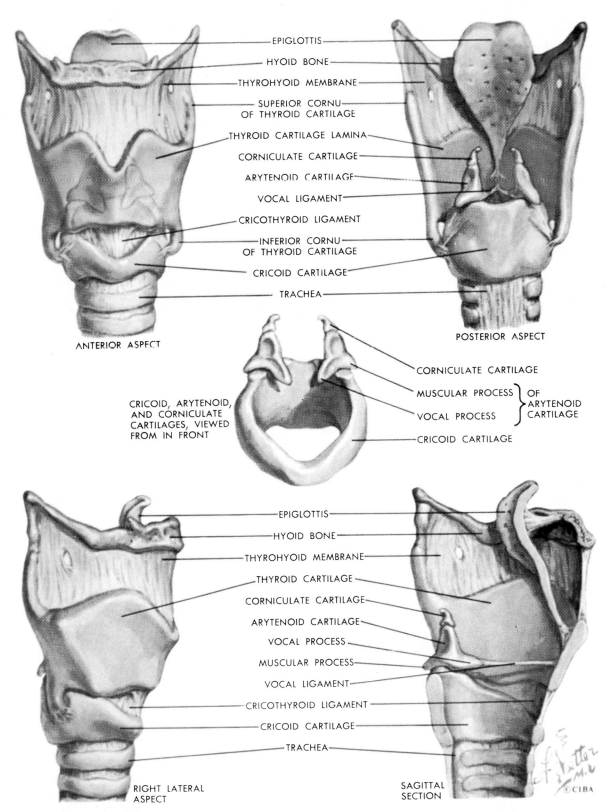

EPIGLOTTIS

HYOID BONE

THYROHYOID MEMBRANE

SUPERIOR CORNU
OF THYROID CARTILAGE

THYROID CARTILAGE LAMINA

CORNICULATE CARTILAGE

ARYTENOID CARTILAGE

VOCAL LIGAMENT

CRICOTHYROID LIGAMENT

INFERIOR CORNU
OF THYROID CARTILAGE

CRICOID CARTILAGE

TRACHEA

ANTERIOR ASPECT

POSTERIOR ASPECT

CRICOID, ARYTENOID,
AND CORNICULATE
CARTILAGES, VIEWED
FROM IN FRONT

CORNICULATE CARTILAGE

MUSCULAR PROCESS

VOCAL PROCESS

OF
ARYTENOID
CARTILAGE

CRICOID CARTILAGE

EPIGLOTTIS

HYOID BONE

THYROHYOID MEMBRANE

THYROID CARTILAGE

CORNICULATE CARTILAGE

ARYTENOID CARTILAGE

VOCAL PROCESS

MUSCULAR PROCESS

VOCAL LIGAMENT

CRICOTHYROID LIGAMENT

CRICOID CARTILAGE

TRACHEA

RIGHT LATERAL
ASPECT

SAGITTAL
SECTION

FIGURE 9–1 ■ Cartilages and ligaments of the larynx. (© Copyright 1964, CIBA Pharmaceutical Company, Division of CIBA-GEIGY Corporation. Reprinted with permission from CLINICAL SYMPOSIA. Illustrated by Frank H. Netter, MD. All rights reserved.)

thyroid cartilage. It forms the base of the larynx and is continuous inferiorly with the first tracheal cartilage. The posterior quadrate lamina, 2 to 3 cm in height, and the narrower anterior arch, 5 to 7 mm in height, form the posterior and anterior boundaries of the lower larynx, respectively.[10] The cricoid is supported from above by the cricothyroid and inferior constrictor muscles attached to the outer surface of the arch and by the cricothyroid ligament attached to the upper rim. The lower rim provides attachment for the stabilizing cricotracheal ligament. On the outer surfaces, at the junction of the arch and the lamina, are facets for articulation with the inferior thyroid horns, forming the synovial cricothyroid joints. The ridges of the lamina afford attachment to the paired longitudinal fibers of the esophagus and a hollow for the origin of the posterior cricoarytenoid muscles. On the upper edge of the lamina are small facets for articulation with the two arytenoid cartilages. The inner surface of the cricoid is smooth and in contact with the mucosal lining of the airway. On CT scans, soft tissue is not normally visible between the inner margin of the cricoid cartilage and the airway below the vocal cords.[11] In older adults, the cricoid cartilage is usually calcified. On CT scans, the lamina has a densely calcified margin and a nonmineralized center. As with the thyroid cartilage, the cricoid cartilage can ossify and surround a marrow-containing cavity.

On MR images, the appearance of the cricoid cartilage varies with the degree of ossification and marrow cavity development. In young adults, the cricoid demonstrates uniform intermediate intensity on T1-weighted sequences. In patients older than 30 years, the medullary cavity of the cricoid lamina is heterogeneous, with mixed high- and low-intensity areas.[9] As fatty marrow replaces hematopoietic marrow, higher signal intensity appears beneath the cortex, corresponding to the low density of fatty marrow on CT. The anterior cricoid arch shows lower signal intensity than the lamina in most individuals, demonstrating new uniform intermediate signal intensity. The cricoid cartilage shows a chemical shift artifact similar to that in the thyroid cartilage when imaged with high field strength magnets. This artifact results from the mismapping of signal at fat-water proton interfaces as a result of the differences in precessional frequencies of water and fat protons at high field strengths.[12] The artifact is seen only along the frequency encoding axis and can create spurious soft tissue asymmetry within the infraglottic larynx. In general, the thyroid and cricoid cartilages show wide variations in signal intensity in patients of the same sex and age. In very broad terms, older males have a higher signal intensity than younger females, but this observation is not of clinical value.

EPIGLOTTIC CARTILAGE

The mobile epiglottis projects upward and backward behind the root of the tongue and contains a thin, curved paddle of elastic cartilage (see Fig. 9–1).

Together with the aryepiglottic folds, the epiglottis forms the inlet to the laryngeal vestibule. Only about one third of the epiglottis has a free margin; this third is covered with mucous membrane both in front and in back. The other two thirds of the epiglottis is within the anterior wall of the laryngeal vestibule. The anterior surface of the free portion of the epiglottis faces the base of the tongue and attaches to it by a median glossoepiglottic fold and to the pharynx by two lateral pharyngoepiglottic folds. The two depressions formed by these three folds are the valleculae. The anterior wall of the inferior two thirds of the epiglottis forms the boundary of the adipose-containing pre-epiglottic space, which is behind the hyoid bone, thyrohyoid membrane, and upper portion of the thyroid cartilage. The laryngeal surface of the epiglottis is concave from side to side and convex from top to bottom. The curvature is maintained by the anterior midline hyoepiglottic ligament and the posterior aryepiglottic ligaments. The stalk of the epiglottic cartilage is firmly attached by the thyroepiglottic ligament to the inner margin of the thyroid cartilage below the notch.

Calcification is not a prominent feature of the epiglottic cartilage. With high-resolution CT scans, discontinuous plaques of calcium can sometimes be seen within the epiglottis. The position of the epiglottic cartilage must otherwise be inferred from its anatomic location.

On MR images, the epiglottic cartilage, composed of elastic cartilage, is intermediate in signal intensity on T1-weighted images and sometimes slightly higher in intensity on T2-weighted and proton density images.

ARYTENOID, CORNICULATE, AND CUNEIFORM CARTILAGES

The two pyramidal arytenoid cartilages sit on and articulate with the superior surface of the lamina of the cricoid cartilage (see Fig. 9–1). Their flat medial surfaces are covered with mucosa. Their concave posterior surfaces give origin to the oblique and transverse arytenoid muscles. The ridged anterolateral surface provides origin for the vocal muscle and thyroarytenoid muscle. Toward the base of each pyramid is an anterior projection called the *vocal process*, from which the vocal ligament extends within the free margin of the true vocal cord. Identification of the level of the vocal process of the arytenoid cartilages is of prime importance in viewing scans of the larynx, because the vocal process precisely identifies the level of the true vocal cords. At this level, the top of the cricoid lamina is still visible between the two arytenoid cartilages.

In adults the arytenoid cartilages are usually densely calcified. In fact, they are frequently the densest portion of the laryngeal skeleton. Their degree of calcification is moderately asymmetric, and on CT one cartilage appears larger than the other in about ten per cent of adults. With the patient in a relaxed state, such as during quiet breathing, the

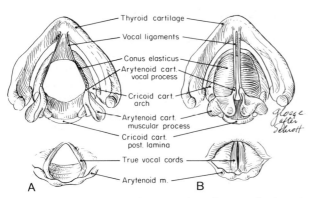

FIGURE 9–2 ■ Movement of arytenoid cartilages with phonation. Views from above the cricothyroid complex *(upper panel)* during quiet breathing *(A)* and phonation *(B)*. Arytenoid cartilages adduct and rotate medially during phonation. (From Mancuso AA, Hanafee WN: Computed Tomography of the Head and Neck. Baltimore, Williams & Wilkins, 1982, p 4. Reprinted with permission.)

arytenoid cartilages are in an abducted position less than 2 cm from the inner margin of the thyroid laminae (Fig. 9–2A). Demonstration of the vocal processes of the arytenoid cartilages is dependent on the spatial resolution of the scan. They can be identified in most people by the use of thin scans. During phonation or a Valsalva maneuver, the arytenoid cartilages adduct and rotate medially, approaching the midline (see Fig. 9–2B).[13, 14]

On MR images, the arytenoid cartilages have a low-intensity cortical rim and a high or intermediate signal intensity center. Signal intensity varies with age and the degree of calcification, ossification, and fat content. At high field strengths, the chemical shift artifact obscuring the thin cortical rim is less noticeable than in the cricoid or thyroid cartilage.[9]

The apex, or superior process, of each arytenoid cartilage, about 5 to 10 mm above the level of the vocal process, is pointed upward and inward and bears the small nodular corniculate cartilages. On CT scans these are normally inseparable from the arytenoid cartilages. The apex of the arytenoid cartilage defines the approximate level of the false vocal cords. On CT the laryngeal ventricles may not be demonstrated, and then differentiation between the true and false vocal cords is not possible.

The insignificant paired cuneiform cartilages are small strengthening rods within the aryepiglottic folds. They are occasionally visible on CT scans as small densities within the aryepiglottic folds, anterior to and slightly above the arytenoid cartilages.

HYOID BONE

The hyoid bone is not anatomically part of the larynx, but because of its intimate contact with the upper airway (see Fig. 9–1), it should be included in any discussion of the larynx. The hyoid is tripartite, with a central body and two wings, each of which contains a greater and lesser horn. The quite massive bar of bone forming the body lies transversely in front of the pre-epiglottic space and valleculae.[15] The

greater horns extend posterolaterally to encompass the lower hypopharynx and the entrances to the piriform sinuses. The larynx is suspended by the thyrohyoid membrane, which attaches the thyroid cartilage to the hyoid bone, and by the hyoepiglottic ligament, which attaches the epiglottis to the hyoid bone. The hyoid bone is in turn stabilized by attachments to the mandible and skull by the stylohyoid ligament and the digastric, stylohyoid, mylohyoid, hyoglossal, and geniohyoid muscles.

The level of the hyoid bone indicates two important anatomic landmarks. It marks the level of the superior extent of the pre-epiglottic space and also the level of the important jugulodigastric nodes in the neck.

At all ages, the hyoid bone is calcified, and on MR the low signal cortical margin surrounds a high signal marrow cavity.

Laryngeal Joints

The larynx is capable of vertical movement as a unit and intrinsic movement by the cricothyroid and cricoarytenoid joints. Both joints are enclosed in well-formed capsules. The cricothyroid joint is synovial and allows the thyroid cartilage to tilt, rotate, and glide with reference to the cricoid cartilage. The cricoarytenoid joint allows the two directions of movement. It allows the arytenoids to rotate around their vertical axes, opening and closing the space between the true vocal cords (the rima glottidis); they can also glide toward or away from each other. These two movements are coordinated so that medial rotation is accompanied by adduction and lateral rotation by abduction.

Laryngeal Membranes and Ligaments

The extrinsic ligaments of the larynx connect the laryngeal cartilages to adjacent structures, and the intrinsic ligaments connect the laryngeal cartilages to one another.

EXTRINSIC LIGAMENTS

The broad thyrohyoid membrane with its medial and lateral condensations of tissue attaches to the superior border of the thyroid cartilage and passes upward behind the body of the hyoid bone (see Fig. 9–1). It is separated from the hyoid by a midline bursa, which facilitates vertical movement of the larynx. The outer surface of the thyrohyoid membrane is immediately behind the infrahyoid strap muscles. Its inner surface forms the anterior boundary of the pre-epiglottic space toward the midline and posterolaterally lies lateral to the outer wall of the piriform sinuses. The thyrohyoid membrane cannot be seen on CT scans, but its position is easily identified between the low-density pre-epiglottic space and the higher density strap muscles. Laryngeal ligaments, more easily identified on MR than on

CT, are generally equal to or lower in intensity than skeletal muscle. The thyrohyoid ligament is imaged as a low-intensity band immediately in front of the high-intensity pre-epiglottic space.

The epiglottis is loosely tethered by the glosso-epiglottic folds and the elastic hyoepiglottic ligament, which runs from the anterior surface of the epiglottis to the upper border of the body of the hyoid bone. The hyoepiglottic ligament is usually visible on CT scans in the midline, traversing the epiglottic space.

The cricotracheal ligament forms the inferior attachment of the larynx. The fibrous membrane of this ligament connects the tracheal cartilages and continues upward to attach to the lower border of the cricoid cartilage.

INTRINSIC LIGAMENTS

The major intrinsic ligament of the larynx is the cricovocal ligament, also known as the *cricothyroid membrane* or *conus elasticus* (see Fig. 9–2). It is formed by two strong but flexible fibroelastic sheets in the shape of a tent open at the back and slit at the top. The strong anterior position attaches the upper edge of the cricoid arch to the inferior border of the thyroid cartilage. The midportion of this part of the membrane is subcutaneous. On MR scans this portion of the conus elasticus appears as a low-intensity band beneath the skin and subcutaneous fat of the anterior neck. The more delicate lateral extensions of the conus elasticus also arise from the superior margin of the cricoid cartilage, but then they arch upward and inward to blend into the vocal ligaments and form the superior free margins of the conus elasticus. The medial surface of the conus elasticus is lined with mucous membrane, continuous with that of the trachea. The lateral surface is medial to the cricothyroid, lateral cricoarytenoid, and thyroarytenoid muscles. Neither the lateral portion of the conus elasticus nor the vocal ligament is identified as a separate structure on MR scans.

The vocal ligaments stretch from the vocal processes of the arytenoid cartilages posteriorly to the inner angle of the thyroid cartilage, a little below the midpoint between the upper and lower borders. Above and parallel to the vocal ligaments are the paired ventricular, or vestibular, ligaments. These ligaments lie within the false vocal cords and are less well defined than the vocal ligaments; they extend from the tubercles on the upper arytenoid cartilages to the angle of the thyroid cartilage, slightly below the notch. The single, cordlike, thyroepiglottic ligament is an elastic prolongation of the epiglottic cartilage. It attaches the stem of the epiglottis to the back of the angle of the thyroid cartilage immediately above the attachment of the ventricular ligaments.

In the posterior larynx, the capsule of the cricoarytenoid joint is strengthened by a posterior cricoarytenoid ligament, which extends from the cricoid cartilage to the medial and dorsal surfaces of the base of the arytenoid cartilage.

Intrinsic Muscles of the Larynx

The intrinsic muscles of the larynx perform two functions: they adjust the aperture of the rima glottis and close off the larynx from the hypopharynx.

The adjuster muscles are grouped around the arytenoid cartilages and the cricoarytenoid joints to affect length, tension, and the degree of adduction of the true vocal cords (Fig. 9–3).[13, 14] Each lateral cricoarytenoid muscle passes from the cricoid cartilage to the muscular process of the ipsilateral arytenoid cartilage, pulling it forward and downward. The posterior cricoarytenoid muscles arise from the posterior surface of the cricoid lamina and attach to the back of the arytenoid cartilage. They abduct the vocal cords. The transverse and oblique arytenoid muscles form a sling between the two arytenoid cartilages, adducting them and, as a result, also adducting the true vocal cords. All of these muscles can be identified on high-resolution CT and MR as individual muscle groups.

The vocal muscles, formed by the lower fibers of the thyroarytenoid muscles, are the only muscles spanning the endolarynx.[15] Each arises from the angle of the thyroid cartilage and the conus elasticus as a broad, thin band within the true vocal cord and paralleling the vocal ligament. Each passes backward to insert into the vocal process, the base, and the anterior surface of the arytenoid cartilage (see Fig. 9–3). By a complicated mechanism, the vocal muscle can both shorten and adduct the vocal cord. On CT scans the vocal muscle cannot be separated from the vocal ligament and paraglottic tissues. On MR scans the vocal and thyroarytenoid muscles blend together as a single intermediate signal intensity unit within the true vocal cord.

The muscular connection between the cricoid and thyroid cartilages is the triangular cricothyroid muscle. It passes from the anterolateral outer surface of the cricoid to the inferior border of the thyroid lamina. By tilting the cricoid cartilage backward, the cricothyroid muscle elongates and increases the tension of the vocal cord.

The sphincter muscles of the larynx are the aryepiglottic, thyroepiglottic, and thyroarytenoid muscles (see Fig. 9–3). Together they form a sling between the epiglottis, thyroid, and arytenoid cartilages. Acting in unison, they constrict the laryngeal inlet by shortening the aryepiglottic folds and pulling the arytenoid cartilages forward and upward toward the epiglottis.[16]

Laryngeal Cavity

The laryngeal cavity extends from the laryngeal inlet above, through the vestibule, false cords, ventricles, true cords, and infraglottic space as far as the inferior border of the cricoid cartilage. The inlet of the larynx is a triangular ovoid set obliquely in the

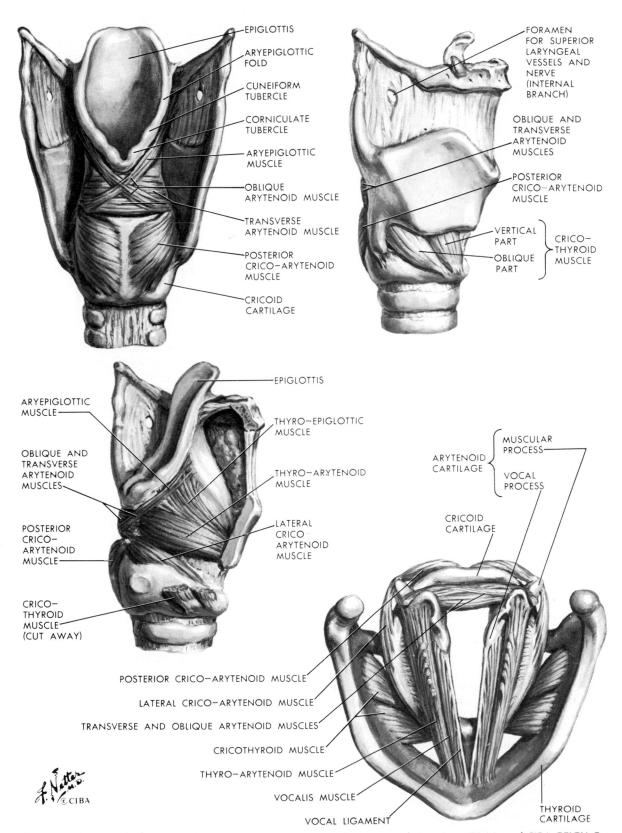

FIGURE 9–3 ■ Intrinsic muscles of the larynx. (© Copyright 1964, CIBA Pharmaceutical Company, Division of CIBA-GEIGY Corporation. Reprinted with permission from CLINICAL SYMPOSIA. Illustrated by Frank H. Netter, MD. All rights reserved.)

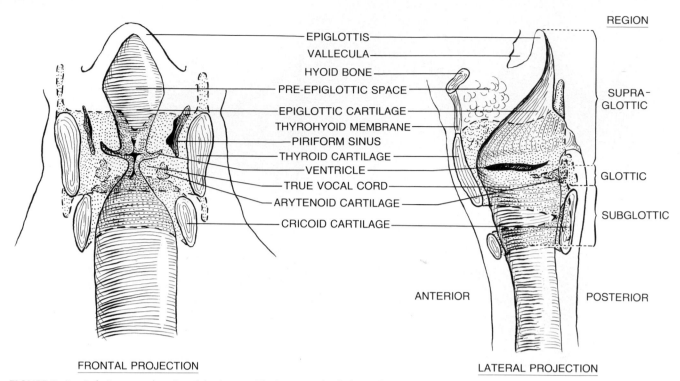

FRONTAL PROJECTION   LATERAL PROJECTION

FIGURE 9–4 ■ Soft tissues and cavity of the larynx. The larynx is divided into three anatomic regions; the largest is the supraglottic region and the smallest is the glottic region.

anterior wall of the hypopharynx. The base of the triangle is formed by the free edge of the epiglottis, the sides by the aryepiglottic folds, and the truncated apex by the arytenoid cartilages and the interarytenoid notch.

For clinical purposes and for the staging of laryngeal cancers, the laryngeal cavity is divided into three regions: the supraglottic, glottic, and infraglottic (Fig. 9–4).[17]

SUPRAGLOTTIC REGION

The supraglottic region consists of the posterior surface of the epiglottis, including its tip; the aryepiglottic folds; the arytenoid cartilages; the ventricular folds (false cords); and the ventricular cavities. The vestibule of the larynx is within the supraglottic region and is bounded by the epiglottic cartilage anteriorly and the aryepiglottic folds laterally. The vestibule is smallest posteriorly, where it is limited by the fold of mucosa between the arytenoid cartilages. During swallowing, the aryepiglottic folds shorten, and the arytenoid cartilages rise to the posterior wall of the epiglottis, closing the upper portion of the vestibule. The ventricular folds form two soft bumpers running from the angle of the thyroid cartilage to the arytenoid cartilages. The ventricular folds have less variety of movement than the true cords, because they do not have many muscle fibers. Inferiorly they merge with the roof of the laryngeal ventricle.

The most inferior extent of the supraglottic region is the keel-shaped laryngeal ventricle between the false and true cords. Immediately beneath the mucosa of the laryngeal ventricle is the thyroarytenoid muscle. Arising as a narrow opening from the anterior recess of the ventricle is the appendix of the laryngeal ventricle. This blind sac of variable size lies between the inner surface of the thyroid cartilage and the ventricular fold. At times it can be large, extending to the upper border of the thyroid cartilage or even through the thyrohyoid membrane to present in the neck as a laryngocele. The appendix of the laryngeal ventricle can be demonstrated in about 40 per cent of laryngograms.[18] On CT scans, especially during phonation, it is seen as an air-containing structure immediately within the anterior third of the thyroid cartilage.

GLOTTIC REGION

The glottic region comprises the true vocal cords (vocal folds) and the anterior and posterior commissures. The inferior extent of this region is not clearly defined, but it is 4 to 10 mm below the free margin of the vocal cords. The vocal folds are tightly bound to the vocal ligaments, which stretch between the junction of the lower third and upper two thirds of the thyroid cartilage at the thyroid angle and the vocal processes of the arytenoid cartilages. The anterior three fifths of the true cords form the membranous portion, and the posterior two fifths form the cartilaginous portion, enveloping the vocal processes of the arytenoid cartilages. The upper surface of the true cords borders on the supraglottic region, and the lower surface merges with the infraglottic region.

Posteriorly the glottic region is bounded by the mucosa between the arytenoid cartilages (the inter-arytenoid notch or posterior commissure).

Lateral and parallel to the vocal ligament is the amazing vocal muscle (see Fig. 9–3), which controls tension, elasticity, and rigidity of the vocal cords. During quiet breathing, the true vocal cords cannot always be precisely distinguished on CT scans. In their abducted position, they blend with the soft tissues of the lateral laryngeal walls. The level of the true cords can always be inferred from the position of the vocal processes of the arytenoid cartilages. CT scans obtained during phonation also demonstrate the normal true cords in apposition in the midline.

On MR images the vocal ligament within the free margin of the vocal cords cannot be defined. The combined vocal-thyroarytenoid muscle, with its low-to-intermediate signal intensity, can be seen in most patients. Lateral to this muscle bundle, a fibrofatty layer interposes between it and the more laterally situated cricoarytenoid muscle within the paraglottic space.

The anterior commissure is the area between the anterior junction of the true and false vocal cords. It is of great clinical significance, because malignant glottic neoplasms tend to both cross the midline and gain access to the infraglottic region at this site.

INFRAGLOTTIC REGION

The infraglottic region extends from the glottis above to the lower margin of the cricoid cartilage. In transverse cross section, the airway is almost perfectly round at this level. Anteriorly the infraglottic region is limited by the mucosa over the lower third of the thyroid cartilage, the cricothyroid membrane, and the anterior arch of the cricoid cartilage. The lateral borders are formed by the conus elasticus and by the lateral arch of the cricoid cartilage. Posteriorly the quadrate lamina of the cricoid cartilage limits the infraglottic space.

Soft Tissues of the Endolarynx

CT and MR precisely reflect the soft tissues contained within the laryngeal cartilages. The amount of soft tissue demonstrated is dependent on the level of the image, the phase of respiration or phonation, and the orientation of the larynx relative to the plane of the scan. For reproducible images, the vocal cords should be parallel to the plane of scanning (see Techniques of Examination).

The most inferior extent of the infraglottic region is within the ring of the cricoid cartilage approximately 15 mm below the level of the true vocal cords. The mucosa of the airway is closely applied to the perichondrium of the underlying cartilage, and no soft tissue is visible at this level on CT or MR scans (Fig. 9–5).[19] Superiorly for a distance of 1 cm, the more massive, posterior, signet portion of the cricoid cartilage maintains its intimate connection to the airway without intervening soft tissue (Fig. 9–6). The inferior border of the thyroid cartilage is 5 to 10 mm below the level of the true cords. MR images at high field strength may demonstrate spurious asymmetric soft tissue in the infraglottic region because of a chemical shift artifact in the axial plane.[9, 20] Interchanging the phase and frequency encoding axes can eliminate this artifact.

Viewed from below upward, soft tissues of the endolarynx appear at a level through the undersurfaces of the true cords (Fig. 9–7). During quiet breathing, the true vocal cords are bordered by the airway medially, the thyroid cartilage anteriorly and laterally, and the arytenoid cartilage and thyroarytenoid tissues posteriorly (Fig. 9–8). As indicated previously, the base and the vocal process of each arytenoid cartilage precisely define the level of each true vocal cord. During quiet breathing, the abducted true vocal cords usually appear symmetric. The distance from the medial margin of the vocal process to the inner margin of the thyroid cartilage is only 5.5 to 9.5 mm, with this distance representing the lateral thickness of the normal tissues of the cords.[19] The posterior portions of the undersurfaces of the true cords are often visible for 5 mm below the level of the vocal processes of the arytenoid cartilages. They invariably appear symmetric and should not be mistaken for an infraglottic mass.

In general the mucosal surfaces of the endolarynx demonstrate intermediate-to-high signal intensity on T1-weighted spin-echo imaging sequences. The mucosa of the upper surface of the vocal cords and the laryngeal ventricles have additional high-intensity foci on T1-weighted images that may be secondary to high concentrations of mucous glands (Fig. 9–9).

At the anterior commissure between the anterior extent of the true vocal cords, the airway is usually bordered by the inner margin of the thyroid angle. When the thyroid angle is acute, 1 to 2 mm of soft tissue are normally seen at the anterior commissure (see Fig. 9–8). As mentioned earlier, the posterior commissure is above the cricoid lamina between the arytenoid cartilages. Soft tissue is not usually visible in this region when the larynx is in a relaxed state.

Phonation, a Valsalva maneuver, or breath holding with the glottis closed causes apposition of the true vocal cords and markedly changes the soft tissues of the glottis (Fig. 9–10). The vocal processes of the arytenoid cartilages move medially an average of 4 to 5 mm as they adduct and medially rotate. On CT scans at soft tissue windows, the true vocal cords can be seen spanning the glottis with a small, slitlike space between them (Fig. 9–11). During phonation, the interarytenoid portion of the airway is nearly circular. With the vocal cords apposed, the anterior and posterior commissures can show compressed soft tissues that should not be mistaken for masses.

When the laryngeal ventricles are visible on high-resolution CT scans (Fig. 9–12), the true and false cords frequently can be distinguished. When they

Text continued on page 358

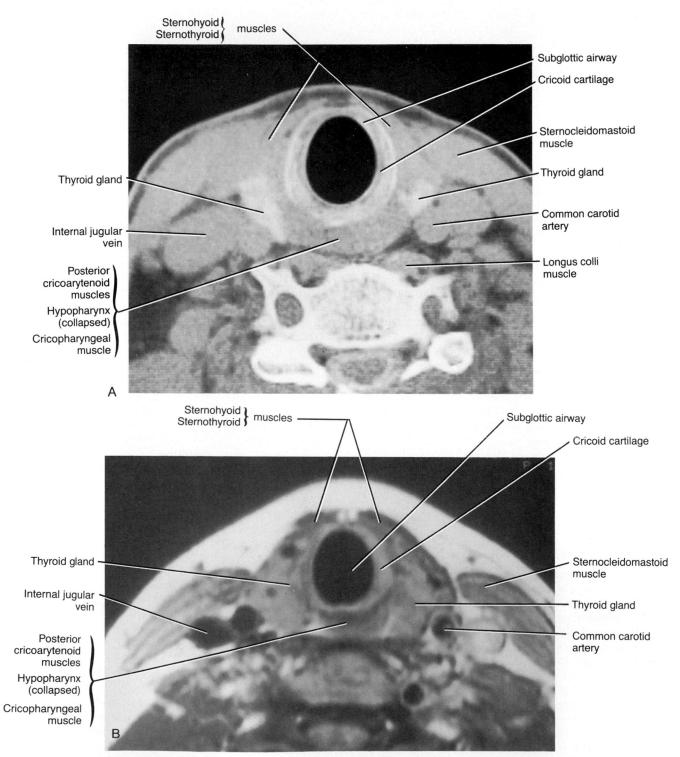

FIGURE 9–5 ■ Low infraglottic level of the normal larynx. *A*, CT scan. *B*, T1-weighted spin-echo MR (1.5 T).

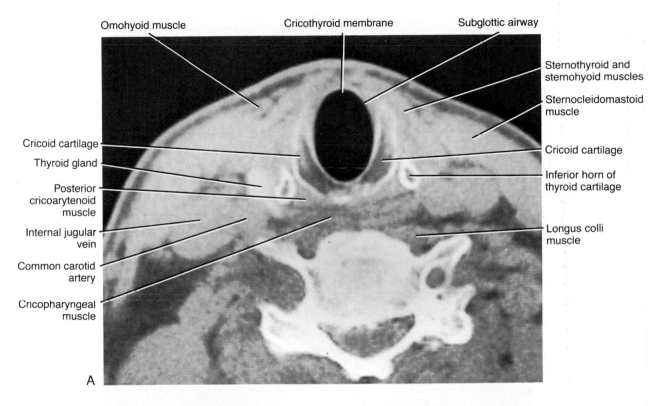

Omohyoid muscle

Cricothyroid membrane

Subglottic airway

Sternothyroid and sternohyoid muscles

Sternocleidomastoid muscle

Cricoid cartilage

Cricoid cartilage

Thyroid gland

Inferior horn of thyroid cartilage

Posterior cricoarytenoid muscle

Internal jugular vein

Longus colli muscle

Common carotid artery

Cricopharyngeal muscle

A

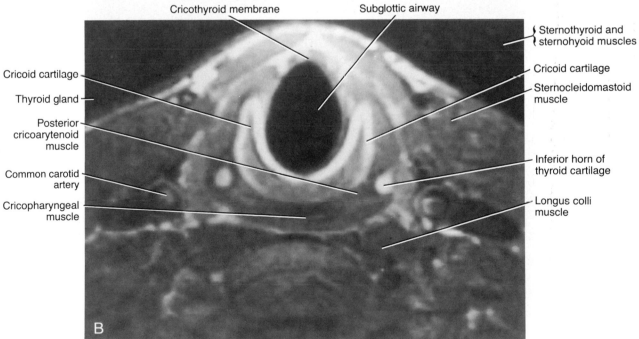

Cricothyroid membrane

Subglottic airway

Sternothyroid and sternohyoid muscles

Cricoid cartilage

Cricoid cartilage

Thyroid gland

Sternocleidomastoid muscle

Posterior cricoarytenoid muscle

Common carotid artery

Inferior horn of thyroid cartilage

Cricopharyngeal muscle

Longus colli muscle

B

FIGURE 9–6 ■ High infraglottic level of the normal larynx. *A*, CT scan. *B*, T1-weighted MR (1.5 T).

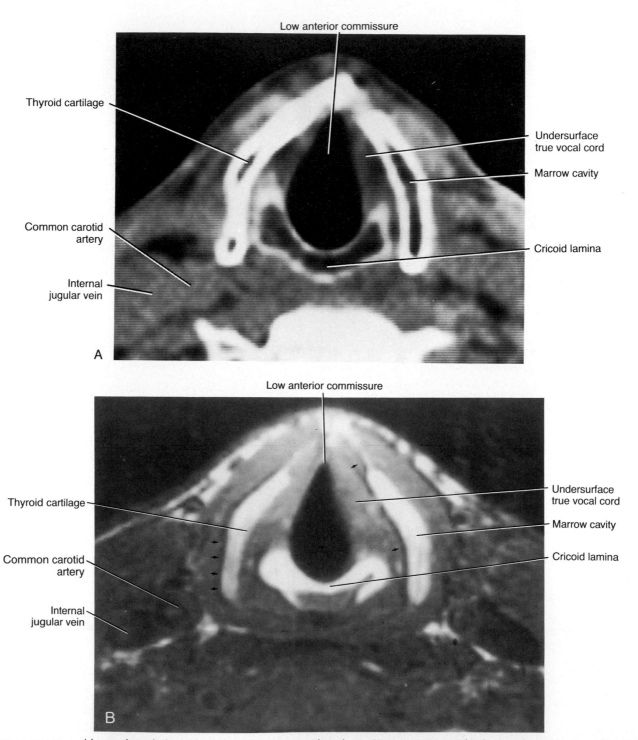

Low anterior commissure

Thyroid cartilage

Undersurface true vocal cord

Marrow cavity

Common carotid artery

Internal jugular vein

Cricoid lamina

A

Low anterior commissure

Thyroid cartilage

Undersurface true vocal cord

Marrow cavity

Common carotid artery

Cricoid lamina

Internal jugular vein

B

FIGURE 9–7 ■ Normal larynx through the undersurface of the true vocal cords. *A,* CT scan. *B,* T1-weighted spin-echo MR image at high field strength. The black line on the inner margin of the left ala of the thyroid cartilage and outer margin of the right ala of the thyroid cartilage *(arrowheads)* is caused by chemical shift artifact.

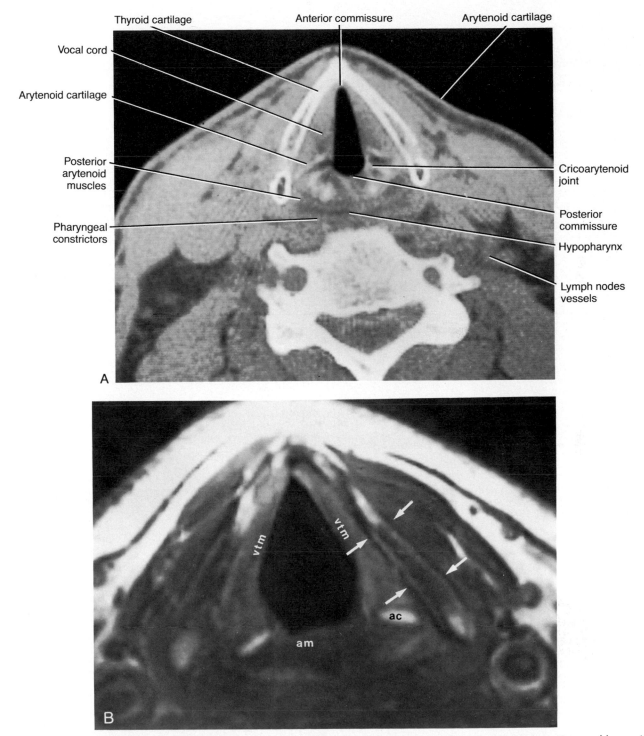

FIGURE 9–8 ■ True vocal cord level of the normal larynx. *A,* CT scan. *B,* T1-weighted (TR, 600; TE, 20) MR scan in a 40-year-old man. Low-intensity vocalis/thyroarytenoid muscle (vtm) is within the true vocal cord. The medullary cavity of the thyroid cartilage shows both high- and intermediate-intensity areas corresponding to fat and hematopoietic marrow or unossified cartilage, respectively. The lateral and medial cortices of the thyroid cartilage *(arrows)* are seen because hematopoietic marrow does not cause a chemical shift artifact. The arytenoid cartilages (ac) are high in signal intensity. The interarytenoid muscle (am) is posterior. (From Sakai F, Gamsu G, Dillon WP, Lynch DA, Gilbert TJ: J Comput Assist Tomogr 14:60, 1990. Reproduced with permission.)

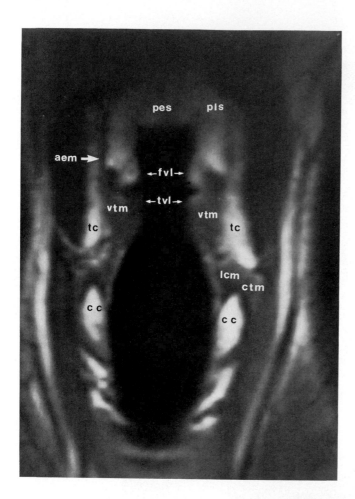

FIGURE 9–9 ■ Coronal T1-weighted (TR, 800; TE, 20) spin-echo MR image obtained with a three-inch circular surface coil. High-intensity fatty marrow is present in the thyroid cartilage (tc) and cricoid cartilage (cc). The cricothyroid (ctm), lateral cricoarytenoid (lcm), and vocalis/thyroarytenoid (vtm) muscles are demonstrated. The low-intensity aryepiglottic muscle (aem) extends superiorly from the thyroarytenoid muscle. The pre-epiglottic space (pes) and paralaryngeal space (pls) are demonstrated. The false vocal cords (fvl) and true vocal cords (tvl) are symmetric. Higher intensity signal in the endolarynx is from the mucosa or submucosal glands. (From Sakai F, Gamsu G, Dillon WP, Lynch DA, Gilbert TJ: J Comput Assist Tomogr 14:60, 1990. Reproduced with permission.)

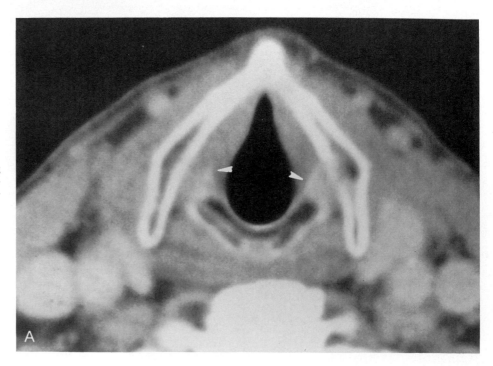

FIGURE 9–10 ■ Normal glottis during quiet breathing and phonation. A, During quiet breathing the arytenoid cartilages (arrowheads) are abducted.

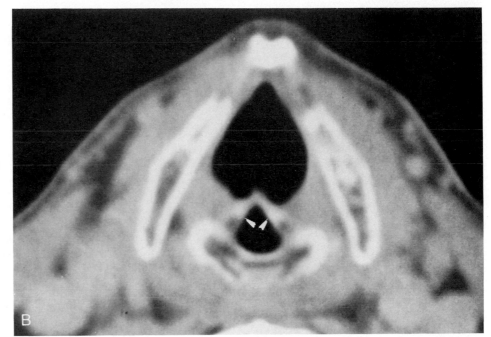

FIGURE 9–10 *Continued B,* During phonation the arytenoid cartilages *(arrowheads)* rotate and adduct.

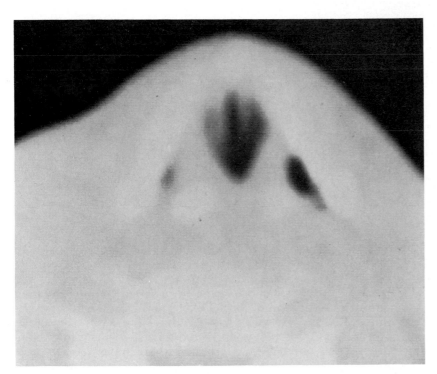

FIGURE 9–11 ■ Normal glottis during phonation, shown at soft tissue window settings. The vocal cords are demonstrated against the laryngeal ventricles in adduction.

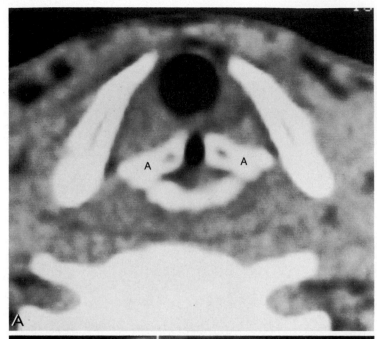

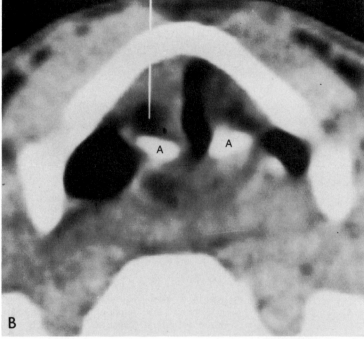

FIGURE 9–12 ■ Normal glottis and laryngeal ventricles. *A,* CT scan at the level of the true vocal cords demonstrates the arytenoid cartilages (A) adducted because of breath holding with the glottis closed. *B,* CT scan 9 mm superior to *A* shows air in the laryngeal ventricles as a low-density area *(vertical marker)* anterior to the arytenoid cartilages.

are not, the true and false cords are inseparable. Mancuso and Hanafee[21] refer to the region 5 to 10 mm above the base of the arytenoid cartilages and their vocal processes as the *transitional zone of the larynx.* At this level, the anterior larynx is still characterized by the airway remaining close to the inner margins of the thyroid cartilage. Laterally the tissues forming the false vocal cords are moderately varied in depth. They maintain a triangular shape and are symmetric from side to side. The CT density of the lateral soft tissues in the transitional zone is low, as these tissues are composed of fat, connective tissues, and a few muscle fibers. The density of the paralaryngeal tissues at this level may also be affected

by partial CT volume averaging of the soft tissues with air in the laryngeal ventricle. On MR scans, the false vocal cords are more intense on T1-weighted images than the true vocal cords because of their abundance of loose areolar tissue and extensive mucous glands.[4, 9] Within the false cord, the upper portion of thyroarytenoid muscle forms a low-intensity broad band crossing the paralaryngeal space. Occasionally one or both of the piriform sinuses extend as far inferiorly as the transitional zone. Then the air-containing apex of the piriform sinus is visible posterolaterally, immediately within the thyroid cartilage.

Posteriorly at the level of the false cords, the

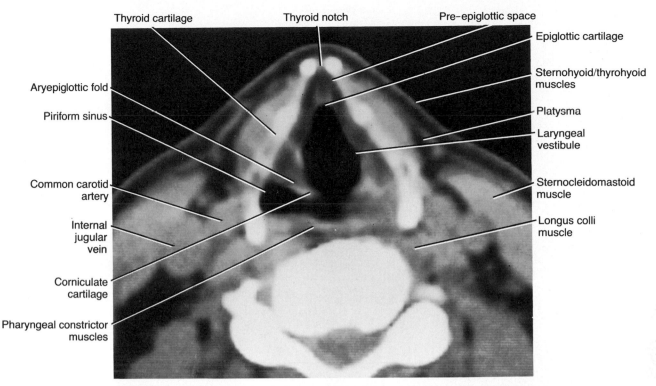

FIGURE 9–13 ■ Normal supraglottic larynx. CT scan is at the level of the thyroid notch.

superior processes of the arytenoid cartilages are still evident (see Fig. 9–12*B*). The posterior soft tissues of the larynx, however, blend with the collapsed hypopharynx and the prevertebral tissues. The distance between the airway and the spine is thus about 10 mm.

The bulk of the endolaryngeal soft tissue is found above the true and false cords. Anteriorly the preepiglottic space is visible 10 to 15 mm above the level of the true vocal cords (Fig. 9–13).[19] The pre-epiglottic space is limited posteriorly by the epiglottic cartilage and anteriorly by the thyroid cartilage, thyrohyoid membrane, and hyoid bone; it extends vertically for 10 to 20 mm. Inferiorly it is narrow, but its anteroposterior diameter rapidly increases to 10 to 15 mm (Fig. 9–14). The space is triangular inferiorly and assumes a crescent shape at the level of the thyrohyoid membrane (Fig. 9–15).

More important than the precise dimensions of the pre-epiglottic space is its fatty density, which is readily apparent on CT. In the midline, the thyroepiglottic ligament can be seen as a higher density, ill-defined structure. On either side, the uniform low density of the pre-epiglottic space measures −20 to −60 Hounsfield units (H).[19] The fatty tissues of the pre-epiglottic space extend laterally into the anterior third of each aryepiglottic fold. On MR the preepiglottic space is moderately inhomogeneous and high in intensity because of a network of fibroelastic tissue coursing within its substance.[22] On T2-weighted images, it shows high intensity and is thus readily identified.

The lateral supraglottic spaces are called the *para-*

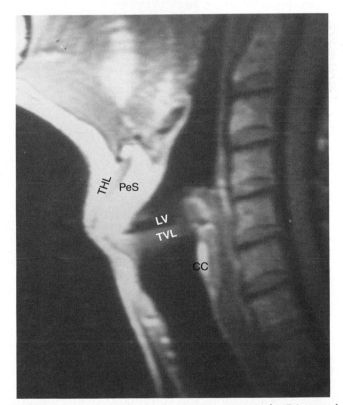

FIGURE 9–14 ■ T1-weighted (TR, 600; TE, 20) sagittal MR image of the larynx and neck slightly to one side of the midline. The pre-epiglottic space (PeS) is high in signal intensity. The laryngeal ventricle (LV) is immediately above the true vocal cord (TVL). The thyrohyoid ligament (THL) runs between the thyroid cartilage and hyoid bone. The signet portion of the cricoid cartilage (CC) contains high-intensity marrow.

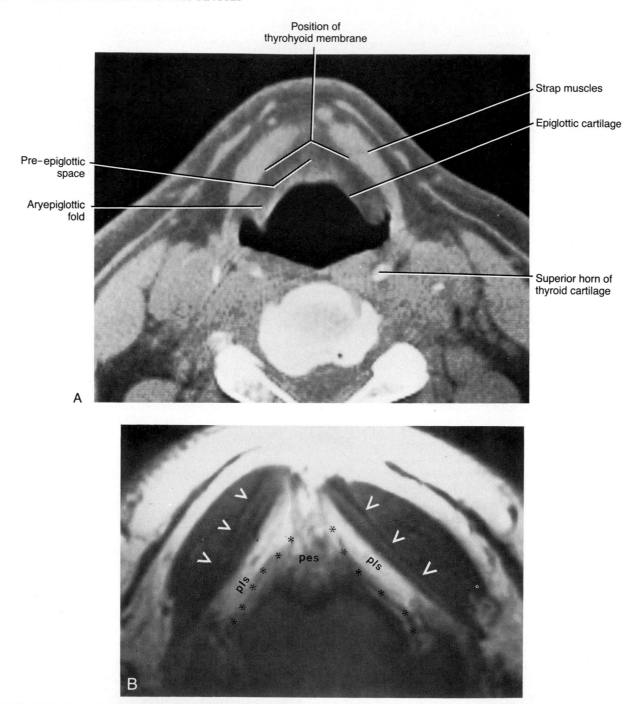

FIGURE 9–15 ■ Normal larynx at the supraglottic level. *A*, CT scan. *B*, T1-weighted MR. The pre-epiglottic space (pes) is separated from the paralaryngeal space (pls) by the quadrangular membrane *(asterisks)*. The thyrohyoid membrane and strap muscles *(arrowheads)* are low in signal intensity. (From Sakai F, Gamsu G, Dillon WP, Lynch DA, Gilbert TJ: J Comput Assist Tomogr 14:60, 1990. Reproduced with permission.)

laryngeal spaces and are limited medially by the quadrangular membrane and laterally by the thyroid cartilage and thyrohyoid membrane. The paralaryngeal spaces extend inferiorly to the level of the false cords. On CT scans they are continuous with the pre-epiglottic space, because the quadrangular membrane is not visible. On MR scans this membrane is seen as a low-intensity narrow band.[23] The paralaryngeal spaces, with their fatty areolar tissues, demonstrate the same MR imaging characteristics as those of the pre-epiglottic space.

The posterior extensions of the paralaryngeal spaces are formed by the aryepiglottic folds. On MR and CT scans the inferior 10 to 15 mm of each fold appears as an obliquely oriented band between the laryngeal vestibule and the piriform sinus. On MR scans the aryepiglottic folds demonstrate high signal intensity. Posteriorly they merge with the collapsed lower hypopharynx in front of the spine. Demonstration of the inferior aryepiglottic folds as distinct structures requires that the piriform sinuses contain air. Each fold is about 5 mm thick in its inferior

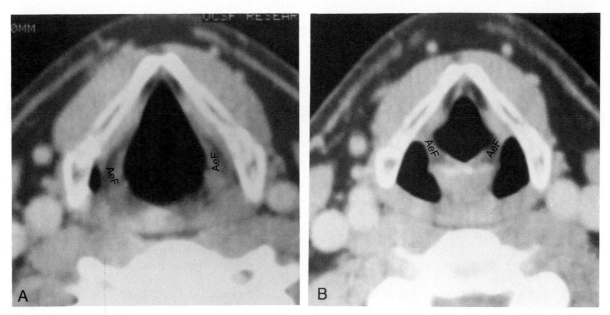

FIGURE 9–16 ■ Normal supraglottic larynx during quiet breathing and phonation. *A,* During quiet breathing, the piriform sinuses are collapsed, and the aryepiglottic folds (AeF) are not well delineated. *B,* At the same level during phonation, the piriform sinuses are distended, and the aryepiglottic folds (AeF) are thrown into relief.

portion and is appreciably thinner during phonation, when the piriform sinuses are distended (Fig. 9–16). A difference in thickness between the two sides of the aryepiglottic folds can be readily appreciated. Anteriorly the folds are continuous with the paralaryngeal space. The upper portion of each aryepiglottic fold is continuous anteriorly with the sides of the

epiglottis (see Fig. 9–15). At this level, the free margins of the aryepiglottic folds form the lateral boundaries of the entrance to the larynx. In front of the epiglottis are the valleculae and the hyoid bone (Fig. 9–17).

The piriform sinuses are between the aryepiglottic folds medially and the inner margin of the posterior

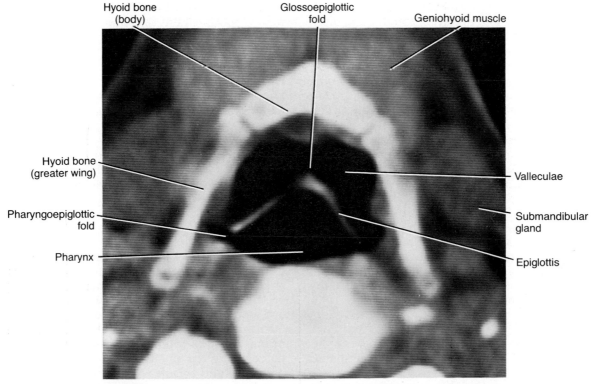

FIGURE 9–17 ■ Normal supraglottic larynx at the level of the hyoid bone and epiglottis.

half of each thyroid lamina. In the transverse plane, the shape of the piriform sinuses varies from triangular to circular to elliptical, but they are generally symmetric from side to side. The entrance to each sinus is from the hypopharynx and is lateral to the laryngeal vestibule (see Fig. 9–15). The lateral margin of each sinus is in intimate contact with the inner margin of the thyroid cartilage (see Figs. 9–12B and 9–16). The presence of any soft tissue between air in the piriform sinus and the inner wall of the thyroid cartilage is abnormal. The inferior extent of each piriform sinus varies between the two sides and among patients. During quiet breathing, the sinuses are partially collapsed and visible from about 15 mm above the true vocal cords.[19] During phonation, the sinuses distend and project downward to the level of the true vocal cords or within 5 mm of them.

Techniques of Examination

Optimal CT and MR scans of a small organ such as the larynx require meticulous attention to the technical details of the examination. Nondiagnostic and even misleading images can be created unless adequate care is taken in such matters as patient positioning and respiratory maneuvers.

Respiration

The structures of the endolarynx are both motile and mobile, and the potential for their distortion during imaging is considerable. The primary examination must be performed with the larynx in a state of complete relaxation (i.e., with the true vocal cords abducted). The patient should be instructed to breathe continuously and quietly through the mouth, without breath holding. If breathing produces artifacts, a second series of scans can be obtained during suspended respiration with the glottis relaxed.

After obtaining a series of scans through the larynx during quiet breathing, an additional series can be obtained during a maneuver that produces adduction of the true cords and distention of the piriform sinuses.[24] Scans during phonation of a low-pitched letter "E" are the easiest to obtain and the most reproducible.[3, 19] During phonation the arytenoid cartilages adduct toward the midline, the piriform sinuses are distended, and the aryepiglottic folds are brought into relief. Scans obtained during a Valsalva maneuver also show adduction of the true cords, but the images from this maneuver are less reproducible because of vertical movement of the larynx.

MR imaging of the larynx is obtained during quiet breathing, as current imaging times preclude imaging during suspended respiration or phonation.

Position

For CT and MR of the larynx the patient should be supine, with a pad between the shoulders to straighten the upper thorax. The arms should be pulled down along the side of the body as far as possible to avoid streak artifacts from the shoulder girdle. A useful adjunct is to have the patient grasp a sheet passed under the feet. The long axis of the larynx should be perpendicular to the plane of the image. The head (orbitomeatal line) is extended 35° to 40° to the vertical axis. For CT a lateral projection radiograph (computed radiograph, digital radiograph, or scout view) should be obtained while the patient phonates. The position of the head can be altered to correctly align the larynx perpendicular to the plane of the scan. The head is then immobilized in this position with tape.

A convenient routine is to start scanning at the lower border of the cricoid cartilage, which is easily palpated or seen on the projection radiograph. Three- or five-millimeter collimation with contiguous scans as far cephalad as the valleculae will encompass the entire larynx, a distance of 6 to 8 cm.

In patients with tumors, the field should be extended cephalad to the angle of the mandible to include the upper internal jugular lymph nodes. With infraglottic tumors, the field is extended caudad to include the trachea and upper mediastinum.

Contrast Material

Intravenous contrast medium has not been shown to assist in the CT diagnosis of lesions within the larynx or piriform sinuses. Detection and assessment of cervical lymph node enlargement is important in the evaluation of laryngeal carcinoma. The neck around the larynx contains numerous arteries and veins; opacification of these vessels is necessary to differentiate them from lymph nodes. The nature of nodal opacification can assist in determining the probability of metastasis (see Chapter 10). Sixty or seventy-six per cent contrast medium should be administered by rapid-drip infusion or bolus injection to a total of 125 to 150 mL (25.25 to 42.3 g of organically bound iodine). The contrast medium infusion should be timed in relationship to scanning in such a way as to maximize intravascular contrast. We have found that a bolus of 50 to 75 mL of 76 per cent contrast medium injected at 2 mL/sec, during rapid sequential scanning with advancement of the scanner table is usually successful in demonstrating the vascular structures of the neck.

Technical Considerations

Improvements in CT scanner capabilities have facilitated imaging of the larynx. Many of the original studies of the larynx were obtained with scan times of 18 sec or longer and had poor spatial resolution and equipment. Fine detail of the larynx was frequently not possible.[1, 2, 25, 26] CT scanners now allow primary magnification with better temporal and spatial resolution of an area the size of the larynx. Rapid, high-resolution scans with 3- to 5-mm slice thickness should always be employed.[11, 27] Reconstruction algorithms that enhance bone detail produce excellent visualizations of the laryngeal cartilages.

Rapid sequential scanning with incrementation of the scanner table improves registration of the scans with less likelihood of the patient moving during the imaging sequence.[11] Images reformatted in the coronal or sagittal plane can be generated from multiple transverse scans, although they do not assist in the diagnosis of laryngeal disease.[3, 28] Direct coronal CT scans of the neck and upper mediastinum can be made using scanners with a large aperture in their gantry.[29] Examination time is reduced, and image quality is better than that with multiplane reformatted images. However, this technique has not gained acceptance.

CT images of the larynx are viewed at settings appropriate for both calcified cartilage and soft tissue. A window level of 65 to 80 H and a window width of 500 H are suitable. Additional images at the level of the vocal cords are viewed at a window level of about −300 H and width of 1000 H to show detail of the soft tissue–air interfaces of the endolarynx.

For MR imaging of the larynx, the resolution required necessitates using surface coils or specially configured saddle-shaped neck coils (see Chapter 10).[4, 11, 23, 30] Spin-echo techniques have been described that employ short echo and repetition times, giving T1-weighted images with satisfactory signal-to-noise ratios.[4, 31] Slice thickness is generally 3 to 5 mm, with 1- to 3-mm interslice gaps. In most circumstances, multisection scans can encompass the larynx and neck with reasonable imaging times. Imaging is generally conducted in the axial plane, whereas coronal and sagittal planes are reserved for circumstances in which additional information is required.

Pathology

Neoplasms

BENIGN NEOPLASMS

True benign neoplasms of the larynx, except for squamous cell papillomas, are uncommon. Benign masses are more frequently non-neoplastic and include cysts, nodules, polyps, granulomas, and hematomas. Without biopsy and histologic examination, many of these non-neoplastic lesions are indistinguishable from neoplasms. Most benign tumors of the larynx are of epithelial connective tissue or neurogenic origin (Table 9–2). They are usually slow growing and tend to recur if incompletely excised.

The CT and MR findings of benign neoplasms have not been extensively described. However, a benign neoplasm may be encountered in a patient suspected clinically of having laryngeal carcinoma. Alternatively, CT and MR scans may be obtained to determine the extent of a known benign neoplasm.

Papillomas ■ Squamous cell papillomas may be single or multiple. They are the most common laryngeal tumor in children and tend to be multiple. In adults they are usually solitary.[32]

Papillomas usually arise in the anterior half of the larynx at the level of the true vocal cords or anterior commissure, and large lesions can cause airway obstruction.[33] Because papillomas do not penetrate deeply into the paralaryngeal tissues, destruction by microelectrocautery, cryotherapy, or laser beam therapy produces good therapeutic results.[34]

Juvenile papillomatosis is an aggressive form of squamous cell papilloma (Fig. 9–18). The papillomas tend to be multiple, and the recurrence rate is high.[32] They spread to the trachea and bronchi in about 5 per cent of cases. If repeated excision does not control the laryngeal lesions, tracheostomy becomes necessary.

Chondromas ■ Eighty per cent of the cartilaginous tumors of the larynx are benign chondromas.[35, 36] Most arise from the inner surface of the posterolateral portion of the cricoid cartilage.[37] Less commonly they originate from the thyroid, arytenoid, or epiglottic cartilages. Symptoms are often insidious, consisting of dyspnea, hoarseness, a sense of fullness in the throat, or a lump in the neck.

Conventional radiographs or xeroradiographs typically show granular or punctate calcifications.[35] CT scans can demonstrate the lesion's site of origin, its cartilaginous component with scattered calcification, distortion of the laryngeal skeleton, and the severity of airway obstruction (Fig. 9–19).[36, 38]

Hemangiomas ■ Hemangioma of the larynx occurs in infants, children, and adults. The adult form is the most common and usually arises on a true vocal cord, but it may be supraglottic or infraglottic.[39] Hemangiomas in infants and children are predominantly infraglottic and of the cavernous type. Approximately 50 per cent of children with laryngeal hemangioma have similar lesions on the skin, espe-

---

TABLE 9–2 ■ Classification of Benign Neoplasms of the Larynx

Epithelial:	Epithelial polyp
	Squamous cell papilloma
	Adenoma
	Oncocytoma (oxyphil adenoma)
	Benign mixed tumor*
Connective tissue:	Fibroma
	Chondroma
	Hemangioma
	Leiomyoma
	Lipoma*
	Rhabdomyoma*
Neurogenic:	Neurilemoma
	Neurofibroma
	Chemodectoma (glomus)*
	Granular cell tumor (myoblastoma)
Hematopoietic:	Plasmacytoma
Miscellaneous:	Hamartoma*
	Adenolipoma*
	Lymphangioma (cystic hygroma)*
	Branchiogenic cyst

Source: Modified from Barney PL: Otolaryngol Clin North Am 3:493, 1970.
*Rare

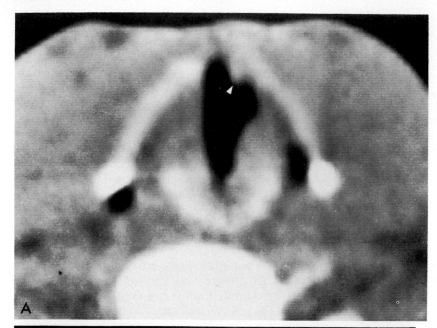

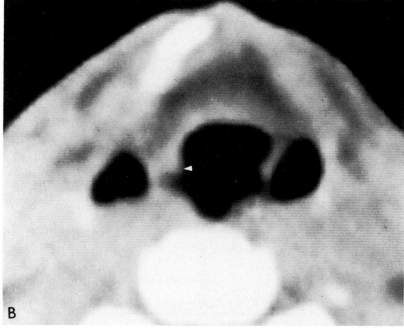

FIGURE 9–18 ■ Juvenile papillomatosis. *A*, CT scan at the level of the true vocal cords shows a papilloma *(arrowhead)* anteriorly on the left side. *B*, Scan 15 mm superior to *A* during phonation, an additional papilloma thickens the right aryepiglottic fold *(arrowhead)*.

cially on the head and neck. Symptoms are usually dyspnea, cough, and hoarseness. When large, these lesions can cause airway obstruction that necessitates tracheostomy. As with other benign tumors, CT scans can assist in determining the origin and extent of laryngeal hemangiomas. The CT findings have not been reported, but in one case that we studied, calcifications within the lesion suggested the correct diagnosis (Fig. 9–20*A*–*C*).

Neurogenic Tumors ■ Neurofibromas and schwannomas of the larynx are rare tumors that may occur at any age. They are slow growing, and symptoms are often insidious. Symptoms relate to the site of origin, which is most commonly an aryepiglottic fold. The CT findings are a nonspecific mass in an aryepi-

glottic fold or on a vocal cord.[40] In a patient with neurofibromatosis, demonstration of a laryngeal mass by CT should suggest the diagnosis of a neurofibroma. Multiple lesions are also suggestive of neurogenic tumors. Malignant neurogenic tumors do not occur in the larynx.

MALIGNANT NEOPLASMS

Understanding the role of CT or MR in the diagnosis and management of laryngeal cancer requires knowledge of the sites of origin, routes of spread, staging, and treatment options for these tumors. Laryngeal cancer accounts for 2 to 5 per cent of all malignant neoplasms.[41] The disease is more common in males than in females by a ratio of 10 to 1, and its

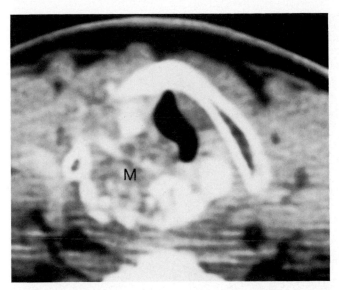

FIGURE 9–19 ■ Chondrosarcoma of the cricoid cartilage. CT scan at the level of the true vocal cords shows a large calcified mass (M) arising from the signet portion of the cricoid cartilage and narrowing the laryngeal vestibule. The tumor has invaded the right true vocal cord and right ala of the thyroid cartilage.

TABLE 9–3 ■ Classification of Malignant Neoplasms of the Larynx

Epithelial:	Squamous cell carcinoma
	Verrucous carcinoma
	Malignant mixed tumor
	Spindle cell carcinoma*
	Adenosquamous carcinoma*
	Basal cell carcinoma*
	Malignant melanoma*
	Adenoid cystic adenocarcinoma*
	Squamous carcinoma with pseudosarcomatous change*
	Adenocarcinoma*
	Oat cell carcinoma*
Connective tissue:	Fibrosarcoma*
	Chondrosarcoma
	Liposarcoma*
	Angiosarcoma*
	Rhabdomyosarcoma*
Hematopoietic:	Reticulosarcoma
	Acute leukemia
	Lymphosarcoma
Miscellaneous:	Metastatic carcinoma*

Source: Modified from Barney PL: Otolaryngol Clin North Am 3:493, 1970.
*Rare

peak incidence is in the fifth, sixth, and seventh decades.[40, 41] The cause of laryngeal cancer remains obscure, although strong associations with alcohol consumption, smoking, and airborne irritants have been demonstrated.[42]

Premalignant Lesions ■ The term *premalignant* refers to a lesion that is reversible or that can develop into frank malignancy. Several epithelial lesions of the larynx can, with time, become the site of laryngeal carcinomas. Keratotic papillomas are warty lesions that probably have malignant potential. Both squamous cell carcinoma and verrucous carcinoma may arise from them. Both acanthosis and pseudoepitheliomatous hyperplasia cause thickening of the laryngeal mucosa but are not known to be associated with malignancy. Leukoplakia, bowenoid dyskeratosis, and chronic laryngeal dyskeratosis are all forms of abnormal laryngeal mucosa. The incidence of malignancy developing from these three conditions is controversial and varies from 3 to 40 per cent.[41, 43] These conditions can be mistaken for carcinoma in situ, which almost certainly progresses to invasive cancer.

Pathology ■ More than 95 per cent of all laryngeal malignancies are squamous cell carcinomas (Table 9–3). They tend to be well differentiated and remain localized; however, once deep infiltration has occurred, they can spread rapidly. The direction and rapidity of spread of a laryngeal cancer depend primarily on its site of origin.

Adenocarcinoma of the larynx is much less common than squamous cell carcinoma. Subgroups of adenocarcinoma are cylindromas and mucoepidermoid carcinomas.[44, 45] Mixed adenosquamous cell carcinoma, oat cell carcinoma, carcinosarcoma, and spindle cell carcinoma are all uncommon. Other malignant tumors of the larynx are rare.

Site of Origin and Classification ■ The site of origin of laryngeal cancer has a direct bearing on its direction and rapidity of spread. Carcinoma of the larynx is classified and staged by its anatomic region of origin and by its site within that region (Table 9–4). The incidence of laryngeal cancer varies for each region. The general range of frequency of laryngeal or piriform sinus cancer according to region is glottic, 50 to 60 per cent; supraglottic, 20 to 30 per cent; piriform sinus, 10 to 20 per cent; and infraglottic, 2 to 5 per cent.[45-47] Extension of tumor to secondarily involve the infraglottic space can occur in up to 25 per cent of cases of glottic cancer.[48]

Staging ■ With appropriate treatment, laryngeal cancer has one of the highest rates of cure of any malignancy arising from an internal organ of the body. Treatment of malignant laryngeal tumor depends on a precise initial staging. Therapy of these neoplasms is directed toward preservation of speech while eradicating all of the tumor.

The staging of laryngeal cancer proposed by the American Joint Committee for Cancer Staging and End-Stage Results Reporting[17] is widely accepted. This system employs the TNM staging classification

TABLE 9–4 ■ Anatomic Classification of Cancer of the Larynx

Region	Site
Supraglottis	Epilarynx
	Posterior surface of suprahyoid epiglottis (including the tip)
	Aryepiglottic fold
	Arytenoid
	Vestibulum
	Infrahyoid epiglottis
	Ventricular bands (false vocal cords)
	Ventricular cavities
Glottis	Vocal cords
	Anterior commissure
	Posterior commissure
Infraglottis	

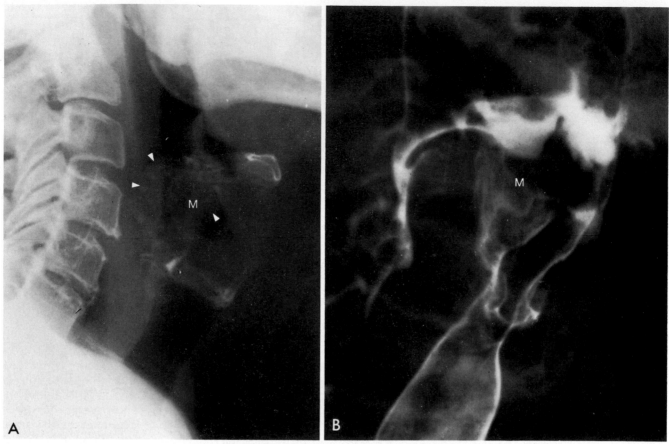

FIGURE 9–20 ■ Hemangioma of the larynx. *A,* Lateral radiograph of the neck shows a mass (M) in the supraglottic region *(arrowheads).* Calcifications are visible within the mass. *B,* Oblique view from a laryngogram confirms the presence of the mass (M).

TABLE 9–5 ■ Classification of Primary Tumor (T)

Primary tumor:	TX	Tumor that cannot be assessed
	T0	No evidence of primary tumor
	Tis	Carcinoma in situ
Supraglottis:	T1	Tumor limited to one subsite of origin with normal vocal cord mobility
	T2	Tumor involves more than one subsite with normal vocal cord mobility
	T3	Tumor limited to larynx with vocal cord fixation and/or involves the postcricoid area, medial wall of piriform sinus, or pre-epiglottic tissues
	T4	Tumor invades through thyroid cartilage and/or extends beyond the larynx to involve oropharynx, soft tissues of neck
Glottis:	T1	Tumor limited to vocal cord(s) with normal mobility (includes involvement of anterior or posterior commissures)
	T1a	One vocal cord
	T1b	Both vocal cords
	T2	Supra- and/or infraglottic extension and/or impaired cord mobility
	T3	Tumor limited to the larynx with cord fixation
	T4	Tumor invades thyroid cartilage and/or extends beyond confines of the larynx
Infraglottis:	T1	Tumor limited to infraglottis
	T2	Tumor extends to vocal cords with normal or impaired cord mobility
	T3	Tumor limited to larynx with cord fixation
	T4	Tumor invades through cricoid or thyroid and/or extends beyond the larynx.

for each of the three anatomic regions of the larynx (Table 9–5) as follows: *T* defines the extent of the tumor based on clinical examinations, endoscopy, and radiologic imaging modalities; *N* defines the status of the regional lymph nodes, usually assessed clinically but with CT and MR able to extend the examination; and *M* denotes the presence or absence of distant metastases, assessed by all available examining modalities.

The primary tumor (T) in each anatomic region is considered in terms of its extent (see Table 9–5). In the diagnostic staging of regional lymph nodes (N), the maximum diameter of the nodal masses is measured, with allowance made for the intervening soft tissue. There are three stages of positive nodes (Table 9–6). Midline nodes are considered ipsilateral. Distant metastases (M) are either present or absent.

Glottic cancer is defined as a malignant tumor originating on the true vocal cords. About 75 per cent of glottic carcinomas arise on the anterior half of the true cord near the anterior commissure, 15 per cent arise near the middle of the cord, and only 10 per cent arise on the posterior third.

Infraglottic cancer originates below the true cords and above a plane through the inferior border of the cricoid cartilage.

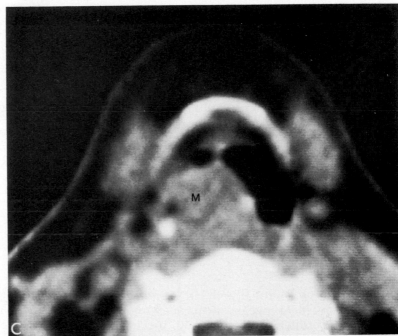

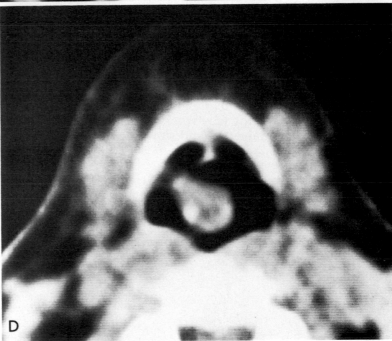

FIGURE 9–20 *Continued* C, CT scan at the level of the thyrohyoid membrane demonstrates the mass (M) extending into the right aryepiglottic fold and compressing the right piriform sinus. *D,* Five millimeters cephalad, the epiglottis and right pharyngoepiglottic fold are thickened. Calcifications are visible within the mass in C and D. Biopsy revealed an hemangioma.

TABLE 9–6 ■ **Classification of Regional Nodes (N)**

NX	Lymph nodes cannot be assessed
N0	No regional node metastasis
N1	Metastasis in a single ipsilateral node 3 cm or less in diameter
N2	Metastasis in a single ipsilateral node between 3 and 6 cm in diameter; multiple ipsilateral nodes, none >6 cm in diameter; or bilateral or unilateral nodes, none >6 cm in diameter
N2a	Metastasis in a single ipsilateral node between 3 and 6 cm in diameter
N2b	Metastasis in ipsilateral nodes, none >6 cm in diameter
N2	Metastasis in bilateral or contralateral nodes, none >6 cm in diameter
N3	Metastasis in a node >6 cm in diameter

Note: Diameter refers to greatest dimension.

Supraglottic cancer arises between the tip of the lingual surface of the epiglottis and the laryngeal ventricles. Of the 20 to 30 per cent of laryngeal cancers that arise in the supraglottic region, 10 per cent originate from the false cords, 8.5 per cent from the epiglottis, 5 per cent from the aryepiglottic folds, 2.5 per cent from the laryngeal ventricles, and 2 per cent from the area of the arytenoid cartilages.[47, 49]

Transglottic cancer is defined as a tumor extending vertically across the laryngeal ventricle to involve the supraglottic and glottic regions.[49, 50] Most arise from the true vocal cords and invade the laryngeal ventricle. Spread of this tumor may be mucosal or by deep penetration of the paralaryngeal tissues.[49]

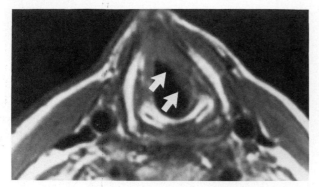

FIGURE 9–21 ■ Left true vocal cord carcinoma extending to the anterior commissure. T1-weighted MR of the glottis demonstrates a left true vocal cord mass *(arrows)* with extension of the tumor to the anterior commissure. Scans at lower levels did not demonstrate infraglottic extension of the tumor.

Dissemination ■ Essential to the interpretation of CT and MR scans of laryngeal cancers is an understanding of their growth potential and their mode of spread. In general, laryngeal carcinomas have defined predilections for their directions of local invasions. Their sites of origin and the normal structural barriers to tumor growth are the main determinants of dissemination. The frequency of nodal metastasis is likewise dependent on the site at which the tumor arises.

Glottic Region ■ Fifty to sixty per cent of laryngeal carcinomas arise from the true vocal cords. They are frequently well differentiated and slow growing. T1 glottic cancers have an excellent prognosis, with cure approaching 95 per cent whether treated by surgery or radiation therapy. Early tumors (T1) are localized, with mobility of the true cords being maintained. The free margins of the true cords do not contain

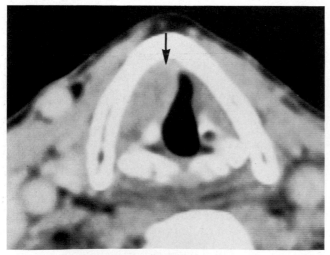

FIGURE 9–22 ■ Squamous cell carcinoma of the left true cord. CT scan of the true vocal cords demonstrates a mass involving the entire length of the right true vocal cord. The right arytenoid cartilage is displaced medially. The distance between the inner margin of the thyroid cartilage and the laryngeal airway is increased, indicating tumor extension to the anterior commissure *(arrow)* but not to the contralateral true cord.

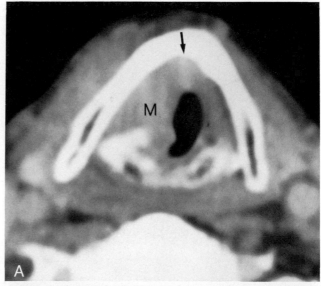

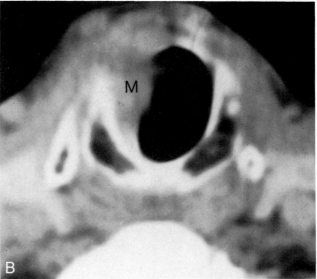

FIGURE 9–23 ■ Squamous cell carcinoma of the right true cord with infraglottic extension. *A,* CT scan of the glottis demonstrates thickening of the right true cord (M) with tumor extension to the anterior commissure *(arrow)*. The right arytenoid cartilage is encased with tumor, causing cordal fixation. *B,* Ten millimeters caudad, the mass (M) within the cricoid cartilage on the right side constitutes infraglottic extension of the tumor.

lymphatics, and nodal metastases are rare with T1 lesions.

CT and MR are probably not indicated for T1 vocal cord lesions and usually show no abnormality. They may show minimal cordal thickening that is indistinguishable from normal variations in cord thickness. The density resolution of CT does not allow for differentiation between tumor tissue and the vocalis muscle; thus detection of tumor depends on the recognition of abnormal thickening or irregularity of the true cord. High-resolution MR can sometimes reveal tumor extension entirely within the true cord (Fig. 9–21).

Glottic cancer spreads anteriorly, posteriorly, inferiorly, or laterally into the paraglottic space. Anterior extension is to the anterior commissure, and CT can demonstrate tumor involvement at this site. The quality of the scan must be excellent and careful attention paid to detect an anterior commissure tumor. In the normal larynx with a wide angle to the thyroid cartilage, the airway is directly behind the thyroid cartilage.[19, 27] The anterior commissure tendon, the point at which the two vocal ligaments attach to the thyroid cartilage, is not normally visible. However, with a narrow thyroid angle, 1 to 2 mm of soft tissue can be present anteriorly. Any additional soft tissue at the anterior commissure is abnormal and indicative of tumor extension to this site (Fig. 9–22). Surgery for tumors that have reached the anterior commissure is more extensive than for glottic tumors, often necessitating an extended hemilaryngectomy. Carcinoma that has reached the anterior commissure can grow in several directions. It can extend inferiorly to the infraglottic space and cricothyroid membrane, contralaterally to the opposite

true vocal cord, superiorly to the pre-epiglottic space, and anteriorly into the thyroid cartilage.

Infraglottic extension of glottic carcinoma is of great importance, because it directly affects staging and therapy. CT is as accurate as direct laryngoscopy for demonstration of infraglottic tumor and is particularly useful for showing the inferior extent of bulky cordal masses.[3, 28] The CT diagnosis of infraglottic carcinoma is made by determining the relationship of the tumor mass to the level of the true vocal cords. With the larynx in a relaxed state during quiet breathing, the level of the true vocal cords is identified by the vocal processes of the arytenoid cartilages. During phonation, the adducted true vocal cords are visible. We allow 5 mm caudal to the level of the vocal processes to encompass the undersurface of the true cords. Any soft tissue within the cricoid cartilage extending further inferiorly is indicative of infraglottic tumor (Fig. 9–23 and 9–24A and B).[3] If the patient's head is not adequately extended, the

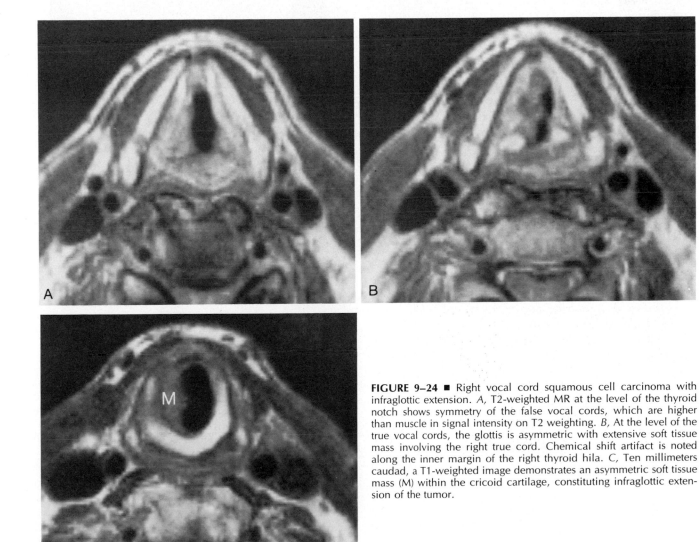

FIGURE 9–24 ■ Right vocal cord squamous cell carcinoma with infraglottic extension. *A,* T2-weighted MR at the level of the thyroid notch shows symmetry of the false vocal cords, which are higher than muscle in signal intensity on T2 weighting. *B,* At the level of the true vocal cords, the glottis is asymmetric with extensive soft tissue mass involving the right true cord. Chemical shift artifact is noted along the inner margin of the right thyroid hila. *C,* Ten millimeters caudad, a T1-weighted image demonstrates an asymmetric soft tissue mass (M) within the cricoid cartilage, constituting infraglottic extension of the tumor.

anterior portions of the vocal cords can project below the arytenoid cartilages and mimic a thickened anterior commissure. MR with high-resolution surface coils and T1-weighted images may be more accurate than CT for detecting infraglottic carcinoma, particularly when coronal images are available. Joffre and colleagues[51] found that MR, rather than CT, could more easily differentiate tumor from the undersurface of the vocal cords.

The thyroid cartilage at the anterior commissure is devoid of perichondrium, which is a natural barrier to tumor spread.[52] Tumor at this site can readily invade the thyroid cartilage and cricothyroid membrane. Dissemination in this direction is not readily detected clinically or endoscopically. The CT finding of thyroid cartilage invasion has a major impact on staging and treatment, because the tumor is then classified as an advanced (T4) lesion.[17] CT scans show a defect in the normally continuous density at the anterior commissure. On MR images, cartilage destruction appears as a defect in the normal low intensity of calcified cartilage and as a loss of the high signal intensity of the subjacent marrow cavity. It must be remembered, however, that variations in the extent of fatty marrow in the thyroid cartilage produce variation in MR signal intensity at this site.

Superior extension of carcinoma from the anterior commissure into the pre-epiglottic space (T2) is difficult to detect endoscopically. CT and MR are the only methods for demonstrating subtle tumor spread in this direction.[3, 4, 31, 53] Tumor within the pre-epiglottic space contrasts markedly with the normal low CT density or high MR intensity of the pre-epiglottic fibroadipose tissue (Fig. 9–25). Once the tumor has gained access to the pre-epiglottic space, it may remain on the ipsilateral side, cross the midline to the contralateral side of the pre-epiglottic space, or extend posteriorly into an aryepiglottic fold.

Glottic cancer commonly spreads to the opposite true vocal cord once the anterior commissure has been infiltrated. This route of spread can usually be detected at endoscopy and confirmed by biopsy of the abnormal-appearing contralateral cord. CT scans can frequently demonstrate contralateral spread (Fig. 9–26), but when both cords are symmetrically thickened, the lack of asymmetry makes detection more difficult.[54]

Posterior extension of glottic cancer is to the arytenoid cartilage, posterior commissure, and cricoarytenoid joint. Spread around the arytenoid cartilage can displace the cartilage medially, and the cartilage will appear adducted on CT scans during quiet breathing. Alternatively the tumor can fix the arytenoid cartilage in the abducted position, making it immobile during phonation (Fig. 9–27). Both of these findings indicate an advanced (T3) tumor. Once the carcinoma has gained access to the posterior commissure, it can cross to the contralateral vocal cord or escape laterally into the tissues of the neck. Tissue medial to the arytenoid cartilage on the same side as a glottic cancer is abnormal and highly suggestive of

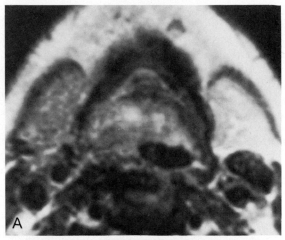

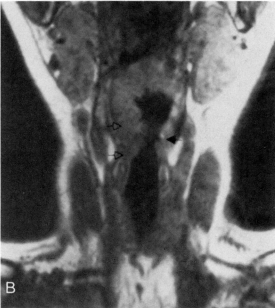

FIGURE 9–25 ■ Extension of right vocal cord tumor to the pre-epiglottic space. *A*, MR scan at the level of the thyrohyoid membrane demonstrates asymmetry of the pre-epiglottic space with thickening on the right side. The normal high-intensity fat within the pre-epiglottic space has been replaced by tumor. *B*, Coronal MR scan demonstrates asymmetry of the larynx. The position of the normal ventricle *(closed arrow)* is shown on the left side. On the right side, tumor *(open arrows)* extends from the level of the true cord superiorly to the pre-epiglottic space.

tumor extension to the posterior commissure. Reactive edema or fibrotic response can also produce thickening at this site. Widening or asymmetry of more than 1 to 2 mm of the distance between the thyroid and cricoid cartilages indicates tumor extension into the lateral cricothyroid space (Fig. 9–28).

Direct lateral extension of glottic cancer is into the paralaryngeal tissues between the conus elasticus and thyroid cartilage. The paralaryngeal space is an important route for tumor infiltration, as it communicates with the pre-epiglottic space anterosuperiorly and with the soft tissue of the neck between the thyroid and cricoid cartilages; glottic tumors can grow in either of these directions. The piriform sinus limits

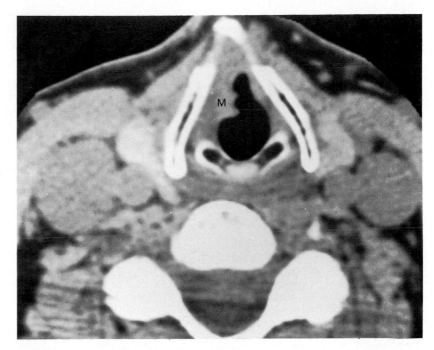

FIGURE 9–26 ■ Right true vocal cord squamous cell carcinoma with contralateral extension. CT scan shows the right glottic mass (M) with extension to the anterior commissure and contralateral anterior third of the left true vocal cord.

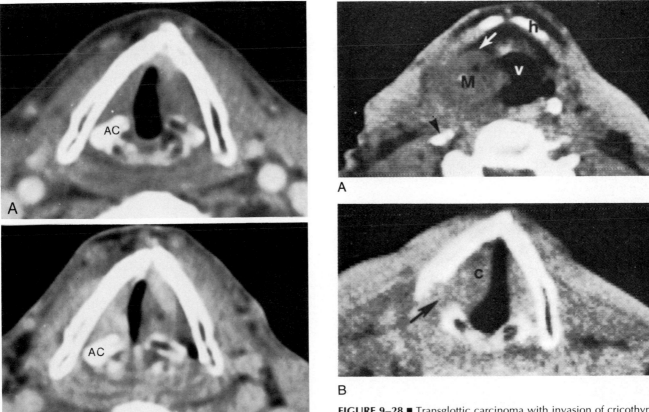

FIGURE 9–27 ■ Right true vocal cord squamous cell carcinoma with cordal fixation. A, CT scan during quiet breathing demonstrates that the normal left true cord has assumed a more midline position than normal. The abnormal right true cord is in an abducted position. The right arytenoid cartilage (AC) shows hyperostosis, possibly as a response to the tumor. B, During phonation, the left arytenoid cartilage has adducted; the right arytenoid cartilage (AC) is immobile. At direct laryngoscopy, a right true cord tumor was found with fixation of the cord.

FIGURE 9–28 ■ Transglottic carcinoma with invasion of cricothyroid space. A, CT scan at the level of the hyoid bone (h) demonstrates a mass (M) obliterating the right piriform sinus and extending to the lateral and posterior pharyngeal wall. The right side of the pre-epiglottic space (arrow) is infiltrated by tumor, which encroaches on the laryngeal vestibule (v). The right superior horn (arrowhead) of the thyroid cartilage is displaced posteriorly. B, CT scan 15 mm caudad at the level of the glottis shows tumor extending into the right cricothyroid space (arrow). The right vocal cord (c) is thickened. (From Archer CR, Sagel SS, Yeager VL, Martin S, Friedman WH: AJR 136:571, 1981. Copyright 1981, American Roentgen Ray Society. Reprinted with permission.)

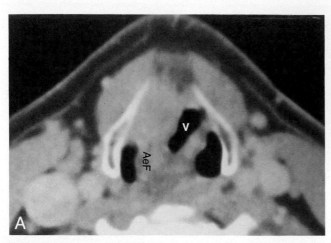
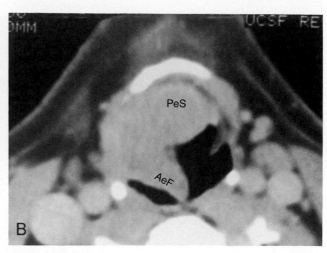

FIGURE 9–29 ■ Supraglottic squamous cell carcinoma with extension into the pre-epiglottic space. *A,* CT scan obtained during phonation demonstrates marked thickening of the right aryepiglottic fold (AeF) with displacement and narrowing of the laryngeal vestibule (V). The piriform sinuses are distended, which aids in defining the extent of tumor. Tumor within the aryepiglottic fold extends around the anterior wall of the right piriform sinuses. *B,* One centimeter cephalad, the upper extent of the right aryepiglottic fold (AeF) is still markedly thickened. The entire pre-epiglottic space (PeS) is replaced by tumor, which was not clinically apparent.

the paraglottic space posteriorly. Encroachment on the anterior wall of the piriform sinus is more easily detected from CT scans obtained during phonation. Carcinoma in the paraglottic space can directly penetrate the thyroid cartilage; its ossified portions offer the least resistance to tumor invasion. The difficulties with detection of cartilage invasion are dealt with later.

CT may underestimate the extent of invasion of the paralaryngeal tissues by glottic cancer.[55–57] Several authors have also shown that an inflammatory reaction and edema around the tumor can cause the extent of tumor to be overestimated on CT.[57] A bulky tumor may also compress adjacent structures, giving a false appearance of tumor invasion. However,

Katsantonis and colleagues[56] have shown that CT tends to underestimate the extent to which carcinomas have reached the anterior commissure and crossed the midline. With laryngoscopy, however, these sites can be observed, and a combination of laryngoscopy and CT has a combined accuracy of more than 90 per cent.

Supraglottic Region ■ Twenty to thirty per cent of laryngeal carcinomas arise in the supraglottic region.[58] The supraglottic region of the larynx develops from the pharyngeal anlage, whereas the glottic and infraglottic regions are derived from the lung and tracheal anlage. The lymphatics of the supraglottic region are abundant and separate from the two inferior regions. They drain laterally and superiorly

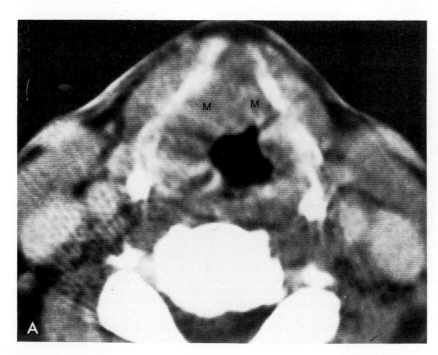

FIGURE 9–30 ■ Supraglottic carcinoma with extension to the pre-epiglottic space, valleculae, and pharyngoepiglottic folds. *A,* CT scan at the level of the thyroid notch demonstrates extensive bilateral tumor (M) in the pre-epiglottic space.

through the thyrohyoid membrane to the jugulodigastric and jugulocarotid nodes (see Chapter 10). Nodal metastases from supraglottic tumors are thus frequent and tend to be high in the neck.

The biologic behavior and surgical treatment of supraglottic cancer have led to the division of this region into two subregions.[59] The *superior subregion* is the epilarynx and consists of the posterior surface of the epiglottis (including the tip), the mucosa over the arytenoid cartilages, and the aryepiglottic folds. Some investigators have used the term *marginal* or *transitional* for epilaryngeal tumors and consider them hypopharyngeal.[47, 60] In the American system of classification, these tumors are included within the lar-

ynx. The *inferior subregion* is the vestibulum and consists of the infrahyoid epiglottis, the false vocal cords, and the superior surfaces of the laryngeal ventricles.

When first diagnosed, supraglottic cancers are usually more advanced than glottic cancers. They frequently metastasize to regional lymph nodes and invade surrounding structures.[41] Epilaryngeal carcinomas infiltrate the valleculae, base of the tongue, walls of the pharynx, infrahyoid epiglottis, pre-epiglottic space, and aryepiglottic folds. Vestibulum tumors infiltrate especially into the lateral paralaryngeal tissues, pre-epiglottic space, and thyroid cartilage. The epiglottic cartilage is fenestrated and

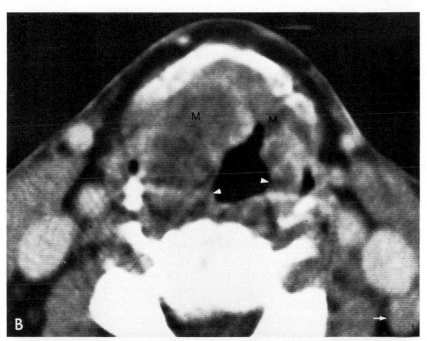

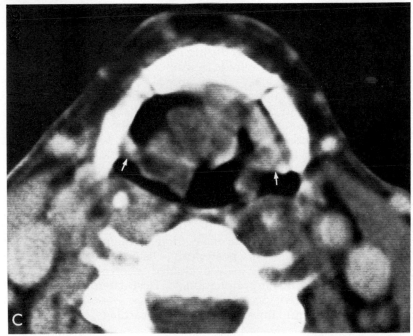

FIGURE 9–30 *Continued B,* Fifteen millimeters cephalad, the mass (M) surrounds the anterior endolarynx, filling the pre-epiglottic space and thickening both aryepiglottic folds *(arrowheads).* An enlarged lymph node is present on the left *(arrow). C,* An additional 10 mm caudad, the tumor invades both valleculae and both pharyngoepiglottic folds *(arrows).*

offers little resistance to tumor spread. Once the pre-epiglottic space and lower vestibulum have been invaded, the carcinoma can spread caudally to the anterior commissure and even to the infraglottic region. Tumors that extend caudally have a propensity for invading the thyroid cartilage.

Because supraglottic cancers frequently are more extensive than clinically suspected, CT can demonstrate deep penetration of these tumors and thereby help in planning appropriate surgery to eradicate the tumor. The pre-epiglottic space is well shown on CT scans, and an increase in its CT density indicates tumor infiltration or edema associated with the tumor (Fig. 9–29).[61, 62] Edema cannot be differentiated from tumor by clinical or radiologic means, including CT scans, and can lead to overinterpretation of the extent of tumor. However, these sites usually are resected or included in the radiation field along with the tumor. The extent of penetration of the pre-epiglottic space and of contralateral spread can be established from CT; both of these are of clinical importance (Fig. 9–30).[3, 63] The normal midline lower CT density of the hyoepiglottic ligament should not be mistaken for tumor. On T1-weighted MR images, the normal pre-epiglottic space is filled with high-intensity fibro-fatty tissue traversed by lower intensity fibroelastic septa. Infiltration of the pre-epiglottic space by intermediate-intensity tumor is readily identified.

Superior extension of cancer into the valleculae can be difficult to detect with CT or MR, unless it is extensive. Because the valleculae are normally asymmetric and their base is in the plane of the scans, they are not well demonstrated on axial scans. Fortunately tumor in this area is easily assessed by endoscopy. Thickening of the median glossoepiglottic and lateral pharyngoepiglottic folds, however, should be recognizable on CT or MR scans.

Extension of marginal tumors into the aryepiglottic folds and to the arytenoid cartilages is well demonstrated on CT scans. During quiet breathing, the piriform sinuses are usually collapsed, and the thickness of the aryepiglottic folds cannot be determined. On CT or MR scans obtained during quiet breathing, infiltration of aryepiglottic folds by tumor frequently cannot be appreciated as a mass effect. CT scans obtained during phonation show distention of the piriform sinuses and thinning of the normal aryepiglottic fold. Phonation thus allows for easier CT demonstration and localization of tumor (Figs. 9–31 and 9–32). Tumor extension into an aryepiglottic fold is recognizable by thickening of the fold and, in its anterior quarter, replacement of fibroadipose tissue by a high-density mass.

Lateral extension of supraglottic tumors is into the paralaryngeal soft tissues (Fig. 9–33). Paralaryngeal tumor is recognizable as a mass that frequently displaces the piriform sinus posteriorly. Distortion of a piriform sinus is more easily evaluated when the sinus is distended during phonation.[3, 24] Deep lateral penetration by tumor occasionally manifests as destruction of a lateral lamina of the thyroid cartilage.

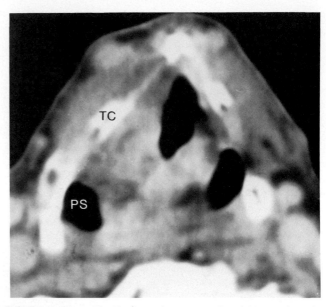

FIGURE 9–31 ■ Marginal carcinoma on the right invading the aryepiglottic fold. CT shows asymmetry of the aryepiglottic folds, with thickening of the right fold and posterior displacement of the right piriform sinus (PS). The right thyroid cartilage (TC) is bowed slightly outward from the tumor.

Infraglottic Region ■ Tumors arising in the infraglottic region are rare, whereas infraglottic extension of cordal or even supraglottic tumors is common.[47, 48, 64] True infraglottic carcinomas disseminate early and widely (Fig. 9–34).[65] Lymphatic spread is through the cricothyroid membrane to the prelaryngeal, pretracheal, and cervical nodes bilaterally. Infraglottic tumors frequently disseminate to the hypopharynx, trachea, and thyroid gland. When CT or MR is used to evaluate infraglottic tumors, the examination should be extended inferiorly to include the lower neck and upper mediastinum. Abnormality within the infraglottic region is particularly well demonstrated with CT because of the absence of normal soft tissue between the cricoid cartilage and airway below the true vocal cords. Any soft tissue in this region is abnormal. With MR, especially at high field strengths, an artifact can produce the appearance of asymmetric soft tissue in the infraglottic region because of chemical shift effects in the axial plane.[9] Interchanging the phase and frequency encoding axes will move this artifact 90°. Direct coronal MR images may demonstrate infraglottic tumor more effectively than transaxial images. Inferior extension of infraglottic tumor to the trachea can be difficult to assess by laryngoscopy but is well seen on CT scans as a mass within the airway. Tumor extension through the cricothyroid membrane into the soft tissues of the neck is seen on CT scans as an abnormal soft tissue mass. Vascular contrast medium can assist in determining the margins of the mass. Superior extension of tumor to the undersurface of the true vocal cords also can be difficult to detect. High-resolution CT images may demonstrate a plane between the tumor and true vocal cords. Alternatively,

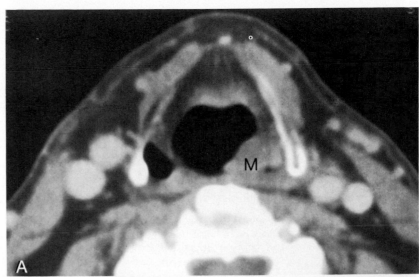

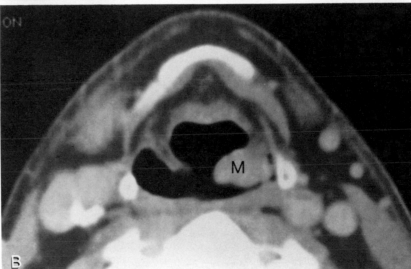

FIGURE 9–32 ■ Left marginal squamous cell carcinoma arising from the edge of the left aryepiglottic fold. *A,* CT scan during quiet breathing demonstrates asymmetry of the aryepiglottic folds, with thickening of the left fold by a mass (M). *B,* CT scan during phonation better demonstrates the mass (M) and narrowing of the left piriform sinus.

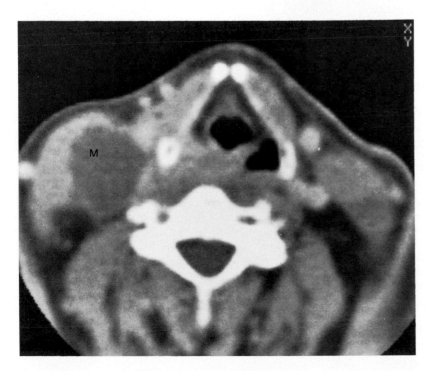

FIGURE 9–33 ■ Right supraglottic tumor with extension into the neck. CT scan shows the tumor having arisen from the right false cord and extending directly into the right side of the neck. A low-density mass (M), demonstrated by intravascular contrast medium, compresses the surrounding vessels.

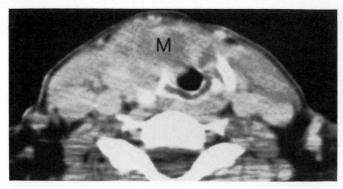

FIGURE 9–34 ■ Primary infraglottic carcinoma invading the neck. CT scan through the infraglottic region demonstrates extensive destruction of the cricoid and thyroid cartilage by a large mass (M), which has extended into the neck on the right side. The infraglottic airway is irregular with tumor between the cricoid cartilage and airway lumen.

MR images obtained in the coronal plane may show a plane of cleavage between the mass and true cords. Destruction of the cricoid cartilage is common with infraglottic tumor,[66] but scans should not be overinterpreted. A normal, thin anterior cricoid arch or tilting of the cricoid cartilage may be misinterpreted as cartilage destruction.

Transglottic Tumors ■ Laryngeal carcinomas that span the laryngeal ventricle to involve both the true and false cords are called *transglottic*.[49, 50, 66] They are advanced tumors, and vocal cord fixation is frequently present. The tumor can originate in the laryngeal ventricle, as do about 2.5 per cent of squamous cell carcinomas of the larynx. Alternatively, transglottic tumors can represent advanced disease that has spread from the glottic or supraglottic region. Dissemination may be superficial and obvious at endoscopy or deep by way of the paralaryngeal soft tissues. The thyroid cartilage and cricothyroid area should be carefully examined, because these tumors have a propensity for lateral invasion into the thyroid cartilage and beyond the confines of the larynx (Fig. 9–35).

Piriform Sinus Tumors ■ Piriform sinus carcinomas are usually classified as being within the inferior hypopharynx and not the larynx. They are discussed here because of their intimate contact with the larynx. Tumors arising in the piriform sinuses have a high incidence of nodal metastases when first seen, because early lymphatic invasion is common into the rich lymphatic supply around the piriform sinuses. Piriform sinus cancers also disseminate by direct infiltration inferiorly into the paralaryngeal tissues, supramedially to the aryepiglottic folds and pre-epiglottic space, and laterally through or around the thyroid cartilage.[63, 66]

Endoscopic observation of the extent of piriform sinus cancer is difficult and frequently underestimates the size of the lesion.[67] CT and MR can appreciably assist the clinical and endoscopic examinations in localizing and staging of the tumor.[1, 3, 4, 63] Soft tissue between the lateral wall of the piriform sinus and the inner margin of the thyroid cartilage is

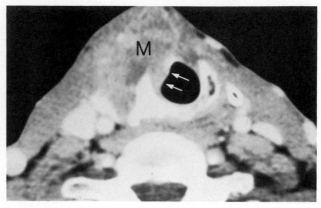

FIGURE 9–35 ■ Transglottic carcinoma with extension into the neck. Primary supraglottic tumor with extension to the infraglottic region. CT demonstrates infraglottic tumor *(arrows)* within the cricoid cartilage. A large soft tissue mass (M) represents tumor extension from the larynx into the neck. The bulky supraglottic component of the tumor prevented endoscopic evaluation. CT demonstrated the inferior extent of the tumor to the level of the first tracheal cartilage.

invariably abnormal (Fig. 9–36). Inferior extension of the tumor is to the level of the false and true vocal cords. Asymmetry of the paralaryngeal soft tissues in this region is the CT finding of spread of tumor in this direction. MR can demonstrate tumor infiltration of paralaryngeal spaces when tumor replaces the high intensity of fat at these sites. The cricothyroid space lateral to the conus elasticus is a potential path for extralaryngeal spread. Abnormal asymmetry in thickness or increased CT density of an aryepiglottic fold is indicative of medial tumor extension. Tumor from a piriform sinus that has extended to the pre-epiglottic space indicates advanced disease (T2). Direct lateral extension of the tumor is common and is indicated by destruction of the lamina of the thyroid cartilage or asymmetry of the soft tissues adjacent to the thyroid cartilage and thyrohyoid membrane. Direct extension of tumor into the soft tissue of the neck often cannot be differentiated on

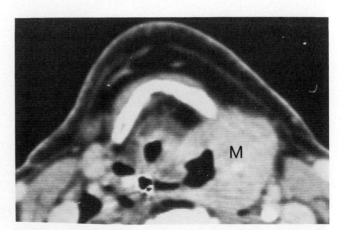

FIGURE 9–36 ■ Left piriform sinus carcinoma. CT at the level of the thyroid cartilage demonstrates a large tumor mass (M) surrounding the left piriform sinus and extending directly into the left side of the neck through the lateral thyrohyoid membrane. Streak artifacts are from a nasogastric tube.

CT scans from matted lymph nodes adjacent to the larynx.

Skeletal Destruction and Distortion ■ Demonstration of cartilage invasion or destruction is important in laryngeal and piriform sinus cancer, because this finding indicates advanced (T4) disease[17] and profoundly affects treatment. Endoscopy cannot demonstrate destruction of cartilage, and radiographs are insensitive for this purpose. The high-density resolution and transverse display of CT make it the most accurate proven method of detecting tumor disruption of the laryngeal skeleton. Because of chemical shift artifacts and the poor visibility of calcified cartilage, MR in our experience has major problems detecting focal cartilage invasion by tumor. Macroscopic cartilage destruction is demonstrated by a defect in the normal low signal intensity of calcified cartilage and a loss in the high signal intensity of the marrow cavity.[8, 58]

The incidence of tumor invasion of the laryngeal skeleton depends on the site of origin of the tumor. Kirchner[66] studied sections of 200 surgically treated larynges and found a marked variation in the incidence of invasion of the laryngeal skeleton. He found that 60 per cent of transglottic, 50 per cent of infraglottic, 45 per cent of piriform sinus, and zero per cent of supraglottic tumors had cartilage invasion. Glottic cancer invaded the thyroid lamina in only ten per cent of cases, usually when infraglottic extension of tumor had occurred. These incidences have been confirmed by several investigators in patients studied by CT.[1, 28, 61, 63] One study[68] reported that chondrosclerosis with increased CT density, as well as chondrolysis with decreased CT density, could be seen in laryngeal cartilages containing tumor. This potentially important observation has not been confirmed.

Marked destruction of the thyroid and cricoid cartilage is readily demonstrated on CT scans (Figs. 9–34, 9–35, and 9–37). Detection of small sites of cartilage invasion by malignant tumor is, however, one of the most difficult aspects of laryngeal CT.[57, 69] For instance, Werber and Lucente,[70] in studying 29 patients with laryngeal carcinoma, found that CT significantly underestimated cartilage invasion. The difficulties with CT are that the upper and lower margins of the thyroid cartilage are curved and normally appear irregular on CT and that the degree and symmetry of normal cartilage calcification or ossification varies among individuals and from side to side.[7, 26, 71] To detect subtle cartilage invasion, high-resolution CT scans are essential. Demonstration of an interruption of the cortex of the cartilage is necessary for a definite diagnosis of tumor invasion. Irregularity of the cortex is nonspecific and can be misleading.[72, 73] Castelijns and colleagues,[69] on the other hand, found that using a combination of spin-echo and protein density images, MR was equal in specificity to CT (88 per cent versus 91 per cent) and more sensitive than CT (89 per cent versus 46 per cent) in detecting cartilage invasion. This important observation requires confirmation, as it is our impres-

sion and that of others, that MR is neither sensitive nor accurate for detecting cartilage invasion. CT or MR detection of cartilage destruction most definitely will define a group of patients at higher risk for recurrence of tumor following radiation therapy.[73a]

Mancuso and Hanafee[74] dealt in detail with distortions of the laryngeal skeleton by laryngeal cancer. They found two types of distortions: deformation of the shape of the thyroid cartilage and disturbance of the normal relationships of the laryngeal cartilages to one another. Neither of these abnormalities is specific for malignant neoplasms, as they also occur with traumatic inflammatory and benign masses, with radiation chondronecrosis, and after surgery.

The thyroid laminae are relatively weak, and their shape can be deformed by bulky masses or abnormal stresses. They can buckle inwardly or bow outwardly. In our experience these distortions do not necessarily signify tumor invasion of the cartilage, and their importance is questionable.

Disturbances in alignment of the cricoid, thyroid, and arytenoid cartilages and of the hyoid bone are common with, but not specific for, laryngeal tumors. The alignment of these cartilages can vary normally with change in patient position and with respiratory maneuvers. Before a diagnosis of abnormal tilting or rotation of the thyroid cartilage or hyoid bone is considered, correct alignment of the head and neck

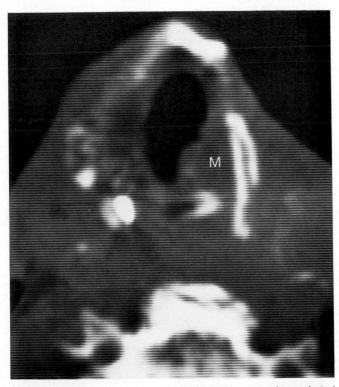

FIGURE 9–37 ■ Transglottic carcinoma extending into the neck and causing cartilage destruction. CT scan shows the endolaryngeal tumor mass (M) with extension into the neck on the left side. The thyroid cartilage is distorted and deformed, with its left outer wall destroyed.

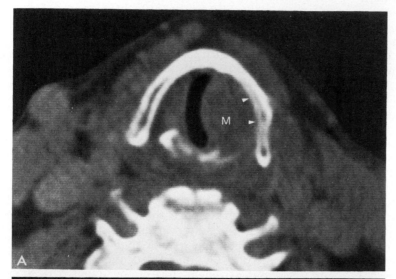

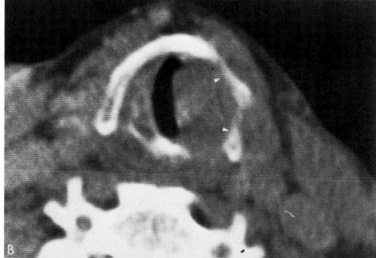

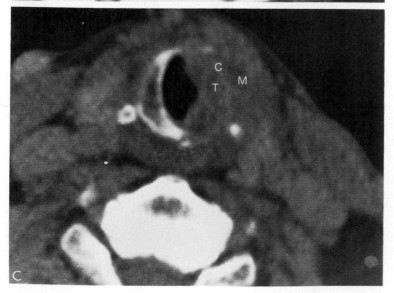

FIGURE 9–38 ■ Destruction of arytenoid and cricoid cartilages and infraglottic extension of carcinoma. *A,* CT scan through the true vocal cords shows a left tumor mass (M) that has destroyed the left side of the cricoid cartilage. The inner margin of the thyroid cartilage *(arrowheads)* is irregular but not definitely invaded. *B,* CT scan 5 mm caudad continues to show the bulky mass with distortion of the thyroid cartilage *(arrowheads)*. The cricoid cartilage should be visible at this level. *C,* CT scan 10 mm caudad demonstrates destruction of the left side of the cricoid cartilage (C). Infraglottic extension of the tumor (T) is present. The mass (M) lateral to the cricoid cartilage represents tumor infiltration into the neck through the crico-thyroid membrane.

must be assured. Bulky masses or cricothyroid joint disruption can cause the thyroid cartilage to tilt forward on the cricoid or to rotate about the long axis of the larynx (Fig. 9–38). Even when real, these distortions do not directly assist in determining tumor extent but may draw one's attention to regions of the larynx that are potentially involved by carcinoma. Frequently, minor buckling or bowing of the thyroid cartilage is caused by previous trauma that may not be remembered by the patient.[75]

The normal vertical distance between the thyroid cartilage and hyoid bone can be increased by a large mass in the pre-epiglottic space. The thyroid cartilage and hyoid bone normally overlap during a Valsalva maneuver or phonation, so both will be demonstrated on the same scan. Failure of the thyroid cartilage to overlap the hyoid bone is a radiographic sign of infiltration of pre-epiglottic space by tumor.[76] Because the tumor itself can be demonstrated with CT or MR, this indirect evidence of pre-epiglottic space invasion is not used for diagnosis. In general, tumor distortion or invasion of the laryngeal skeleton should not be diagnosed unless an adjacent mass is visible.

Cordal Fixation ■ Endoscopically determined immobility of a true cord is defined as *cordal fixation*. The significance of this finding was first recognized in 1959 by Lenz and colleagues.[77] Patients with laryngeal tumors that cause cordal fixation generally have a lower survival rate than those with laryngeal tumors and vocal cord motility.[78] The failure rate for radiation therapy when there is cordal fixation is high, and in most situations, simple hemilaryngectomy is inadequate for eradication of the tumor. Total laryngectomy or extended vertical hemilaryngectomy is the usual surgical procedure for removal of a tumor with cordal fixation.

The American Joint Committee Staging System classifies tumors with cordal fixation as advanced (T3) lesions.[17] Five focal mechanisms[79] can cause cordal fixation from laryngeal tumor:

1. Complete replacement of the thyroarytenoid muscle by tumor can immobilize the true vocal cord.
2. Lateral extension of tumor to the thyroid cartilage can bind and immobilize the vocal cord, although the thyroarytenoid muscle is not replaced by tumor.
3. A bulky tumor involving the true cord can prevent it from moving, without either of the first two mechanisms being operational.
4. Infraglottic tumor, particularly posteriorly, can fix the vocal cord to the cricoid cartilage.
5. Finally, cricoarytenoid joint invasion by tumor can freeze the joint and immobilize the true vocal cord.

Immobility of the vocal cord is readily confirmed by a combination of CT performed during quiet breathing and phonation.[3, 24] Two patterns of abnormality may be seen. Either the arytenoid cartilage is in an abducted position during quiet breathing and is not adducted during phonation (see Fig. 9–27), or it remains adducted during both quiet breathing and phonation. However, these findings alone are not specific, because vocal cord paralysis from damage to the recurrent laryngeal nerve can have the same CT scan patterns of abnormality.[80]

CT can accurately demonstrate the mechanism of cordal fixation in most instances.[81] Tumor mass infiltrating the arytenoid cartilage and the cricoarytenoid joint is the most common finding. CT scans are extremely accurate in showing posterior infraglottic extension of the tumor within the cricoid cartilage, seen as a soft tissue mass below the level of the true vocal cords. Occasionally CT distortion of the laryngeal skeleton from prior trauma can explain an immobile cord in a patient with a carcinoma. We have seen several patients with cordal tumors in whom CT indicated cordal fixation that had not been detected at indirect laryngoscopy; while repeat endoscopy confirmed the CT findings.

Regional Lymph Node Metastases ■ The most important determinant of the survival of patients with laryngeal cancer is the presence of carcinoma in the regional lymph nodes. Survival decreases approximately 40 per cent when cervical lymph nodes contain tumor and are palpable. The incidence of nodal metastases varies with the degree of histologic differentiation and the growth pattern of the tumor, as well as with the tumor's location and size. The highest correlation of the metastatic rate is with the location of the primary tumor.[45, 82]

Small (T1) glottic tumors have an incidence of nodal metastases of only zero to two per cent. When the tumor has spread locally to the anterior commissure, infraglottic region, or posterior commissure (T2 lesions), the incidence of regional metastases increases to 5 to 16 per cent. Occult metastases occur in approximately 5 per cent of patients. When tumor extends to the infraglottic region, lymph nodes around the thyroid gland and upper trachea may contain metastatic deposits.

Supraglottic cancers are often larger than glottic cancers when first discovered, and the supraglottic region has a more abundant lymphatic supply than the glottis. The incidence of nodal metastases is 20 to 50 per cent (see Fig. 9–38), half of which are not clinically palpable.

Primary infraglottic carcinomas are rare but tend to metastasize to regional nodes; with an incidence of approximately 25 per cent. As with infraglottic extension of glottic tumors, primary infraglottic tumors can metastasize to the upper mediastinal nodes.

Transglottic cancer is advanced disease, reflected in its high incidence of metastasis. Regional tumor metastases are found at neck exploration in 40 to 50 per cent of patients with transglottic cancer, and 30 per cent of the time the metastases are occult and not palpable.

Piriform sinus tumors are also usually advanced when first diagnosed. The incidence of regional metastases is 50 to 75 per cent, with up to 40 per cent being occult. Supraglottic and piriform sinus tumors metastasize upward to the jugulodigastric lymph nodes; therefore this area should always be included in the imaging examination.

CT and MR provide detailed assessment of the cervical lymph nodes. Mancuso and colleagues[83] found that CT was highly sensitive in detecting cervical lymph node enlargement from laryngeal carcinoma. In several instances in their study, CT was able to show nonpalpable lymph nodes. Cervical lymph nodes must be distinguished from adjacent blood vessels. Rapid sequential scanning with incrementation of the table and high concentrations of intravascular contrast medium (Fig. 9–39) is best for imaging cervical nodes. One technique is to use a slow bolus injection of 50 to 75 mL of contrast medium at a rate of 2 mL/sec and to begin scanning after 20 mL have been injected. The injection is continued throughout the imaging sequence. CT and MR are about equal in their ability to demonstrate enlarged lymph nodes.[8] Extracapsular extension of tumor is recognized by an indistinct margin to the node.

In the patient with laryngeal cancer, enlarged lymph nodes may not necessarily contain cancer; in one group of patients with supraglottic cancer, 45 per cent of the palpable nodes were found histologically to be benign.[84] Mancuso and colleagues[83] have described the positions of the cervical lymph nodes and diagnostic criteria for discriminating malignant involvement of nodes from reactive hyperplasia (see Chapter 10).

Treatment and Prognosis ■ The treatment of laryngeal cancer is by radiotherapy, surgery, or a combination of the two.[41, 45, 47, 85–87] Several surgical procedures may be employed for laryngeal cancer (Table 9–7), and the choice varies with the preference of the physician and the type of tumor. If cervical lymph nodes are palpable, a neck dissection is usually

TABLE 9–7 ■ **Surgical Procedures for Cancer of the Larynx**

Partial laryngectomy by laryngofissure
Partial lateral laryngectomy
Partial frontal-lateral laryngectomy
Lateral hemilaryngectomy
Partial laryngectomy by pharyngotomy
Epiglottidectomy
Partial horizontal laryngectomy
Total laryngectomy

Source: Modified from English GM: Malignant neoplasms of the larynx. In English GM (ed): Otolaryngology. Hagerstown, MD, Harper & Row, 1976, p 536.

indicated. The approach in an individual patient requires determination of the precise site and extent of tumor. Therapy differs for each anatomic region of the larynx.

Glottic Region ■ The cure rate for T1 tumors of the glottis is 85 to 95 per cent using either irradiation or surgery.[88] In most instances irradiation is preferred, because vocal function is better preserved. T2 glottic cancers have a 60 to 80 per cent cure rate with irradiation, and surgery can salvage most of the failures of radiotherapy. In more advanced lesions, such as infraglottic extension of the tumor, or invasion of the arytenoid cartilage, hemilaryngectomy is an alternative to irradiation.

The choice of treatment for T3 glottic lesions with cordal fixation remains controversial. The surgical approach can be extended hemilaryngectomy or total laryngectomy.[89, 90] Alternatively, radiotherapy has been used with early assessment of the response of the tumor.[47, 87] If CT demonstrates deep infiltration of a T3 tumor with cartilage destruction or infraglottic extension, an aggressive surgical approach is usually indicated. The cure rate for T3 lesions is about 70 per cent when there are no palpable neck nodes. The larger and more extensive the cervical lymphadenopathy, the worse the prognosis. T4 glottic cancer is

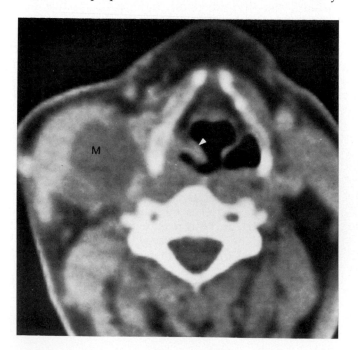

FIGURE 9–39 ■ Tumor within cervical lymph nodes. CT scan at the level of the thyroid notch demonstrates thickening of the right aryepiglottic fold *(arrowhead)* caused by tumor. The bulky low-density mass (M) on the right is caused by carcinoma within lymph nodes.

treated by total laryngectomy or by irradiation followed by total laryngectomy. The cure rate is about 50 per cent if there are no nodal metastases and considerably lower if palpable nodes are present.

Supraglottic Region ■ Early T1 and T2 carcinomas are not commonly found in the supraglottic larynx but are amenable to treatment by irradiation.[47, 87] The cure rate is 75 to 85 per cent when surgery is used to salvage the failures from irradiation.

Larger T2 and T3 lesions are treated by irradiation, surgery, or radiotherapy followed by supraglottic laryngectomy or total laryngectomy. The cure rate is 60 to 70 per cent and decreases with the presence of palpable cervical lymph nodes. The CT demonstration of tumor invasion of the thyroid cartilage, of the pre-epiglottic space, or through the thyrohyoid membrane indicates the need for an aggressive surgical approach.

Infraglottic Region ■ Because infraglottic cancers can be difficult to evaluate by endoscopy, CT can appreciably assist in defining their inferior extent. In general, infraglottic cancer that is small and does not extend inferiorly more than 1 cm below the vocal cord can be treated by hemilaryngectomy. More extensive tumors require total laryngectomy.

Transglottic Tumors ■ Transglottic cancer can be treated by hemilaryngectomy in selected instances of smaller tumors. Tumors that are bilateral, impair vocal cord motility, extend to the infraglottic region for more than 5 to 8 mm, or invade cartilage require total laryngectomy. CT and MR can demonstrate clinically undetected cartilage invasion, as well as extension to the contralateral pre-epiglottic space or to the infraglottic region. Under these circumstances, total laryngectomy is indicated to reduce the risk of recurrence. Clinically undetected nodal enlargement can also be demonstrated by CT and MR and indicates the need for neck exploration.

Non-Neoplastic Lesions

The larynx can be affected by a variety of congenital, inflammatory, connective tissue, and idiopathic diseases. CT can show the size and extent of the disease process and detail the cross-sectional area and adequacy of the airway. Laryngeal CT is usually not capable of tissue characterization and cannot differentiate among edema, inflammation, and neoplasia.

GRANULOMATOUS DISEASES

Both infectious granulomatous and noninfectious granulomatous diseases can involve the larynx. In general, biopsy is required for diagnosis because the gross appearances are nonspecific.

Sarcoidosis is a systemic inflammatory disorder characterized by a granulomatous lesion containing noncaseating epithelioid tubercles. The incidence of laryngeal involvement is only 1.3 per cent of patients with sarcoidosis, and very rarely is the larynx the only site of disease.[91, 92] Patients with laryngeal sarcoid present with hoarseness, cough, dysphasia, and dyspnea. Upper airway obstruction can occur.[93] The larynx becomes diffusely edematous, often with the epiglottis and supraglottic larynx most severely affected. The true vocal cords are less frequently involved, but neuritis of the recurrent laryngeal nerve can result in unilateral vocal cord paralysis.[91] Laryngoscopy reveals mucosal changes consisting of edema, erythema, nodules, and masslike lesions. We have seen one case of sarcoidosis in which CT scans showed marked thickening of the epiglottis and aryepiglottic folds. The glottis in this case showed diffuse thickening (Fig. 9–40). Treatment for laryngeal sarcoidosis consists of systemic steroids with local steroid injections and, in selected cases, surgical excision.

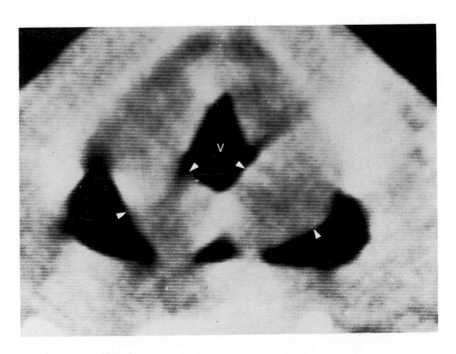

FIGURE 9–40 ■ Laryngeal involvement with sarcoidosis. CT scan through the supraglottic larynx demonstrates symmetric thickening of the aryepiglottic folds *(arrowheads)* with encroachment on the laryngeal vestibule (V). Biopsy revealed noncaseating sarcoid granulomas.

Tuberculosis of the larynx occurs almost exclusively in patients with active pulmonary tuberculosis. Symptoms are hoarseness, cough, and pain that frequently radiates to one ear. Constitutional symptoms and dysphasia are evident in less than 50 per cent of patients.[94, 95] Most commonly involved are the epiglottis and posterior laryngeal structures, areas that are readily visible with indirect laryngoscopy.[95] The diagnosis is usually made by direct laryngoscopy and biopsy. In some cases the vocal cords are predominantly involved and may have the appearance of an exophytic carcinoma. CT shows a diffuse thickening and increased density of the paralaryngeal and pre-epiglottic tissues. The epiglottis and aryepiglottic folds are likewise thickened. Encroachment on the laryngeal airway may be evident, although severe compromise of the airway seldom occurs. The CT appearance is nonspecific and cannot differentiate laryngeal tuberculosis from other diffuse granulomatous processes of a diffusely infiltrating circumglottic carcinoma. Involvement of the cervical lymph nodes is common.

Other chronic granulomatous diseases caused by specific infectious agents can also involve the larynx. With most of them, additional areas of the upper airway are affected simultaneously or prior to laryngeal involvement. Scleroma of the larynx (rhinoscleroma) is caused by the bacillus *Klebsiella rhinoscleromatis* (von Frisch bacillus).[96] It is a chronic granulomatous disease of central and southern Europe and South America, but the incidence of scleroma is increasing both in the United States and in other countries. The nose is the most commonly involved site, but the larynx, pharynx, trachea, and bronchi can also be affected without nasal involvement. Acute laryngeal obstruction can occur in the initial, exudative stage. Untreated, the disease progresses to proliferative and cicatricial stages, resulting in stenosis throughout the upper respiratory tract.

Tertiary or congenital syphilis of the larynx can produce "punched-out" ulcers or nodular infiltration. Healing is accompanied by deforming scar formation and may necessitate surgical intervention.

Mycotic infections of the larynx are rare and are usually associated with disease at other sites.[96] Symptoms include hoarseness, hemoptysis, and cough. Laryngeal histoplasmosis is mostly seen with the mucocutaneous form of the disease. Endoscopy reveals a nodular granulomatous mass or ulceration. Laryngeal blastomycosis can also show nodular granulation and ulcerations. Pulmonary disease is usually evident, as well as skin lesions. Coccidioidomycosis rarely involves the supraglottic larynx, and its appearance is similar to that of the other mycotic infections. Candidiasis of the larynx is usually seen in immunocompromised patients or as a superinfection in patients receiving systemic antibiotics. Pain and dysphasia are the common symptoms, although respiratory obstruction can occur from sloughing of the thick membranous exudate, which can be observed at endoscopy.

Nonspecific posttraumatic granulomas of the larynx are common; they are caused by endotracheal intubation and are bilateral in 50 per cent of cases.[97] Their typical location is along the free margins of the true vocal cords in their posterior third, adjacent to the vocal processes of the arytenoid cartilages. They may also occur along the lower borders of the aryepiglottic folds. The CT finding of these granulomas is a focal thickening of the involved region, often with increased CT density of the adjacent tissues. This appearance is not specific and should not be mistaken for tumor.

COLLAGEN VASCULAR DISEASES

The collagen vascular diseases form an overlapping group of conditions in which fibrinoid necrosis of the walls of small vessels is a constant finding. They are multisystem disorders, and the larynx is frequently involved. Symptoms can include hoarseness, dyspnea, dysphasia, odynophagia, and respiratory obstruction.

Rheumatoid diseases affect the larynx in up to 40 per cent of patients who have generalized rheumatoid disease.[98, 99] Rheumatoid synovitis of the cricoarytenoid joints is the most common cause of symptoms and can lead to ankylosis and subluxation. Indirect or direct laryngoscopy shows decreased vocal cord motion. Neuritis of the recurrent laryngeal nerve can also cause decreased vocal cord movement and must be differentiated from cricoarytenoid arthritis. Lawry and co-workers[100] studied 45 patients with moderately severe rheumatoid arthritis. They found abnormalities in more than 50 per cent, even when symptoms were absent. The most frequent finding was a paramedian location of a true vocal cord, indicating reduced lateral mobility at the cricoarytenoid joint. Other findings included reduced motion of a vocal cord, thickening of the true vocal cords, an abnormal position of an aryepiglottic fold, and partial or total subluxation of an arytenoid cartilage. Rheumatoid nodules and polyps have been described on the vocal cords but are rare. CT shows localized masses in addition to the other features of rheumatoid disease.

Cricoarytenoid arthritis, mucosal ulcerations, scarring, and laryngeal stenosis can also be found in systemic lupus erythematosus, progressive systemic sclerosis, polyarteritis, and Wegener's granulomatosis. In all of these conditions, laryngeal involvement is part of the systemic disease.

POLYPS AND CYSTS

Laryngeal polyps and cysts are most frequently posttraumatic. Their appearance on CT can be confused with laryngeal carcinomas, but an understanding of their typical sites and appearances can suggest the correct diagnosis.

Fibrous or fibroangiomatous polyps are among the most common lesions encountered in the larynx.[101] They are a form of traumatic laryngitis and are seen most often in singers and professional speakers. These nodular masses characteristically occur on the free margin of the true vocal cords at the junction of the anterior and middle thirds and are frequently bilateral. Occasionally vocal polyps are diffusely situated on the vocal cords. Surgical removal may be indicated in patients unresponsive to voice therapy.

Saccular (congenital) cysts of the larynx constitute only two to three per cent of all congenital anomalies of the larynx[102] and may develop in infancy or in later life. The most common saccular cyst arises in an aryepiglottic fold and is presumed to result from maldevelopment of the appendix of the laryngeal ventricle.[103] When distended with mucus, these cysts can be up to 6 or 7 cm in diameter. They originate in the paralaryngeal tissue at the level of the false cords and enlarge along planes of least resistance. They are particularly well demonstrated on CT scans. If the cysts extend upward, they will thicken the anterior aryepiglottic fold or bulge into the anterior wall of the laryngeal vestibule. If directed anteromedially, they can extend through the pre-epiglottic space and present as a mass in the ipsilateral valleculae. Occasionally a cyst grows laterally through the thyrohyoid membrane and appears as a mass in the side of the neck (Fig. 9–41). On CT scans the thin cyst wall and uniform low density cyst contents are readily apparent. With the aid of serial scans, the position of the cyst within the larynx can be determined and a correct diagnosis made.

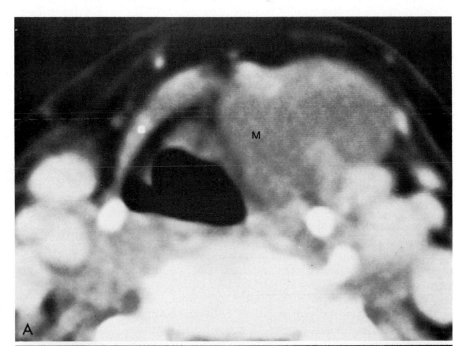

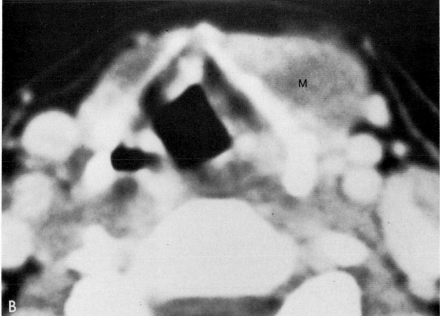

FIGURE 9–41 ■ Congenital saccular cyst of the larynx. *A,* CT scan at the level of the thyrohyoid membrane demonstrates a low-density cystic mass (M) within the pre-epiglottic space on the left and extending into the neck. *B,* One centimeter caudad, the external laryngeal component of the cyst (M) is visible. The left piriform sinus is obliterated.

Congenital cysts also occur along the tracts of the primitive second, third, and fourth branchial clefts. Although they do not involve the endolarynx, cysts arising from the third and fourth clefts can pierce the thyrohyoid membrane and communicate with a piriform sinus (see Chapter 10).[104]

Thyroglossal duct cysts, like branchial cleft cysts, are not intrinsic to the larynx but can impinge on laryngeal structures. The thyroglossal duct extends downward in the midline from the base of the tongue, in front of the hyoid bone and thyroid cartilage, as far as the isthmus of the thyroid gland. Cysts can occur anywhere along the course of the duct tract but are most common around the hyoid bone. Those arising below the hyoid bone bulge into the pre-epiglottic space to displace the epiglottic cartilage posteriorly. On CT scans the uniform low density of these lesions is readily apparent.[36] The density of the cyst varies with its protein content.[105] Midline positioning of a cyst strongly favors the diagnosis of a thyroglossal duct cyst.

LARYNGOCELE

In adults the normal appendix, or saccule, of the laryngeal ventricle measures only 5 to 15 mm in length. In apes such as the orangutan, the laryngeal appendix is much larger than in humans and can even extend into the axilla. In about 30 per cent of adults, the laryngeal appendix is normally visible on CT scans obtained during phonation as a round air density structure immediately medial to the cartilage of the thyroid lamina at the junction of its anterior and middle thirds.

A laryngocele, or laryngeal aerocele, is an enlargement and elongation of the normal ventricular appendix. More than 90 per cent of laryngoceles present in adult life when the ventricular appendix is obstructed or occasionally infected.[106] They are bilateral in almost 25 per cent of cases. Occupations that are associated with increased intralaryngeal pressure, such as the blowing of wind instruments, probably predispose to the development of laryngoceles.

Laryngoceles are classified into three types: internal, external, and mixed.[107] Internal laryngoceles are confined to the soft tissues of the larynx. Similar to saccular cysts of the larynx, they can extend anterosuperiorly into the pre-epiglottic space and even as far cephalad as the valleculae. They can also project posterosuperiorly into an aryepiglottic fold and present as a submucosal supraglottic mass.

External laryngoceles expand laterally through the thyrohyoid membrane posterior to the thyrohyoid muscles. This is a relatively weak area in which the superior laryngeal vessels and internal laryngeal nerve penetrate the membrane.

Laryngoceles are called *mixed* when cystic spaces are present both internal and external to the thyroid cartilage. The mixed type is the most common laryngocele, followed by the internal and then the external type. In almost 20 per cent of cases, a laryngeal tumor, usually a carcinoma, is found in conjunction with a laryngocele (Fig. 9–42).

With few exceptions, the clinical and radiographic diagnosis of an uncomplicated laryngocele is straightforward. Conventional radiographs may reveal an air-containing space within the paralaryngeal tissue, pre-epiglottic space, or aryepiglottic fold or lateral to the thyrohyoid membrane. If the laryngocele contains liquid and air, one or two air-fluid levels are visible. CT scans show an air- or fluid-filled structure and the exact location of both internal and external laryngoceles (Fig. 9–43).[108, 109] Occasionally a large excavating laryngeal carcinoma can superficially resemble a laryngocele.[103]

If the neck of the laryngocele is obstructed by chronic inflammation or by a tumor and the laryngocele becomes filled with mucus, CT scans show a circumscribed, uniform, fluid-density mass arising above the level of the false cord and extending superiorly.[110] The density varies from that of water to that of soft tissue. The CT appearance of a fluid-filled laryngocele is indistinguishable from that of a lateral saccular cyst, to which laryngoceles are embryologically related.[111] Direct laryngoscopy is indicated in all patients with a laryngocele to exclude a ventricular tumor.

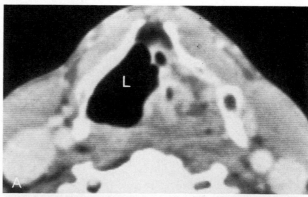
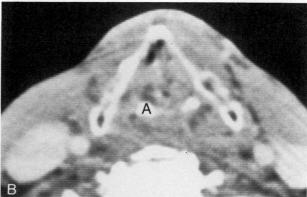

FIGURE 9–42 ■ Right laryngocele with small right vocal cord tumor. *A,* CT scan at the level of the thyroid notch demonstrates a large, right-sided, air-containing space representing a laryngocele (L). *B,* Ten millimeters caudad at the level of the true vocal cords, the right arytenoid cartilage (A) is displaced medially by a tumor localized to the upper surface of the right true cord. At endoscopy, the orifice of the right laryngeal appendix was obstructed by the tumor.

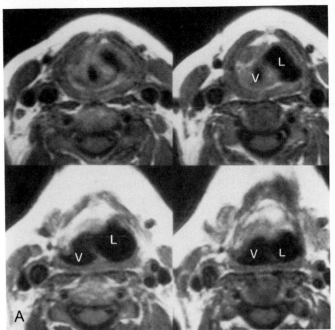

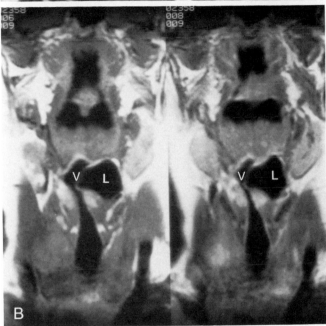

FIGURE 9–43 ■ Internal laryngocele. A, Serial MR images demonstrate an air-containing space on the left side extending superiorly from the level of the glottis. The laryngocele (L) displaces and narrows the laryngeal vestibule (V). B, Two adjacent coronal MR images demonstrate the relationship of the laryngocele (L) to the laryngeal vestibule and vocal cords.

Trauma

Trauma to the larynx is uncommon but increasing in frequency; recent interest in this injury has stimulated improved methods of diagnosis and treatment. A complete understanding of the types of injury that can affect the larynx, their significance, and their management is essential for the interpretation of the CT scans.

Acute trauma to the larynx may be internal or external. Internal trauma from intubation rarely results in severe damage to the larynx. Radiation or inhalation of noxious gases and liquids (e.g., smoke, steam, acids, caustics, and corrosives) causes various degrees of mucosal damage, edema, and formation of granulation tissue.[112] CT can be a useful adjunct to endoscopy; and internal trauma is revealed as a marked supraglottic swelling in the acute phase with stenosis occurring in the chronic phase. External trauma is either penetrating or blunt in nature. Penetrating injuries are usually evaluated clinically, and exploratory surgery is frequently indicated.

BLUNT LARYNGEAL INJURY

Blunt injury to the larynx is caused by compression of the neck against the spine by an object that does not penetrate the soft tissues. In children and adolescents, blows from bats or sticks and colliding with objects while bicycle riding are the most frequent causes of blunt injury. In adults, dashboard and steering wheel injuries are the most common.

Symptoms can be severe or subtle. Voice change varies from hoarseness to aphonia. Cough is evidence of laryngeal irritation. Hemoptysis and pain are nonspecific findings. Dyspnea and symptoms of airway compromise usually indicate serious structural damage.

Physical examination of the neck may reveal the type of laryngeal injury; sometimes it is limited by the presence of severe edema or hematoma. Extensive subcutaneous emphysema may be present, indicating a mucosal tear. There may be palpable distortion of the laryngeal cartilages or an appreciably displaced fracture of the thyroid cartilage.[113] Loss of the normal prominence of the cricoid cartilage strongly suggests a fracture at the infraglottic level.

Although it is frequently difficult to clinically assess the extent of laryngeal injury, every effort should be made to determine the extent of laryngeal injury and initiate early therapy to avoid poor functional results.[114, 115] Improved function will result if acute fractures are reduced within 7 days after injury, thus reducing the incidence of chronic laryngeal stenosis.

Endoscopy should be undertaken early and radiographic studies obtained as soon as an adequate airway has been secured. The usual radiographic examinations include frontal and lateral views of the soft tissues of the neck and radiographs of the cervical spine.[112] Concomitant injuries to the cervical esophagus should also be considered.

CT OF THE INJURED LARYNX

CT has greatly extended the noninvasive assessment of the injured larynx with precise demonstration of disruption of the laryngeal cartilages and soft tissues. The established indications for exploratory surgery[116, 117] are the same clinical circumstances in which CT scanning can assist in the evaluation of the patient.[118, 119]

Airway Obstruction ■ Trauma sufficient to cause compromise of the airway usually results in secondary stenosis. A prompt surgical approach is indicated.

Subcutaneous Emphysema ■ Extensive subcutaneous emphysema is indicative of a mucosal tear large enough to warrant surgical closure.

Exposed Cartilage ■ Endoscopic visualization of exposed fragments of cartilage usually indicates disruption of the laryngeal skeleton and a need for surgical repair of the larynx.

Fractured Cricoid Cartilage ■ Cricoid fractures are frequently associated with acute airway obstruction and necessitate tracheostomy. Inadequate treatment of infraglottic injuries frequently leads to chronic stenosis.[120]

Fistulous Tracts ■ Endoscopic or CT evidence of a false passage or fistulous tract from the larynx is uncommon and does necessitate surgical repair.

Arytenoid Disruption ■ Avulsion or dislocation of the arytenoid cartilages requires repositioning in the acute phase of the injury. Arytenoid dislocations are frequently associated with damage to the true or false cords, and restoration of vocal function may not be achieved even with surgical repair.[120]

CLASSIFICATION OF INJURIES

Laryngeal Edema, Hematoma, Minor Lacerations ■ Swelling of the endolaryngeal soft tissues can occur without skeletal damage. At the supraglottic level, blood and edema fluid can distend the fibrofatty tissues of the pre-epiglottic space and aryepiglottic folds (Fig. 9–44). The CT density of these structures

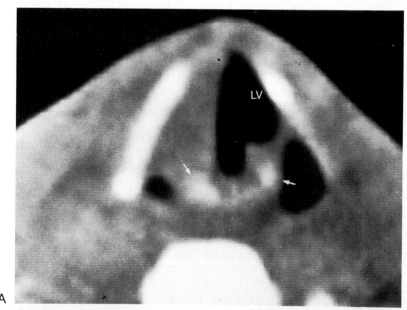

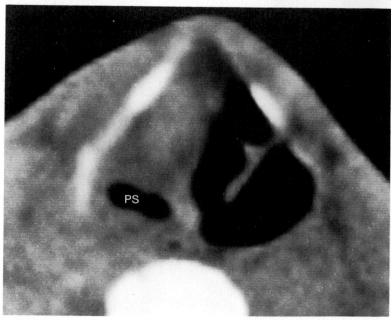

FIGURE 9–44 ■ Hematoma and edema of the right endolarynx following neck trauma. *A,* CT scan at the level of the glottis during phonation shows the arytenoid cartilages *(arrows)* adducted. The right piriform sinus is compressed. The right true cord is thickened. The left laryngeal ventricle (LV) is normal. *B,* CT scan during phonation at the level of the thyroid notch shows posterior displacement of the right piriform sinus (PS) with hematoma between the piriform sinus and thyroid cartilage. The right aryepiglottic fold is thickened. No cartilage damage was found.

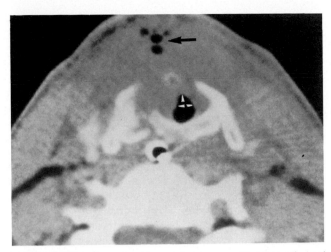

FIGURE 9–45 ■ Extensive laryngeal damage with gas in the soft tissues of the neck. CT scan shows disruption of the thyroid and cricoid cartilages. Extensive subglottic hematoma is present (arrowheads). Gas is visible in the neck anteriorly (arrow). At surgery, a large mucosal tear was found in the anterior larynx.

will be increased. CT scans can also show swelling of the true and false cords.

Careful attention should be directed to the positions of the arytenoid cartilages. Scans obtained during both quiet breathing and phonation are important. Motion of the arytenoids and function of the true vocal cords can be limited by the mass effect of a hematoma or by dislocation at the cricoarytenoid joint.

At the infraglottic level, blood or edema tends to spread around the airway below the vocal cords within the cricoid cartilage. This is readily shown on CT scans as soft tissue density within the cricoid cartilage.

CT is an excellent method for demonstrating gas within the soft tissues of the larynx and neck (Fig. 9–45). This finding of gas is an indication for careful endoscopy to exclude significant mucosal lacerations and skeletal exposure.

In general, CT extends the clinical examination by providing information about the cartilaginous structures, soft tissues, and airway.[119] When conservative management is being considered for soft tissue injury of the larynx, CT scans can confirm that the cartilages are not damaged and the airway is adequate.

Skeletal Injuries and Extensive Soft Tissue Laceration ■ With severe laryngeal injuries, CT scans are the most precise noninvasive method for determining the sites of soft tissue swelling and skeletal disruption. Skeletal injuries of the larynx are classified regionally as supraglottic, glottic, infraglottic, or transglottic. Although two or more regions are frequently involved, this classification serves for descriptive purposes.

Supraglottic Injury ■ Patients with supraglottic injuries typically have early onset of airway obstruction and difficulty in swallowing. Skeletal injuries of the supraglottic larynx involve the thyroid and epiglottic cartilages. A vertical paramedian fracture of the thyroid cartilage is the most common type of injury,

although transverse, oblique, or comminuted fractures can all occur.[117] With transverse fractures, the upper fragment tends to be displaced superiorly and posteriorly (Fig. 9–46). Extensive soft tissue damage and lacerations of the true and false cords and of the aryepiglottic folds are frequently associated with transverse fractures. CT scans will demonstrate marked swelling of the soft tissues. Mucosal lacerations should be suspected if gas is shown in the soft tissues.

A common supraglottic injury is avulsion of the epiglottic cartilage from the thyroid cartilage. This occurs when the thyroepiglottic ligament is ruptured, causing bleeding around the base of the epiglottis, which is displaced posteriorly and superiorly. The injury can be suspected from CT scans by an increase in the depth and density of the inferior pre-epiglottic space. The displaced epiglottic cartilage frequently can be seen. However, CT cannot reliably differentiate avulsion of the epiglottis from hematoma and edema of the pre-epiglottic space without rupture of the thyroepiglottic ligament. With a transverse or vertical fracture of the thyroid cartilage, avulsion of the epiglottic cartilage should be considered.

When damage to the lower aryepiglottic folds is extensive, the capsule of the cricoarytenoid joint may be damaged. An arytenoid cartilage may then dislo-

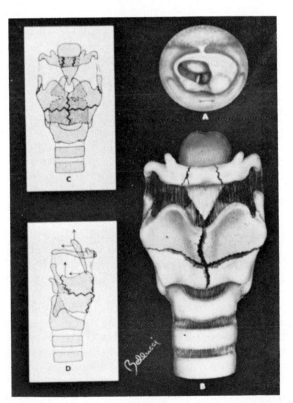

FIGURE 9–46 ■ Schema of transverse and vertical fractures of the thyroid cartilage. A, Endoscopy shows marked soft tissue swelling of the supraglottic region. B, Schema shows thyroid cartilage and hyoid bone fractures in multiple directions. C and D, Schemata demonstrate superior fragments of the thyroid cartilage and epiglottis displaced posteriorly and superiorly. (From Ogura JH, Heeneman H, Spector GJ: Can J Otolaryngol 2:112, 1973. Reprinted with permission.)

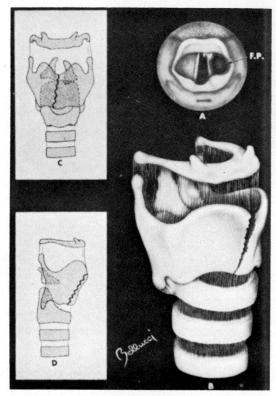

FIGURE 9–47 ■ Glottic injury. *A,* Endoscopy reveals a mucosal tear, or false passage (F.P.), and exposed cartilage. *B,* Schema shows that vertical paramedian fractures of the thyroid cartilage are most common. *C and D,* Schemata demonstrate that the alignment of the larynx is usually normal. (From Ogura JH, Heeneman H, Spector GJ: Can J Otolaryngol 2:112, 1973. Reprinted with permission.)

cate, usually in a posterosuperior direction. Careful attention should be given to the position and mobility of the arytenoid cartilages and true vocal cords.[121]

Glottic Injury ■ As with trauma to other portions of the larynx, glottic injuries usually result from compression of the larynx against the cervical spine. Parasagittal, transverse, oblique, and comminuted fractures of the thyroid cartilage are frequently associated with damage to the true and false cords and the anterior commissure (Fig. 9–47). Posterior displacement of fragments of the thyroid cartilage may be evident on CT scans at the glottic level (Fig. 9–48). The thyroarytenoid muscles within the true cords can rupture or be avulsed, with lacerations of the cords and aryepiglottic folds.

CT shows soft tissue swelling of the glottis with narrowing of the airway. One or both arytenoid cartilages frequently have subluxated or dislocated in an anterior or anterosuperior direction (Fig. 9–49). Careful evaluation of the cartilaginous fragments seen on CT may reveal the displaced arytenoid cartilage. Detection of air in the swollen soft tissues of the larynx or neck is suggestive of a mucosal laceration and an indication for careful endoscopy.

Loss of function and mobility of the true vocal cords may result from one or more of several causes; CT may assist in determining which of the following is present: dislocation of one or both arytenoid car-

tilages, avulsion of a true vocal cord, edema of the true vocal cords, or injury to the recurrent laryngeal nerve.

Dislocation of an arytenoid cartilage may be detected by means of endoscopy or suspected from an abnormal position on CT scans. There are no specific findings on CT of an avulsed true vocal cord, but marked soft tissue swelling will be manifest.

Infraglottic Injury ■ The hallmark of infraglottic injury to the laryngeal skeleton is one or more fractures of the cricoid cartilage (Fig. 9–50). Airway obstruction is common and is usually severe and immediate. Detection of cricoid fractures is most important. Morgenstein[122] showed that infraglottic injuries, unless repaired, frequently result in instability, chronic scarring, and stenosis of the larynx. The cricoid cartilage is the only complete cartilaginous ring in the airway, so fractures from compression tend to occur in two places. Direct frontal force fractures the cricoid cartilage anteriorly and posteriorly, whereas oblique force produces ipsilateral and contralateral fractures.

Fractures of the anterior arch of the cricoid ring can usually be suspected clinically from a loss of the normal prominence of the cricoid; however, soft tissue swelling and subcutaneous emphysema can obscure this finding. CT can readily demonstrate fragments of the cricoid cartilage and their impingement on the airway (Fig. 9–51). Reduction in the anteroposterior diameter of the cricoid cartilage with distortion of its normal round shape is strong evidence of a comminuted cricoid fracture. With severe blunt trauma, multiple fragments may be evident. The cricopharyngeal muscles attach to the lateral margins of the cricoid cartilage. With anterior and posterior fractures, the cricoid cartilage can appear sprung open. The fragments are retracted posterolaterally, contributing to the decrease in the anteroposterior diameter of the airway.

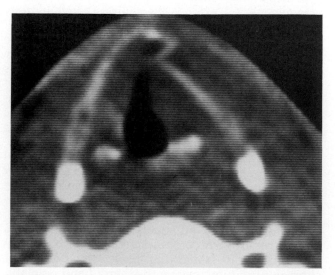

FIGURE 9–48 ■ Fracture of the thyroid cartilage from prior trauma. CT scan demonstrates deformity of the right thyroid cartilage without surrounding edema, indicating the injury is old.

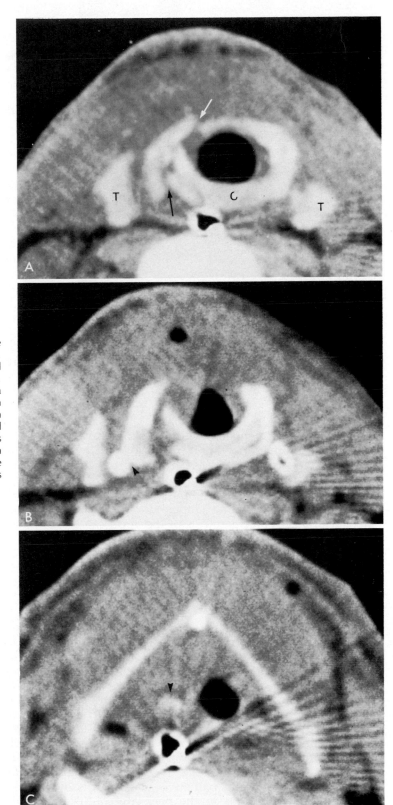

FIGURE 9–49 ■ Comminuted fracture of the cricoid cartilage with edema, hemorrhage, and a dislocated arytenoid cartilage. *A,* CT scan through the infraglottic region shows a comminuted fracture *(arrow)* involving the right side of the cricoid ring (C). The dense lateral structures are the thyroid gland (T). Edema or hematoma is visible within the cricoid cartilage. *B,* Ten millimeters cephalic to *A,* a fracture of the right inferior horn of the thyroid cartilage *(arrowhead)* is present. The thyroid cartilage is tilted. Edema of the neck is present with bubbles of gas, indicating severe injury and a mucosal tear. *C,* CT scan 15 mm cephalad continues to show marked edema of the endolarynx. A dislocated arytenoid cartilage *(arrowhead)* is demonstrated.

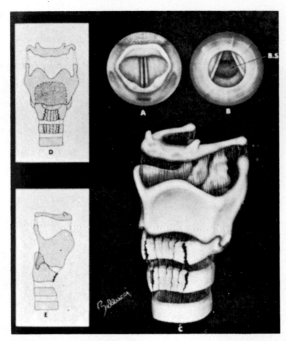

FIGURE 9–50 ■ Schema of cricoid fracture of subglottic injury. *A* and *B*, Endoscopy shows bilateral vocal cord paralysis with a blind sac (B.S.) visible if the vocal cords are wedged apart. *C*, Schema shows presence of fractures of the anterior arch of the cricoid cartilage and first tracheal ring. *D* and *E*, Schemata show that the cricoid cartilage is displaced posteriorly, leading to loss of cricoid prominence. (From Ogura JH, Heeneman H, Spector GJ: Can J Otolaryngol 2:112, 1973. Reprinted with permission.)

Fractures of the cricoid cartilage are frequently found in conjunction with fractures of the thyroid cartilage and disruption or separation of the cricoarytenoid joint. Careful scrutiny of all the CT scans can reveal these various components of the injury. Frequently, concomitant damage to the recurrent laryngeal nerves and paralysis of the vocal cords are present. Demonstration of a fracture involving the posterior half of the cricoid cartilage should suggest injury to the recurrent laryngeal nerve.

Injury directed to the cricothyroid membrane results in stenosis of the upper infraglottic region.[113] Narrowing of the airway is from posterior displacement of the thyroid cartilage with the cricoid cartilage remaining in normal position. Careful examination of the serial scans through the larynx shows narrowing and loss of alignment of the larynx in the infraglottic region.

Complete avulsion of the trachea from the larynx is a rare, severe infraglottic injury. Most patients die immediately; early diagnosis is essential in those who survive long enough to reach a hospital. Airway obstruction is progressive, and vocal cord paralysis resulting from injury to the recurrent laryngeal nerves is frequent. The patient is usually aphonic, and prominent features in the neck are contusion, swelling, and subcutaneous emphysema. The avulsed trachea retracts downward toward the sternum, and the larynx retracts upward and, in many instances, rotates around its axis. The displaced, obliquely situated cricoid cartilage produces a confusing appearance on CT scans. Associated cricoid fractures and disruption of the cricothyroid joints further distort laryngeal structures. A high index of suspicion for this injury is necessary to suggest the diagnosis from CT and to advocate immediate further investigation.

Indications for CT and MR of the Larynx

The ability of CT and MR to image the anatomy of the larynx and diseases that involve it has been extensively documented. CT and MR provide detailed images of the deep tissues and laryngeal skeleton. Structural and functional information is available and is important for diagnosis. In most circumstances, CT or MR is used to determine the extent of a lesion and to explain abnormal vocal cord function. Endoscopy and biopsy remain the main methods of diagnosis. Whether MR will replace or complement CT is still to be determined.

The most common use for CT and MR imaging of the larynx is to determine the extent of laryngeal and piriform sinus cancer. Small (T1) glottic and supraglottic tumors, treatable with radiotherapy, frequently do not benefit from additional study. In larger (T2 or greater) and ulcerating tumors, CT can detect deep penetration of soft tissues, invasion of the laryngeal skeleton, and presence of lymphadenopathy. Whenever endoscopy has not adequately visualized the inferior extent of the tumor, CT or MR should be undertaken. Tumors, even if small, that have caused cordal fixation should be studied with these imaging modalities. Marginal supra- and infraglottic tumors with a propensity for metastasis to regional lymph nodes will benefit from an imaging staging procedure.

Only recently have detailed correlative histologic studies demonstrating the limitations of CT in the assessment of tumor been undertaken. Additional studies with MR are still required. Laryngeal tumors can elicit an inflammatory and edematous response at their periphery; CT and MR may overestimate the extent of the tumor. When treatment involves radiation therapy, this may not be significant; however, when planning surgery, overestimation of the size and extent of the tumor may be critical. Both CT and MR clearly demonstrate moderate and major degrees of destruction of the laryngeal skeleton. However, if laryngeal neoplasms invade cartilage at the microscopic level (which is significant for recurrence), they will remain undetected by these techniques.

Infiltrative neoplasms extending into the soft tissues are not visible on CT or MR. This limitation is a problem mainly with vocal cord neoplasms, which can be well evaluated endoscopically.

The role of CT and MR in detecting recurrent tumor in irradiated sites remains difficult and controversial. Good clinical evaluation with endoscopy and

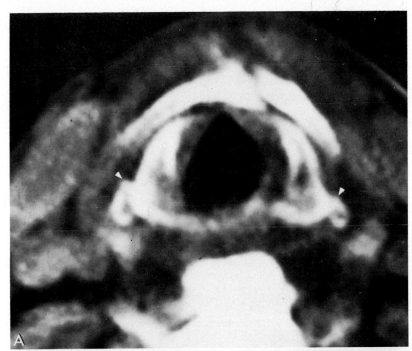

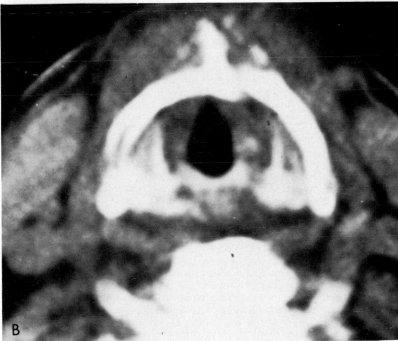

FIGURE 9–51 ■ Fractures of the cricoid and thyroid cartilages. *A,* CT scan through the infraglottic region shows anterior and posterior fractures of the cricoid cartilage with reduction in anteroposterior dimension. Fractures of the thyroid cartilage anteriorly and its inferior horns *(arrowheads)* are demonstrated. *B,* Ten millimeters cephalic to *A,* thyroid cartilage fragments can be seen anterior to the main cartilage within the neck.

biopsy of suspicious areas are still the primary methods of handling this situation.

In the evaluation of blunt, nonpenetrating laryngeal trauma in which surgery is a consideration, CT combined with endoscopy has a definitive place. The information provided on skeletal injury and soft tissue gas can greatly assist surgery planning.

Most non-neoplastic lesions of the larynx are adequately evaluated by clinical examination, laryngoscopy, and biopsy. When bulky masses distort the airway and limit endoscopic visualization, CT or MR frequently shows the adequacy of the airway and the inferior margins of the disease.

References

1. Mancuso AA, Calcaterra TC, Hanafee WN: Computed tomography of the larynx. Radiol Clin North Am 16:195, 1978.
2. Ward PH, Hanafee W, Mancuso AA, Shallit J, Berci G: Evaluation of computerized tomography, cinelaryngoscopy, and laryngography in determining the extent of laryngeal disease. Ann Otol 88:454, 1979.
3. Gamsu G, Webb WR, Shallit JB, Moss AA: CT in carcinoma of the larynx and piriform sinus: value of phonation scans. AJR 136:577, 1981.
4. Teresi LM, Lufkin RB, Hanafee WN: Magnetic resonance imaging of the larynx. Radiol Clin North Am 27:393, 1989.
5. Lockhart RD, Hamilton GF, Fyfe FW: Anatomy of the Human Body. London, Faber & Faber Ltd., 1959, pp 535–541.

6. Gray H: The respiratory system. In Goss CM (ed): Anatomy of the Human Body. Philadelphia, Lea & Febiger, 1966, p 1127.
7. Yeager VL, Lawson C, Archer CR: Ossification of the laryngeal cartilages as it relates to computed tomography. Radiology 151:11, 1984.
8. Lufkin RB, Hanafee WN, Wortham D, Hoover L: Larynx and hypopharynx: MR imaging with surface coils. Radiology 158:747, 1986.
9. Sakai F, Gamsu G, Dillon WP, Lynch DA, Gilbert TJ: Magnetic resonance imaging of the larynx at 1.5 Tesla. J Comput Assist Tomogr 14:60, 1990.
10. Gray H: The respiratory system. In Goss CM (ed): Anatomy of the Human Body. Philadelphia, Lea & Fibiger, 1966, p 1128.
11. Silverman PM, Korobkin M: High resolution computed tomography of the normal larynx. AJR 140:875, 1983.
12. Dwyer AJ, Knop RH, Hoult DI: Frequency shift artifact in MR imaging. J Comput Assist Tomogr 9:16, 1985.
13. Pressman JJ, Kelemen G: Physiology of the larynx. Physiol Rev 35:506, 1955.
14. Ardran GM, Kemp FH: The mechanism of the larynx, I: the movements of the arytenoid and cricoid cartilages. Br J Radiol 39:641, 1966.
15. Last RJ: Anatomy: Regional and Applied, 5th ed. Edinburgh, Churchill Livingstone, 1972, p 573.
16. Ardran GM, Kemp FH: The mechanisms of the larynx, II: the epiglottis and closure of the larynx. Br J Radiol 40:372, 1967.
17. Beahrs OH, Hensen DE, Hutter RVP, Myers MH (eds): American Joint Committee for Cancer Staging and End-Results Reporting: Manual for Staging of Cancer, 2d ed. Philadelphia, JB Lippincott, 1988, pp 39–41.
18. Bassett LW, Hanafee WN, Canalis RF: The appendix of the ventricle of the larynx. Radiology 120:571, 1976.
19. Gamsu G, Mark AS, Webb WR: Computed tomography of the normal larynx during quiet breathing and phonation. J Comput Assist Tomogr 5:353, 1981.
20. Kikinis R, Wolfensberger M, Boesch C, Martin E: Larynx: MR imaging at 2.35 T. Radiology 171:165, 1989.
21. Mancuso AA, Hanafee WN: Computed Tomography and Magnetic Resonance Imaging of the Head and Neck, 2d ed. Baltimore, Williams & Wilkins, 1985, pp 246–247.
22. Wortham DG, Hoover LA, Lufkin RB, Fu YS: Magnetic resonance imaging of the larynx: a correlation with histologic sections. Otolaryngol Head Neck Surg 94:123, 1986.
23. Castelijns JA, Doornbos J, Verbeeten B Jr, Vielvoye GJ, Bloem JL: MR imaging of the normal larynx. J Comput Assist Tomogr 9:919, 1985.
24. Di Guglielmo L, Vadala G, Galioto G, Dore R, Semplici P, et al: Computerized tomography in the study of malignant tumors of the larynx. Radiol Med (Torino) 70:294, 1984.
25. Mancuso AA, Hanafee WN, Juillard GJF, Winter J, Calcaterra TC: The role of computed tomography in the management of cancer of the larynx. Radiology 124:243, 1977.
26. Archer CR, Friedman WH, Yeager VL, Katsantonis GP: Evaluation of laryngeal cancer by computed tomography. J Comput Assist Tomogr 2:618, 1978.
27. Sagel SS, AufderHeide JF, Aronberg DJ, Stanley RJ, Archer CR: High resolution computed tomography in the staging of carcinoma of the larynx. Laryngoscope 91:292, 1981.
28. Scott M, Forsted DH, Rominger CJ, Brennan M: Computed tomographic evaluation of the laryngeal neoplasms. Radiology 140:141, 1981.
29. van Waes PFGM, Zonneveld FW: Direct coronal body computed tomography. J Comput Assist Tomogr 6:58, 1982.
30. Lufkin RB, Hanafee WN: Application of surface coil to MR anatomy of the larynx. AJR 145:483, 1985.
31. Hoover LA, Wortham DG, Lufkin RB, Hanafee WN: Magnetic resonance imaging of the larynx and tongue base: clinical applications. Otolaryngol Head Neck Surg 97:245, 1987.
32. Shaw H: Tumors of the larynx. In Ballantyne J, Groves J (eds): Scott-Brown's Diseases of the Ear, Nose and Throat, 4th ed, Vol 4. London, Butterworths, 1979, pp 423–426.
33. Ogura JH, Thawley SE: Cysts and tumors of the larynx. In Paparella MM, Shumrick DA (eds): Otolaryngology, 2d ed, Vol 3. Philadelphia, WB Saunders, 1980, pp 2507–2508.
34. Lyons GD, Lousteau RJ, Mouney DF: CO_2 laser laryngoscopy in a variety of lesions. Laryngoscope 86:1658, 1976.
35. Weber AL, Shortsleeve M, Goodman M, Montgomery W, Grillo HC: Cartilaginous tumors of the larynx and trachea. Radiol Clin North Am 16:261, 1978.
36. Aspestrand F, Kolbenstvedt A, Boysen M: CT findings in benign expansions of the larynx. J Comput Assist Tomogr 13:222, 1989.
37. Singh J, Black MJ, Fried I: Cartilaginous tumors of the larynx: a review of literature and two case experiences. Laryngoscope 90:1872, 1980.
38. Shulman HS, Noyek AM, Steinhardt MI: CT of the larynx. J Otolaryngol 11:395, 1982.
39. English GM: Benign neoplasms of the larynx. In English GM (ed): Otolaryngology. Hagerstown, MD, Harper & Row, 1976, pp 528–529.
40. Schaeffer BT, Som PM, Biller HF, Som ML, Arnold LM: Schwannomas of the larynx: review and computed tomographic scan analysis. Head Neck Surg 8:469, 1986.
41. Harrison DFN: Carcinoma of the larynx. Br Med J 2:615, 1969.
42. Kissin B, Kaley MM, Su WH, Lerner R: Head and neck cancer in alcoholics: the relationship to drinking, smoking, and dietary patterns. JAMA 224:1174, 1973.
43. McGavran MH, Bauer WC, Ogura JH: Isolated laryngeal keratosis. Laryngoscope 70:932, 1960.
44. Batsakis JG: Tumors of the Head and Neck: Clinical and Pathological Considerations, 2d ed. Baltimore, Williams & Wilkins, 1979.
45. Million RR, Cassisi NJ (eds): Larynx. In Management of Head and Neck Cancer: A Multidisciplinary Approach. Philadelphia, JB Lippincott, 1984, p 315.
46. Ogura JH, Spector GJ: The larynx. In Nealon TF (ed): Management of the Patient with Cancer. Philadelphia, WB Saunders, 1976, pp 206–238.
47. Lederman M: Radiotherapy of cancer of the larynx. J Laryngol Otol 84:867, 1970.
48. Norris CM: Laryngectomy and neck dissection. Otolaryngol Clin North Am 2:667, 1969.
49. Tucker GF Jr: The anatomy of laryngeal cancer. Can J Otolaryngol 3:417, 1974.
50. Kirchner JA: One hundred laryngeal cancers studied by serial section. Ann Otolaryngol 78:689, 1969.
51. Joffre P, Giron J, Fraga J, Serres-Cousine O, Senac JP, et al: MRI/CT x-ray comparison in the preoperative evaluation of cancer of the larynx: apropos of 46 cases. J Radiol 69:387, 1988.
52. Tucker GF, Alonso WA, Tucker JA, Cowan M, Druck N: The anterior commissure revisited. Ann Otol 82:625, 1973.
53. Mancuso AA, Hanafee WN: A comparative evaluation of computed tomography and laryngography. Radiology 133:131, 1979.
54. Mancuso AA, Hanafee WN: Computed Tomography and Magnetic Resonance Imaging of the Head and Neck, 2d ed. Baltimore, Williams & Wilkins, 1985, pp 256–257.
55. Reid MH: Laryngeal carcinoma: high-resolution computed tomography and thick anatomic sections. Radiology 151:689, 1984.
56. Katsantonis GP, Archer CR, Rosenblum BN, Yeager VL, Friedman WH: The degree to which accuracy of preoperative staging of laryngeal carcinoma has been enhanced by computed tomography. Otolaryngol Head Neck Surg 95:52, 1986.
57. Hoover LA, Calcaterra TC, Walter GA, Larsson SG: Preoperative CT scan evaluation for laryngeal carcinoma: correlation with pathological findings. Laryngoscope 94:310, 1984.
58. Silverman PM, Bossen EH, Cole TB, Korobkin M, Halvorsen RA: Carcinoma of the larynx and hypopharynx: computed tomographic-histopathologic correlations. Radiology 151:697, 1984.
59. English GM: Malignant neoplasms of the larynx. In English GM (ed): Otolaryngology. Hagerstown, MD, Harper & Row, 1976, p 536.

60. Fletcher GN, Hamberger AD: Cause of failure in irradiation of squamous cell carcinoma of the supraglottic larynx. Radiology 111:697, 1974.

61. Parsons CA, Chapman P, Counter RT, Grundy A: The role of computed tomography in tumours of the larynx. Clin Radiol 31:529, 1980.

62. Gregor RT, Michaels L: Computed tomography of the larynx: a clinical and pathologic study. Head Neck Surg 3:284, 1981.

63. Larsson S, Mancuso A, Hoover L, Hanafee W: Differentiation of pyriform sinus cancer from supraglottic laryngeal cancer by computed tomography. Radiology 141:427, 1981.

64. Kirchner JA, Cornog JL, Holmes RE: Transglottic cancer: its growth and spread within the larynx. Arch Otolaryngol 99:247, 1974.

65. Stell PM, Tobin KE: The behaviour of cancer affecting the subglottic space. Can J Otolaryngol 250:620, 1974.

66. Kirchner JA: Two hundred laryngeal cancers: patterns of growth and spread as seen in serial section. Laryngoscope 87:474, 1977.

67. Kirchner JA: Pyriform sinus cancer: a clinical and laboratory study. Ann Otol Rhinol Laryngol 84:793, 1975.

68. Lloyd GAS, Michaels L, Phelps PD: The demonstration of cartilaginous involvement in laryngeal carcinoma by computerized tomography. Clin Otolaryngol 6:171, 1981.

69. Castelijns JA, Gerritsen GJ, Kaiser MC, Valk J, van Zanten TEG, et al: Invasion of laryngeal cartilage by cancer: comparison of CT and MR imaging. Radiology 166:199, 1987.

70. Werber JL, Lucente FE: Computed tomography in patients with laryngeal carcinoma: a clinical perspective. Ann Otol Rhinol Laryngol 98:55, 1989.

71. Hatley W, Evison G, Samuel E: The pattern of ossification in the laryngeal cartilages: a radiological study. Br J Radiol 38:585, 1965.

72. Schild JA, Valvassori GE, Mafee MF, Bardawil WA: Laryngeal malignancies and computerized tomography: a correlation of tomographic and histopathologic findings. Ann Otol Rhinol Laryngol 91:571, 1982.

73. Mafee MF, Schild JA, Valvassori GE, Capek V: Computed tomography of the larynx: correlation with anatomic and pathologic studies in cases of laryngeal carcinoma. Radiology 147:123, 1983.

73a. Castelijns JA, Golding RP, van Schaik C, Valk J, Snow GB: MR findings of cartilage invasion by laryngeal cancer: Value in predicting outcome of radiation therapy. Radiology 174:669, 1990.

74. Mancuso AA, Hanafee WN: Computed Tomography and Magnetic Resonance Imaging of the Head and Neck, 2d ed. Baltimore, Williams & Wilkins, 1985, pp 254–256.

75. Hanson DG, Mancuso AA, Hanafee WN: Pseudomass lesions due to occult trauma of the larynx. Laryngoscope 92:1249, 1982.

76. Jing BS: Roentgen examination of laryngeal cancer: a critical evaluation. Can J Otolaryngol 4:64, 1975.

77. Lenz M, Okraineta C, Berne AS: Radiotherapy of cancer of the larynx. In Pack GT, Ariel IM (eds): Treatment of Cancer and Allied Disease. New York, PB Hoeber, 1959, p 542.

78. Vermund H: Role of radiotherapy in cancer of the larynx, as related to the T.N.M. system of staging. Cancer 5:485, 1970.

79. Kirchner JA: Clinical significance of fixed vocal cord. Laryngoscope 81:1029, 1971.

80. Agha FP: Recurrent laryngeal nerve paralysis: a laryngographic and computed tomographic study. Radiology 148:149, 1983.

81. Mancuso AA, Tamakawa Y, Hanafee WN: CT of the fixed vocal cord. AJR 135:529, 1980.

82. McGavran MH, Bauer WC, Ogura JH: The incidence of cervical lymph node metastases from epidermoid carcinoma of the larynx and their relationship to certain characteristics of the primary tumor. Cancer 14:55, 1961.

83. Mancuso AA, Maceri D, Rice D, Hanafee WN: CT of cervical lymph node cancer. AJR 136:381, 1981.

84. Cummings CW: Incidence of nodal metastasis in T2 supraglottic carcinoma. Arch Otolaryngol 99:268, 1974.

85. Ogura JH, Henneman H: Conservation surgery of the larynx and hypopharynx—selection of patients and results. Can J Otolaryngol 2:11, 1973.

86. Wang CC: Part III: cancer of the larynx: radiation therapy. CA 26:212, 1976.

87. Moss WT, Brand WN, Battifora H: Radiation Oncology, 5th ed. St Louis, CV Mosby, 1979.

88. Ogura JH, Sessions DG, Spector GJ: Analysis of surgical therapy for epidermoid carcinoma of the laryngeal glottis. Laryngoscope 85:1522, 1975.

89. Lesinski SG, Bauer WC, Ogura JH: Hemilaryngectomy for T3 (fixed cord) epidermoid carcinoma of larynx. Laryngoscope 86:1563, 1976.

90. Bryce DP, Ireland PI, Rider WD: Experience in the surgical and radiological treatment of 500 cases of carcinoma of the larynx. Ann Otolaryngol 72:416, 1963.

91. Caldarelli DD, Friedberg SA, Harris AA: Medical and surgical aspects of the granulomatous diseases of the larynx. Otolaryngol Clin North Am 12:767, 1979.

92. Carasso B: Sarcoidosis of the larynx causing airway obstruction. Chest 65:693, 1974.

93. Bower JS, Belen JE, Weg JG, Dantzker DR: Manifestations and treatment of laryngeal sarcoidosis. Am Rev Respir Dis 122:325, 1980.

94. Proctor DF: Laryngeal tuberculosis in the negro. Am Rev Tuberc 47:582, 1943.

95. Travis LW, Hybels RL, Newman MA: Tuberculosis of the larynx. Laryngoscope 86:549, 1976.

96. Friedmann I: Granulomas of the larynx. In Paparella MM, Shumrick DA (eds): Otolaryngology, 2d ed, Vol 3. Philadelphia, WB Saunders, 1980, pp 2459–2461.

97. Friedmann I: Granulomas of the larynx. In Paparella MM, Shumrick DA (eds): Otolaryngology, 2d ed, Vol 3. Philadelphia, WB Saunders, 1980, p 2449.

98. Pearson JEG: Rheumatoid arthritis of the larynx. Br Med J 2:1047, 1957.

99. Bridger MWM, Jahn AF, van Nostrand AWP: Laryngeal rheumatoid arthritis. Laryngoscope 90:296, 1980.

100. Lawry GV, Finerman ML, Hanafee WN, Mancuso AA, Fan PT, Bluestone R: Laryngeal involvement in rheumatoid arthritis: a clinical, laryngoscopic, and computerized tomographic study. Arthritis Rheum 27:873, 1984.

101. Salmon LFW: Chronic laryngitis. In Ballantyne J, Groves J (eds): Scott-Brown's Diseases of the Ear, Nose and Throat, 4th ed, Vol 4. London, Butterworths, 1979, pp 395–401.

102. Holinger PH, Brown WT: Congenital webs, laryngoceles, and other anomalies of the larynx. Ann Otol Rhinol Laryngol 76:744, 1967.

103. Bachman AL: Benign, non-neoplastic conditions of the larynx and pharynx. Radiol Clin North Am 16:273, 1978.

104. Hansberger HR, Mancuso AA, Muraki AS, Byrd SE, Dilton WP, et al: Branchial cleft anomalies and their mimics: computed tomographic evaluation. Radiology 152:739, 1984.

105. Reede DL, Bergerson RT, Som PM: CT of thyroglossal duct cysts. Radiology 157:121, 1985.

106. Canalis FF, Maxwell DS, Hemenway WG: Laryngocele—an updated review. J Otolaryngol 6:191, 1977.

107. Landing BH, Dixon LG: Congenital malformations and genetic disorders of the respiratory tract. Am Rev Respir Dis 120:151, 1979.

108. Silverman PM, Korobkin M: Computed tomographic evaluation of laryngoceles. Radiology 145:104, 1982.

109. Glazer HS, Mauro MA, Aronberg DJ, Lee JKT, Johnston DE, Sagel SS: Computed tomography of laryngoceles. AJR 140:549, 1983.

110. Mancuso AA, Hanafee WN: Computed Tomography and Magnetic Resonance Imaging of the Head and Neck, 2d ed. Baltimore, Williams & Wilkins, 1985, pp 268–269.

111. DeSanto LW: Laryngocele, laryngeal mucocele, large saccules, and laryngeal saccular cysts: a developmental spectrum. Laryngoscope 84:1291, 1974.

112. Greene R, Stark P: Trauma of the larynx and trachea. Radiol Clin North Am 16:309, 1978.

113. Templer JW: Trauma to the larynx and cervical trachea. In English GM (ed): Otolaryngology. Hagerstown, MD, Harper & Row, 1976, p 555.

114. Montgomery WW: The surgical management of supraglottic and subglottic stenosis. Ann Otol Rhinol Laryngol 77:534, 1968.
115. Ogura JH, Powers WE: Functional restitution of traumatic stenosis of the larynx and pharynx. Laryngoscope 74:1081, 1964.
116. Ogura JH, Henneman H, Spector GJ: Laryngo-tracheal trauma: diagnosis and treatment. Can J Otolaryngol 2:112, 1973.
117. Brandenburg JH: Management of acute blunt laryngeal injuries. Otolaryngol Clin North Am 12:741, 1979.
118. Mancuso AA, Hanafee WN: Computed tomography of the injured larynx. Radiology 133:139, 1979.
119. Stanley RB Jr: Value of computed tomography in management of acute laryngeal injury. J Trauma 24:359, 1984.
120. Cohn AM, Larson DL: Laryngeal injury: a critical review. Arch Otolaryngol 102:166, 1976.
121. Dudley JP, Mancuso AA, Fonkalsrud EW: Arytenoid dislocation and computed tomography. Arch Otolaryngol 110:483, 1984.
122. Morganstein KM: Treatment of the fractured larynx: use of a new grafting technique. Arch Otolaryngol 101:157, 1975.

CHAPTER 10

THE NECK

WILLIAM P. DILLON ▪ *ANTHONY A. MANCUSO*

Anatomy

The neck is separated from the floor of the mouth by the mylohyoid muscle, which originates from the myloid line of the mandible and runs obliquely and inferiorly to insert into the hyoid bone.[1] The inferior extent of the neck is the thoracic inlet, an oblique plane from the suprasternal (jugular) notch to the first thoracic vertebra. For descriptive purposes and for the interpretation of CT and MR images, it is useful to divide the neck into several compartments (Fig. 10–1).

The visceral compartment of the neck is the most anterior and contains the structures of the aerodigestive tract, including the larynx, hypopharynx, trachea, and esophagus. The thyroid and parathyroid glands also lie within the visceral compartment. The infrahyoid strap muscles arise from the laryngeal skeleton and insert on the anterosuperior chest wall, forming the anterior boundary of the visceral compartment. More laterally, the sternocleidomastoid muscles extend from their relatively posterior origin on the mastoid process of the temporal bone to their insertion on the sternum and clavicle. The sternocleidomastoid muscles are prominent landmarks in cross-section images of the neck, and although their course is quite oblique, they are for the most part seen laterally. Most important, they overlie the ca-

rotid sheaths, which are the major components of the paired lateral compartments and which are lateral to the viscera of the neck.

The cervical spinal cord, the spine, and the surrounding musculature posteriorly form a fourth posterior compartment. The submandibular salivary glands straddle the mylohyoid muscle and are therefore contained within the floor of the mouth as well as the upper neck.

Visceral Compartment

In the upper neck, the larynx and hypopharynx occupy the visceral compartment. (These structures are described in detail in Chapter 9.) Figures 10–2A to E and 10–3A to D show the CT appearance of normal variations in the anatomic relationships of structures in the visceral compartment of the lower and upper neck. Figure 10–4 demonstrates the MR appearance on T1-weighted images of this region in the axial, coronal, and sagittal planes.

The cricoid cartilage is a major landmark for the infrahyoid neck. It is a complete cartilaginous ring, and its appearance depends on its degree of ossification. A rounded, somewhat elliptic, soft tissue density just posterior to the middle portion of the cricoid lamina represents the cricopharyngeal muscle and upper cervical esophagus (see Figs. 10–2C and D

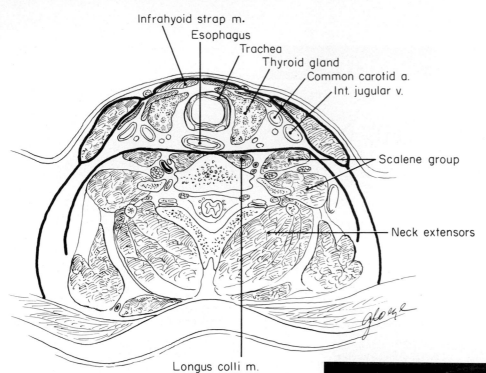

Infrahyoid strap m.
Esophagus
Trachea
Thyroid gland
Common carotid a.
Int. jugular v.

Scalene group

Neck extensors

Longus colli m.

FIGURE 10–1 ■ Schema of the neck. Heavy black lines show an investing layer of deep cervical fascia and prevertebral fascia. Topographically, the neck is separated into the visceral compartment, located anteriorly around the midline; two lateral compartments, mainly containing the structures within the carotid sheath; and the posterior compartment, containing the cervical spine and its surrounding muscles. (From Mancuso AA, Hanafee WN: Computed Tomography of the Head and Neck. © 1982, The Williams & Wilkins Company, Baltimore. Reprinted by permission.)

FIGURE 10–2 ■ Normal anatomy between the thoracic inlet and the midneck. CT scans, during intravenous contrast infusion, are from several patients. A, CT scan through the thoracic inlet shows the subclavian vein (SV) and subclavian artery (SA) as they enter the thorax below the clavicle (C) and above the first rib (R). Visceral compartment of the neck is represented by the trachea (Tr) and esophagus (E) in the midline. Brachiocephalic vessels surround the airway. B, CT scan at a level above the thoracic inlet. High-density thyroid gland (Th) is distinguished from surrounding tissues. Esophagus (E) lies behind trachea (Tr). Small enhancing structures behind the thyroid gland and in front of longus colli muscles (LC) are thyrocervical vessels. Parathyroid glands are located within the small fatty space just lateral to the esophagus and behind the thyroid gland (asterisks). Common carotid artery (C) and jugular vein (J) lie lateral to the thyroid gland and anterior to the scalene muscle (SM).

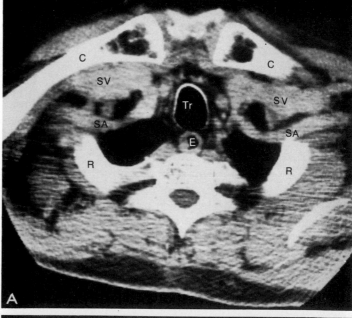

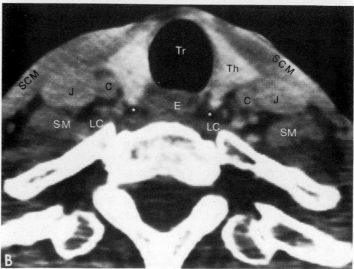

396

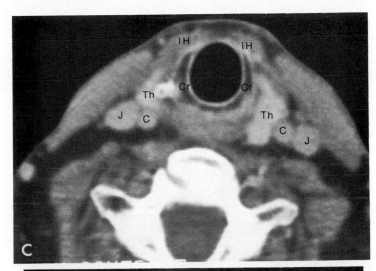

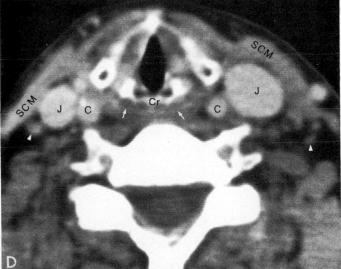

FIGURE 10–2 *Continued* The sternocleidomastoid muscle (SCM) lies anterolaterally. *C*, CT scan through the infraglottic larynx shows the upper pole of the thyroid gland (Th) lateral to the cricoid cartilage (Cr). Carotid artery (C) and jugular veins (J) are well opacified. Infrahyoid strap muscles (IH) are anterolateral to the cricoid cartilage.

D, CT scan through the true vocal cords. The visceral compartment is composed of the larynx and postcricoid portion of cervical esophagus. Cricopharyngeal muscle *(arrows)* is posterior to cricoid cartilage (Cr). Sternocleidomastoid muscles overlie paired lateral carotid sheaths. Asymmetry in size of jugular veins (J) is common and can be even greater than shown. Small, nonenhancing densities posterior to jugular vein and carotid artery (C) are normal lymph nodes *(arrowheads)*.

E, CT scan through midneck at the level of midsupraglottic larynx. The visceral compartment is formed by the supraglottic larynx (L) and piriform sinuses (PS). Small normal nodes are found around the carotid sheath. Infrahyoid strap muscles (IH) border the larynx anteriorly. Longus colli muscles (LC) occur anterior to lateral masses of the cervical spine; the scalene muscle group (SM) is directly lateral.

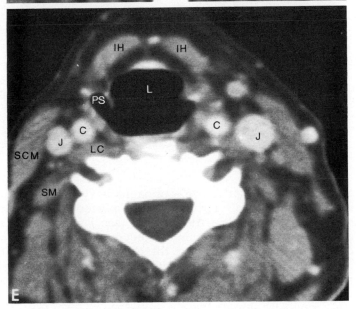

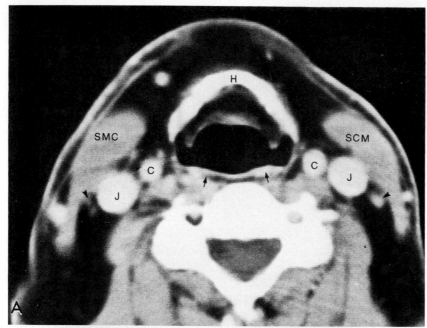

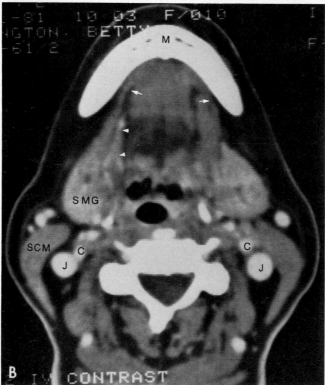

FIGURE 10–3 ■ Normal anatomy of the midneck and lower face, showing both the parotid and submandibular salivary glands. *A*, CT scan through supraglottic larynx at level of the hyoid bone (H). The visceral compartment is composed of the supraglottic larynx and piriform sinuses. Fat within the prevertebral space lies between the cervical spine and pharyngeal constrictor *(arrows)*. Carotid sheath structures are visible within the fat beneath the sternocleidomastoid muscle (SCM). Small nodes *(arrowheads)* are visible near the carotid artery (C) and jugular veins (J). *B*, CT scan through the lower oropharynx and floor of mouth. The mandible (M) is anterior. Mylohyoid muscle *(arrows)* separates the mouth from the upper neck. The jugular vein (J) has changed from its lateral and anterior location low in the neck to posterior to the carotid (C) artery higher in the neck. A small posterior triangular node is visible on the right behind the jugular vein. Submandibular glands (SMG) enhance homogeneously and to a slightly greater degree than surrounding muscles. Lingual vessels lie medial to the submandibular gland within the floor of mouth *(arrowheads)*.

and 10–4*A*). Inferiorly, the esophagus is visible as a slightly smaller soft tissue density, posteriorly indenting the trachea in the midline (see Fig. 10–2*A* and *B*). At the thoracic inlet, the esophagus frequently deflects to the left of the midline. Below the cricoid cartilage, the incomplete rings of the upper trachea are prominent landmarks in the center of the visceral compartment. The posterior wall of the trachea is usually slightly convex anteriorly because the cartilaginous rings are incomplete posteriorly, at the tracheoesophageal interface. The trachea normally re-

mains midline through the lower neck and into the thoracic inlet and upper mediastinum. On CT, the tracheal rings and laryngeal cartilages may be poorly visible if they are incompletely mineralized. On MR, the laryngeal cartilages have a varied appearance, dependent upon their degree of ossification and the extent of yellow marrow conversion that has occurred. Unossified cartilage is almost isointense to muscle on T1-weighted images (see Fig. 10–4*C*). As ossification occurs, the cartilage develops a cortical margin and central medullary cavity. The latter pro-

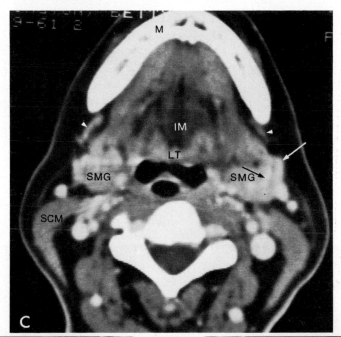

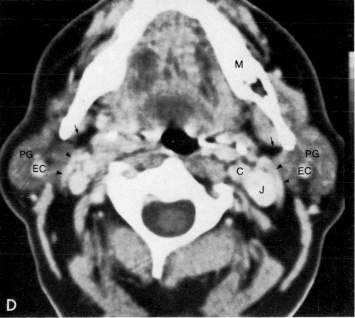

FIGURE 10–3 *Continued* ■ *C*, CT scan, slightly cephalad, shows numerous branches of facial artery and vein coursing through and around the submandibular gland (SMG), especially on the left *(arrows)*. Nonenhancing structures anterior to glands probably represent small, normal-sized lymph nodes *(arrowheads)*. Submandibular glands enhance fairly homogeneously. The interface between the base of the tongue and submandibular glands is usually visible as a result of differences in contrast enhancement. Normal-enhancing lingual tonsil (LT) extends into intrinsic muscles (IM) of the base of the tongue. *D*, CT scan through the midoropharynx. Parotid glands (PG) wrap around the angle and ramus of the mandible (M). Their deep lobes abut a region of low CT density, indicating parapharyngeal space *(arrows)*. Mandibular vein and external carotid artery (EC) are within the substance of the gland. Digastric muscle *(arrowheads)* separates the parotid gland from the jugular vein (J) and carotid artery (C).

gressively converts from red to fatty marrow, yielding an increase in signal intensity with advancing age (see Figs. 10–4*A*, *B*, *D*, and *E*).

The thyroid and parathyroid glands are at the level of and immediately below the lower margin of the cricoid cartilage. The lobes of the thyroid gland are usually evident as wedge-shaped areas of increased CT density on either side of the trachea in the lower neck (see Fig. 10–2*B*). The upper poles of the thyroid gland can usually be seen along the posterolateral margins of the cricoid cartilage near its articulations with the inferior horns of the thyroid cartilage (see Fig. 10–2*C*). After intravenous infusion of iodinated contrast medium, the thyroid gland becomes much more dense than on unenhanced CT scans. On MR scans, the thyroid gland has a slightly higher signal

intensity than muscle on T1-weighted images (see Fig. 10–4*C*) and increases in signal on T2-weighted images. The normal parathyroid glands are rarely visible on CT or MR scans of the neck; however, the inferior thyroid arteries and veins can usually be seen in the fat posterior to each lobe of the thyroid gland and anterior to the longus colli muscles (see Fig. 10–2*B*). These tiny vessels are less than 5 mm in diameter and represent the anatomic location of the normal inferior parathyroid glands.

Lateral Compartments

The carotid sheaths and their surrounding fat form the two lateral compartments of the neck. The internal jugular vein lies posterior to the carotid artery in

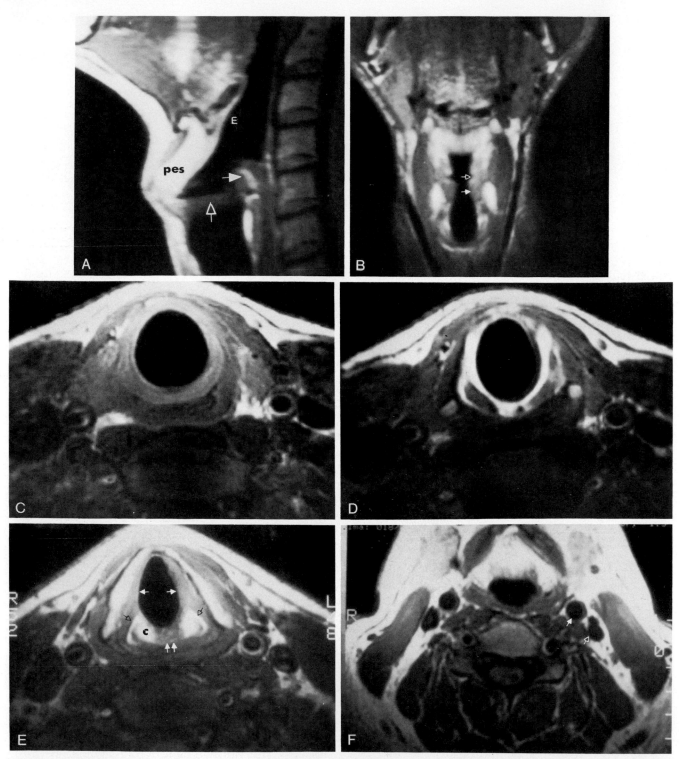

FIGURE 10–4 ■ Normal MR anatomy of the neck (TR 600, TE 20). *A*, Sagittal MR scan of the floor of mouth, base of tongue, and larynx. The prominent landmarks are the epiglottis (E) the pre-epiglottic space (PES), the arytenoid cartilages *(arrow)*, and the vocal cords *(open arrow)*. *B*, Coronal T1-weighted image through the larynx demonstrates the normal symmetric thyroarytenoid muscles *(solid arrows)*, and the laryngeal ventricle *(open arrows)*. *C*, Axial T1-weighted scan through the cricoid cartilage in a 20-year-old male. The unossified cricoid cartilage demonstrates a signal intensity slightly higher than that of muscle. There is no fat in the marrow of the cricoid. *D*, Axial T1-weighted scan through the cricoid cartilage in a 40-year-old male. The cricoid has become ossified. The medullary cavity has both low-intensity marrow, representing hematopoietic marrow, and high intensity, representing fatty marrow.

E, Axial T1-weighted scan through the vocal cords. The thyroid cartilage forms a shield anterior to the vocal cords. At this level, the thyroarytenoid muscle constitutes the inferior margin of the vocal cord process *(arrows)*. Posteriorly, the arytenoid cartilages *(open arrows)* rest on the superior surface of the cricoid cartilage (C). The interarytenoid muscle *(double arrow)* can be seen between the two arytenoid cartilages. *F*, Axial T1-weighted scan through the base of the epiglottis. The pre-epiglottic space is between the epiglottis and the anterior strap muscles. The middle and inferior constrictor muscle surround the airway posteriorly. To each side of the airway, the carotid artery *(closed arrow)* and the internal jugular vein *(open arrow)* are in their typical positions. The jugular vein forms the anterior boundary of the posterior triangle of the neck.

400

the upper neck but becomes progressively more lateral to the artery in the middle neck and lies somewhat anterior to the artery in the lower neck (see Figs. 10–2B to E, 10–3A to D, and 10–4C to F). The jugular fossa lies posterior to the carotid canal at the base of the skull, whereas the deep venous structures lie superficial to the brachiocephalic arteries in the lower neck and upper mediastinum. The common carotid artery bifurcates at approximately the level of the hyoid bone. Numerous tributaries enter the internal jugular vein, and CT and MR both show these as rounded densities around the carotid sheath. On CT they are indistinguishable from enlarged lymph nodes unless the vessels are opacified with contrast material. On MR, signal void from flowing blood within vessels allows their differentiation from solid nodes without the use of contrast medium (see Fig. 10–4E and F).

The deep cervical or internal jugular lymph nodes are divided into three groups: upper, middle, and lower (Fig. 10–5A). The most prominent node in the upper deep cervical group is the jugulodigastric

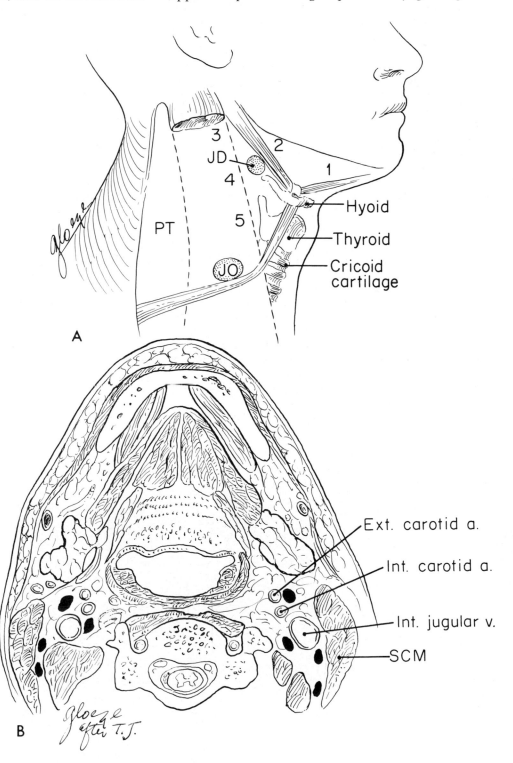

FIGURE 10–5 ■ Lymph nodes of lateral compartments of the neck. A, Schema of various lymph node groups: (1) submental; (2) submandibular; (3–5) upper, middle, and deep cervical groups. Jugulodigastric (JD) and jugulo-omohyoid (JO) nodes are of specific importance. The jugulodigastric node is below the posterior belly of the digastric muscle. The posterior triangle (PT) nodes lie along spinal accessory nerves. B, Typical locations of deep cervical lymph nodes (in black) in relation to the carotid sheath and surrounding muscles. SCM = sternocleidomastoid muscle. (From Mancuso AA, Hanafee WN: Computed Tomography of the Head and Neck. © 1982, The Williams & Wilkins Company, Baltimore. Reprinted by permission.)

node, which is located where the posterior belly of the digastric muscle crosses the internal jugular vein.[1] The jugulo-omohyoid node is located at the crossing of the jugular vein and omohyoid muscle[1] and is therefore at the junction of the upper and middle deep cervical groups. The spinal accessory nodes lie in the fat of the posterior triangle behind the internal jugular vein. The retropharyngeal lymph nodes are not accessible to physical examination. They lie medial to the internal carotid artery, and extend from the level of the thyroid bone to the base of the skull.[1]

Three other groups of nodes in the neck are less often studied by CT or MR. The submental nodes, between the anterior bellies of the digastric muscles, are usually palpable. The submandibular nodes surround the submandibular gland and lie just below and lateral to the plane of the mylohyoid muscle; their territory extends from the middle of the mandibular ramus to the mandibular angle. The intraparotid and periparotid nodes lie within and around the parotid gland.

Normal deep cervical nodes appear on CT as discrete densities near the internal jugular vein (Fig. 10–5B).[2] On MR nodes have an intermediate signal intensity on T1-weighted images (see Fig. 10–4F) and increase in signal intensity with T2-weighting. They are usually 5 to 10 mm or less in diameter, with the exception of the jugulodigastric node, which can normally be up to 11 or 12 mm in longest diameter. Normal submandibular, submental, and periparotid nodes, lying near the mandible or their respective salivary glands, have a CT appearance similar to that of deep cervical nodes. On CT or MR, normal lymph nodes do not show peripheral (capsular) enhancement after intravenous infusion of contrast medium;[2] however, diffuse homogeneous enhancement is typical of benign, reactive adenopathy.

The ninth through twelfth cranial nerves exit the skull base at or near the jugular foramen, remaining with the carotid sheath for at least part of its course through the neck. These nerves can be reliably identified on T1-weighted scans through the posterior fossa. The recurrent laryngeal nerve travels with the minor neurovascular bundle (inferior thyroid artery and vein) to pierce the cricothyroid membrane and enter the lower portion of the larynx. The articulation of the inferior horn of the thyroid cartilage with the cricoid ring marks the entry site of the recurrent laryngeal nerve. The phrenic nerve lies anterior to the scalene muscle group and is therefore considered with the posterior compartment of the neck.

Posterior Compartment

The cervical vertebrae are surrounded by two major muscle groups: a group of extensor muscles located posterior to the transverse processes of the cervical vertebrae, and a much smaller flexor group anterior to the transverse processes. The flexor muscles include the longus colli, longus capitis, rectus capitis, and scalene muscles (see Fig. 10–1). The longus colli and longus capitis muscles lie anterior to the vertebral bodies and should not be mistaken for vascular or lymphatic structures on CT or MR scans of the upper neck. These small muscles are symmetric and form elliptic densities that contact the anterolateral aspect of the vertebral bodies. Lower in the neck, their position assists in identifying the minor neurovascular bundle on CT scans.

The parathyroid glands lie along the course of the minor neurovascular bundle in the fat space bordered by the thyroid gland anteriorly, the longus colli muscle posteriorly, and the carotid artery laterally (Fig. 10–6; also see Figs. 10–1 and 10–4). The scalene muscles arise from the transverse processes of the

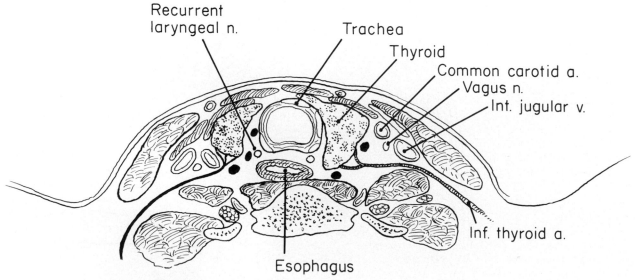

FIGURE 10–6 ■ Cross section through the lower neck. Anatomy of the thyroid and parathyroid glands relative to structure in the visceral compartment. Usual parathyroid locations (in black) are shown relative to the inferior thyroid artery and recurrent laryngeal nerve. (From Mancuso AA, Hanafee WN: Computed Tomography of the Head and Neck. © 1982, The Williams & Wilkins Company, Baltimore. Reprinted by permission.)

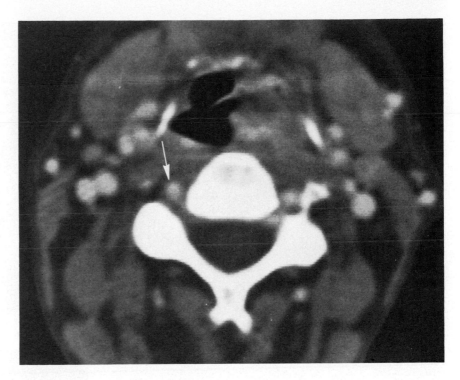

FIGURE 10–7 ■ Posterior pharyngeal wall carcinoma. CT scan at the level of the hyoid bone shows the relationship of the vertebral artery *(arrow)* to the lateral masses. Contrast enhancement within the epidural space is not prominent. (Higher in the neck, normal epidural enhancement between the bony spinal canal and the dural sac is more pronounced.) Also shown is the relationship of the neural foramina to soft tissues of the neck and various vessels.

cervical vertebrae and sweep laterally with a gradual posterior curve. The levator scapulae muscles lie posterior to the scalene muscles. The phrenic nerve courses anterior to the anterior scalene muscle.

A detailed knowledge of the fascial planes is not required to interpret CT or MR scans of the neck. It is sufficient to understand that all of the musculature already described lies within a compartment that is limited anteriorly by the prevertebral fascia (see Fig. 10–1). Posteriorly, the extensor muscle group is surrounded by the trapezius muscle, itself surrounded by the investing layer of deep cervical fascia. Anteriorly and laterally, the investing layer of deep cervical fascia envelops the sternocleidomastoid muscle and courses anterior to the strap muscles (see Fig. 10–1). The platysma can be seen on CT and MR scans as a thin layer within the subcutaneous fat (see Fig. 10–4B to F). Although it has no clinical significance, it should not be mistaken for normal or abnormally thickened fascia within the neck.

The cervical vertebrae, epidural space, dural sac, and cervical spinal cord are regularly visible on CT and MR scans of the neck (see Fig. 10–4). Intravenous injection of contrast medium usually produces CT enhancement of the epidural venous plexus, the venous plexus within the extensor muscle groups, the dura, and the vertebral arteries (Fig. 10–7). CT or MR scans with high spatial resolution clearly define the relationship of lesions in the neck to the cervical neural foramina, the cervical vertebral bodies, and the epidural space and cervical spinal cord. Abnormalities arising from any of these structures can often be identified and distinguished from secondary involvement. MR studies frequently are more useful than CT in depicting these relationships, especially when involvement of neural structures is suspected.

Salivary Glands

The parotid and submandibular salivary glands bridge the anatomic compartments of the neck. Their unique position in the neck and varied pathology require separate consideration. The parotid gland in most patients contains a considerable amount of fat mixed with glandular tissue, which results in an intermediate density on CT and intensity on MR (Figs. 10–8A to D and 10–9). The gland wraps posteriorly around the mandibular condyle and angle of the mandible, its deep lobe projecting medial to the mandible to abut the parapharyngeal space lateral to the nasopharynx and oropharynx (Fig. 10–3D). CT scans through this region show the external carotid artery and retromandibular vein as two rounded, relatively high-density structures running through the gland posterior to the mandible. On MR, these structures are usually seen as signal voids; however, slow flow within the vein may result in increased signal owing to even-echo rephasing or entry slice phenomena (see Fig. 10–9).

The posterior belly of the digastric muscle is visible as an oblong density as it leaves its origin on the mastoid tip. It courses lateral to the carotid sheath on its way to insert on the hyoid bone (see Figs. 10–3D, 10–5A, and 10–9). The facial nerve is often visible on CT and MR as it exits the stylomastoid foramen. MR and CT scans depict the facial nerve as a low signal intensity, round structure surrounded by fat just medial to the origin of the posterior, digastric muscle. As it enters the parotid gland, the facial nerve separates the gland into deep and superficial portions (see Fig. 10–9). The parotid gland can be studied by CT combined with sialography by injection of contrast medium into Stensen's duct[3–5] or by

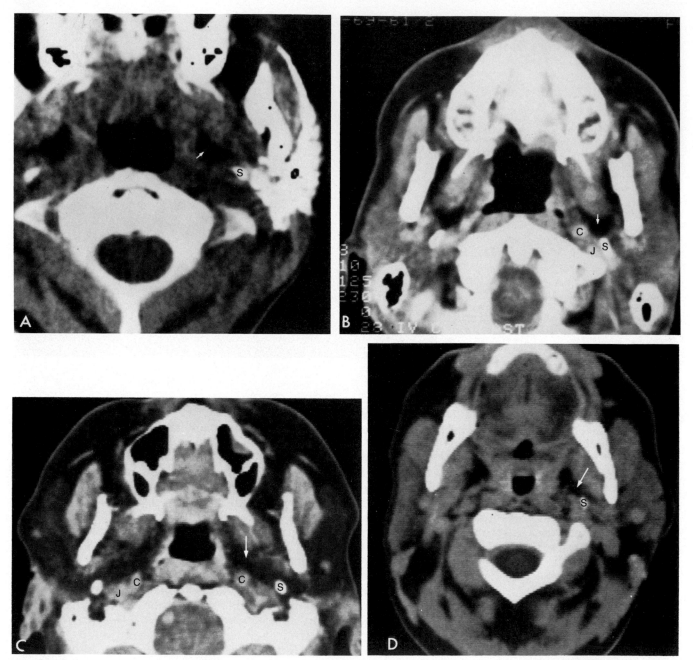

FIGURE 10–8 ■ Variable appearance of the normal parotid gland, depending on its fat content. *A,* CT scan after the left parotid duct has been filled with contrast material, shows the gland in greater detail than without contrast. *B* to *D,* Appearance of the parotid gland varies with its relative content of fat and glandular tissue. Even without injection of contrast material into the parotid duct, the gland is seen. Difference in density between the deep parotid lobe and the parapharyngeal space *(arrows)* is sufficient to distinguish the two. S = styloid process; J = jugular vein; C = internal carotid artery.

CT after injection of intravenous contrast medium. Currently, most authors have abandoned CT sialography in favor of MR or contrast-enhanced CT.

The submandibular gland straddles the posterior edge of the mylohyoid muscle and therefore resides partly in the floor of the mouth and partly in the upper neck (see Fig. 10–3B and C).[1] The major portion of the gland lies below the mylohyoid muscle in the neck. The submandibular glands are visible on CT and MR scans from approximately the angle of the mandible to the level of the hyoid bone, and one gland is usually larger than the other. These glands are more homogeneous and denser than the parotid glands because they contain less fat.[1] Normally, the CT density and MR intensity of the submandibular glands approach that of the surrounding musculature. However, on T2-weighted MR images, the glands often have a higher signal intensity than muscle.

After intravenous injection of iodinated contrast medium, the submandibular and parotid glands both show slight capsular enhancement. With a bolus of

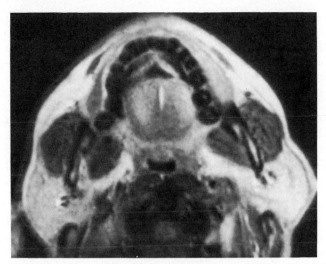

FIGURE 10–9 ■ Normal T1-weighted image through the parotid glands. Note that the parotid glands have a high signal intensity, presumably owing to fat. The parotid glands are located posterior to the mandible and have a superficial portion and a deeper portion, divided by the plane of the external carotid artery and the facial nerve. Occasionally, the facial nerve can be detected on MR studies within the parotid glands as an area of lower signal intensity.

intravenous contrast material, some internal architecture of both the parotid and submandibular glands can become visible. This enhancement may be from opacification of the branching vessels in the gland, concentration of the iodine in the gland, or excretion of iodine into the ductal systems. A ramifying pattern can be seen on CT within the gland during peak intravascular concentrations of contrast medium and for approximately 5 to 10 min afterwards. This has not been shown to assist in diagnosis, but does identify the normal glandular architecture. The branching pattern is usually more prominent in the submandibular gland but also can be seen within the fatty CT density of the parotid gland. The retromandibular vein and external carotid artery are visible on CT scan as prominent high-density structures in the parotid gland after a bolus of contrast medium.

Techniques of Examination

CT

For CT examination of the neck excluding the larynx, the head should be in a neutral (slightly extended) position. For standardization, the inferior ramus of the mandible may be brought perpendicular to the scanner table by a slight extension of the chin. Mild extension of the head does not produce clinically significant alterations in the anatomic display. Extreme flexion or hyperextension of the neck should however be avoided. For CT examination of the larynx, the neck should be moderately hyperextended to bring the central axis of the larynx perpendicular to the plane of the scan. A digital or projection radiograph obtained in the lateral position is ex-

tremely useful for accurate localization of the levels for the CT scans. The patient's shoulders should be relaxed and the technician should pull them as far down as possible. The head should be immobilized. A molded radiographic sponge placed beneath the head and upper neck can maintain a satisfactory position.

With CT scan times under 5 sec, it is usually satisfactory to allow the patient to breathe quietly during the examinations; however, suspending respiration can reduce scan artifacts in the neck and the floor of the mouth. The patient must not move or swallow while scanning is in progress.

The neck can be adequately surveyed by obtaining 3- to 5-mm-thick scans, at 5-mm intervals. The examination should include the abnormal area as well as areas into which the disease might extend. If more than a survey study is required, thinner sections at close intervals should be obtained through the region of interest. For example, for studying the parotid or submandibular glands, contiguous sections 3 to 4 mm thick should be employed. Similar intervals and scan thicknesses should be used for detailed studies of the thyroid and parathyroid glands. Thinner sections and closer intervals can be used if the findings on a survey examination indicate the need for more refined detail.

Direct coronal scans are sometimes used to study the submandibular and parotid glands. A preliminary digital projection radiograph is especially useful in planning direct coronal examinations. It is usually necessary to tilt the gantry so that the plane of scanning is as nearly coronal as possible. CT examination of the parotid gland in the direct coronal plane often avoids dental fillings, which can render transaxial CT scans of the parotid region uninterpretable. Direct coronal scans are usually preferred, as they may be helpful in studying the relationship of adenopathy to the submandibular and parotid glands; the same localizing and gantry-tilting maneuvers are necessary for a high-quality study. Sagittal and coronal reformations are, in general, cumbersome to perform and contribute little diagnostic information that is not apparent on the transaxial scans. Occasionally, reformations can show the superior and inferior extent of a lesion that extends from the neck, through the thoracic inlet, and into the upper mediastinum.

Most CT studies of the neck require the injection of intravenous contrast medium. A rapid injection provides the highest intravascular concentration of iodine.[6, 7] Contrast medium opacifies the many branching vessels in the neck, allowing distinction from enlarged lymph nodes or masses.[2, 8, 9] Opacification can also provide important information about the boundaries of masses, their vascularity, and their relationship to surrounding structures.[2, 3, 8, 9] The thyroid gland is enhanced after intravenous injection of contrast material, which helps in its precise localization.

A simple bolus injection offers no advantage over

rapid-drip infusion and, in fact, may produce nausea, which generally delays the examination during the time of maximal intravascular opacification. Our technique includes an infusion of 30 to 50 mL of contrast medium followed rapidly by the remainder of 150 mL of 60 per cent contrast medium as a rapid-drip infusion. This requires that a 19-gauge needle be placed in a large antecubital vein and that the bottle of contrast material be elevated maximally. Alternatively, a power injector may be used to inject 0.5 mL per sec for 2 to 3 min. Scanning begins after approximately 25 mL of contrast material has been infused. Opacification of the intravascular space is maximal from the time when 50 mL of the contrast material has been infused until 5 to 10 min after the entire 150 mL has been administered. The examination should be timed so that the area of interest is being studied during this period. Infusion of additional contrast material may be required; however, it should be done only if there is no contraindication to an increased load of contrast material (e.g., decreased renal function or diabetes). The rapid-drip infusion may be augmented by injecting a 30- to 40-mL bolus and rescanning a particular area. It is seldom necessary to augment the initial rapid-drip infusion if the area of interest is studied during maximal opacification.

Indications for contrast infusion include suspected or known lymphadenopathy; delineating the extent of mass lesions within the neck, especially the relationship to the carotid sheath; determining the vascularity of a neck mass; determining the extent of thyroid gland masses; searching for parathyroid adenomas in the neck or the anterior mediastinum; and examining the parotid or submandibular salivary glands.

CT scans after rapid intravenous infusion of contrast medium can show masses both inside and outside the salivary glands. Compared with CT, MR appears to provide equivalent diagnostic benefit in the evaluation of the parotid glands.[10] CT after intravenous infusion of contrast material, or MR are sufficient for studying both parotid and submandibular masses. To avoid artifacts from dental fillings, which often make images through the lower portion of the parotid gland nondiagnostic, a projection digital radiograph should be obtained. The patient's head and the scanner gantry should be angled to as near a coronal plane as possible before infusing the contrast material. If the study is not helpful, contrast material can be injected into the parotid duct to show the gland in greater detail (see Fig. 10–8A). Injection of the submandibular gland duct is often tedious and excessively time consuming. These patients can be studied either by the rapid-drip infusion technique, by conventional sialography, or by MR.

MR

In order to maximize its diagnostic value, both T1- and T2-weighted sequences usually are required, frequently in more than one plane. This is acceptable either when there is a confined region of interest or when the study can provide the answer to a well-defined clinical question (for example, Is there a lesion of the thoracic inlet producing a brachial plexopathy? or What is the extent of a known lymphangioma of the neck?). In a more complex situation, CT or ultrasound may be more effective. For instance, in a patient with squamous cell carcinoma of the oropharynx, a complete CT study should include the full extent of the primary tumor, bone windows of the mandible, and a detailed staging of the cervical nodes. MR imaging, although capable of producing the same information, is invariably more time consuming. Although unenhanced MR examinations are advantageous for many clinical situations, enhanced MR scans with intravenous paramagnetic contrast agents (gadolinium-DTPA) often produce better depiction of the morphology of certain lesions, such as abscesses in the deep spaces of the head and neck.[11-13] A potential drawback with gadolinium-DTPA is the possibility of obscuring the interface between enhancing pathology and fat (both have high signal intensity) on T1-weighted images. Fat saturation techniques are useful in overcoming this difficulty.

An MR examination of the neck is accomplished best with a localized, contoured receiver coil. A volume coil is preferred to a flat surface coil, but the changing contours of the head-neck and neck-shoulder junctions make it difficult to design a coil with optimal geometry for all cases. Some remarkable advances have been made utilizing contoured Helmholtz's pairs. Such coils allow one to study the lower craniofacial region as well as the entire neck without changing the coil. Receiver coil development has lagged behind the rest of MR technology, but these coils are now available to most users. In general, the limited penetration and restricted coverage of flat surface coils impede their effectiveness and make their use impractical except in selected cases.

Two-dimensional Fourier transform techniques with Radiofrequency (Rf)–refocused spin-echo pulse sequences form the basis of the MR examination. These should use flow compensation techniques, such as gradient moment nulling, to reduce motion degradation. In addition to being effective in eliminating temporal phase shift artifacts induced by moving blood or cerebrospinal fluid, this technique can also reduce swallowing- and respiratory-induced motion artifacts, but at the expense of a reduced number of slices (coverage). In the neck, Rf presaturation pulse techniques are useful for eliminating entry-slice signal from the lumina of patent vessels and for reducing phase shift artifacts. Presaturation pulses are routinely positioned above and below an area of interest in order to saturate incoming arterial and venous flow. Gradient-echo MR angiography techniques generate qualitative flow-related information. This improves identification of the major vascular structures in the neck, better illustrating their separation from or compromise by adjacent pathologic processes. At present, gradient-echo imaging remains adjunctive, and it is reserved for specific circumstances, such as suspected carotid artery disease and vascular masses.

The axial plane is used most frequently in the study of the head and neck. Coronal views are particularly helpful for evaluating the thoracic inlet, supraclavicular region, and brachial plexus and for showing the relationship of laterally situated masses to the neural axis. Sagittal views are occasionally useful in imaging masses that are near the midline or affect the spinal cord. Table 10–1 lists a general outline of protocols for MR of the neck.

Pathology

Mass lesions of the neck can originate at several sites. We will consider these lesions according to the compartment in which they are found or the organ from which they arise, rather than according to an etiologic classification (Table 10–2).

Visceral Compartment

THYROID GLAND

The thyroid gland anlage descends from the base of the tongue (foramen cecum) to the base of the neck. Persistence of a portion of this tract results in a thyroglossal cyst. Thyroid tissue may occur anywhere along this tract. Approximately 65 per cent of thyroglossal cysts are infrahyoid, 20 per cent are suprahyoid, and 15 per cent occur at the level of the hyoid bone.[14] These masses usually occur on or near the midline, are firm but somewhat fluctuant, and

TABLE 10–1 ■ Protocols for MR of the Neck

FOV:	18–24 cm
Slice Thickness:	3–5 mm (3 mm in selected region of interest)
Acquisition Matrix:	256 × 192 or 256 × 256

UPPER AND MIDNECK: NEURAL AXIS INVOLVEMENT UNLIKELY
Acquisition No.

1	Sagittal, T1-weighted (500–700/20–30)
2	Axial, T2-weighted, dual-echo (2000–3000/30/80 msec)
3, 4	Axial, coronal T1-weighted, with pulse sequence optimized for desired contrast through pathology of interest
5	Another plane, contrast-enhanced as necessary

LOW NECK, THORACIC INLET, BRACHIAL PLEXUS
Acquisition No.

1	Sagittal, T1-weighted (500–700/20–30)
2	Coronal, T1-weighted (500–700/20–30)
3	Axial, coronal, or sagittal dual-echo 2000/30–100*
4	Optional postcontrast coronal T1-sequence

NECK: NEURAL AXIS PROBABLY INVOLVED
Acquisition No.

1	Sagittal, T1-weighted (500–700/20–30)
2, 3	Axial, T1-weighted, with and without contrast (500–700/20–30), same for paramedian coronal
4	Repeat most informative plane with T2-weighted images, dual-echo 2000/30–100*
5	Optional plane, pulse sequence, gradient-echo

*Echo delay time (TE) range allows for selection of spin-density and T2-weighted pair of images as desired.

TABLE 10–2 ■ Indications for CT and MR Scans of the Neck

DETERMINATION OF THE EXTENT OF PRIMARY AND SECONDARY NEOPLASMS OF THE NECK
1. Mass of unknown origin: for preoperative differential diagnosis (MR = CT)
2. Suspected benign tumors (MR > CT)
   Neuromas
   Branchial cleft cysts
   Laryngoceles
3. Thyroid masses
   Extent of benign masses (goiter) (MR > CT)
   Stage known malignancy (nodes and deep invasion) (MR = CT)
4. Malignancies of the aerodigestive tract and nodes (? MR)
   Stage primary tumor (MR > CT)
   Stage cervical metastases (MR − CT)
   Detect recurrent tumor (MR > CT)
   Search for unknown primary neoplasms presenting as nodal metastases (MR > CT)

EVALUATION OF BONY ABNORMALITIES OF THE CERVICAL SPINE
1. Neoplasms (CT > MR)
2. Fractures (CT > MR)
3. Dislocations (CT > MR)
4. Congenital anomalies (CT > MR)

LOCALIZATION OF FOREIGN BODIES IN THE SOFT TISSUES, HYPOPHARYNX, OR LARYNX AND ASSESSMENT OF AIRWAY INTEGRITY AFTER TRAUMA (CT > MR)
1. Foreign body localization
2. Laryngeal trauma

can often be correctly diagnosed from the physical findings. The diagnosis is confirmed by CT when a well-circumscribed, thin-walled, fluid-containing structure is localized either directly in the midline or within the infrahyoid strap muscles (Fig. 10–10 and 10–11).

One of the most important functions of CT is to detail the extent of the cyst relative to the hyoid bone and base of the tongue. Frequently, the cyst extends up and through the hyoid bone. The entire thyroglossal duct tract from the foramen cecum to the cyst must be removed to prevent recurrence. If the cyst is going to recur, it will usually do so within 4 months of surgical excision.[15] Rarely, other cystic lesions of the neck, such as cystic hygroma, occur within the visceral compartment. CT scans can distinguish the origin of some of these masses and can differentiate thyroglossal duct cysts from branchial cleft cysts or external components of laryngoceles.

Although MR imaging can easily depict cystic masses as well, it seems to offer little advantage over CT. Indeed, if the protein concentration is elevated, a reduction in the T1 and T2 relaxation times may result in an appearance that is similar to a solid lesion. Thyroglossal duct cysts typically are multiloculated and very bright on T2-weighted images (Fig. 10–12). Sagittal MR is ideal for showing the full extent of these lesions relative to the tongue base. The body of the hyoid sometimes is difficult to identify with MR imaging, but a cystic component of the lesion extending through it and into the tongue base is extremely easy to demonstrate on heavily T2-

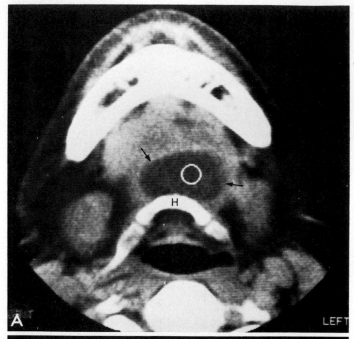

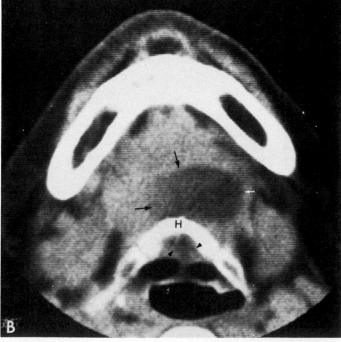

FIGURE 10–10 ■ A thyroglossal duct cyst. *A,* CT scan shows a rounded area of low attenuation, representing a thyroglossal duct cyst *(arrows)* limited to the soft tissues of tongue and floor of mouth. No extension posterior to the hyoid bone (H) is visible. *B,* CT scan at a slightly cephalad level shows a mass anterior to the hyoid bone (H) *(arrows)* and a component of the cyst posterior to it *(arrowhead).*

weighted images. The sagittal and axial planes are most useful (Fig. 10–12).

Thyroid nodules are clinically apparent in 4 to 7 per cent of patients. Once detected, thyroid scintigraphy is usually performed to assess the nodule's biological activity. "Hot," or biologically active, thyroid nodules are composed of functioning thyroid disease, whereas "cold," or inactive, nodules do not contain functioning tissue. The most common "cold" solitary thyroid nodule is adenomatous hyperplasia, which can be either cystic or solid. The other common causes of low-uptake ("cold") thyroid nodules on scintigrams include adenomas, cysts, involutional nodules, carcinoma, and focal thyroiditis. The uncommon causes of "cold" thyroid nodules include lymphomas, metastases, granulomas, abscesses, and parathyroid tumors. Between 5 and 20 per cent of solitary thyroid nodules are malignant. However, "cold" nodules on thyroid scintigraphy in a multinodular thyroid have only a 1 to 4 per cent incidence of malignancy. Also, 20 to 25 per cent of solitary thyroid nodules by scintigraphy are multinodular by ultrasound. A "cold" thyroid nodule detected by scintigraphy is cystic by ultrasound in 11 to 20 per cent of patients. Thus, all "cold," or low-uptake, lesions should be evaluated by ultrasound.

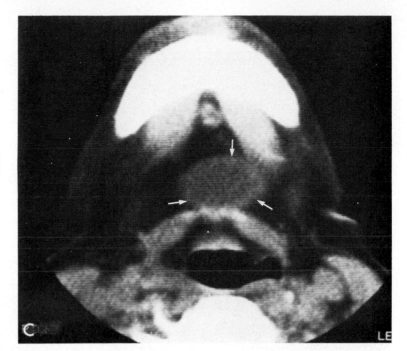

FIGURE 10–10 *Continued* ■ *C,* CT scan 20 mm caudad shows continuation of the cyst *(arrows)* below the hyoid bone.

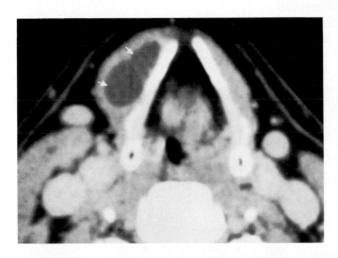

FIGURE 10–11 ■ A thyroglossal duct cyst. CT scan following contrast material injection demonstrates a well-defined cystic mass within the right thyroid strap muscles, adjacent to the right thyroid lamina *(arrows)*. The position of this mass within the strap muscles is typical for a thyroglossal duct cyst. The cysts are usually located at or below the hyoid bone and are a cystic remnant of the thyroglossal duct tract.

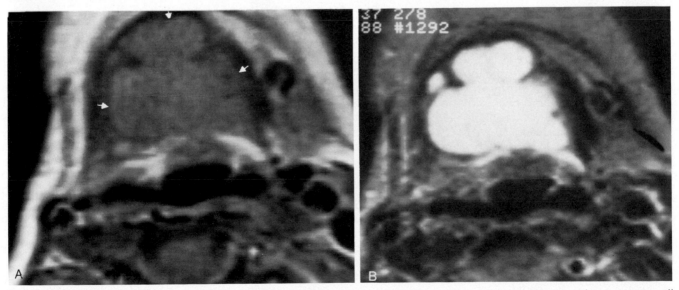

FIGURE 10–12 ■ Thyroglossal duct cyst. *A,* Axial T1-weighted MR scan through the floor of the mouth demonstrates a low-intensity, well-circumscribed mass *(arrows)* separating the muscles of the anterior belly of the digastric muscle. The mass is located superior to the hyoid bone. *B,* Axial T2-weighted MR scan through the same location as *A* (TR 2000, TE 85). The smooth margins of the mass and its high signal intensity are consistent with the diagnosis of thyroglossal duct cyst. A sagittal scan is helpful for determining its extent within the tongue.

409

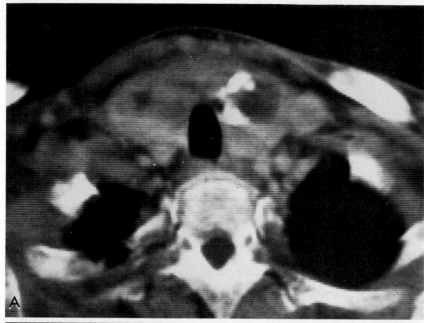

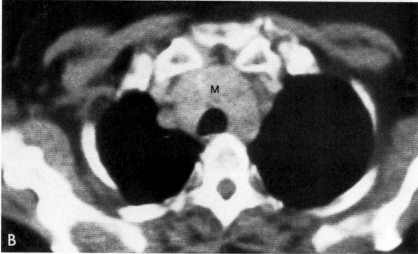

FIGURE 10–13 ■ Thyroid masses. *A*, CT scan shows the typical appearance of a thyroid gland enlarged by multiple adenomas in various states of degeneration and calcification. *B* to *D*, Scans show thyroid goiter extending into the mediastinum. Scan *B* shows a mass (M) at the thoracic inlet. Scans before *(C)* and after *(D)* contrast medium infusion show the exact extent of caudad extension into the middle mediastinum of the enlarged thyroid gland (M).

Thyroid ultrasound is primarily used to determine the cystic or solid nature of a palpable thyroid nodule, the presence of multiple nodules, response to therapy, and as a screening study in patients who have had prior head and neck radiation. A transducer of the highest frequency available is used to examine the neck: 5 MHz at least, 10 MHz if possible. Ultrasound is used to assess the echogenicity and homogeneity of the gland, its size and volume, the size and number of nodules, and their characteristics (i.e., cystic or solid).

Most thyroid cysts are not true cysts. The fluid is usually straw-colored, chocolate-colored, or hemorrhagic and contains elevated levels of thyroid hormone whether or not the patient has hyperthyroidism. An important work on thyroid cancer by Solbiati and colleagues[16] concluded that cystic masses in the thyroid were rarely malignant; mixed lesions had a malignant potential of 4 per cent; hyperechoic lesions, 3 per cent; isoechoic lesions, 22 per cent; and hypoechoic lesions, 71 per cent.

Patients being examined for suspected multiple endocrine neoplasia syndrome may have medullary thyroid cancer as well as parathyroid hyperplasia. Medullary thyroid carcinoma is associated with an elevated calcitonin level and represents between 1 and 3 per cent of thyroid cancers. It can be sporadic or familial, and the treatment is total thyroidectomy.

Ionizing radiation increases the incidence of both benign and malignant thyroid nodules. After radiation exposure, thyroid cancer can be the cause of 30 to 50 per cent of thyroid nodules. Neck irradiation in childhood is associated with a 7 per cent rate of thyroid cancer in later life. Ultrasound shows no distinction between benign or malignant lesions unless local invasion is demonstrated, and aspiration is appropriate for this diagnosis.

With the advent of color-coded ultrasound, some differentiation between thyroid and parathyroid lesions can be made. Thyroid lesions tend to be vascular if over 0.5 cm in size, whereas parathyroid lesions are more apt to develop vascularity at 1 cm.

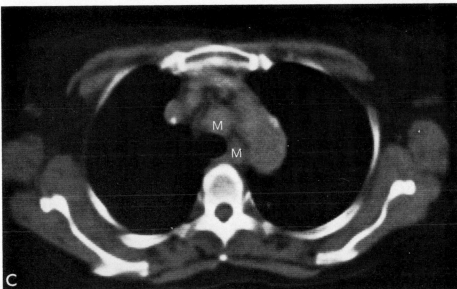

FIGURE 10–13 *Continued*

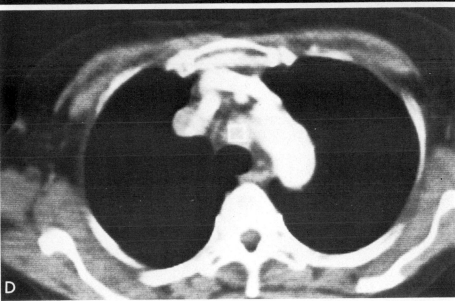

Benign masses of the thyroid gland are extremely common, and imaging is frequently pivotal in their management. Most masses of the thyroid gland are benign, and ultrasound remains the mainstay of anatomic imaging of the thyroid gland, whereas radionuclide imaging provides useful functional information. In patients with a large, adenomatous thyroid gland causing obstruction of the airway (Fig. 10–13A), CT scans can show its extension both behind the trachea and into the superior mediastinum (Fig. 10–13B to D). This information is valuable to the surgeon in planning resection. The organ of origin of a lower neck mass can be unclear, and MR or CT scans will show whether it arises from the thyroid.

CT can assist in planning surgery for a thyroid malignancy. Aggressive thyroid malignancies invade the trachea, larynx, and esophagus. Invasion may be suspected clinically or may not readily be demonstrated by imaging studies (Fig. 10–14A and B). CT scans can show invasion of these viscera, as well as regional nodal metastases. However, if ultrasound and physical examination show the malignancy clearly limited to the thyroid bed, preoperative CT is not warranted.

The role of MR in the evaluation of thyroid disease has been reviewed in detail.[17] MR offers superb soft tissue contrast but has no other functional advantages over ultrasound and scintigraphy. Its present role appears limited to the assessment of muscle involvement by invasive thyroid tumors and the identification of recurrent thyroid carcinomas. MR can possibly characterize tissue in the thyroid bed after surgical excision and may be valuable for differentiating fibrosis from recurrent tumor.[18] It can also detect tracheal or esophageal invasion in the

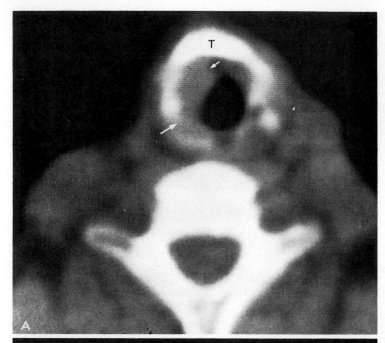

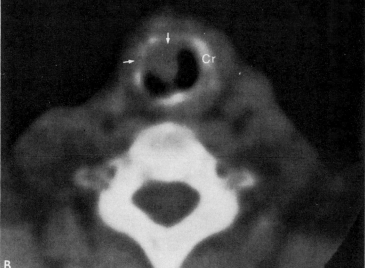

FIGURE 10–14 ■ Thyroid carcinoma 15 years after bilateral radical neck dissections and total thyroidectomy. *A,* CT scan through subglottic regions shows a mass within the infraglottic larynx (*arrows*). Visualization of thyroid cartilage (T) at this level is abnormal and due to distortion of the larynx. *B,* CT shows the mass (*arrows*) extending to the junction of larynx and trachea. Cricoid cartilage (Cr) is visible. Surgery confirmed a recurrent tumor.

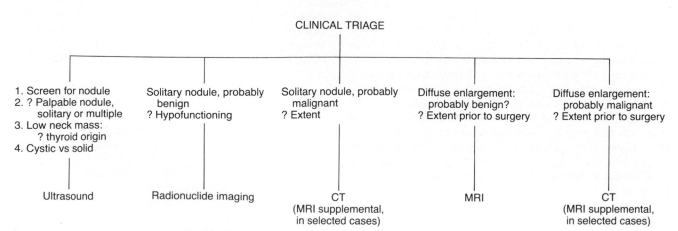

FIGURE 10–15 ■ Imaging algorithm for thyroid-related masses. Clinical triage leading to a well-formulated issue in which imaging may alter clinical disposition. (Modified from Mancuso A, Dillon W: Radiol Clin North Am 27:407, 1989.)

untreated patient and with recurrence of tumor. An algorithmic approach to thyroid masses is offered in Fig. 10–15.

PARATHYROID GLANDS

Congenital lesions of the parathyroid glands are rare. Parathyroid cysts are usually visible posterior to the lower pole of the thyroid gland and are best evaluated by ultrasound.

Imaging studies are usually directed toward the parathyroid glands for the evaluation of hyperparathyroidism. Adenomas are by far the most common lesions of the parathyroid glands that require treatment. Parathyroid carcinomas are rare, and as their clinical presentation does not differ significantly from that of parathyroid adenomas, they can be considered together. Noninvasive lateralization of cervical parathyroid adenomas can permit unilateral neck dissection in patients with primary hyperparathyroidism. High-resolution ultrasonography can detect 71 to 78 per cent of parathyroid adenomas,[19–22] whereas CT can localize 50 to 77 per cent.[23, 24] MR results equal those of ultrasound in the initial evaluation of hyperparathyroidism, offering little advantage in this setting. However, following surgery MR is superior for detecting ectopic parathyroid glands in patients who have persistent hyperparathyroidism.[18]

In one study comparing ultrasound, thallium scintigraphy, and MR in patients with recurrent or persistent hyperparathyroidism after surgery,[25] MR accurately localized an abnormal gland in 75 per cent of cases evaluated prospectively and in 86 per cent evaluated retrospectively. These figures were improved to 80 and 92 per cent, respectively, when MR was combined with thallium scintigraphy.

The ease of examination and accuracy of ultrasonography make it the preferred initial technique for examining the parathyroid glands (Fig. 10–16A and B). Transducers of 7.5 to 10 MHz are those of choice. Parathyroid adenomas are typically oval, hypoechoic lesions oriented in a craniocaudad direction, often

posterior to the thyroid, and less echo-producing than the thyroid. About 10 per cent of parathyroid glands are intrathyroidal. Larger adenomas show variations in echogenicity, extent of cystic change, and contour. Primary hyperparathyroidism is from enlargement of one parathyroid gland in about 80 per cent of instances. However, 3 to 5 per cent of patients with primary hyperparathyroidism have several abnormal glands. About 60 to 80 per cent of parathyroid adenomas can be detected by sonography. About 15 per cent of patients with primary hyperparathyroidism have primary parathyroid hyperplasia with several glands affected. The glands are small and often are difficult to image with sonograms.

Four to 5 per cent of patients with primary hyperparathyroidism have a parathyroid cyst or parathyroid cancer. Parathyroid cancer can appear identical to parathyroid adenoma, but, typically, the patient has a markedly elevated serum calcium level. Ten per cent of parathyroid glands are ectopic, either in the neck or in the mediastinum, often in the thymus. These lesions cannot be seen with ultrasonography. Nuclear scintigrams, using thallium and technetium, or MR are the advocated techniques for detection of mediastinal parathyroid glands.

When an ultrasound examination does not demonstrate a mass in the usual parathyroid locations, CT or MR scans of the lower neck and the superior and anterior mediastinum may show a parathyroid mass (Fig. 10–17A and B). Ultrasonograms often fail to demonstrate parathyroid adenomas at the upper pole of the thyroid gland, probably because of their proximity to the larynx,[21] and CT or MR may help to detect adenomas at this site (Fig. 10–17C). When CT is used to detect parathyroid adenomas, a bolus injection of contrast material is essential.[24, 26, 27] About 20 per cent of parathyroid adenomas enhance after a bolus injection of iodinated contrast material (Fig. 10–17C). Cervical lymph nodes, tortuous vessels, thyroid masses, and even a collapsed esophagus can be mistaken for a parathyroid tumor. Streak artifacts, limited spatial resolution of some scanners, and im-

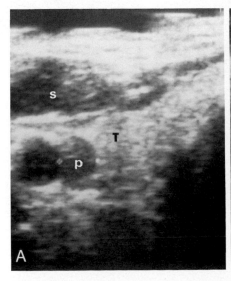
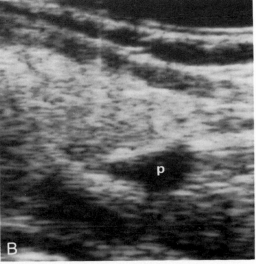

FIGURE 10–16 ■ Ultrasound scan of parathyroid adenoma. *A,* Transverse view with a 10-MHz transducer through the thyroid gland (T) and strap muscle (S). The carotid artery (C) is located adjacent to the hypoechoic parathyroid adenoma (p). *B,* A longitudinal scan through the thyroid gland demonstrates the oblong-appearing, hypoechoic parathyroid adenoma (p) located at the inferior-posterior border of the thyroid gland. (Courtesy of Gretchen A. W. Gooding, MD, San Francisco, CA.)

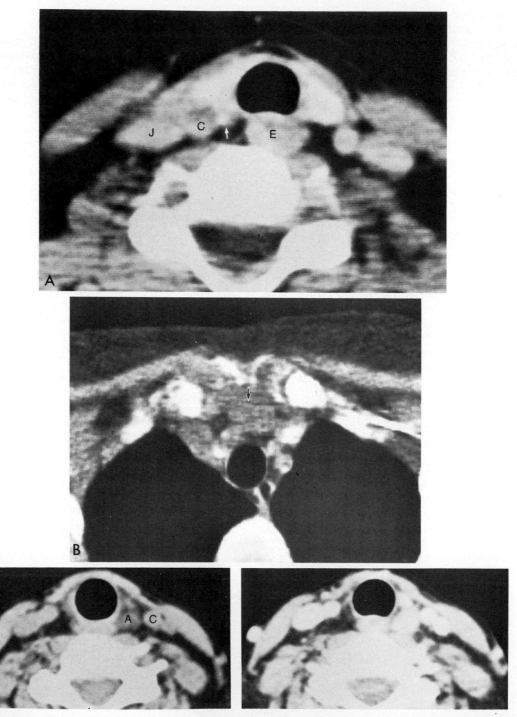

FIGURE 10–17 ■ Parathyroid adenomas in four patients. *A,* CT scan shows small parathyroid adenoma *(arrow)* medial to the carotid artery (C) and jugular vein (J) and lateral to the esophagus (E). *B,* CT scan shows an ectopic, mediastinal adenoma *(arrow).* Ultrasound examination of the neck was normal in this patient. *C,* CT scan at the level of the cricoid cartilage before contrast medium infusion (left) shows a parathyroid adenoma (A) medial to carotid artery (C). During bolus injection of contrast (right), the adenoma has enhanced markedly. *D* and *E,* T1-weighted (TR 600/20) *(D)* and T2-weighted (TR 2000, TE 80 ms) *(E)* sequences demonstrate a large parathyroid adenoma in the typical location, adjacent to the trachea (T) and inferior to the thyroid gland. The thyroid adenoma (asterisk) has the usual low intensity on T1- and high intensity on T2-weighted images. (*C,* Courtesy of D.D. Stark, MD, Boston, MA; *D,* Courtesy of Charles B. Higgins, MD, San Francisco, CA.)

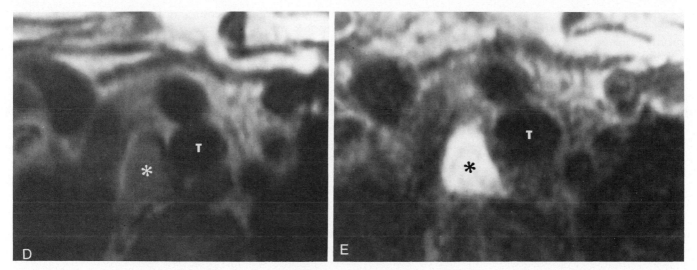

FIGURE 10–17 *Continued*

age unsharpness from magnification can all cause difficulties with interpretation of CT.[28]

Parathyroid adenomas usually show a low signal intensity on T1-weighted MR images and a high signal intensity on T2-weighted sequences, although variations do occur.[17] Enhancement following gadolinium-DTPA may be a useful adjunct to diagnosis (Fig. 10–17*D* and *E*).

ESOPHAGUS

Abnormalities of the cervical esophagus are seldom studied by CT. Occasionally, a Zenker's diverticulum mimics a lateral neck mass for which CT might be indicated (Fig. 10–18). Usually, the symptoms of a Zenker's diverticulum clearly relate to swallowing, and the presence of this lesion is confirmed by an esophagogram. CT and MR are valuable for assessing malignancies of the cervical esophagus or hypopharynx that have extended inferiorly to involve the postcricoid region. Both types of scans can show the extent of the lesion and the presence of either cervical or mediastinal adenopathy. At present CT is more accurate than MR for staging lymph nodes and detecting early capsular penetration.

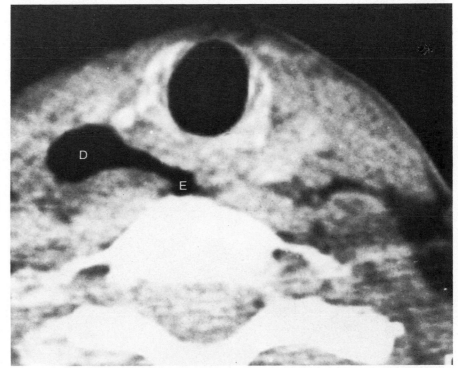

FIGURE 10–18 ■ Zenker's diverticulum. CT scan shows Zenker's diverticulum (D) extending from the region of cricopharyngeal muscle and upper cervical esophagus (E) into lateral soft tissues of the neck.

LARYNX

Recurrent laryngeal nerve palsy and, less commonly, phrenic nerve dysfunction may be due to a variety of causes that can originate in the neck. Often, a specific cause is not discovered, and the dysfunction is considered idiopathic or viral in nature. A structural lesion causing paresis of a vocal cord or hemidiaphragm is usually sought before the diagnosis of idiopathic dysfunction is accepted.

Before CT and MR became available, the course through the neck of the vagus, recurrent laryngeal, or phrenic nerve could not be studied effectively. At present, the path of the vagus nerve from the thoracic inlet and the upper mediastinum to the skull base can be evaluated by CT, even if the nerves themselves cannot be seen (Fig. 10–19A and B). Careful

imaging along the course of the minor neurovascular bundle and scrutiny of the fascial planes anterior to the anterior scalene muscles are important. Adequate clinical history and good neurologic examination is valuable in determining the appropriate imaging study.[29] For instance, if both the larynx and palate are immobile, MR or CT of the skull base is required. However, if the palate functions normally, CT should be directed to the larynx, thoracic inlet, and upper mediastinum. Alternatively, MR can be employed, but a body coil, with some disadvantages, is required to image both neck and mediastinum. In the mediastinum and thoracic inlet, the aortic-pulmonic window on the left and the origin of the right subclavian artery on the right are important areas to examine for recurrent laryngeal nerve lesions. CT of the neck

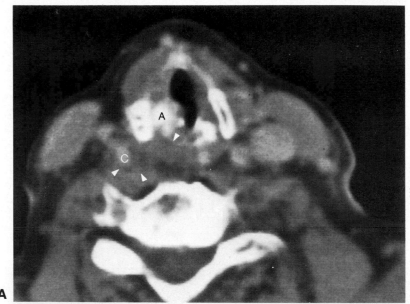

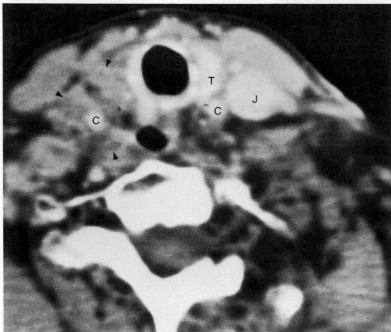

FIGURE 10–19 ■ Paralyzed vocal cord in a patient with metastatic breast carcinoma. *A,* CT scan through true vocal cord shows superior and medial displacement of right arytenoid cartilage (A) and a relatively paramedian position of the true cord and base of the aryepiglottic fold. Marked asymmetry is present in soft tissues of the postcricoid region and surrounding the right carotid sheath. Tissue planes are also obliterated *(arrowheads).* *B,* A scan 15 mm caudad, at the level of the cricoid cartilage, shows marked asymmetry in deep soft tissue planes. The carotid artery (C) is surrounded by abnormal tissue, and the right jugular vein (J) does not opacify *(arrowheads).* Planes between the carotid sheath and esophagus are obliterated, and the esophagus is retracted to the right. The thyroid (T) on the right side is replaced by abnormal tissues. Metastatic disease was not clinically evident.

should be scrutinized with special attention to the tracheoesophageal groove below the larynx and the carotid sheath above the larynx. In recurrent laryngeal nerve paralysis, CT scans of the larynx show that the affected true vocal cord lies in a paramedian position and should not be mistaken for pathology of the true cord itself. CT scans during both phonation and breath-holding maneuvers demonstrate abnormal mobility of the affected cord.

In our experience, CT has proved more useful than MR for patients with known malignancies and recent onset of symptoms consistent with phrenic or recurrent laryngeal nerve dysfunction. Nonpalpable metastatic disease in the neck has been found to be the cause in many instances (Fig. 10–19B).[23]

Lateral Compartments

CONGENITAL MASSES

Masses of developmental origin in the lateral compartments of the neck are frequently either hygromas or second branchial cleft cysts. These masses usually differ considerably in their clinical, morphologic, and anatomic presentation.

BRANCHIAL CLEFT CYST

The branchial arches consist of five mesodermal bars separated by clefts covered by epithelium. Each cleft is in intimate contact with a pharyngeal pouch. As the embryo develops, the arches and clefts form the muscles, nerves, and cartilages of the lower face and neck. The second arch grows caudad to overlap the third and fourth arches. The second, third, and fourth clefts open into a common chamber called the cervical sinus. Defective involution of this sinus results in the formation of a bronchial anomaly. Branchial cleft cysts in the lateral compartments are the most common and arise from the second branchial cleft or the cervical sinus. Cysts of the first branchial cleft are rare and manifest as parotid or periparotid masses. Third branchial cleft cysts are extremely unusual and are located in the lower pharynx near the piriform sinuses. Patients usually have a long history of a slowly enlarging, fluctuant neck mass. Pain in the region of the mass is unusual unless there is superimposed inflammation or hemorrhage.

Second branchial cleft cysts usually present as a unilocular cyst projecting anterolaterally in the neck (Fig. 10–20A and B).[30] The sternocleidomastoid muscle usually is displaced posterolaterally, and the carotid sheath and its structures are displaced posteromedially. These cysts occasionally manifest deep to the sternocleidomastoid muscle and posterior to the carotid sheath. If the diagnosis can be suspected clinically, MR is a good way to study the extent of the cyst and to confirm the diagnosis (Fig. 10–20A and B). Unfortunately, these lesions frequently manifest clinically as inflammatory masses or masses suggestive of adenopathy. In this event, needle biopsies are often inconclusive and compatible with a node containing a large area of cystic necrosis.

Neither CT nor MR can discriminate between fluid collections and surrounding cellulitis (Fig. 10–20C). If adenopathy is suspected, CT is preferred, unless fat saturation MR imaging is available. CT provides better images for evaluation of the internal morphology of surrounding lymph nodes and can search efficiently for a potential primary tumor.[11, 31–34]

On MR, branchial cleft cysts typically will appear cystic with either a thin or thick enhancing wall, depending on whether there has been prior inflammation (Fig. 10–20A and B). The signal characteristics of the cyst fluid may vary on T1-weighted sequences from hypointense to slightly hyperintense relative to muscle. The cyst contents are very bright on T2-weighted images (Fig. 10–20B). Surrounding cellulitis often is slightly hyperintense relative to fat, on T2-weighted images.

CT scans show branchial cleft cysts as very well circumscribed, usually thin-walled, masses containing low-density fluid (Fig. 10–20C). Their round appearance and the CT density of their fluid content suggest a cyst. They neither obliterate the surrounding tissue nor invade surrounding structures. Large cysts may displace the carotid sheath, the sternocleidomastoid muscle, or the larynx. Irregularity and excessive thickness or marked contrast enhancement of the wall suggest inflammation in the cyst. Rarely, branchial cleft cysts have malignancies in their walls.[14]

All branchial cleft cysts have a fistulous tract that extends to the hypopharynx and usually opens into one of the following: a piriform sinus, vallecula, or glossopharyngeal sulcus. Most of the length of the tract is usually not visible on CT, but the portion between the internal and external carotid arteries can sometimes be imaged. Clinically, it may not be possible to differentiate between an external laryngocele that extends from the appendix to the laryngeal ventricle and a branchial cleft cyst. This distinction is easily made by CT, which can demonstrate the internal component of a laryngocele within the paralaryngeal space and its extension through the thyrohyoid membrane.

CYSTIC HYGROMA

The only other common congenital cystic mass in the neck is a cystic hygroma. It is composed of dilated lymphatic channels and is a type of lymphangioma. Cystic hygromas are almost exclusively seen in children, although in rare instances, they may first be diagnosed in adulthood. Therapy is usually surgical and is aimed at cosmesis or relieving airway obstruction. These lesions are diffuse and appear as a septated network of interconnected loculations of high and low density on CT scans. Their diffuse and insinuating characteristics make it difficult to delineate the normal fascial planes within the neck.

Lymphangioma-cystic hygroma usually occurs in the posterior lateral compartments of the neck. Involvement of virtually all the deep spaces of the craniofacial region and neck can occur, and extension

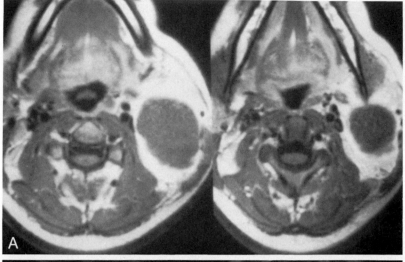

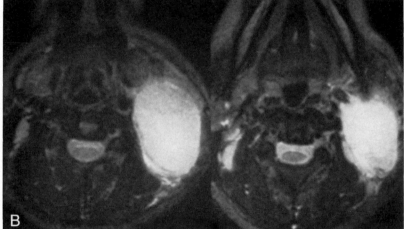

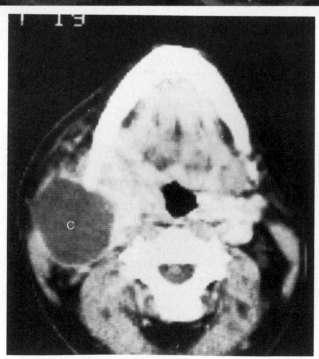

FIGURE 10–20 ■ Branchial cleft cyst. *A*, Axial T1-weighted images (after gadolinium injection) through the midoropharynx (TR 600/20). A cystic mass in the left neck is interposed between the sternocleidomastoid muscle and the submandibular gland. The mass has a peripheral enhancing border and a low-density center. This position and appearance is most typical of a second branchial cleft cyst with inflammatory changes in its periphery. A neck abscess and necrotic lymph node metastasis could look similar. *B*, T2-weighted (TR 2000, TE 80) images. The cyst increases in signal intensity. *C*, CT scan of a typical branchial cleft cyst in the lateral compartment of the neck. The extent of the mass in relationship to the surrounding structures is demonstrated.

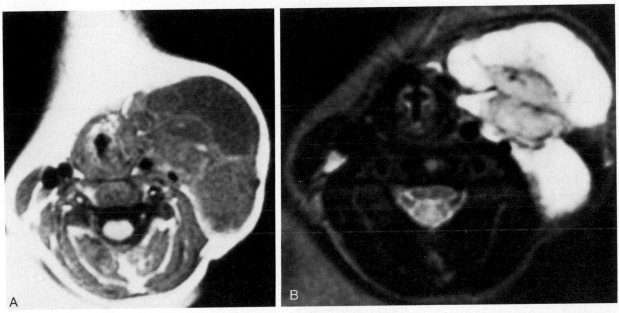

FIGURE 10–21 ■ Cystic hygroma. *A,* Axial T1-weighted (TR 600, TE 20) image. A well-defined, septated mass is seen in the left of the neck, adjacent to the larynx. The mass has several different intensities associated with different protein concentrations. *B,* Axial T2-weighted (TR 2000, TE 80) image. Hyperintense signal is associated with the cystic components of the mass. A central hypointense area probably relates to an area of high protein content or hemorrhage. Notice that the mass insinuates among normal tissues. This is typical for cystic hygroma. (Branchial cleft cysts are generally smaller in size, whereas thyroglossal duct cysts occur more toward the midline.)

into the mediastinum or along the chest wall is not uncommon. Cystic hygromas can become extremely large and can extend superiorly to the parotid region or inferiorly to the axilla. Extension within the deep planes of the neck to the parapharyngeal space can reach to the infratemporal fossa and the base of the tongue. This tumor can also extend into the thoracic inlet and superior mediastinum.

The clinical diagnosis almost never is in question in the newborn, although it may be in older individuals. MR is clearly the best way to map the full extent of these masses (Fig. 10–21*A* and *B*). Lymphangiomas or cystic hygromas usually are multiseptated. The cystic spaces may be large or small. They characteristically are extremely bright on T2-weighted images and less intense than muscle on T1-weighted images, unless they are complicated by hemorrhage, infection, or prior surgery. Hemangiomas occasionally are difficult to distinguish clinically from lymphangiomas. CT may hold a minor advantage for this purpose, if phleboliths are present or if intravenous contrast is used (see later).

OTHER PARENCHYMAL CYSTS

Thymic cysts are rare and can appear identical to branchial cleft cysts. Branchial cleft cysts, however, seldom extend below the clavicle, whereas this is a common characteristic of thymic cysts.[14, 35] Parathyroid cysts are rare and typically located posterior to the thyroid gland. Thyroglossal duct cysts should not be mistaken for branchial cleft cysts on CT, as the course and location of thyroglossal duct cysts differ from those of branchial cleft cysts.

HEMANGIOMA

Benign hemangiomas involving the head and neck have a distribution similar to that described for cystic hygromas. In fact, cystic hygromas may have hemangiomatous elements, and the converse is also true. Most hemangiomas are present at birth or develop during infancy. Hemangiomas may be located in the skin or deep tissues. Deep hemangiomas are frequently poorly circumscribed and are locally invasive. These lesions often involve multiple structures or spaces within the head and neck. CT after infusion of intravenous contrast material may show the extent of the lesion if a significant vascular component is present (Fig. 10–22*A* and *B*). However, these lesions may exhibit little or no enhancement. MR demonstrates a confluent mass with prolonged T1 and T2 relaxation times.[36] If the diagnosis is in question on MR, CT may demonstrate phleboliths. Treatment of lesions is for cosmesis and to relieve airway obstruction.

INFLAMMATORY MASSES

There is no reported experience comparing CT and MR in the evaluation of inflammatory neck masses. In fact, the reported experience with MR evaluation of neck abscesses, cervical adenitis, and other masses mimicking inflammatory lesions is limited.[37–39] CT currently remains the primary imaging study for evaluating patients with inflammatory neck masses. CT can differentiate abscess from cellulitis clearly and rapidly.[11, 12] It shows the full extent of abscesses, allowing the surgeon to appreciate the spaces that require drainage. MR can also clearly differentiate

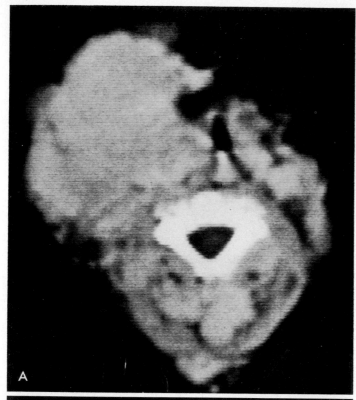

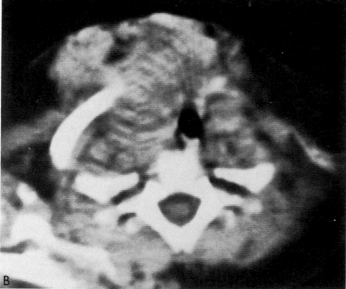

FIGURE 10–22 ■ Hemangioma of the face and neck in an 18-month-old child with stridor. *A,* CT scan of the larynx shows a large right-sided mass displacing the larynx to the left. *B,* After intravenous infusion of contrast medium, the mass is still visible at the level of the clavicle. Enhancement of the mass has occurred with contrast. (Ring densities are artifacts.)

cellulitis from a drainable fluid collection. Both abscesses and cellulitis may be bright on heavily T2-weighted images, potentially obscuring the margin between an abscess and the related cellulitis. Gadolinium-enhanced T1-weighted images appear able to differentiate between these processes. More experience with MR in deep-space infections should clarify this point. On T1-weighted images, pus-filled cavities should easily be differentiated from edematous fat but may be isointense to surrounding musculature. There may also be difficulty on MR in detecting small collections of gas or small foreign bodies, both of which are detected readily by CT. MR aptly demon-

strates jugular thrombosis and thrombophlebitis. When this is the presumptive diagnosis of a neck mass, MR is a reasonable first choice, although ultrasound and CT both are capable of confirming this clinical diagnosis.

Tuberculous adenitis is not an uncommon cause of a neck mass in several regions of the United States and the world.[40] Imaging studies frequently demonstrate extensive adenopathy. The internal jugular and spinal accessory nodal groups are usually both involved. Individual nodes usually are frankly necrotic, with thick, indistinct margins. Nodes frequently are matted into conglomerate masses. MR shows these nodes; however, its potential limitations for assessing inflammatory disease have been discussed.

Intravenously administered gadolinium-DTPA may help in the evaluation of inflammatory neck masses. Although an enhancing necrotic mass is not specific for an abscess, this appearance is indicative of a maturing abscess or necrotic tumor and can help differentiate the mass from surrounding edema. On MR an enhancing margin is helpful in delineating the interfaces between abscess and muscle. However, without fat-suppressing techniques, gadolinium-DTPA is likely to decrease the contrast between an enhancing rim of a mass and surrounding fat on T1-weighted images. The role of MR, with and without paramagnetic contrast, in the evaluation of inflammatory neck masses requires further clarification with clinical experience.

BENIGN NEOPLASMS

Benign neoplastic lesions in the lateral compartments are rare and usually arise from the structures in and about the carotid sheath or from the mesenchymal elements that surround them. The most common tumors are schwannomas and paragangliomas.

NON-NEOPLASTIC VASCULAR MASSES

On physical examination, a pulsatile neck mass can be a highly vascular mass or a tumor of vascular origin or can consist of transmitted pulsations to a mass. Imaging should precede needle biopsy in the evaluation of such lesions. Ultrasound can differentiate between a prominent carotid bifurcation and a significant lesion. MR, CT, or both are usually performed, unless the patient goes directly to angiography for clinical reasons. Pulsatile masses virtually always present in the lateral compartment, except for the rare vertebral artery aneurysm and arteriovenous malformation. Standard spin-echo MR pulse sequences, as well as gradient-echo sequences, can demonstrate intracranial, thoracic, and abdominal aneurysms and dissections; they can be applied to similar lesions in the neck. The role of MR in the evaluation of atherosclerotic plaques in the cervical carotid arteries is experimental.

Aneurysms vary in their appearance, based on the presence of thrombosis and the rate and turbulence of blood flow within them. Depending on the methods of flow compensation used, the lumen may contain bright signal or flow void. Gradient-echo techniques show increased signal in areas of rapid flow. Similarly, a combination of two-dimensional (2D) or three-dimensional (3D) spin-echo and gradient-echo pulse sequences can be used to evaluate vascular malformations and, perhaps, lesions with slower flow, such as hemangiomas.

The diagnosis in patients suspected of having jugular thrombosis or thrombophlebitis can be confirmed by ultrasound. If additional imaging is required to identify a possible etiology such as abscess or tumor, CT or MR may be appropriate.

MR can show intraluminal thrombosis, but flow-related phenomena are complex, and care is necessary not to mistake flow-related artifacts for thrombus. This error is avoided either by altering the plane of study and using long TR/TE sequences or by using a combination of a short TR/TE sequence, presaturation pulses, and short flip-angle gradient-echo images. The appearance of thrombus varies considerably with its age and the pulse sequences being used. In general, on standard spin-echo pulse sequences, intraluminal clot is slightly hyperintense to muscle on T1-weighted images and very bright on T2-weighted pulse sequences. Flow-sensitive gradient-echo imaging (flip angle 30° to 60°, TR 30 to 50 ms, TE < 15 ms) usually demonstrates thrombosed vessels as lower signal compared with the high signal of blood in patent vessels.

NEOPLASMS OF THE NECK

Neoplasms of the neck, apart from nodal metastases, are unusual. Some manifest clinically as a neck mass, whereas others are discovered during an examination for complaints such as dysphagia or vocal cord paresis, for Horner's syndrome, or for a pharyngeal mass detected on physical examination.[29]

Carotid body tumor is probably the most common benign tumor in a lateral compartment. The diagnosis is usually suspected clinically; however, differentiation from other anterior and lateral neck masses is important for deciding on further evaluation by angiography or surgical neck exploration. CT of a carotid body tumor typically shows a well-circumscribed mass at or above the carotid bifurcation. Intravascular contrast material shows a well-circumscribed mass with a homogeneously dense pattern of enhancement (Fig. 10–23A to C). Carotid body tumors rarely extend to the base of the skull, whereas tumors of the glomus jugular and glomus vagal commonly do involve the base of the skull in and about the carotid bulb.[14]

Some investigators choose MR as the primary examination for suspected carotid body tumors. This variety of paraganglioma typically lies at the carotid bifurcation and splays the internal and external carotid arteries. On T2-weighted spin-echo sequences, paragangliomas 2 cm or greater in diameter usually show a "salt and pepper" appearance caused by vessels with absent signal, within the increased signal from tumor and stroma (Fig. 10–24).[41] On T1-weighted spin-echo MR, branching tubular areas of signal void are found as expressions of the hypervascularity of the tumor. Gradient-echo pulse sequences can confirm the presence of rapidly flowing blood. The glomus vagal variant of paraganglioma may also manifest as a neck mass, and imaging is useful for showing the full cephalocaudal extent of the mass; this is important because large lesions in elderly patients frequently are treated with radiotherapy rather than surgery.

MR can also be used to survey patients for multiple paragangliomas, but its sensitivity relative to angiography in this regard is unknown. Paragangliomas

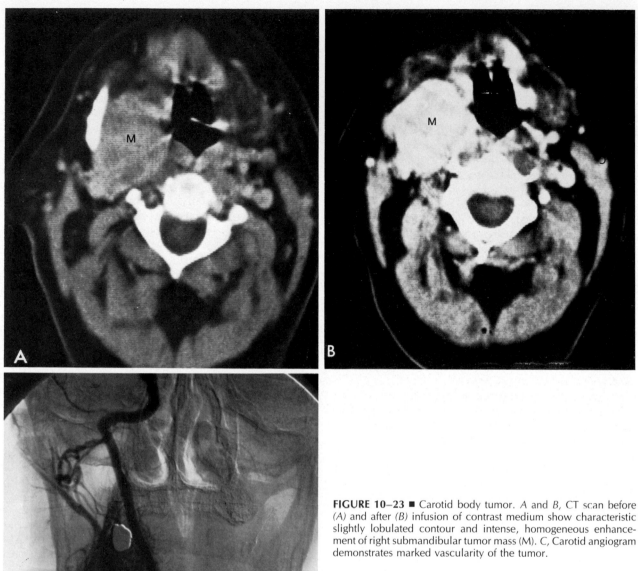

FIGURE 10–23 ■ Carotid body tumor. *A* and *B*, CT scan before *(A)* and after *(B)* infusion of contrast medium show characteristic slightly lobulated contour and intense, homogeneous enhancement of right submandibular tumor mass (M). *C*, Carotid angiogram demonstrates marked vascularity of the tumor.

occasionally invade the jugular vein, and MR shows the spread to this site by a more graphic and simpler means than arteriography and venography.

MR is the appropriate examination for evaluation of lesions arising from or involving the neural axis. It should be used in patients presenting with vocal cord paresis, Horner's syndrome, and brachial plexopathy of uncertain etiology. It should also be used to evaluate palpable masses involving the deep musculature of the posterior neck, or in the unusual circumstance when needle biopsy suggests a neural

tumor. When a mass presents as a submucosal retropharyngeal or lateral pharyngeal bulge and squamous cell carcinoma is considered unlikely, MR is the best initial imaging study. These circumstances occur infrequently but are occasions when MR may prove to be definitive and is the only imaging examination that is necessary.

In general, tumors of neural origin are round or elliptic and are well circumscribed. On T1-weighted images, they tend to be isointense to muscle and are clearly brighter than fat on T2-weighted images. They

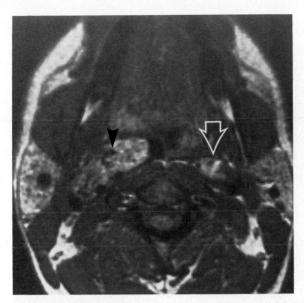

FIGURE 10–24 ■ Bilateral carotid body tumors. Axial T2-weighted MR scan (TR 2000/80) demonstrates bilateral heterogenous masses in the carotid space. These masses have internal flow voids typical of paraganglioma (*arrowheads* and *arrow*). The masses also have a salt-and-pepper appearance from the tumor matrix (high signal intensity) and vessels (low signal intensity).

may have a surrounding thick wall.[42] Sarcomas of neural origin may be more aggressive appearing, with ill-defined margins. Gadolinium-DTPA can show perineural extension of these masses proximally to the nerve roots and even into the spinal cord—proximal disease that usually is not seen on CT or MR without intravascular contrast.

Tumors of neural origin presenting in the neck can arise from the vagus, spinal accessory, or hypoglossal nerves. These usually present as masses in the lateral compartment. It is difficult to diagnose this unusual etiology for a neck mass without a biopsy. Because the common cause of these masses is nodal disease, CT may be obtained first. On MR, the morphology of these tumors is the same as their counterparts in other locations. On CT, they will enhance less intensely than paragangliomas and will sometimes have a relatively low density center (Fig. 10–25A to C).

The most common tumor of mesenchymal origin in the neck is a lipoma. Small, not obviously encapsulated, lipomas may be difficult to separate from normal fat on MR or CT. These lesions typically are isointense or slightly hyperintense to normal fat on T1- and T2-weighted images. Liposarcomas should show focal areas of altered signal intensity, usually hypointense to fat on T1- and slightly hyperintense to fat on T2-weighted images.

Benign lesions of mesenchymal origin otherwise are rare. Rhabdomyoma or rhabdomyosarcoma of the sternocleidomastoid or other muscles may manifest as a neck mass in the pediatric age group. In adults the musculoaponeurotic fibromatoses (desmoid tumors) may involve the sternocleidomastoid or other muscles. MR is the best way to map the

extent of these masses. In these and in rhabdomyomas, T2-weighted images usually are most informative because of the better tumor-to-muscle contrast. T1-weighted images may be necessary to show the extent of infiltration of surrounding fat. Other sarcomas, such as malignant fibrosis histiocytoma, can occur in virtually any compartment.

Rarely, primary or metastatic tumors of the cervical spine manifest as a neck mass. These usually produce neck pain or a neurologic deficit before causing a palpable mass, and MR is the primary imaging examination after plain radiographs. CT may be necessary in some cases for better characterization of an osseous lesion.

LYMPHADENOPATHY

A reasonable body of literature, primarily from North America and Europe, substantiates the value of CT in the staging of metastases to the cervical lymph nodes from squamous cell carcinoma arising in the head and neck.[11, 31, 33, 43] A few reports have described metastatic disease from a clinically occult head and neck squamous cell carcinoma.[32, 34, 43] With the exception of anecdotal impressions, there is no significant reported experience with MR for staging cervical metastases. The accurate appraisal of cervical metastatic disease is very important for the prognosis and management of patients with squamous cell carcinoma of the head and neck. Modern CT with optimal technique can

1. Routinely detect metastatic foci in nodes 6 to 15 mm (or larger) in diameter
2. Detect multiple enlarged nodes when only one node is clinically palpable
3. Detect multiple levels of neck involvement when only one level is clinically positive or when the neck is clinically normal
4. Demonstrate occult contralateral nodal disease when nodes are palpable only on one side
5. Show capsular penetration of metastases in nodes as small as 10 mm
6. Show extranodal extent of tumor and help predict likelihood of fixation to the carotid artery, floor of the neck, and structures in the visceral compartment
7. Detect metastases in the retropharyngeal area, tracheoesophageal groove, and other deep, usually nonpalpable nodal groups

Intravenous contrast medium should always be used to distinguish nodes from the numerous branching vessels within the neck. Contrast enhancement may also help determine whether capsular or extranodal extension of the tumor is present.[2, 8, 33, 44] Some nodes less than 15 mm in diameter show a thin rim of contrast enhancement (Fig. 10–26), a finding that suggests capsular enhancement of metastatic nodes. A thick, ill-defined rim of contrast enhancement in an enlarged node usually signifies extracapsular extension of tumor. Obliteration or

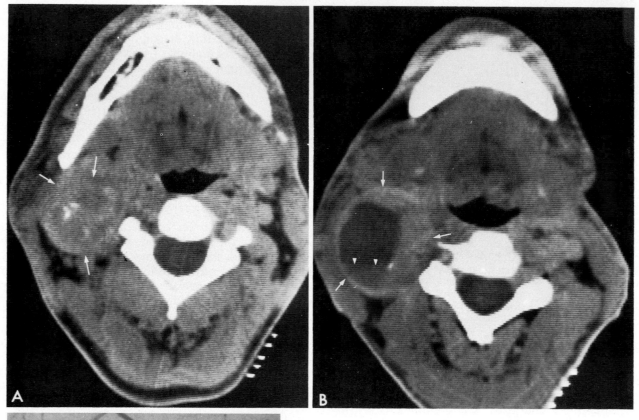

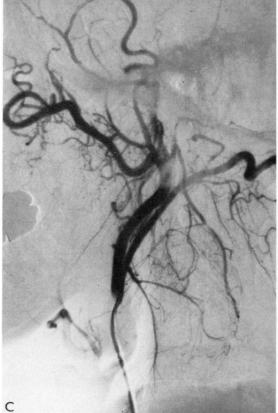

FIGURE 10–25 ■ Vagus nerve neurilemoma in a 37-year-old man who has had a neck mass for 4 years. *A* and *B,* CT scans show a well-circumscribed mass with peripheral enhancement. Punctate areas of calcification and central necrosis surround the carotid sheath *(arrows).* In *B,* a fluid-debris level is visible *(arrowheads).* These findings are nearly pathognomonic for a neurilemoma. *C,* Arteriogram shows a hypovascular mass displacing the internal and external carotid artery branches.

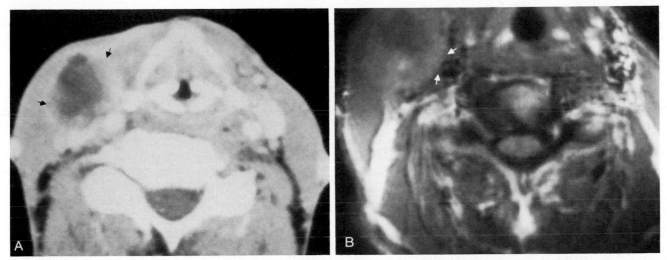

FIGURE 10–26 ■ Squamous cell carcinoma metastatic to the cervical lymph nodes, without carotid artery invasion. *A,* Contrast-enhanced CT scan at the level of the glottis shows a mass lateral to the carotid sheath *(arrows).* Peripheral enhancement is present. The mass proved to be a metastatic tumor to the cervical nodes that has not invaded the carotid artery. *B,* T1-weighted MR scan (600/20). The interface between the nodal mass and the carotid artery *(arrows)* is more clearly depicted than with CT. Less than 10 per cent of the carotid artery wall is effaced. This generally indicates an absence of invasion of the carotid wall by the tumor, although such an invasion is often difficult to detect.

edema of the fat planes surrounding lymph nodes and swelling of the adjacent neck muscles also indicate extracapsular extension of tumor (Fig. 10–26*A*).

Once the tumor has extended beyond the lymph node capsule and into the soft tissues of the neck, it may become attached to the carotid artery. If a cleavage plane between the nodal mass and the carotid artery is visible, attachment to the carotid artery can be excluded. Unfortunately, if the tissue planes between the carotid artery and nodes are not visible, it cannot be ascertained whether the tumor abuts on, adheres to, or has invaded the carotid artery. MR and ultrasound have been shown to be more reliable than CT for this evaluation (Fig. 10–26; see also Fig. 10–27). When a nodal mass obliterates these tissue planes, a carotid artery graft may be needed during surgery. Nodal masses can also obliterate the tissue planes overlying the scalene muscles, which implies fixation to the brachial plexus. However, it is frequently difficult to determine whether the tumor mass merely adheres to or actually encases these nerve sheaths. This distinction is important, because tumor encasement of the brachial plexus by a nodal mass is a definite contraindication to radical dissection. The larger the mass, the more likely is fixation to these important structures; but proximity and obliteration of tissue planes do not necessarily imply that the tumor is attached to an adjacent structure.

One of the most important contributions of CT or MR to the evaluation of cervical lymph nodes is assessment of the high, deep cervical, and retropharyngeal lymph nodes, which are beyond the range of physical examination or other imaging techniques. These nodes are most often enlarged in patients with recurrent tumors after initial treatment.[14] Strict criteria for evaluating these nodes are not available because it is difficult to obtain pathologic confirmation

of their involvement with tumor. CT-guided fine-needle aspiration may make pathologic correlation possible in the future. The degree of symmetry between the two sides can be important in detecting enlargement of high, deep cervical and retropharyngeal nodes. Adenopathy in these regions may man-

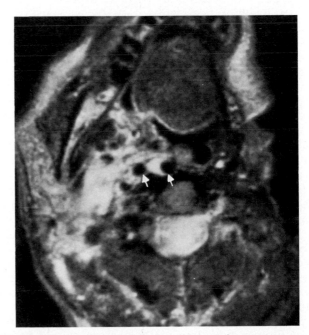

FIGURE 10–27 ■ Invasion of the carotid artery by metastatic squamous cell carcinoma in a patient with recurrent squamous cell carcinoma to the right neck. Status was post left hemiglossectomy and mandibular resection for squamous cell carcinoma of the tongue. Axial T2-weighted MR (2000/80) shows a high signal intensity mass located in the right parapharyngeal and carotid spaces. The mass surrounds the internal and external carotid arteries *(arrows).* At surgery, the carotid arteries were found to be encased and invaded by neoplasm.

ifest as obliteration of the tissue planes around the internal carotid artery and jugular veins rather than as discrete masses. Once tumor has involved these lymph nodes, it may extend cephalad to the base of the skull.[14]

CT has proved especially valuable in patients who have been treated with either surgery or radiation for lymphoma or carcinoma involving the head and neck and who return with either neck pain or neurologic symptoms referable to the cervical cord or brachial plexus.[44] CT can demonstrate recurrent tumor in the deep cervical and retropharyngeal nodal groups, as well as direct extension into the soft tissues of the neck and to the epidural space. Radiation fibrosis, however, may appear similar in density to recurrent or residual tumor. The larger the initial primary tumor, the more likely that a mass of fibrous tissue will remain at the tumor site after treatment.

MR presently is considered adjunctive to CT for the detection of cervical metastases.[11, 37–39, 43] Its main limitation, assuming high-quality images, is the depiction of small metastatic foci in normal-sized nodes.[11, 37–39] CT is capable of this, giving CT superiority over clinical examination in staging cervical metastases.[31, 33, 43] Fat-saturation MR techniques in conjunction with gadolinium-DTPA may improve the diagnostic capability of MR. Size criteria are relatively unimportant for detecting metastases to lymph nodes, because most nodes over 1 cm in diameter are palpable in the untreated neck of almost all patients. Thus, size criteria alone are not adequate to detect abnormal nodes with CT or MR.

MR has not been shown to be as sensitive as contrast-enhanced CT for detecting early capsular penetration or subtle extranodal spread in fat surrounding the nodes or along neurovascular bundles (for example, around the external carotid artery branches). MR certainly is a useful adjunct for showing the extent of gross extranodal spread of tumor relative to the carotid artery and deep neck musculature (see Figs. 10–26 and 10–27). Ultrasound and MR are proving complementary to CT in demonstrating the relationship of nodal disease to the carotid arteries,[45] and important in deciding whether to sacrifice the carotid artery encased by tumor or to treat the patient with preoperative radiation, followed by surgery with carotid artery preservation.

MR shows more ability than CT to distinguish fibrosis from recurrent tumor in patients treated with radiation for neck cancer.[11, 38] This is as true in the neck as it is elsewhere in the body. Active granulation tissue, however, can have the same MR imaging characteristics as recurrent or residual tumor. In squamous cell carcinoma of the neck, one can assume that fibrosis with low water content should be evident on MR three to four months after completion of successful therapy. Increased signal within areas of fibrosis after this time is highly suggestive of recurrent tumor. End-stage fibrosis (dehydrated scar) should be isointense or hypointense to muscle on *both* T1- and T2-weighted images. Following radia-

tion, deeper tissues and muscles infiltrated by tumor and surrounding the upper aerodigestive tract should return to normal or show a similar pattern of radiation fibrosis.

The mucosa of the larynx, nose, sinuses, and pharynx, can show persistently bright signal caused by mucositis and edema for months and even years following radiation. These surfaces, excluding the paranasal sinuses, are best evaluated clinically. MR imaging can detect suggestive sites of recurrent tumor that could be biopsied by needle aspiration, using CT localization. This method reduces sampling errors caused by placing needles in the fibrotic portion of the residual mass. Neither imaging studies nor biopsy are infallible in detecting and confirming residual tumor; however, these techniques can help select patients who require careful imaging and clinical follow-up. This is particularly important in patients in whom early detection of recurrence can lead to cure.

The limitations of MR for staging cervical metastases unfortunately restrict its effectiveness in the evaluation of patients with squamous cell carcinomas of the upper aerodigestive tract. The same does not hold true for sinonasal cancers because of their low rate of cervical metastatic disease. Precise nodal staging in patients with nasopharyngeal tumor is less critical than at other primary sites. MR is superior to CT for detecting and staging the local extent of nasopharynx tumors, making MR the preferred imaging study.[11, 46]

In our experience, appropriately performed MR is better than CT for showing infiltrating masses in the nasopharynx, tonsillar region, and tongue base. Patients with neck masses that are either positive on biopsy for squamous cell carcinoma or are clinically suggestive of nodal metastases should be studied with contrast-enhanced MR, using fat-suppression techniques. High-resolution, thin-section CT is an acceptable alternative. This approach has proved valuable for directing the endoscopist to a site most likely to yield a positive biopsy. Twenty to thirty per cent of carcinomas not apparent on initial clinical examination by an experienced head and neck surgeon, can be detected by CT if the imaging and interpretation are of high quality.[33] Some of these tumors can be confirmed endoscopically because of the localization provided by CT or MR. In about 15 to 20 per cent of all cases, the mass seen on CT, MR, or both is not endoscopically palpable or visible, but blind biopsy is positive. In other patients, a small mucosal primary lesion is discovered by the endoscopist. In many patients with metastases to neck nodes, the primary carcinoma goes undetected and is assumed to be small and hidden in the squamous cell–lined crypts of tonsillar tissue within Waldeyer's ring. In some patients, CT suggests an etiology other than enlarged nodes for the neck mass.[33] In others it can suggest that the adenopathy is either reactive or caused by lymphoma. The number of patients in each of these categories varies, depending on patient

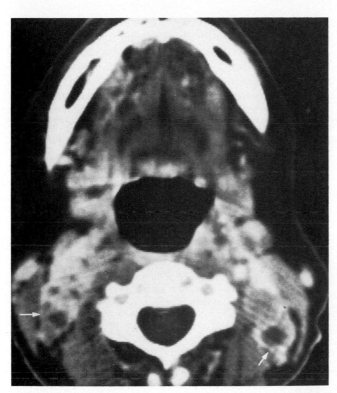

FIGURE 10–28 ■ Carcinoma of the nasopharynx. CT scan shows metastasis both to deep cervical nodes and to the posterior triangle (spinal accessory) nodes *(arrows).*

selection and the experience of the observer. History, age, physical findings, and the results of needle biopsy can alter the imaging approach to a neck mass of unknown etiology. Faster MR scanning techniques combined with paramagnetic contrast agents may

become the preferred imaging technique for some situations. This shift in imaging modalities requires additional efficacy studies.

The lymph nodes in the posterior triangle of the neck lie posterior to the jugular vein and can project into the space between the sternocleidomastoid and trapezius muscles. Metastases to these lymph nodes are less frequent, except for nasopharyngeal carcinoma, which has an incidence of up to 30 per cent of metastasis to the posterior compartment (Fig. 10–28).[14] Lymphomas are the next most common group of malignancies that involve the nodes of the posterior triangle (Fig. 10–29).

Occasionally, malignancies arising in the upper aerodigestive tract extend directly into the area around the carotid sheath, and it may be impossible to distinguish direct extension of tumor from nodal metastases. Direct extension tends to remain medial to the carotid sheath, whereas nodal metastasis is often lateral and slightly anterior or posterior to the jugular vein. Direct extension of tumor into the lateral neck compartment is most commonly seen with carcinomas of the piriform sinus and the postpharyngeal wall but may also occur in tumors arising in the larynx and from the base of the tongue. Thyroid and cervical esophageal malignancies also occasionally extend into a lateral compartment of the neck. Surprisingly, large extensions of these tumors may not be detectable on physical examination or they may be palpable only as a "vague fullness" in the neck. Other primary malignancies of the neck usually arise from mesenchymal elements. Low-grade fibrous histiocytoma and malignant fibrous histiocytoma are the most common of these infrequent primary tumor malignancies.

FIGURE 10–29 ■ Lymphoma with large bilateral submandibular nodal masses. CT scan after intravenous contrast infusion shows multiple discrete nodes on the right and a large nodal mass *(arrowheads)* on the left. The mass on the left cannot be separated from the left submandibular salivary gland. Smaller nodes within the posterior triangle on the left and right *(arrows)* show a thin rim of enhancement.

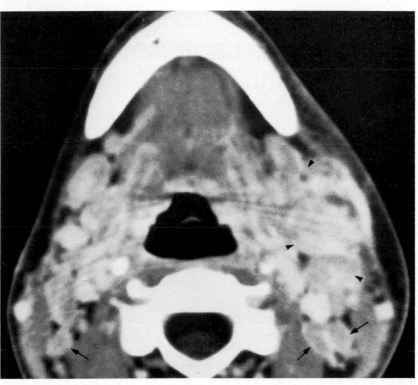

Posterior Compartment

Masses in the posterior compartment are unusual and most often are of mesenchymal or neural origin. They can be confused with abnormalities arising in other compartments of the neck, but CT or MR scans can clearly identify their site of origin. Likewise, malignant masses can extend from the other compartments of the neck to involve the neural and bony elements in the posterior compartment. These exten-sions may not be apparent from the clinical evaluation and radically alter the therapeutic approach.

Experience with lesions in this compartment is largely anecdotal. We have seen several patients with expansile lesions of the cervical vertebral column, either aneurysmal bone cysts or osteoblastomas, involving the lateral masses of the cervical vertebrae and mimicking neck masses or tumors of salivary gland origin. The most common benign lesions in

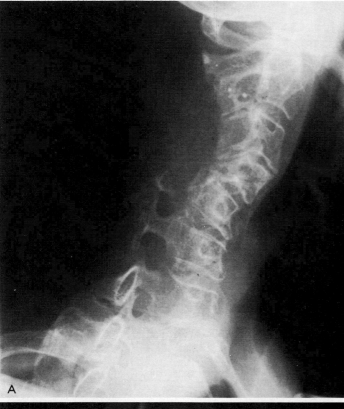

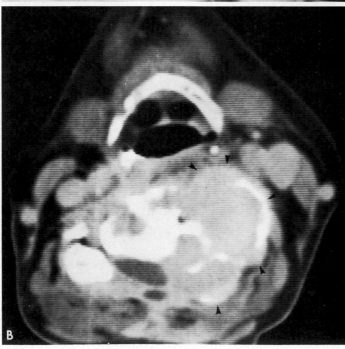

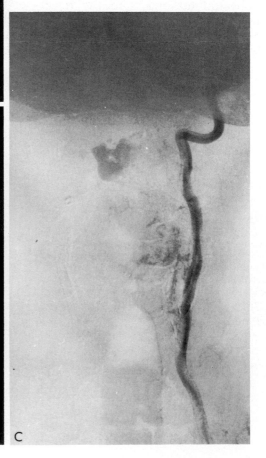

FIGURE 10–30 ■ Cervical neurofibroma. *A,* Oblique radiograph of the cervical spine shows the combined effects of a large neurofibroma and prior surgery. *B,* CT scan shows the extent of the neurofibroma *(arrowheads),* its relationship to the dural sac, and its growth through the neural foramina. Expansion and destruction of skeletal structures is from progressive tumor growth. *C,* Left vertebral artery angiogram shows moderate vascularity, which correlates with opacification visible on CT scan. (Courtesy of T.H. Newton, MD, San Francisco, CA.)

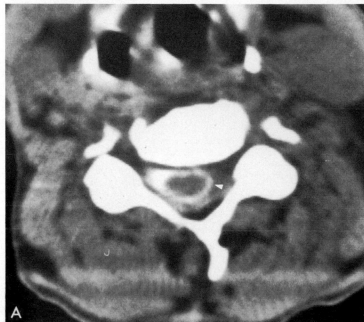

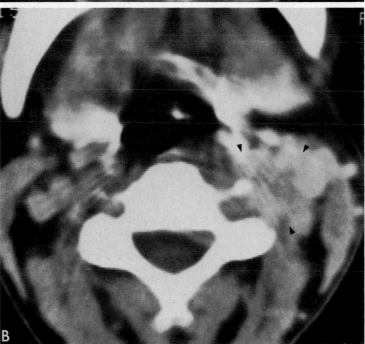

FIGURE 10–31 ■ Two patients with lymphoma. *A,* CT at the level of the larynx shows obliteration of the epidural space and displacement of the opacified dural sac and spinal cord *(arrowhead).* No direct extension from neck nodes or bony involvement. *B,* CT after intravenous administration of the contrast material shows a clinically occult nodal mass *(arrow heads).*

the posterior compartment of the neck are of neurogenic origin. They usually involve the spinal cord and extend through the neural foramina into the neck or arise from the brachial plexus (Fig. 10–30*A* to *C*). In patients with malignant cervical adenopathy and neurologic symptoms or neck pain after treatment, CT can demonstrate otherwise occult nodal masses with extranodal extension or spread directly to the epidural space (Fig. 10–31).

Congenital lesions of the posterior compartment usually do not manifest as neck masses, except for meningomyeloceles. In these patients, the diagnosis is clinically obvious, and MR is the imaging examination for confirmation of the diagnosis.

Salivary Glands

PAROTID GLAND

CT can evaluate suspected parotid masses and determine whether a palpable mass is intrinsic or extrinsic to the gland.[2–5] CT and, more importantly, MR can also determine the relationship of an intrinsic mass to the facial nerve and at times can suggest whether the mass is benign or malignant.

Frequently, masses suspected of being within the parotid gland are in fact external to the gland. The location of the mass in relation to the parotid gland markedly alters the diagnostic and therapeutic approach to the lesion. The surgical procedure for an

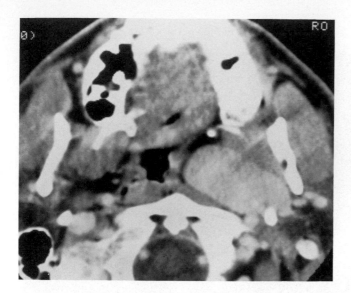

FIGURE 10–32 ■ A benign mixed cell tumor. Axial CT scan following contrast administration demonstrates a well-circumscribed mass within the left parapharyngeal space. The mass is well demarcated from the adjacent parotid gland, and medially displaces the mucosal surface of the oropharynx.

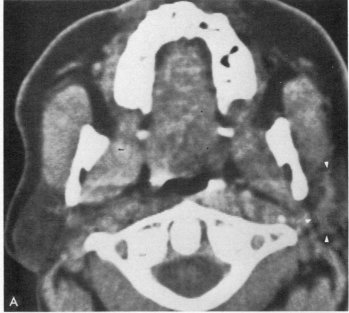

FIGURE 10–33 ■ Adenoid cystic carcinoma of the parotid gland. *A,* CT scan at level of soft palate shows left parotid is abnormal *(arrowheads)* compared with normal right side. *B,* Two cm higher, CT scan through lower nasopharynx shows the left periparotid region diffusely infiltrated by tumor *(arrowheads)*. Decrease in bulk of the pterygoid (PM) and masseter (M) muscles reflects abnormality in the motor division of the fifth cranial nerve. Surgery showed tumor extension to the skull base at the foramen ovale, stylomastoid foramen, and jugular fossa.

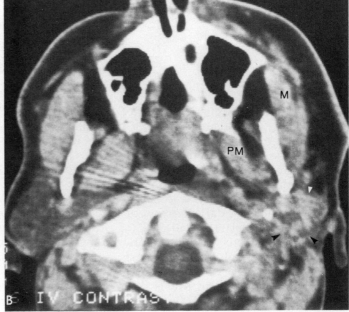

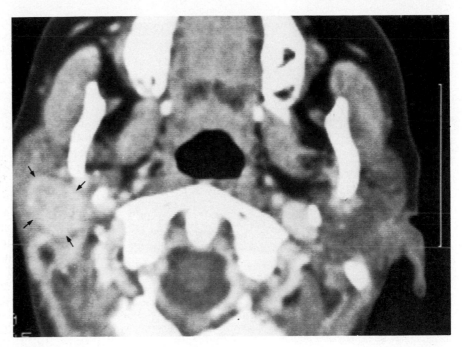

FIGURE 10–34 ■ Benign mixed tumor of the parotid gland. CT scan shows a well-circumscribed mass *(arrows)* in the medial portion of superficial lobe of right parotid gland. The deep lobe is normal.

intrinsic parotid mass external to the facial nerve is a superficial parotidectomy that encompasses the mass completely and places the facial nerve at least risk. The facial nerve is at greater risk of surgical injury with a mass medial to the plane of the nerve itself.

Masses medial to the parotid gland within the parapharyngeal space can displace the parotid gland laterally and create the impression of an intrinsic parotid lesion. CT or MR can often show the correct origin of these masses. A mass arising primarily in the parapharyngeal space is most likely to be a benign pleomorphic adenoma of accessory salivary tissue (Fig. 10–32). Paragangliomas or neuromas arising within the carotid sheath can also laterally displace the parotid gland. Nasopharyngeal or oropharyngeal carcinomas that are primarily submucosal occasionally extend into the parapharyngeal space and similarly displace the gland. The diagnostic approach to each of these lesions and their management differs from those for an intrinsic parotid mass.

Masses extrinsic and lateral to the parotid gland are usually enlarged periparotid lymph nodes. Enlargement is usually due to a reactive response to infections in the scalp and face. Other possibilities include metastases from parotid malignancies and lymphoma. When CT shows that the mass is clearly extrinsic and lateral to the gland, the patient can usually be managed conservatively, with observation and antibiotics. When the benign nature of the lesion is uncertain, aspiration or excisional biopsy are necessary.

A detailed discussion of the pathology of intrinsic parotid lesions is beyond the scope of this text; the pathology text by Batsakis is an excellent resource.[14] Approximately 85 per cent of parotid masses are benign. Benign mixed tumors (pleomorphic adeno-mas) and Warthin's tumors are the most common benign tumors. Mucoepidermoid carcinoma and adenoid cystic carcinoma are the two most common malignancies.[14]

The CT findings in malignant tumors include irregular margins or extension of tumor masses beyond the confines of the gland and obliteration of surrounding tissue planes (Fig. 10–33A and B). Malignant adenopathy may also be present. Benign lesions are usually smooth and well circumscribed (Fig. 10–34), although a specific tissue diagnosis should never be attempted from CT appearances alone.

Lymphoma may present as either an intraparotid mass, or periparotid adenopathy, or diffuse infiltration of the gland. When lymphoma is within the periparotid lymph nodes, it is usually associated with regional or disseminated disease. An infiltrating pattern is seen in the rare primary salivary gland lymphoma.

MR now offers several advantages over CT in the assessment of salivary gland neoplasms. First, tumors can be distinguished from surrounding normal tissues by morphologic derangement and changes in signal intensity (Fig. 10–35). Although most benign lesions are of high signal intensity on T2-weighted images, many cellular malignancies will demonstrate lower signal intensity on T2-weighted images.[47] Second, multiplanar MR imaging can assess critical structures, such as the facial nerve, external auditory canal, and skull-base. Finally, the intraparotid course of the facial nerve can be traced from its landmarks more easily on MR than on CT.[48, 49]

SUBMANDIBULAR GLAND

The patient with a clinically suspected submandibular gland mass presents the same diagnostic problem as the patient with a suspected parotid mass.

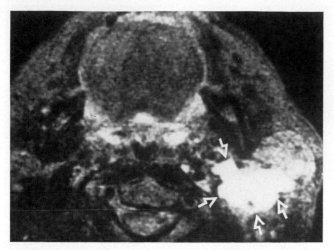

FIGURE 10–35 ■ Adenocarcinoma of the parotid gland. Axial T2-weighted image (2000/80) demonstrates a mass with high signal intensity involving the middle and deep portions of the parotid gland and extending into the left parapharyngeal space *(arrows)*. The irregularities of this mass and its diffuse hyperintensity are typical of a malignant tumor of the parotid gland. Highly malignant tumors may occasionally be isointense with parotid gland tissue.

The mass can be intrinsic or extrinsic to the gland, and the diagnosis and management differ accordingly. Extrinsic masses originate almost exclusively in periglandular lymph nodes that abut on the gland. CT after intravenous infusion of contrast medium can differentiate between enlarged nodes and intrinsic submandibular gland masses, which are usually malignant.[14] Rarely, bony lesions of the mandible or lesions arising from the base of the tongue manifest clinically as submandibular gland masses, and CT or MR can readily diagnose these abnormalities. Enlarged periglandular lymph nodes are frequently excised, because the surgical approaches to intrinsic and extrinsic masses of the submandibular gland not of nodal origin are similar, and the CT findings may not alter treatment. When CT or MR demonstrates that the lesion is an enlarged lymph node, a conservative approach similar to that followed in periparotid adenopathy may be indicated. The combination of an intrinsic submandibular gland mass and enlarged nodes suggests malignancy.

Thoracic Inlet

MR is an outstanding modality for displaying masses at the thoracic inlet or for evaluation of patients with signs and symptoms that suggest a lesion in this area, such as the neurologic complaints that relate to brachial plexopathy, Horner's syndrome, and vocal cord paresis (vagus nerve).[11, 29, 50–52] MR also is applicable for evaluating the thyroid gland and cervical esophagus, so masses arising from these structures can be differentiated from other lesions that arise in the region.

The anatomy of the brachial plexus and thoracic inlet has been described (see Chapters 2 and 5). Several investigators have shown that the course of the roots, trunk, and cords of the brachial plexus can be traced on good quality MR studies in virtually all patients.[50–52] This certainly is true in our experience.

The cervicothoracic junction is a region of changing body contours and anatomic relationships that present a challenge to optimal Rf coil design. This is compounded by the variety of body habitus among patients. A contoured Helmholtz pair or some variant of this design probably is the best receiver coil to study the thoracic inlet and low neck. Contoured surface coils are limited because of significant roll-off of MR signal, either anteriorly or posteriorly, depending on where these flat segments of the surface receivers are placed. Standard body coils can be used, but the lower signal-to-noise ratio with these large-volume coils limits resolution, making MR studies performed with them a suboptimal compromise.

On standard T1-weighted spin-echo images, the nerve roots of the brachial plexus are seen as tubular structures of slightly higher signal intensity than surrounding scalene muscle groups. The plexus then parallels the course of the subclavian artery into and within the axilla. The contrast between the nerve roots and muscles is improved on long TR, short TE (for example, 2000/30) pulse sequences while retaining good contrast between the plexus elements and fat.[50, 52] Axial and coronal T1-weighted images are the starting point for evaluating the thoracic inlet. Sagittal images also may be useful for cross-section evaluation of the distal brachial plexus. T2-weighted images are used selectively. Gradient-echo techniques are likely to prove useful in distinguishing normal vessels and vascular abnormalities from other pathologies.

The types of abnormalities that occur at the thoracic inlet reflect its junctional position between the body and neck. It is prone to involvement by diseases that spread from above and below the clavicles and those that arise in the supraclavicular fossa and at the inlet itself. Many patients who have lower neck pain and inconclusive findings suggesting brachial plexopathy have normal imaging studies. Patients with similar complaints and a history of cancer however are at high risk for a demonstrable mass. In this clinical setting, one can expect to find an infiltrating mass about 50 per cent of the time. Asymmetry of deep tissue spaces in the supraclavicular fossa within the scalene muscle group is an important sign of abnormality. Subtle thickening of the tissue planes around the subclavian vessels and within the epidural space is an additional important finding that is easily overlooked unless one maintains a high index of suspicion. These lesions usually are most obvious on T1-weighted images and tend to blend with fat with increasing T2 weighting. The most common cause of an infiltrating mass around the brachial plexus is recurrent breast or lung cancer, although many other primary sites can metastasize to this area.

Use of MR for evaluation of both primary and recurrent thyroid malignancies and for the preoperative determination of the relationships of large goiters has been discussed. MR can also help evaluate the submucosal and extraluminal extent of esophageal cancer. In all of these circumstances, both T1- and T2-weighted images are obtained because various combinations of tumor-muscle and tumor-fat contrast are necessary.

The most common congenital lesion at the thoracic inlet is a lymphangioma–cystic hygroma. These tumors typically have an extremely bright multiseptated appearance on T2-weighted images. MR imaging is excellent for showing the full extent of these lesions in the neck and their extension into the chest wall and mediastinum. Third and fourth branchial cleft cysts are rare.

The inflammatory and vascular abnormalities that occur at the thoracic inlet basically are the same as those discussed for the other regions on the neck. The same benefits and limitations in differential diagnosis apply here as they do elsewhere in the neck, but because there are more major vessels in this region, MR has a significant advantage over CT if a vascular etiology is suspected clinically.

MR may also be useful in the evaluation of traumatic brachial plexopathy. Its role relative to myelography and CT has yet to be defined.

References

1. Last RJ: Anatomy: Regional and Applied, 5th ed. Edinburgh, Churchill-Livingston, 1982.
2. Mancuso AA, Hanafee WM: Computed Tomography of the Head and Neck. Baltimore, Williams & Wilkins, 1982.
3. Carter B, Karmody CS: Computed tomography of the face and neck. Semin Roentgenol 13:257, 1978.
4. Som PM, Biller HF: The combined CT sialogram. Radiology 135:387, 1980.
5. Stone D, Mancuso AA, Rice D, Hanafee WN: CT parotid sialography. Radiology 138:393, 1981.
6. Ono N, Martinez CR, Fara JW, Hodges FJ III: Diatrizoate distribution in dogs as a function of administration rate and time following intravenous injection. J Comput Assist Tomogr 4:174, 1980.
7. Young SW, Noon MA, Marincek B: Dynamic computed tomography time-density study of normal human tissue after intravenous contrast administration. Invest Radiol 16:36, 1981.
8. Mancuso AA, Maceri D, Rice DM, Hanafee WN: CT of cervical lymph node cancer. AJR 136:381, 1981.
9. Miller EM, Norman D: The role of computed tomography in the evaluation of neck masses. Radiology 133:145, 1979.
10. Casselman JW, Mancuso AA: Major salivary gland masses: comparison of MR and CT. Radiology 165:183, 1987.
11. Mancuso AA, Hanafee WN: Computed Tomography and Magnetic Resonance Imaging of the Head and Neck, 2nd ed. Baltimore, Williams & Wilkins, 1985.
12. Nyberg D, Jeffrey RB, Brant-Zawadzki M, Dillon WP: Computed tomography of cervical infections. J Comput Assist Tomogr 9:288, 1985.
13. Crawford SC, Harnsberger HR, Lufkin RB, Hanafee WN: The role of gadolinium-DTPA in the evaluation of head and neck lesions. Radiol Clin N Am 27:219, 1989.
14. Batsakis JG: Tumors of the Head and Neck. Clinical and Pathological Considerations, 2nd ed. Baltimore, Williams & Wilkins, 1979.
15. Bennett KE, Orgron CH, Williams GR: Is the treatment for thyroglossal duct cyst too extensive? Am J Surg 152:602, 1986.
16. Solbiati L, Votterrani L, Rizzato G, Bazzocchi M, Busitacci P: The thyroid gland with low-uptake lesions: evaluation by ultrasound. Radiology 155:187, 1985.
17. Higgins CB, Auffermann W: MR imaging of thyroid and parathyroid glands: a review of current status. AJR 151:1095, 1988.
18. Auffermann W, Clark DH, Thurnher S, Galante M, Higgins CB: Recurrent thyroid carcinoma: characteristics on MR images. Radiology 168:753, 1988.
19. Van Heerden JA, James EM, Kasell PR, Charboneau JW, Grant CS, et al: Small-part ultrasonography in primary hyperparathyroidism. Ann Surg 195:774, 1982.
20. Simeone JF, Mueller PR, Ferrucci JT, van Sonnenberg E, Wang CA, et al: High-resolution real-time sonography of the parathyroid gland. Radiology 141:745, 1981.
21. Scheible W, Deutsch AL, Leopold GR: Parathyroid adenoma: accuracy of preoperative localization by high resolution real-time sonography. J Clin Ultrasound 9:325, 1981.
22. Kalovidouris A, Mancuso AA, Sarti D: Static grey-scale parathyroid ultrasonography: is high-resolution real-time technique required? Clin Radiol 34:385, 1983.
23. Sommer B, Welter HF, Spelsberg F, Scherer U, Lissner J: Computed tomography for localizing enlarged parathyroid glands in primary hyperparathyroidism. J Comput Assist Tomogr 6:521, 1982.
24. Whitley NO, Bohlman M, Connor TB, McCrea ES, Mason GR, et al: Computed tomography for localization of parathyroid adenomas. J Comput Assist Tomogr 5:812, 1981.
25. Auffermann W, Gooding GAW, Okerlund M, Clark OH, Thurnher S, et al: Diagnosis of recurrent hyperparathyroidism: comparison of MR and other imaging techniques. AJR 150:1027, 1988.
26. Reed D: Personal communication. May 1981.
27. Stark DD, Moss AA, Gooding GAW, Clark OH: Advances in parathyroid CT scanning. Radiology 148:297, 1983.
28. Adams JE, Adams PH, Mamtora H, Isherwood I: Computed tomography and the localization of parathyroid tumors. Clin Radiol 32:251, 1981.
29. Jacobs CJ, Harnsberger HR, Lufkin RB, Osborn AG, Smoker WR, et al: Vagal neuropathy: evaluation with CT and MR imaging. Radiology 164:97, 1987.
30. Harnsberger HR, Mancuso AA, Muraki A, Byrd SE, Dillon WP, et al: Brachial cleft anomalies and their mimics: computed tomographic evaluation. Radiology 152:739, 1984.
31. Friedman M, Shelton VK, Mafee M, Bellity P, Grybauskas, et al: Metastatic neck disease. Evaluation by computed tomography. Arch Otolaryngol 110:443, 1984.
32. Mancuso AA, Hanafee WN: Elusive head and neck carcinomas beneath intact mucosa. Laryngoscope 93:133, 1983.
33. Mancuso AA, Harnsberger HR, Muraki AS, Stevens MH: Computed tomography of cervical and retropharyngeal lymph nodes: normal anatomy, variants of normal, and application in staging head and neck cancer. Parts I and II. Radiology 148:709, 1983.
34. Muraki AJ, Mancuso AA, Harnsberger HR: Metastatic cervical adenopathy from tumors of unknown origin: the role of CT. Radiology 152:749, 1984.
35. Merino DS, Fishman EK, Zerhouni EA: Computed tomography and magnetic resonance imaging of thoracic cyst. J Comput Tomogr 12:220, 1988.
36. Itoh K, Nishimura K, Togashi K, Fugisawa J, Nakanoy K, et al: MR imaging of cavernous hemangioma of the face and neck. J Comput Assist Tomogr 10:831, 1986.
37. Dooms GC, Hricak H, Crooks LE, Higgins CB: Magnetic resonance imaging of the lymph nodes: comparison with CT. Radiology 153:719, 1984.
38. Glazer HS, Neimeyer JH, Balfe DM, Devineni VR, Emami B, et al: Neck neoplasms: MRI. Parts I and II. Initial evaluation and post-treatment evaluation. Radiology 160:343, 1986.
39. Stark DD, Moss AA, Gamsu G, Clark OH, Gooding GA, et al: Magnetic resonance imaging of the neck. Parts I and II. Normal anatomy and pathologic findings. Radiology 150:4447, 1984.
40. Reede DL, Bergeron RT: Cervical tuberculous adenitis: CT manifestations. Radiology 154:701, 1985.
41. Olsen WL, Dillon WP, Kelly WM, Norman D, Brant-Zawadzki

M, et al: Magnetic resonance imaging of paragangliomas. AJR 148:201, 1987.

42. Som PM, Braun IF, Shapiro MD, Reede DL, Curtin HD, et al: Tumors of the parapharyngeal space and upper neck: MRI characteristics. Radiology 164:823, 1987.

43. Som PM: Lymph nodes of the neck. Radiology 165:593, 1987.

44. Harnsberger HR, Mancuso AA, Muraki A, Parkin JL: The upper aerodigestive tract and neck: CT evaluation of recurrent tumors. Radiology 149:503, 1983.

45. Gooding GA, Langdon AW, Dillon WP, Kaplan MJ: Malignant carotid artery invasion: sonographic detection. Radiology 171:435, 1989.

46. Teresi LM, Lufkin RB, Vinuela F, Dietrich RB, Wilson GH, et al: MR imaging of the nasopharynx and floor of the middle cranial fossa. Parts I and II. Normal anatomy and malignant tumors. Radiology 164:811, 1987.

47. Som PM, Biller HJ: High-grade malignancies of the parotid gland: identification with MR imaging. Radiology, 173:823, 1989.

48. Teresi LM, Kolin E, Lufkin RB, Hanafee WN: MR imaging of the intraparotid facial nerve: normal anatomy and pathology. AJR 148:995, 1987.

49. Millon SJ, Daniels DL, Meyer GA: Gadolinium-enhanced magnetic resonance imaging in temporal bone lesions. Laryngoscope 99:257, 1989.

50. Kellman GM, Kneeland JB, Middleton WD, Cates JD, Pech P, et al: Magnetic resonance imaging of the supraclavicular region: normal anatomy. AJR 148:77, 1987.

51. Kneeland JB, Kellman GM, Middleton WD, Cates JD, Jesmanowicz A, et al: Diagnosis of diseases of the supraclavicular region by use of MRI. AJR 148:1149, 1987.

52. Kneeland JB, Krubsack AJ, Lawson TL, Wilson SD, Collrer BD, et al: Enlarged parathyroid glands: high-resolution local coil MRI. Radiology 162:143, 1987.

INDEX

Note: Page numbers in *italics* indicate figures; those followed by *t* indicate tables.

ISBN 0-7216-4358-2

90038

9 780721 643588